Periodontal Manifestations of Local and Systemic Diseases

George Laskaris • Dimitris Tatakis • Eleana Stoufi

Periodontal Manifestations of Local and Systemic Diseases

Color Atlas and Text

Second Edition

Springer

George Laskaris
Ass. Professor Emeritus of Oral Medicine
Medical School, University of Athens
Athens, Greece

Visiting Professor, University of London
Private Practice
Athens, Greece

Dimitris Tatakis
The Ohio State University
Columbus, OH, USA

Eleana Stoufi
Harvard School of Dental Medicine (HSDM)
Boston, USA

Private Practice
Athens, Greece

ISBN 978-3-031-10830-3 ISBN 978-3-031-10828-0 (eBook)
https://doi.org/10.1007/978-3-031-10828-0

This Springer imprint is published by the registered company Springer Nature Switzerland AG
The registered company address is: Gewerbestrasse 11, 6330 Cham, Switzerland

Foreword

Being familiar with the first edition of this *Color Atlas and Text* on periodontal manifestations of local and systemic diseases, I could not imagine seeing the appearance of an even more detailed and extended edition. Not surprisingly, several new disease entities have been added. A separate chapter is devoted to the dental biofilm as a risk factor for systemic diseases, such as cardiovascular diseases, pulmonary diseases, diabetes mellitus, and low birthweight infants. Ample attention has been paid to periodontal diseases that may be associated with a vast number of systemic diseases.

The structure of the book with 46 chapters is well chosen. The text is concise and supported by high-quality pictures. A selected list of references is provided at the end of each chapter. Altogether, the authors have to be congratulated with this unprecedented second edition.

At first sight, this scholarly Atlas and Text seems mainly to be useful for Periodontologists and specialists in the field of Oral Medicine. However, in view of the well-structured and accessible text, and the use of abundant clinical pictures, this masterpiece can also be strongly recommended for the general Dentists and all other healthcare workers who are involved in the diagnosis and management of periodontal diseases.

Professor Emeritus Oral Pathology, ACTA Dental School
Amsterdam, The Netherlands

Isaäc van der Waal

Foreword

Readers of this comprehensive atlas will gain invaluable practical knowledge of the systemic diseases that manifest to practitioners in the periodontal setting. Periodontists and student alike will have at their fingertips the most up-to-date information needed to understand the important relationship between periodontal and systemic health.

As providers of patient care, we constantly need to be aware of advances in knowledge to stay at the forefront of clinical practice. By gaining a solid understanding of how complex medical problems manifest in the oral cavity, and particularly the periodontium, we are better equipped to offer our patients the best evidence-based information to improve their oral and overall health.

Periodontal Medicine and Oral Medicine both have their roots in oral pathology. The forefathers of periodontics and oral medicine were physicians, including Gottlieb, Orban, and Goldman. With this in mind, Drs. Laskaris (Oral Medicine), Tatakis (Periodontology), and Stoufi (Oral Medicine) have focused on oral medicine issues that impact the periodontium. The second edition of this comprehensive atlas has been greatly expanded to cover a vast range of systemic disorders that present with gingival or periodontal lesions. The authors highlight, by example, the importance of the periodontal and oral medicine team in the diagnosis and management of patients with complex medical problems.

Professor George Laskaris and Professor Dimitris Tatakis are both active clinicians, teachers, and researchers in oral medicine and periodontology, respectively, who have extensive experience and a special interest in periodontal manifestations of systemic disease. Both are widely published experts in this field.

Now, more than ever, oral health practitioners need to keep up to date of new discoveries and developments in oral health management. This atlas greatly expands the possibilities for learning and teaching.

Thomas E. Van Dyke

Diplomate, American Board of Periodontology
Vice President and Senior Member of Staff,
The Forsyth Institute
Professor of Oral Medicine, Infection and Immunity,
Faculty of Medicine,
Harvard University,
Cambridge, MA, USA

In Memoriam & Dedication

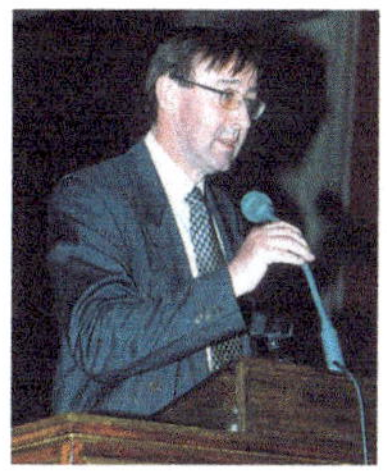

Crispian Scully 1945–2017

It is with the deepest sorrow for the loss of **Professor Crispian Scully** an exceptional scientist, beloved friend, and invaluable collaborator.

I therefore dedicate this volume, as a tribute to his memory and as an expression of my admiration that goes well beyond words for the man and his work in the field of Oral Medicine. I bow with immense respect before the memory of a man who honored his country and who adorned with his achievements the edifice of international science; a true spiritual and intellectual leader.

We worked together for over 35 years and during this time an unbreakable golden bond of friendship and scientific collaboration developed that generated the inspiration for the first edition of this book in 2003. His participation in innumerable scientific activities such as lectures, seminars, congresses, research papers, books, and discussions of difficult clinical problems helped educate and inspire generations of young scientists in my home country. He was a motive force that helped Oral Medicine flourish in Greece and for this we owe him a great debt.

Crispian Scully was driven by and served in outstanding manner seven fundamental qualities. He was an exceptional **Scientist**, an inspiring **Teacher**, a prolific **Writer**, a remarkable **Clinician**, a worthy **Researcher**, an excellent **Manager** but above all a **Virtuous Man**, shining with the greatest blessing that can be bestowed on a man according to Aristotle (384–322 BC) His achievements and the memory of his perceptive, ever questioning mind will continue to guide us.

George Laskaris MD, DDS, PhD

Introduction to Oral Medicine

Oral Medicine is an important, rapidly developing dental specialty around the world that recognizes and cultivates the close relation between oral and systemic health. On the other hand, the spectrum of oral diseases is wide and includes diseases of oral mucosa and gingiva, lip disorders, salivary gland and jaw diseases, temporomandibular joint disorders, orofacial pain, taste changes, malodor, and mainly oral manifestations of systemic diseases. Oral diseases may be *common or rare, local* or *systemic, acute* or *chronic, innocent* or *serious, life-changing* or *life-threatening*. Oral Medicine Specialist should collaborate with several *Medical* and *Dental specialties* and the *general Dentists* as well.

A particular scientific relation exists between Oral Medicine and Periodontology, as in several local and systemic diseases the periodontal tissue can be involved in varying degrees of severity. It is important to keep in mind that periodontal lesions may be the earliest signs of systemic diseases. Early recognition of this fact expedites the diagnostic process and therapy of the disease to the benefit of the patients, including saving their lives in cases of life-threatening diseases.

The volume at hand was written, taking into account the complexity of the subject, with a two-fold purpose in mind:

- To aid the oral medicine and periodontology practitioner as well as the general dentists in making the correct diagnosis.
- To facilitate the planning and implementation of the optimal therapy for the clinical problem at hand, always adhering to the highest moral principles and standards of patient care.

The final aim is the prevention, diagnosis, and treatment of diseases of the mouth.

The Diagnostic Decision

From the point of view of clinical examination, the mouth presents several advantages to the examiner:

- It is an open cavity readily accessible and amenable to all modalities of clinical examination.
- Biopsies of lesions are easily obtained.
- The patient can do self-examination.
- Early diagnosis of oral lesions is achieved during visits to the dentist.

However, diagnostic difficulties occur for the following reasons:

- There is a great variety of lesions affecting the oral cavity that are associated with a wide spectrum of local and systemic diseases.

- There is overlapping and variety of expression of the elementary lesions themselves.
- There is frequent modification of the elementary oral lesions by local factors, such as foods, dentures, saliva, and teeth.

The diagnostic approach follows codified diagnostic and differential diagnostic rules.

Diagnosis

- Detailed medical history
- Clinical evaluation of oral lesions
- Examination and evaluation of skin and mucosal lesions elsewhere in the body
- Evaluation of symptoms and signs in other organs and systems
- Recording of medication intake prior to the beginning of the present illness
- Grouping of probable disease entities based on clinical criteria
- Re-evaluation of symptoms and signs in cases of doubt regarding the diagnosis
- If necessary, communication with the patient's family physician
- Performance of biopsy if necessary
- Study of the obtained tissue specimens by an experienced Pathologist
- Evaluation of the pathology report in light of the clinical diagnosis
- Repetition of the biopsy if necessary
- Laboratory workup as needed
- Confirmation of diagnosis
- Re-examination and repeat evaluation of the patient after initiation of therapy

Differential Diagnosis

- Beginning of symptoms and signs of the disease
- Duration (acute, subacute, chronic)
- General symptoms (fever, pain, malaise, anorexia, weight loss, arthralgias, etc.)
- Primary lesions (macule, papule, blister, bulla, pustule, plaque, nodule, etc.)
- Secondary lesions (erosion, ulcer, crust, scar)
- Color of the lesions (white, red, black, brown, yellow)
- Localization (tongue, buccal, palate, floor of the mouth, gums, lips)
- Coexistence with skin lesions, mucosa, and organs elsewhere in the body
- Biopsy and histopathology
- Other laboratory tests (microbiology, immunology, hematology, molecular, imaging studies)

Therapeutic Decision

The rules and principles that must be adhered to are presented below in codified form.

Therapeutic Approach

- Before the initiation of any form of therapy the diagnosis must be firmly established.
- Therapy without diagnosis is as a rule ineffective and on occasion may prove deleterious, even life-threatening to the patient.
- Medications are administered if and only if it is absolutely necessary and the expected benefits outweigh the probable risks caused by their use.

- A successful therapy depends heavily on the choice of the appropriate drug and the compliance of the patient with the instructions of use of the medication.
- For every medicine that the clinician uses, he must be thoroughly familiar with the mode of action, indications, and interactions with other drugs, side effects, contraindications for its use, form of the drug, precise dose, and schedule of administration. The clinician always chooses the drug with the best therapeutic effect, the least side effects, and the lowest cost.
- The clinician is extra careful when using new medications.
- Dentists should abstain from the treatment of oral diseases with a serious prognosis and refer patients to specialists in Oral Medicine or related specialty.
- The local therapy of oral lesions should be undertaken in collaboration with a specialist.
- Patients with oral diseases with a serious prognosis in the acute phase should always be hospitalized.

The Hippocratic (460–377 B.C.) aphorism "to benefit or do not harm" must always be the beacon of every physician before making a diagnostic or therapeutic decision.

George Laskaris

Introduction to Periodontology

Periodontology is the specialty of Dentistry which encompasses the prevention, diagnosis, and treatment of diseases of the supporting and surrounding tissues of the teeth or their substitutes and the maintenance of the health, function, and esthetics of these structures and tissues. The supporting tissues of the teeth, referred to as the periodontium, include the gingiva, alveolar bone, cementum, and the periodontal ligament. Dental implants, serving as tooth substitutes, are lacking periodontal ligament and cementum but are surrounded by alveolar bone and gingiva or alveolar mucosa.

Periodontal diseases and conditions, which include a wide spectrum of clinical entities, as this book attests, have been known to humankind for millennia. Periodontitis, the destructive form of disease identified exclusively in the periodontium, has been found in early humans from diverse prehistoric cultures and has been identified as one of the most common diseases affecting ancient and present-day populations. Many of the ancient cultures of the historical era described diseases such as necrotizing ulcerative gingivitis and periodontitis, practiced oral hygiene, and were aware of the importance of keeping teeth clean. However, meaningful progress towards characterization of periodontitis as a disease entity, its possible etiology, and effective treatment approaches did not materialize until the nineteenth century, a period of time when many scientific advances took place.

The mouth, despite being the subject of independent study and clinical practice, is not disconnected from the rest of the body. Just as many systemic diseases can manifest in the oral cavity, disease processes, whether infectious, inflammatory, or neoplastic in nature, that initiate in oral tissues may spread via vascular networks and non-vascular routes to distant sites in the body. The term "Periodontal Medicine" has been used to describe how periodontal infection and/or inflammation may impact extraoral health. In the last few years, significant new evidence has been presented that bolsters the contribution of periodontal diseases to systemic disease processes. These findings underscore the fact that keeping the mouth healthy is important for maintaining general health and well-being.

From a professional perspective, the specialty of Periodontology was organized and started to evolve in the USA after two pioneering female periodontists, Grace Rogers Spalding and Gillette Hayden, founded the American Academy of Periodontology in 1914. In the 1940s and 1950s, several national periodontal societies were established around the world. Periodontology was formally granted specialty status by the American Dental Association in 1949, when it recognized the American Board of Periodontology, incorporated in 1940, as the official specialty Board to certify periodontists. In the 73 years since this formal recognition, the specialty has seen tremendous advancements and progressive expansion of its scope to include dental implant placement and implant site development, among other procedures.

One aspect of the specialty that has remained constant over the years is the interest and involvement in the diagnosis and treatment of oral pathologies, clinical activities that many periodontists worldwide perform on a daily basis. Periodontology is historically considered to be the discipline that gave rise to the specialty of Oral Medicine. With this background, it is no surprise that the two specialties intersect, especially in the context of oral manifestations, and more specifically periodontal manifestations, of various systemic and oral diseases. The fact that the gingiva is often a primary site for such manifestations provides a sound basis for this strong interdisciplinary interaction. Timely interdisciplinary care, exemplified by the active collaboration between the general dentist, the periodontist, and the oral medicine specialist, is the only way to offer our patients the best possible treatment and safeguard their oral and systemic health and well-being.

This textbook serves to emphasize this unique interface and to support the diagnostic and therapeutic efforts of practitioners who find themselves in this realm. By offering practical clinical information, this volume will allow readers to review what they have learned previously and to explore new knowledge. Because, as G.V. Black stated, "the professional person has no right to be other than a continuous student."

Dimitris Tatakis

Preface to the Second Edition

Oral Medicine and Periodontology are two challenging clinical dental specialties whose respective scientific focus on diseases of the oral mucosa and of the periodontal tissues is maintained sharp and constant by the needs and expectations of our patients. However, the two individual specialties intersect where patients with periodontal manifestations of oral diseases are concerned. A strong scientific interaction between Oral Medicine and Periodontology is needed to allow us to keep properly serving the needs of patients and enhancing the care we provide, especially in the face of constantly emerging new biomedical information and an expanding knowledge base.

Although there are several excellent papers and chapters in Periodontology and Oral Medicine/Oral Pathology textbooks, no other books specifically focused on the periodontal manifestations of oral and systemic diseases had been available in this form. This book aimed to fill this gap.

Nineteen years have elapsed since the first edition of this book, wherein remarkable scientific advances have been made in this field, followed by fundamental changes, thus necessitating this new edition.

The latest classification scheme for periodontal and peri-implant diseases and conditions, published in 2018 and adopted by the American Academy of Periodontology and the European Federation of Periodontology, represents a strong impetus for the increased interest in this field. This new classification, which encompasses both dental biofilm-induced diseases and non-dental biofilm-induced periodontal conditions and diseases, has expanded the number of clinical entities previously considered and illustrates the broad spectrum of pathological processes that can manifest in the periodontium. The breadth and complexity of the scientific information concerning all these diseases can be challenging for the clinician and underscore the need for a concise and useful source that combines pertinent knowledge from Periodontology and Oral Medicine.

In this 2023 edition of the book, we closely followed both the classification of periodontal diseases related to dental biofilm and the vast spectrum of local and systemic diseases that affect the periodontal tissues, oral mucosa, and other organs and systems. This classification is schematically captured as a "tree" (Fig. 1). A concerted effort has been made to cover the broad range of local and systemic diseases that can affect the periodontal tissues.

In this context, the second edition of the book has been almost entirely rewritten, expanded, and updated to include new clinical information and to adapt to contemporary publishing and scientific standards. New chapters and types of diseases have been added and over 50% of the pictorial material has been renewed and enriched with high-quality color images. In addition, significant advances made over the last 20 years in diagnostic methods, for example, histopathology, immunology, biochemistry, genetics, and others, have been included. This provides the reader with a concise, comprehensive, and reliable book.

According to Hippocrates (460–377 B.C.), "…the wise should consider that health is the greatest of human blessings."

It is certain that when one considers human health, the mouth commands a leading position, as it is associated with unique functions and fundamental pleasures of life: *taste, speech, love, every verbal expression of human affection,* and *social and professional interactions*. From this

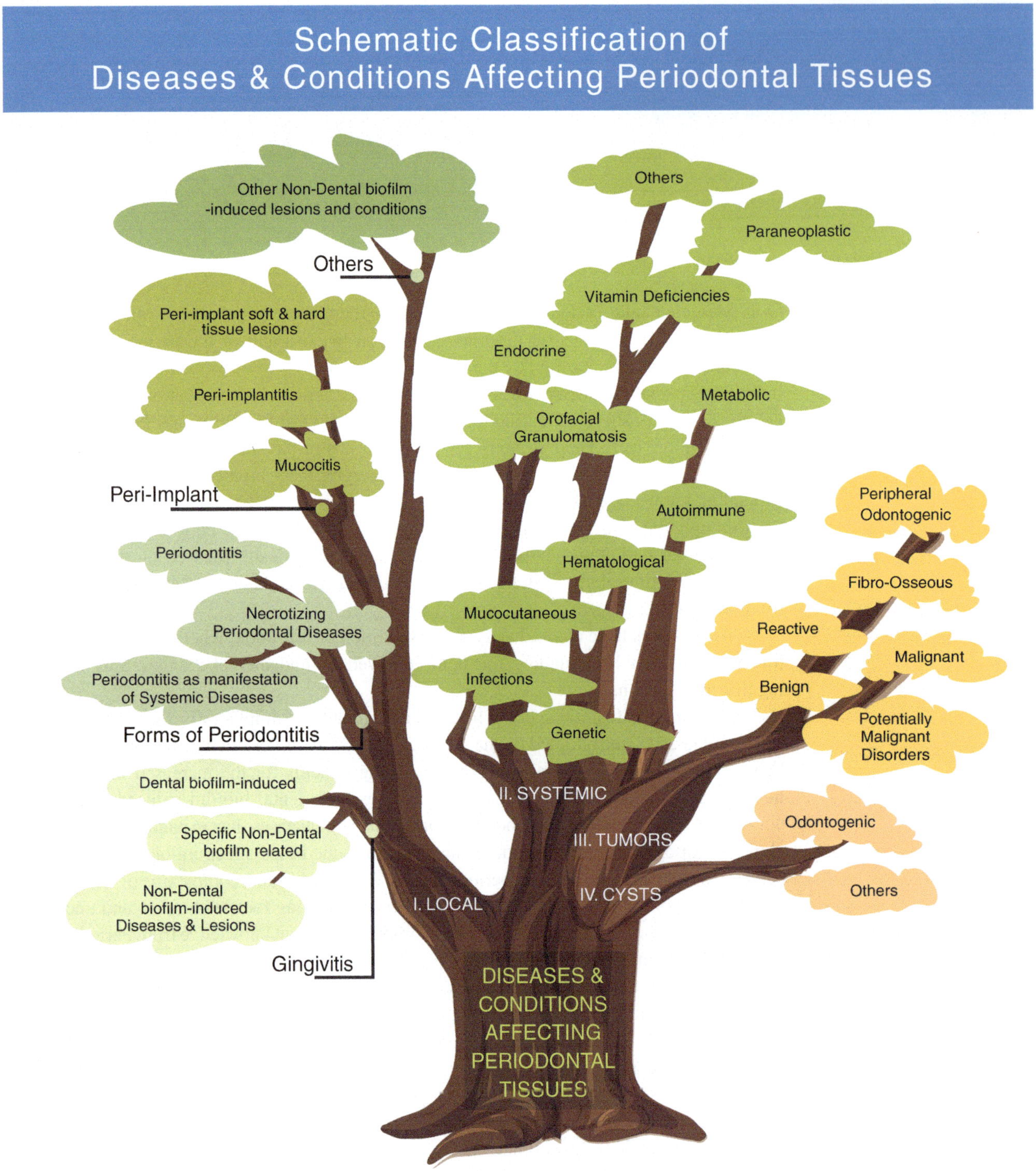

Fig. 1 A panoramic drawing of updated classification of diseases and conditions affecting the periodontal tissues in the form of a "tree," providing a quick framework to the Periodontologists, specialists in Oral Medicine, general Dentists, and the students of Dentistry. © George Laskaris

viewpoint, general Dentists and Dental Specialists are placed in a prominent position and, at the same time, are being entrusted with the responsibility to ensure the key mission of *prevention-diagnosis-treatment* and finally *function restoration* of this critical organ, the *mouth*, whenever it is being affected.

We hope that the second edition of this book will make a valuable contribution to this mission, as it has the noble goal of helping to maintain oral and general health at the highest of standards. General Dentists, Periodontists, Oral Medicine Specialists, Dental students, and other healthcare providers can acquire basic and current information, which in combination with the high-quality clinical images constitute a practical and easy-to-use book.

It is our expectation that Oral Medicine and Periodontology, individually and combined, as in this textbook, will continue to offer new perspectives in the delivery of oral and general health services and further benefit the global community.

George Laskaris
Dimitris Tatakis
Eleana Stoufi

Acknowledgments

The completion of this book could not have been possible without the assistance of many individuals who kindly contributed to this effort in different ways. Their contributions are sincerely appreciated and gratefully acknowledged. However, we would like to express our deep appreciation and indebtedness particularly to the following:

We are especially grateful to Professor and Researcher ***Nikos Soukos*** (USA) for his suggestions on the text and his thorough final critical review, as well as to Professor ***Stathis Papavassiliou*** *(Greece)* for his suggestions on the text. Any errors are the sole responsibility of the authors.

Our special thanks go to Professor ***Isaäc van der Waal*** (the Netherlands) and to Professor ***Thomas E. Van Dyke*** (USA) for the excellent forewords.

The great majority of images come from the vast collection, of more than 130,000 color slides of Professor Laskaris and fewer from late Professor Scully's, Professor Tatakis' and Dr. Stoufi's archives.

Several colleagues, listed below, contributed to this edition by providing images from their own collection, which undoubtedly enhanced the quality of this book. We would like to express our sincere gratitude to all of them for their support.

List of contributors

Prof. Oslei Paes de Almeida (Brasil) Figs. 29.1, 29.7, 29.8, 30.1, 30.2, 30.3, 42.21
Dr. Ghada Alzamel (Saudi Arabia) Fig. 25.58
Dr. Wilson Delgado Azanero (Peru) Fig. 26.13
Prof. Marilia Heffer Cantisano and Geraldo Oliveira Silva junior (Brasil) Fig. 34.25
Prof. Iain LC Chapple (UK) Figs 25.57, 25.59, 25.60
Prof. Kamile Erciyas (Turkey) Figs. 25.81, 25.82
Dr. Mark G. Hochberg (USA) Fig. 25.24
Dr. John Koutlas (USA) Figs. 25.7, 25.52
Dr. Dimitris Malamos (Greece) Figs. 13.7, 13.8, 14.9, 20.16
Dr. Andreas Parashis (Greece) Figs. 5.4, 5.5, 10.1, 10.4, 10.5, 10.6
Prof. Stephen Porter (UK) Fig. 25.91
Dr. Yeshwant Rawal (USA) Figs. 34.24, 46.9
Prof. Karla Mayra Rezende (Brazil) Figs. 25.1, 25.2, 25.3, 25.4
Prof. Lida Toomarian (Iran) Fig. 25.65
Drs. Sergio Verdu, Paula Mastrotta, Gabriella Nalli (Argentina) Fig. 25.64
Prof. Isaäc van der Waal (the Netherlands) Figs. 25.70, 25.71

The Division of Periodontology, College of Dentistry, The Ohio State University (USA), provided access to its clinical image archive, which was a valuable source of material.

Wickepedia Commons Fig. 10.3. https://upload.wikimedia.org/wikipedia/commons/f/ff/EnamelPearl.JPG. Creator: Wicketcity License: CC BY-SA 4

Our special thanks go to the staff of Springer Verlag publisher for their valued assistance, support, and excellent cooperation during this project. Among the Springer staff, we especially appreciate **Ms. Allison Wolf's** leading role in bringing this book to fruition. Special thanks to Lilly Oikonomou (Greece) for her IT support.

Last but not least, we wish to recognize and thank our spouses **Vivi Laskari, Wei Tatakis,** and **Spyros Dimas** for their support, patience, and understanding during the time that was required for researching, writing, and finalizing this volume.

Contents

About the Authors

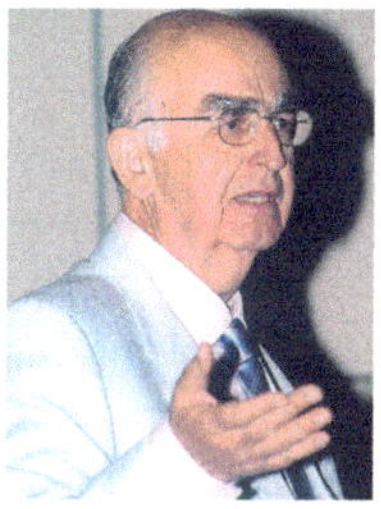

George Laskaris, D.D.S., M.D., Ph.D., (University of Athens), completed his postgraduate studies in Dermatology at the University Hospital "A. Sygros"—Athens and in Oral Medicine at the University of London and the University of Bristol. He received his PhD from the University of Athens and has been Associate Professor of Oral Medicine at the Medical School, University of Athens, and Visiting Professor at the University of London. He established the Oral Medicine department at the University Hospital of Dermatology "A. Sygros" and was head of the clinic (1971–2008).

He is Member of the WHO committee for the classification of Oral Manifestations on AIDS (1990–1995). Over 850 scientific publications and has delivered over 1000 presentations. He has published 11 books in Greek and 5 in English (*Color Atlas of Oral Diseases* 4th ed., *Pocket Atlas of Oral Diseases* 3rd ed., *Color Atlas of Oral Diseases in Children and Adolescents*, *Treatment of Oral Diseases* by Thieme, *Periodontal Manifestations of Local and Systemic Diseases* 2nd ed. by Springer) which have been translated 26 times into 12 more languages [French, Italian, Spanish, Portuguese, Croatian, Russian, Turkish, Portuguese (Brazil), Spanish (17 countries in Latin America), Indonesian, Korean, Chinese].

Two English books, a) *Color Atlas of Oral Diseases*, by Thieme now in 4th edition and b) *Pocket Atlas of Oral Diseases* by Thieme now in 3rd edition, are international best medical sellers. He has also contributed with chapters in 23 Greek and 3 English books.

Book Awards

The Greek book, Oral Medicine: Diagnosis and Treatment, received an award from the National Greek Academy in 2013.

The English book Color Atlas of Oral Diseases 2nd ed., was awarded in 1995 by the British Medical.

Association at an international book competition. The book is now at the 4th edition and is considered as the Bible of Oral Medicine all over the world.

In 2005, the Russian Academy of Health Sciences presented an award for the books Color Atlas of Oral Diseases and Periodontal Manifestations of Local and Systemic Diseases, 1st ed., translated in Russian.

The book Color Atlas of Oral Diseases, 2nd edition, was awarded by the Greek Association of Dermatology-Venereology in 1996.

He was also awarded for all English books by the Medical School, University of Athens in 2003.

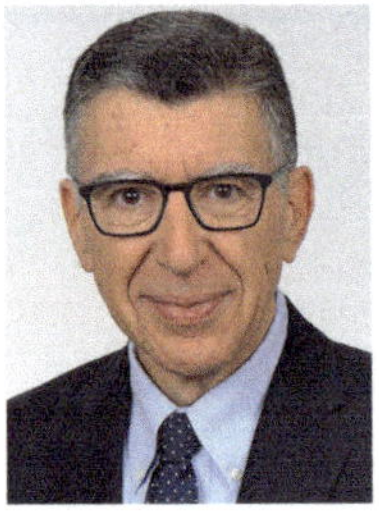

Dimitris Tatakis, DDS, PhD attended the University at Buffalo (SUNYaB) and received his Periodontics certificate and his Ph.D. degree in Oral Biology, after completing his dental education at the University of Athens. He is a Diplomate of the American Board of Periodontology, a Fellow of the International College of Dentists, and a Fellow of the American Association for Dental, Oral, and Craniofacial Research. He currently serves as Professor and Director of the Advanced Education Program in Periodontics and Director for Global Initiatives at The Ohio State University College of Dentistry and as examiner for the American Board of Periodontology. He serves on the Editorial Board of several publications, including the *Journal of Clinical Periodontology* and the *Journal of Periodontology*.

His research interests include wound healing and periodontal surgical outcomes. He has authored over 170 peer-reviewed scholarly articles, several book chapters, and co-authored the new second edition of the book *Periodontal Manifestations of Local and Systemic Diseases* (2023). His research has been recognized with the E. Bud Tarrson Research Award in Oral Plastic Surgery (2004) and the R. Earl Robinson Periodontal Regeneration Award (2015). He is the recipient of the American Academy of Periodontology Outstanding Periodontal Educator Award (2019), and he lectures nationally and internationally.

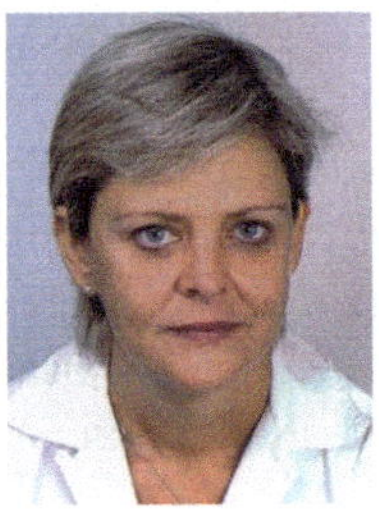

Eleana Stoufi, D.M.D. (University of Athens), M.Sc., (Harvard University), Ph.D. completed her postgraduate studies in Oral Medicine and Oral Pathology at Harvard University of Boston, USA, and received her Ph.D. from the University of Athens. She is Part time Lecturer at Harvard School of Dental Medicine and Honorary Associate Professor at the University of Rwanda where she has served as HRH (Human Resources for Health) Harvard faculty member for 4 years (2016–2019) teaching the Oral Medicine/Oral Pathology curriculum. She is Head of the Oral Medicine department of the "Euroclinic Hospital" in Athens and has been scientific Associate of the Dental School, University of Athens. She has served as Scientific Director of a 2-year program for "Oral Cancer Prevention" sponsored by the EC, the Greek Ministry of Health and the Greek Dental Association (2015–2016). Since 2019 she is member of the National Committee of the Greek Ministry of Health for strategic campaign against smoking, and since 2020 she is elected Secretary of the Scientific Committee of the Greek Dental Association. Since 2022 has been external contributor of the FDI tobacco cessation project task team. She has over 40 scientific publications and over 200 presentations at national and international meetings. She is the co-author of the book *Pocket Atlas of Oral Diseases* in Greek (2019).

Part I

The Periodontium in Health

1 The Normal Periodontium

Contents

This chapter will review the normal periodontium (anatomy and physiology), the etiology and pathogenesis of gingivitis and periodontitis, and the diagnosis of periodontal diseases.

Anatomy

Periodontal Tissues

The following tissues, in order of encounter from the vestibular or oral aspect, constitute the periodontium and support the teeth: gingiva, alveolar bone, periodontal ligament, and cementum. Under ideal healthy conditions, the gingiva is the only clinically observable periodontal tissue and the tissue on which most of the pathological manifestations occur. Cementum may be clinically observable under common conditions where the tooth root is exposed, such as in gingival recession. Clinical exposure of the alveolar bone occurs in pathological conditions or in the course of post-operative healing; in the latter cases, the exposure is temporary. Because of the significance of the gingiva as the tissue on which most diseases and conditions manifest themselves, the emphasis in this introductory chapter will be on the gingiva.

Clinical Features of the Gingiva

The gingiva, i.e., the keratinized mucosa that covers the teeth and the alveolar bone, is demarcated from the alveolar mucosa by the mucogingival junction (MGJ) (Figs. 1.1, 1.2, 1.3, 1.4 and 1.5). In health, the gingiva should have a light or salmon pink color, compared to a much darker or

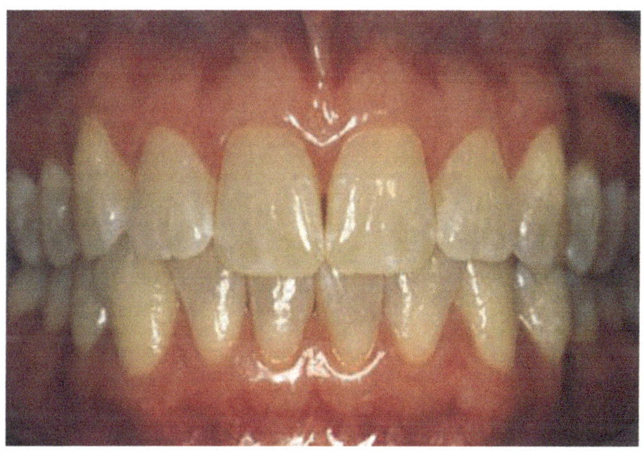

Fig. 1.1 Normal periodontium. Gingiva appears with a typical salmon pink color

G. Laskaris et al., *Periodontal Manifestations of Local and Systemic Diseases*, https://doi.org/10.1007/978-3-031-10828-0_1

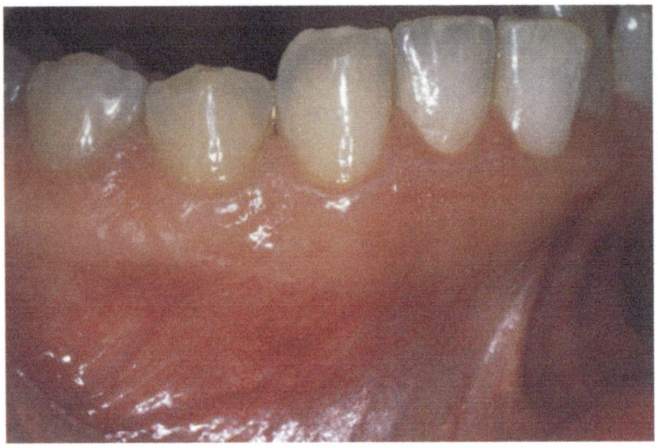

Fig. 1.2 Normal periodontium. Note stippling of attached gingiva

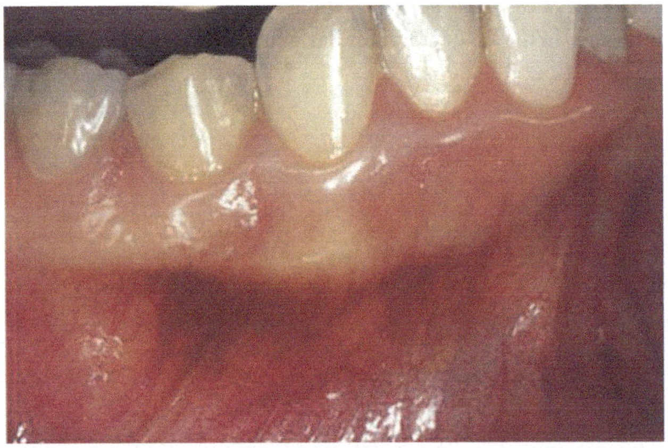

Fig. 1.3 Normal periodontium. The mucogingival junction is demonstrated by iodine staining of the alveolar mucosa (same case as Fig. 1.2)

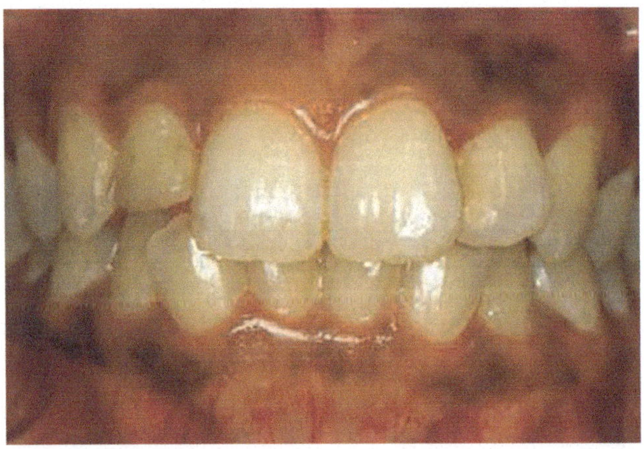

Fig. 1.4 Normal periodontium. Normal pigmentation in an individual with moderate skin pigmentation. Note stippling of attached gingiva

red color for the alveolar mucosa (Figs. 1.1 and 1.2). Depending on the extent of skin pigmentation of the individual, the gingiva may also display significant pigmentation (Fig. 1.4), which may vary in color from light tan to dark brown.

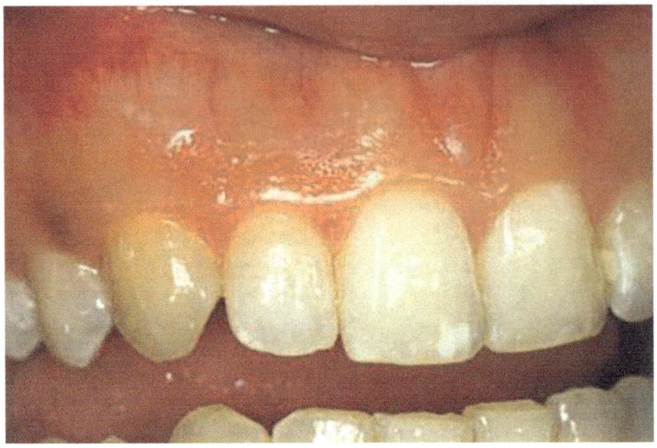

Fig. 1.5 Normal periodontium. The free and attached gingiva and the gingival groove are evident, particularly on the incisors

The gingiva is divided into free, marginal, and attached gingiva (Fig. 1.5). The free gingiva constitutes the movable, most coronal portion of the tissue. The attached gingiva is the immovable portion that extends to the MGJ. In less than 50% of gingiva examined, a shallow groove runs parallel to the gingival margin and delineates the free from the attached gingiva (Fig. 1.5). This gingival groove is located 1–2 mm apical to the gingival margin and its formation appears to depend on the organization of the underlying connective tissue collagen fibers. The attached gingiva often exhibits stippling (orange peel-like appearance) of the surface, most evident on the facial aspect of maxillary anterior teeth (Figs. 1.2 and 1.4). In periodontally healthy subjects, the buccolingual dimension (thickness) of facial gingiva ranges between 0.8 mm (mandibular canines) and 1.5 mm (mandibular second molars). The apicocoronal dimension (width) of the attached gingiva ranges between 1 and 10 mm and varies by site. It is narrowest on the lingual aspect of mandibular incisors, the facial aspect of mandibular canines and first bicuspids, and the facial aspect of maxillary first bicuspids. It is the widest on the facial of maxillary incisors and the lingual of mandibular molars.

Histology of the Gingiva

The gingiva consists of epithelium and connective tissue (Fig. 1.6). The gingival epithelium, according to location and histological characteristics, can be divided into three types: oral, sulcular, and junctional epithelium.

The oral epithelium (OE) lines the surfaces facing the oral cavity. The OE is thick, stratified, orthokeratinized, or parakeratinized, with elongated, narrow rete pegs (projections). The epithelium is separated from and linked to the underlying connective tissue by a basement membrane (basal lamina). The underlying lamina propria is dense and firmly attached to the periosteum without distinct submucosa.

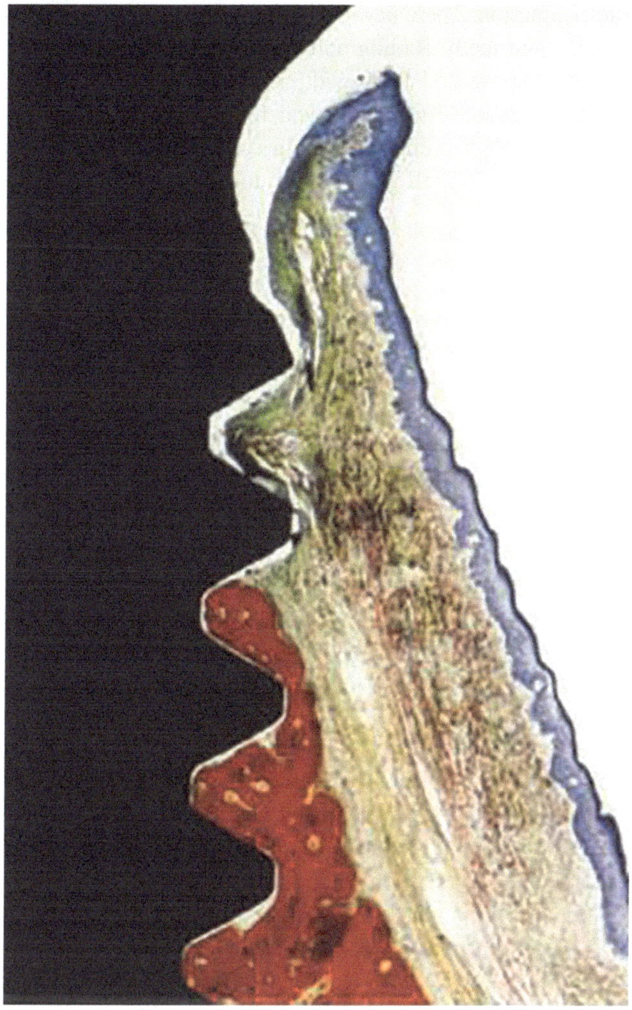

Fig. 1.6 Animal histology of gingiva around a titanium dental implant. The epithelium is stained blue, the connective tissue is green, and the alveolar bone is red

The connective tissue of the gingiva is primarily composed of fibroblasts, collagen and elastin fibers, vasculature and neuronal processes. Other cells normally present include mesenchymal and immune system cells, e.g., monocytes, macrophages, neutrophils, lymphocytes, and plasma cells. The collagen fibers of the gingival connective tissue are either randomly scattered in the extracellular ground substance or organized in characteristically oriented bundles. These bundles are named based on the location and direction of the fibers. Circular, dentogingival, dentoperiosteal, and transseptal fibers are the main groups described.

The sulcular epithelium is non-keratinized with shallow pegs, lines the sulcus, and faces the tooth. Its stratified structure resembles that of oral epithelium, except for the lack of complete keratinization. It continues into the junctional epithelium, which is the epithelial tissue attached to the tooth (enamel, cementum, or dentine) and located at the bottom of the sulcus.

The junctional epithelium (JE), whose length is typically 1–3 mm, is a non-keratinized, stratified epithelium that is only one to two layers thick at its apical end and a few layers thick at its coronal end, i.e., at the base of the sulcus. The connective tissue underlying the JE is highly vascularized. Beneath the JE, inflammatory cell infiltrates, predominantly neutrophilic in nature, can be observed even in clinically healthy gingiva. This inflammatory infiltrate present under conditions of clinical health underscores the fact that periodontal health is accompanied by a physiological level of immune surveillance that is compatible with tissue homeostasis.

The distance between the depth of the gingival sulcus, i.e., the most coronal limit of the JE, and the alveolar crest has been called "biologic width," a term that has now been replaced by "*supracrestal tissue attachment.*" The supracrestal tissue attachment consists of the JE (epithelial attachment) and the supracrestal connective tissue, i.e., the length of connective tissue attachment located apical to the junctional epithelium and coronal to the alveolar crest. The supracrestal tissue attachment varies significantly between sites and individuals and reportedly ranges from 0.75 to 4.3 mm, while the epithelial attachment and the connective tissue attachment ranges are 0.3–3.3 mm and 0.3–1.8 mm, respectively. The mean values reported in histological studies are 1.1 mm for epithelial attachment and 0.8 mm for connective tissue attachment. The results of clinical studies are consistent with the histological findings, i.e., in health, the supracrestal tissue attachment averages 2 mm (±0.7 mm) in apicocoronal length. The supracrestal tissue attachment may be significantly greater in teeth successfully treated for periodontitis or following root coverage procedures.

Alveolar Bone

The alveolar bone structure is similar to that of bone elsewhere in the body. The alveolar bone proper is the thin compact bone forming the walls of the tooth socket, and radiographically corresponds to the structure called lamina dura (Fig. 1.7); it is the bone that anchors the periodontal ligament fibers (Sharpey's fibers, see below). The wall of the alveolus shows numerous openings that allow the passage of vessels and nerve fibers (Fig. 1.7).

Under ideal conditions, the crest of the interdental bone is located 1–2 mm apical to the cementoenamel junction (CEJ) of the adjoining teeth. The shape and location of the crest depend on the width of the interdental space and the relative position of the CEJs.

The buccal and lingual compact bone plates of the alveolar process surround trabecular bone. The trabeculation pattern of this bone varies widely and depends on functional conditions. Like all other bones, alveolar bone undergoes

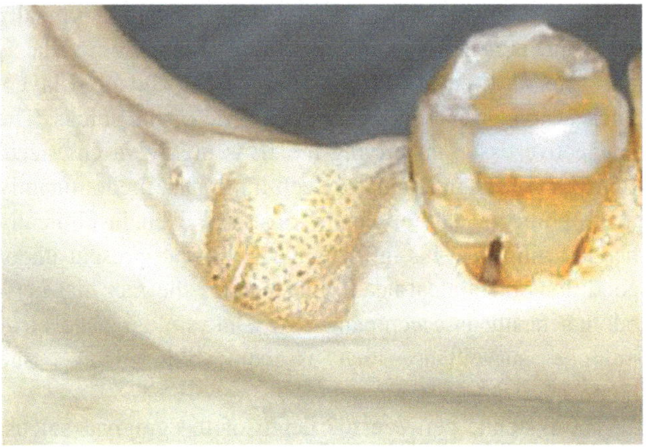

Fig. 1.7 Alveolar bone. The alveolar bone proper (socket wall) and its numerous openings are evident

constant remodeling, which entails both bone formation and bone resorption. Systemic (metabolic) bone diseases, as well as drugs altering bone metabolism, may affect alveolar bone in a manner similar to their effects on long bones.

Periodontal Ligament

The periodontal ligament (PDL) is a specialized loose connective tissue located between the alveolar bone and the tooth. PDL is the tissue that attaches the tooth (cementum) to the alveolar bone. It is a highly vascularized and innervated tissue with considerable adaptive capacity in response to mechanical stimulation. This property can probably be attributed to the very high turnover rate of the PDL connective tissue. The PDL contains precursor cells that give rise to bone-forming (osteoblasts) and cementum-forming (cementoblasts) cells. In addition to the above connective tissue cellular elements, PDL contains epithelial cells, the epithelial rests of Malassez. These remnants of the enamel organ (Hertwig's epithelial root sheath) are thought to contribute to cyst formation. Studies suggest that the epithelial rests may have functions related to the development of PDL innervation, the maintenance of PDL homeostasis, protection from root resorption and ankylosis, and regeneration of periodontal tissues.

The principal collagen fibers of the PDL are organized in characteristically oriented bundles: the dentoalveolar crest group, the horizontal group, the oblique group, the apical group, and the interradicular group. The principal PDL fibers that are embedded in the alveolar bone and in cementum are called Sharpey's fibers.

The space between the tooth and alveolar bone that is occupied by the PDL (PDL space/width) can vary, on average, from 0.08 mm for impacted teeth to 0.2 mm for teeth under function. There is wide variation however among individuals and teeth. Radiographic assessment helps visualize the PDL space and PDL width changes, which can occur either in response to mechanical forces (e.g., during orthodontic tooth movement) or as a consequence of diseases that significantly affect collagen turnover (e.g., systemic sclerosis).

Cementum

Although part of the tooth structure, cementum is also considered a tissue of the periodontium, as it helps attach the tooth to the gingiva and the alveolar bone. Cementum (and/or dentine) is clinically exposed when the gingival recession is present (Fig. 1.8). It may also be exposed, and accessible, after pocket formation following disease.

Cementum is found in two forms: acellular and cellular. Acellular cementum, as the name implies, does not contain embedded cementoblasts (cementocytes). It covers the cervical portion of the root and extends apically to a varying extent. The thickness of acellular cementum varies from a few microns near the cervix up to 200 μm towards the apex. Cellular cementum contains embedded cementocytes and thus resembles bone in structure. Cellular cementum thickness increases with age and may reach several millimeters. Although it shares structural characteristics with bone, unlike bone, cementum lacks vasculature, exhibits continuous apposition throughout life, and does not normally undergo remodeling. Pathological resorption may occur under several different conditions, including excessive mechanical stimulation. Such resorption may be followed by repair, i.e., deposition of cellular cementum.

Cementum may also be visualized in radiographs, especially when significantly increased in thickness (hypercementosis).

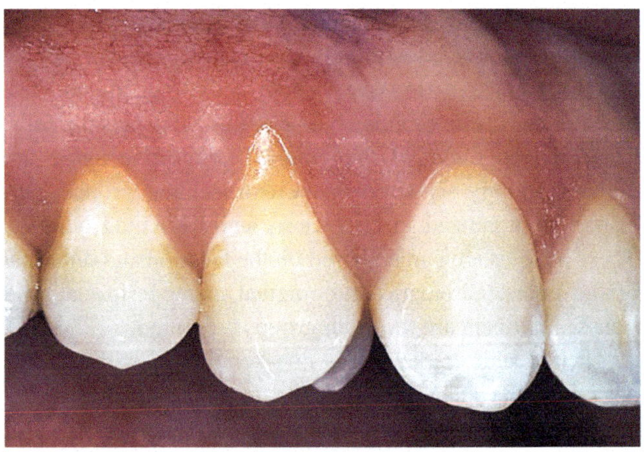

Fig. 1.8 Clinically evident cementum and/or dentine because of recession in the premolar area

Vasculature and Innervation

As previously alluded, several periodontal tissues exhibit a high degree of vascularization. The gingiva receives its blood supply from supraperiosteal vessels as well as vessels emerging from the alveolar bone. The gingival blood vessels are typically arterioles, small veins, and capillaries. Underlying the sulcular and junctional epithelium is a rich plexus of arterioles and venules. The rich vascular network of the gingiva, which expands with proliferating capillaries during chronic inflammation, is considered one of the reasons why the gingiva is the oral soft tissue most commonly affected by metastatic tumors.

The PDL is the other highly vascularized periodontal tissue, with vessels originating from the alveolar bone and the dental (periapical) vasculature. The PDL vessels predominantly run parallel to the long axis of the tooth and are located closer to the bone surface than the cementum.

The gingiva is supplied by nerve fibers stemming from the trigeminal nerve (second and third division). These fibers reach the gingiva either from the supraperiosteal area (like the vessels) or through the coronal portion of the PDL.

The PDL is richly innervated by fibers originating either in the trigeminal ganglion or the mesencephalic trigeminal nucleus. These demonstrate differential distribution along the root. Ruffini-like nerve endings provide the PDL with mechanoreceptor function. Besides Ruffini-like endings, lamellated corpuscles and free nerve endings have been described in the PDL.

Biochemistry and Physiology

In animal studies, the quantitative composition of clinically healthy gingiva has been reported to be 39% epithelium, 5% infiltrated connective tissue (ICT), and 56% non-infiltrated connective tissue (NCT). The inflammatory infiltrate in ICT is composed of polymorphonuclear leukocytes (neutrophils, PMNs), monocytes and macrophages, lymphocytes, and plasma cells.

Water accounts for 66% of the gingival tissue, while collagen fibers occupy 70% of the NCT volume and only 18% of the ICT volume, indicative of the significant loss of collagen associated with inflammation of the gingiva. This loss of collagen clinically translates to the "transformation" of a very firm, dense, and resilient tissue (healthy gingiva) to a soft, edematous, and spongy one.

Although collagen type I is the most abundant collagen type present in the connective tissue, with collagen type III being the second most prevalent type, other collagen types (e.g., IV, V, VI, and XII) are also found in the periodontium. Collagen types I and III constitute the bulk of the gingival fibers, while type V collagen filaments run parallel to the main fibers. In PDL, type I collagen is the main constituent of the principal fibers, although types III, V, VI, and XII are also present. Type I and III collagens are the principal component of the organic matrix of cementum and alveolar bone.

Besides collagen, glycosaminoglycans (e.g., dermatan sulfate, heparan sulfate, chondroitin sulfate, hyaluronate) and other extracellular matrix proteins (e.g., fibronectin, elastin, tenascin) contribute to the formation of the organic matrix. The organic matrix of the mineralized tissues contains several nonfibrous proteins such as osteopontin and bone sialoprotein-II. The organic matrix of alveolar bone and cementum also contains growth factors (biologically active protein molecules) which may be significant for tissue repair and regeneration. Examples of such polypeptides include platelet-derived growth factors (PDGFs), fibroblast growth factors (FGFs), transforming growth factors (TGFs), and bone morphogenetic proteins (BMPs).

The gingiva has a high turnover rate. It has been estimated that the turnover time for gingival epithelium is 10–12 days, while the reported half-life of mature collagen is approximately 10 days in the lamina propria of the gingiva.

When subclinical inflammation is present in the gingiva, a fluid appears in the gingival crevice. This gingival crevicular fluid (GCF) is an exudate, with a composition that represents roughly a 30% dilution of serum. Besides serum proteins, GCF contains cellular elements, including PMNs and epithelial cells, and proteins produced locally in the gingiva, e.g., immunoglobulins synthesized and released by locally residing plasma cells. GCF also contains bacteria and their products, even when the gingiva is clinically healthy.

Microbiology and the Role of Microorganisms in the Pathogenesis of Periodontal Disease

Colonization of the oral cavity with microorganisms occurs during birth or soon thereafter, through contact. Establishment of common plaque species such as *Streptococcus sanguis* is evident after tooth eruption. Studies have shown that pathogenic plaque bacteria, whether cariogenic or periodontopathogenic, are transmitted from parents to children.

The classic experimental gingivitis studies of Löe and coworkers in the 1960s provided clinical proof that dental plaque is the etiological factor for gingivitis, a reversible condition. Subsequently, human epidemiological studies and animal experiments showed that plaque accumulation is a factor that leads to the development of periodontitis, which is an irreversible destructive disease manifesting with attachment loss and bone loss.

The development of bacterial plaque, as it accumulates and matures, progresses from a supragingival collection of aerobic or facultative, Gram-positive cocci and nonmotile rods, to a subgingival aggregation of anaerobic, Gram-negative, motile rods and other morphotypes. The organization of dental plaque in a biofilm, defined as a "matrix-enclosed bacterial populations adherent to each other and/or to surfaces or interfaces," has special implications for the survival and management of the oral flora, especially in relation to the pathogenesis and treatment of periodontitis.

The normal flora, or the flora that is compatible with periodontal health, comprises primarily Gram-positive facultative microorganisms. *Streptococcus sanguis*, *S. mitis*, *Actinomyces naeslundii*, *A. viscosus*, and *Veillonella parvula* are the predominant species, among many others.

The development of gingivitis is associated with an increase in Gram-negative species. Species associated with gingivitis include *Fusobacterium nucleatum*, *Treponema denticola*, *Prevotella intermedia*, *Campylobacter rectus*, *Actinomyces*, and *Veillonella*.

In periodontitis, the subgingival flora is characterized by a significant shift to Gram-negative anaerobic species, such as *Porphyromonas gingivalis*, *Tannerella forsythia* (formerly *Bacteroides forsythus*), *Aggregatibacter* (formerly *Actinobacillus*) *actinomycetemcomitans*, *Campylobacter rectus*, *P. intermedia*, *Eikenella corrodens*, and *Treponema* species. A few of these bacteria have been more strongly implicated in certain forms of periodontitis, e.g., *A. actinomycetemcomitans* in localized aggressive periodontitis (now classified as periodontitis with molar-incisor pattern, see section "Diagnosis of Periodontal Diseases"). Certain species exhibit strong associations with each other, such as *P. gingivalis*, *T. forsythia*, and *T. denticola*; these bacteria are often found together ("Red complex") and have been strongly associated with severe periodontitis.

The use of novel open-ended molecular methods for the detection of bacteria present in periodontal diseases has expanded the spectrum of species associated with gingivitis and periodontitis to include many previously uncultivated and/or unidentified bacteria. Such studies indicate that one person may be harboring nearly 300 species of oral bacteria. Limited evidence has also suggested that certain viruses and protozoa (*Entamoeba gingivalis*) may also contribute to disease pathogenesis.

Recent evidence indicates that transition from health to disease is characterized by a change in the abundance of species already present rather than acquisition of new ones; this imbalance among the members of the biofilm is called dysbiosis. New evidence also suggests that specific bacterial functions (e.g., motility, proteolysis, etc.) may be more critical determinants of disease than the presence of a particular species. It has been recently proposed that the organized subgingival plaque biofilm mimics a human tissue, both structurally and functionally, and thus can have complex interactions with the periodontal tissues of the host.

In the context of the significance of the subgingival biofilm and its dysbiosis in periodontal disease pathogenesis, it should be noted that evidence suggests that it is the host-derived inflammation that creates an environment leading to microbial dysbiosis, and this induced dysbiosis is sustaining the inflammatory state of the host tissues.

Pathology: Immunological Mechanisms

Pathology and Clinical Correlates

Quantitative analysis of human gingival biopsies from experimental gingivitis and periodontitis studies has led to the description of four histopathological stages in the development of the disease.

The *initial lesion* develops within 4 days of the first exposure to plaque and is characterized by acute inflammation, vasculitis, migration of PMNs, alteration in the coronal aspect of the junctional epithelium (JE), and loss of collagen around blood vessels. The clinical feature of this stage is increased gingival crevicular fluid flow.

The *early lesion* has, in addition to the features of the initial lesion, the following characteristics: accumulation of lymphocytes, altered (damaged) fibroblasts, further loss of interstitial collagen, and proliferative changes in the basal cell layer of JE. The collagen loss in the infiltrated area may be as high as 70%. The predominance of lymphocytes is the distinguishing feature of this stage, which develops within 7 days of the beginning of plaque accumulation and is clinically evident as gingivitis.

As time progresses, the early lesion evolves into the *established lesion*, which clinically corresponds to developed gingivitis. This stage is characterized by continued presence of inflammation, appearance of plasma cells and immunoglobulins in the tissue, connective tissue loss, and severe changes in the JE. The duration of the established lesion is indeterminate; chronic gingivitis may persist for a long time as such, without ever progressing to periodontitis.

The *advanced lesion* corresponds clinically to periodontitis and has, in addition to the features of the established lesion, the following characteristics: alveolar bone loss, pocket formation (attachment loss), distant fibrosis, and altered plasma cells.

Increased flow of GCF is the first clinical sign to appear during the development of gingivitis. GCF flow correlates well with the degree of histological inflammation. Another clinical sign of gingival inflammation is bleeding on probing. Bleeding sites, when compared to non-bleeding sites, exhibit significantly higher levels of inflammation. The absence of bleeding on probing is a reliable clinical sign of periodontal stability.

Immunological Mechanisms: Immunopathogenesis

The epithelium of the gingiva forms the first natural barrier of the periodontium against microorganisms and foreign substances. The pathogenic potential of certain bacteria implicated in periodontitis, such as *P. gingivalis*, appears to be related, at least in part, to their ability to invade epithelial cells.

PMNs are an essential component of the innate or nonspecific immune response against bacteria. Systemic conditions associated with periodontal involvement, such as diabetes, and cyclic neutropenia among others, are characterized by qualitative or quantitative PMN defects. Hereditary PMN disorders result in severe susceptibility to bacterial infections, in general, and periodontal infections, in particular.

Although PMNs are critical for periodontal health, evidence also suggests that these cells may be responsible, at least partly, for some of the tissue destruction encountered in periodontal diseases; in GCF or diseased gingiva from periodontitis patients, the collagenase present is predominantly of PMN origin. This has led to the pursuit of pharmacological anti-collagenase interventions.

Besides PMNs, macrophages and natural killer (NK) cells are also cellular contributors to innate immune responses. Upon their migration from the vessel into the tissues, monocytes differentiate into macrophages, which contribute to pathogen elimination by phagocytosis. Hereditary defects in monocyte function, such as leukocyte adhesion deficiency syndromes, may lead to severe periodontal involvement (e.g., severe periodontitis in children).

The adaptive or specific immune response relies on lymphocyte function. The gingiva contains significant numbers of the various lymphocyte classes and subclasses, distributed in the lamina propria and the infiltrated gingival connective tissue. Lymphocytes are categorized according to their function into B lymphocytes (B cells) and T lymphocytes (T cells). B cells, when appropriately stimulated, differentiate into plasma cells. The presence of high numbers of plasma cells in the infiltrated connective tissue is considered characteristic of long-standing periodontal pathology. T cells are classified as cytotoxic T cells and helper T cells. T helper cells have been classified into two major phenotypes, Th1 and Th2 cells, based on their functional properties, including the profile of cytokines produced. Some of the cytokines (see below) lead to pronounced inflammatory reactions, while others suppress inflammatory processes. The overall characteristics of the gingival immune (inflammatory) response to plaque bacteria appear to depend on the balance between Th1 and Th2 responses. Genetic predisposition to the development of responses with an exacerbated inflammatory component may lead to greater tissue destruction, i.e., severe periodontitis.

Severe immunodeficiencies, such as the congenital lack of both T and B cells, lead to lethal infections. Acquired immunodeficiencies, such as the severe depletion of T cells following HIV infection (AIDS), are also characterized by high susceptibility to infection, including the development of necrotizing periodontitis.

Cytokines, protein factors produced by cells that affect other cells, have emerged as critical components in the immune response to plaque and the ensuing periodontal tissue destruction. Experimental periodontitis studies indicate that interleukin-I (IL-1) and tumor necrosis factor-alpha (TNF-α) play a major role in the development of local inflammatory infiltrates and the accompanying alveolar bone loss. Interleukin-8 (IL-8) and monocyte chemoattractant protein-1 (MCP-1) are two cytokines that direct recruitment of PMNs and monocytes, respectively, to specific tissue sites such as the junctional epithelium and the subepithelial connective tissue. It appears that pathogens, such as *P. gingivalis*, may have the ability to inhibit local IL-8 production, which results in lack of PMN recruitment and consequently enables the pathogen to thrive. More recently, newer members of the IL-1 superfamily have been implicated in periodontal pathogenesis, through their pro-inflammatory (IL-18, IL-33, IL-36α, IL-36β, IL-36γ) or anti-inflammatory (IL-1Ra, IL-36Ra, IL-37) activities. A lack of interleukin-10 (IL-10), a cytokine with significant anti-inflammatory properties, leads to more severe periodontal bone loss, as indicated by animal studies. The relative local balance between pro-inflammatory (IL-1, IL-36, TNF) and anti-inflammatory (IL-1Ra, IL-36Ra, IL-10) cytokines may determine the severity of inflammation and tissue destruction. The use of anti-cytokine medications, whether biologics (antibodies, e.g., adalimumab, tocilizumab) or small molecules (e.g., baricitinib), to treat systemic diseases such as rheumatoid arthritis has been shown to reduce inflammation in the periodontium, without effects on plaque levels.

Lipid molecules with pro-inflammatory activities such as the arachidonic acid metabolites (prostaglandins, thromboxanes, and leukotrienes) have been shown to be involved in inflammatory processes that lead to significant tissue remodeling or tissue destruction. The processes in question may be physiological (e.g., orthodontic tooth movement) or pathological (e.g., gingivitis, periodontitis) in nature. The use of nonsteroidal anti-inflammatory drugs (NSAIDs), whose mechanism of action includes inhibition of prostaglandin synthesis, prevents the development of experimental gingivitis and halts the tissue damage associated with periodontitis. New evidence suggests that various host-derived lipid mediators that naturally drive the resolution of inflammation (collectively called specialized pro-resolving mediators; e.g., resolvin E1, benzo-lipoxin A4, and maresin 1) can arrest the disease process, reverse the microbial dysbiosis, and also result in regeneration of lost periodontal structures.

Collectively, these findings suggest that control of the various inflammatory processes can prevent, limit, and/or reverse the tissue destruction associated with periodontitis, as well as curtail the systemic effects of periodontitis.

Diagnosis of Periodontal Diseases

Periodontal Examination

The periodontal examination should include a written medical and dental history, a patient interview, and a clinical and radiographic examination. As with all procedures, the patient should provide his/her consent to the examination process.

Self-Reported Medical and Dental History, Patient Interview

Self-Reported Medical History

This textbook is a testament to the fact that numerous systemic conditions have important manifestations in the periodontium, in general, and the gingiva, in particular. Therefore, the significance of a complete medical history cannot be overstressed. The use of a written/digital questionnaire to assess medical/dental history is essential. It should include a review of systems, with an emphasis on diseases known to affect the periodontal tissues and on conditions that may interfere with or complicate treatment. It should also elicit information on pertinent social/environmental factors (e.g., use of tobacco products, recreational drugs, occupational exposure to hazardous materials). Relevant medications should be listed, with a check/circle option. Open-ended questions regarding health conditions and medications, both prescription and over-the-counter ones, should also be included.

Self-Reported Dental History

Identification of previous periodontal involvement and treatments, oral hygiene practices, and other relevant dental conditions and treatments (e.g., tooth extractions, orthodontic treatment, removable partial dentures) that may impact periodontal health should be included.

Patient Interview

During the interview process, the patient's chief complaint should be established. Then medical and dental histories are reviewed. Details regarding the timing and reasons behind any significant findings in the medical (e.g., specific drug treatment) or dental (e.g., time and reason for previous tooth extractions) history should be elicited. The interview process should be structured in a manner that helps ascertain the patient's dental/periodontal IQ (intelligence quotient) and treatment expectations. At the end of the interview, the oral health care provider should have a clear view of the patient's relevant or contributory past medical and dental history, of the need for any further medical clearance or consultation, and possibly of the need for medical or dental specialist referral.

Clinical Examination

The clinical examination should include recording of vital signs (blood pressure, pulse) and examination of extraoral and intraoral tissues. The extraoral exam should include evaluations of the skin and appendages, of the lips, of the temporomandibular joints (TMJ) and assessment of possible lymph node involvement. The intraoral examination should include visual assessment of all structures. Where necessary, tactile assessment (palpation) should also be performed. If indicated by the patient's chief complaint/medical history or by clinical findings, additional vital signs (e.g., temperature and respiration rate) should be recorded.

The proper examination of the periodontium requires charting of the clinical parameters described below on appropriate form(s). The examination should start with visual assessment of the gingiva, alveolar mucosa, and teeth (Figs. 1.1 and 1.2). Deviations from normal color and surface anatomy or structure are recorded. In some patients, this may require the removal of loose debris, food particles, plaque accumulations, or excessive supragingival calculus from certain areas. The presence of such material is recorded, as well as the presence of factors that lead to plaque retention. Such factors may be iatrogenic, as in inadequate restorative treatments (e.g., amalgam overhangs, open crown margins), pathological, as in carious lesions, and anatomical/developmental in nature, such as deep radicular grooves, enamel projections, and enamel hypoplasia. Although visual inspection may provide abundant information, the proper detection of these plaque retentive factors requires detailed examination with a sharp explorer.

After the visual assessment, periodontal probing is performed. Typically, probing should be recorded in six sites per tooth (mid-buccal, distobuccal, distolingual, mid-lingual, mesiolingual, and mesiobuccal). However, the entire circumference of the tooth should be probed for proper examination and data collection. Using a periodontal probe with appropriate length marks, the depth of the gingival sulcus is measured to the nearest mm (probing depth: PD). In periodontal health (absence of bleeding on probing, no attachment loss), the probing depth varies between 0.5 and 4.5 mm, depending on the site and the individual (Fig. 1.9). It should be pointed out that evidence from histological studies indicates that the clinical probing depth does not necessarily correspond to the histological sulcus (or pocket) depth. This is because the tip of the probe may easily penetrate through the sulcular or junctional epithelium, depending on the applied force, the dimensions (e.g., diameter) and shape of the instrument, and the inflammatory status of the tissues.

From a practical standpoint, probing is what is usually performed and recorded. Should one need to have more detailed

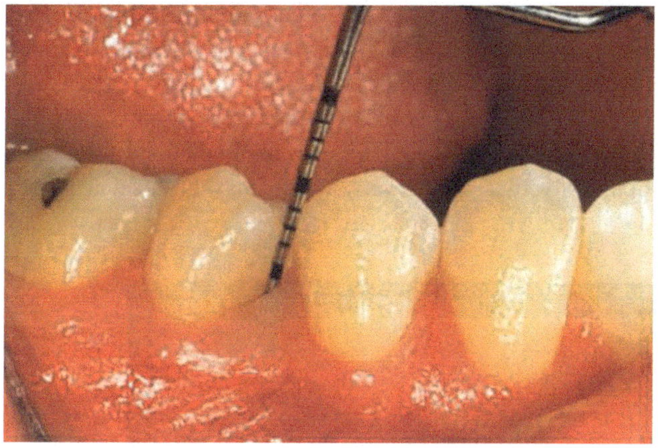

Fig. 1.9 Periodontal probing. The probe is held parallel to the long axis of the tooth

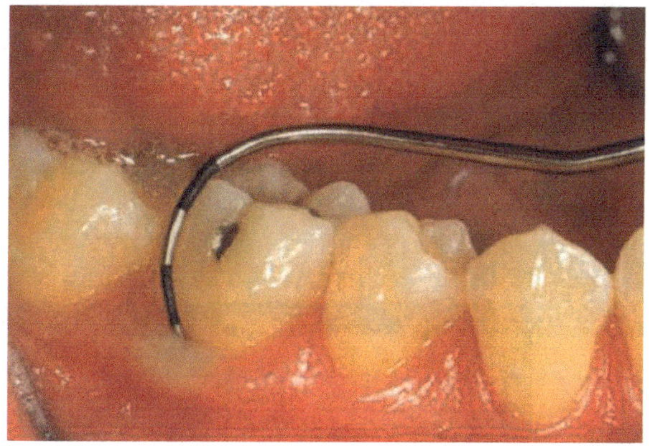

Fig. 1.10 Furcation examination. The curved probe is used to detect furcation involvement

information, then clinical attachment level (CAL) measurements will be required. Concurrently with PD, the distance from the free gingival margin (GM) to the cementoenamel junction (CEJ) is measured (GM-CEJ). This measure, in conjunction with the PD, allows determination of the clinical attachment level (CAL). The formula used is CAL = PD+(GM-CEJ). In the presence of marginal tissue recession, i.e., when GM is apical to CEJ, the GM-CEJ distance is added to PD; in this manner, in sites with gingival recession, CAL equals the sum of PD and recession (GM-CEJ). When the GM is exactly at the CEJ, the GM-CEJ distance is zero; in such cases CAL equals PD. When the GM is coronal to the CEJ, the GM-CEJ measurement is given a negative value; therefore, for such sites CAL equals PD minus the GM-CEJ distance.

The amount of CAL is used to determine the severity of periodontitis (e.g., slight, moderate, and severe, or Stage I, II, and III/IV, for CAL levels of 1–2, 3–4, and 5, respectively). During probing, sites exhibiting bleeding on probing (BOP) or presence of purulent exudate (pus) are also recorded.

Probing should be performed with the probe held parallel to the long axis of the tooth (Fig. 1.9). In the interproximal areas, the probe needs to be slightly angulated to reach the deepest site under the contact point. When calculus is present, the probe should be gently guided past the deposit to reach the bottom of the pocket. In sites with significant calculus deposits, probing may be difficult or impossible and result in inaccuracies. In addition, coexistent severe gingival inflammation may render probing unfeasible due to patient pain sensitivity. In such cases, debridement and/or anesthesia may be necessary prior to periodontal probing and charting.

Furcation involvement and tooth mobility should be assessed and recorded. Furcation involvement is evaluated using a curved periodontal probe (Fig. 1.10). Furcations are usually classified as Class I, II, or III, depending on the degree of involvement, i.e., loss of attachment in the interradicular area in a horizontal direction. Tooth mobility is classified as 1, 2, or 3, depending on increasing severity. Typically, each tooth is held between two hard instruments

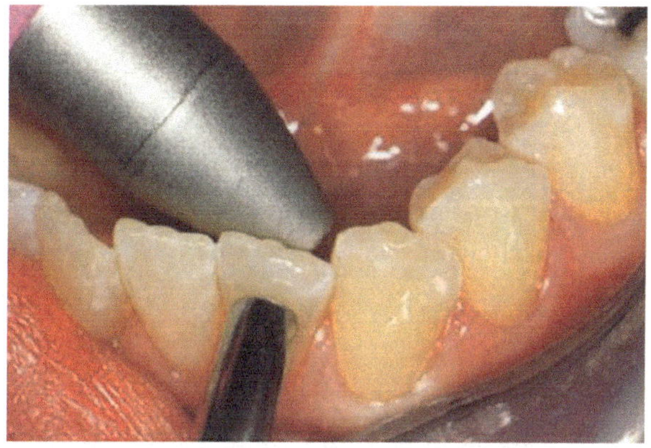

Fig. 1.11 Determination of tooth mobility. The tooth is held between the two instruments

and pushed in a labiolingual (and apical) direction to determine mobility (Fig. 1.11).

The radiographic examination (see section "Radiographic Examination") provides a two-dimensional depiction of the alveolar crest levels around the teeth. However, should the practitioner desire detailed information regarding the osseous anatomy, e.g., prior to surgical treatment planning, then bone sounding may be performed. Bone sounding, which requires anesthesia, consists of probing through the gingiva (or mucosa) until resistance from the bone is met. Bone sounding allows the health care provider to clinically identify the shape and dimensions of osseous defects (e.g., intrabony defects) without reflecting a flap. It helps corroborate and expand on the information provided by the radiographic examination and is useful in planning the surgical treatment of periodontal defects.

Radiographic Examination

The radiographic evaluation is an integral part of the periodontal examination, as radiographic findings complement and corroborate clinical findings. The purpose of the periodontal radiographic examination is to determine the level of the alveolar bone crest and to identify changes in the hard (bone and teeth) and soft (PDL) periodontal tissues that cannot be visualized clinically. Radiographs also help identify calculus deposits, inadequate restorations (overhangs, etc.), and carious lesions on teeth.

The best determination of alveolar bone levels is made from a fullmouth set of periapical and bitewing radiographs of diagnostic quality (Fig. 1.12). Ideally, vertical bitewing radiographs should be taken. In periodontal health, the alveolar crest level is located 1–2 mm apical to the CEJ; the interdental crest is also parallel to a line connecting the CEJs of two adjacent teeth. In cases of severe periodontitis, only vertical bitewing radiographs will allow depiction of the interdental alveolar crest levels, which may be located several

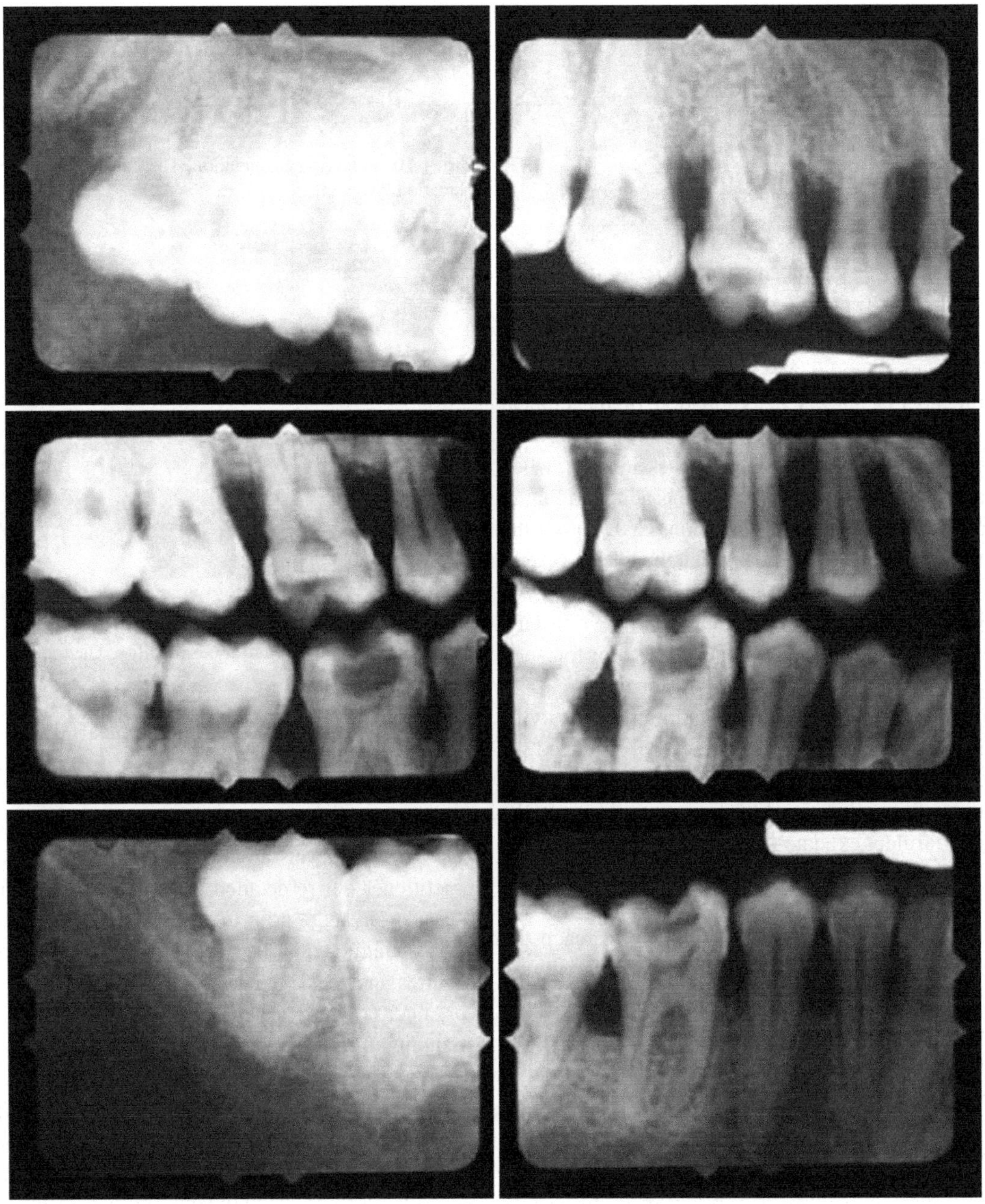

Fig. 1.12 Radiographic examination. Periapical and bitewing radiographs of the right sextant. The patient, a 24-year-old, systemically healthy, non-smoker, female, exhibits moderate to severe bone loss. Calculus deposits are evident on the bitewing radiographs. The patient was diagnosed with generalized aggressive periodontitis (Stage III, Grade C, generalized periodontitis)

millimeters apical to the CEJ (Fig. 1.12). Depending on the presence of specific lesions, additional types of radiographic assessment, e.g., panoramic radiographs, occlusal radiographs, or Cone-beam computed tomography (CBCT) scans, may be necessary to properly diagnose the case and treatment plan surgical approaches.

Diagnosis

At the end of the periodontal examination, the oral health care provider should reach a working (clinical) diagnosis based on the history, symptoms, and signs present. He or she should ascertain the need for any laboratory tests or medical and dental specialist referrals that may be necessary for the definitive diagnosis and management of the case.

In 2017, the American Academy of Periodontology and the European Federation of Periodontology jointly organized a World Workshop to revisit the 1999 classification of periodontal diseases. As a result of this effort, a new classification scheme for periodontal and peri-implant diseases and conditions was adopted and published in 2018 (Table 1.1). This new classification scheme, which is far more inclusive than previous ones, features the following major categories: (a) under Periodontal Health, Gingival Diseases, and Conditions: Periodontal Health and Gingival Health; Gingivitis, dental biofilm-induced; Gingival diseases, non-dental biofilm-induced; (b) under Periodontitis: Necrotizing Periodontal

Table 1.1 Classification of periodontal and peri-implant diseases and conditions (modified from Caton et al. 2018)

1. Periodontal health, gingival diseases, and conditions
(a) Periodontal health and gingival health
• Clinical gingival health on an intact periodontium
• Clinical gingival health on a reduced periodontium
– Non-periodontitis patient
– Stable periodontitis patient
(b) Gingivitis—Dental biofilm-induced
• Associated with dental biofilm alone
• Mediated by systemic or local risk factors
• Drug-influenced gingival enlargement
(c) Gingival diseases—Non-dental biofilm-induced
• Genetic/developmental disorders
• Specific infections
• Inflammatory and immune conditions
• Reactive processes
• Neoplasms
• Endocrine, nutritional, and metabolic diseases
• Traumatic lesions
• Gingival pigmentation
2. Periodontitis
(a) Necrotizing periodontal diseases
• Necrotizing gingivitis
• Necrotizing periodontitis
• Necrotizing stomatitis
(b) Periodontitis as manifestation of systemic diseases
Classification of these conditions should be based on the primary systemic disease (in accordance with the International Statistical Classification of Diseases and Related Health Problems (ICD) codes)
(c) Periodontitis
• Stages: Based on severity and complexity of management
– Stage I: Initial periodontitis
– Stage II: Moderate periodontitis
– Stage III: Severe periodontitis with potential for additional tooth loss
– Stage IV: Severe periodontitis with potential for loss of the dentition
• Extent and distribution: Localized; generalized; molar-incisor distribution
• Grades: Evidence or risk of rapid progression, anticipated treatment response
– Grade A: Slow progression rate
– Grade B: Moderate progression rate
– Grade C: Rapid progression rate

(continued)

Table 1.1 (continued)

3. Periodontal manifestations of systemic diseases and developmental and acquired conditions
(a) Systemic diseases or conditions affecting the periodontal supporting tissues
(b) Other periodontal conditions
• Periodontal abscesses
• Endodontic-periodontal lesions
(c) Mucogingival deformities and conditions around teeth
• Gingival phenotype
• Gingival/soft tissue recession
• Lack of gingiva
• Decreased vestibular depth
• Aberrant frenum/muscle position
• Gingival excess
• Abnormal color
• Condition of the exposed root surface
(d) Traumatic occlusal forces
• Primary occlusal trauma
• Secondary occlusal trauma
• Orthodontic forces
(e) Prostheses and tooth-related factors that modify or predispose to plaque-induced gingival diseases/periodontitis
• Localized tooth-related factors
• Localized dental prostheses-related factors
4. Peri-implant diseases and conditions
(a) Peri-implant health
(b) Peri-implant mucositis
(c) Peri-implantitis
(d) Peri-implant soft and hard tissue deficiencies

Diseases; Periodontitis as a Manifestation of Systemic Disease; Periodontitis; (c) under Other Conditions Affecting the Periodontium: Systemic diseases or conditions affecting the periodontal supporting tissues; Periodontal Abscesses and Endodontic-Periodontal lesions; Mucogingival Deformities and Conditions; Traumatic Occlusal Forces; Tooth and Prosthesis Related Factors; and (d) under Peri-Implant Diseases and Conditions: Peri-Implant Health; Peri-Implant Mucositis; Peri-Implantitis; Peri-Implant Soft and Hard Tissue Deficiencies. Of all the conditions listed, dental biofilm-induced gingivitis and periodontitis are the two most prevalent periodontal diseases.

References

1. Caton JG, Armitage G, Berglundh T, et al. A new classification scheme for periodontal and peri-implant diseases and conditions–introduction and key changes from the 1999 classification. J Clin Periodontol. 2018;45(Suppl 20):S1–8.
2. Alpiste-Illueca F. Dimensions of the dentogingival unit in maxillary anterior teeth: a new exploration technique (parallel profile radiograph). Int J Periodontics Restorative Dent. 2004;24:386–96.
3. Ancuța C, Chirieac R, Ancuța E, et al. Exploring the role of Interleukin-6 receptor inhibitor tocilizumab in patients with active rheumatoid arthritis and periodontal disease. J Clin Med. 2021;10(4):878. Published 2021 Feb 20. https://doi.org/10.3390/jcm10040878.
4. Armitage GC. Development of a classification system for periodontal diseases and conditions. Ann Periodontol. 1999;4:1–6.
5. Bao X, Wiehe R, Dommisch H, Schaefer AS. *Entamoeba gingivalis* causes oral inflammation and tissue destruction. J Dent Res. 2020;99:561–7.
6. Bartold PM, Narayanan AS. Molecular and cell biology of healthy and diseased periodontal tissues. Periodontol. 2006;40:29–49.
7. Berglundh T, Armitage G, et al. Peri-implant diseases and conditions: consensus report of workgroup 4 of the 2017 world workshop on the classification of periodontal and Peri-implant diseases and conditions. J Clin Periodontol. 2018;45(Suppl 20):S286–91.
8. Bosshardt DD, Selvig KA. Dental cementum: the dynamic tissue covering of the root. Periodontol 2000. 1997;13:41–75.
9. Byers MR, Dong WK. Comparison of trigeminal receptor location and structure in the periodontal ligament of different types of teeth from the rat, cat, and monkey. J Comp Neurol. 1989;279:117–27.
10. Chapple ILC, Mealey BL, Van Dyke TE, et al. Periodontal health and gingival diseases and conditions on an intact and a reduced periodontium: consensus report of workgroup 1 of the 2017 world workshop on the classification of periodontal and Peri-implant diseases and conditions. J Clin Periodontol. 2018;45(Suppl 20):S68–77.
11. Darveau RP, Curtis MA. Oral biofilms revisited: a novel host tissue of bacteriological origin [published online ahead of print, 2021 mar 10]. Periodontol 2000. 2021;86(1):8–13. https://doi.org/10.1111/prd.12374.
12. Deng ZL, Szafrański SP, Jarek M, Bhuju S, Wagner-Döbler I. Dysbiosis in chronic periodontitis: key microbial players and interactions with the human host. Sci Rep. 2017;7:3703.

13. Eger T, Muller HP, Heinecke A. Ultrasonic determination of gingival thickness. Subject variation and influence of tooth type and clinical features. J Clin Periodontol. 1996;23:839–45.
14. Fowler C, Garrett S, Crigger M, Egelberg J. Histologic probe position in treated and untreated human periodontal tissues. J Clin Periodontol. 1982;9:373–85.
15. Graves DT, Delima AJ, Assuma R, Amar S, Oates T, Cochran D. Interleukin-1 and tumor necrosis factor antagonists inhibit the progression of inflammatory cell infiltration toward alveolar bone in experimental periodontitis. J Periodontol. 1998;69:1419–25.
16. Greenstein G, Polson A, Iker H, Meitner S. Associations between crestal lamina dura and periodontal status. J Periodontol. 1981;52:362–6.
17. Hajishengallis G, Chavakis T, Lambris JD. Current understanding of periodontal disease pathogenesis and targets for host-modulation therapy. Periodontol. 2020;84(1):14–34. https://doi.org/10.1111/prd.12331.
18. Hajishengallis G, Lamont RJ. Polymicrobial communities in periodontal disease: their quasi-organismal nature and dialogue with the host. Periodontol. 2021;86(1):210–30. https://doi.org/10.1111/prd.12371.
19. Hassell TM. Tissues and cells of the periodontium. Periodontol 2000. 1993;3:9–38.
20. Hirshberg A, Buchner A. Metastatic tumours to the oral region. An overview. Eur J Cancer B Oral Oncol. 1995;31B:355–60.
21. Jepsen S, Caton JG, et al. Periodontal manifestations of systemic diseases and developmental and acquired conditions: consensus report of workgroup 3 of the 2017 world workshop on the classification of periodontal and Peri-implant diseases and conditions. J Clin Periodontol. 2018;45(Suppl 20):S219–29.
22. Kim DM, Bassir SH. When is cone-beam computed tomography imaging appropriate for diagnostic inquiry in the management of inflammatory periodontitis? An American Academy of periodontology best evidence review. J Periodontol. 2017;88:978–98.
23. Kumar PS, Griffen AL, Moeschberger ML, Leys EJ. Identification of candidate periodontal pathogens and beneficial species by quantitative 16S clonal analysis. J Clin Microbiol. 2005;43:3944–55.
24. Lamster IB, Smith QT, Celenti RS, Singer RE, Grbic JT. Development of a risk profile for periodontal disease: microbial and host response factors. J Periodontol. 1994;65:511–20.
25. Madianos PN, Papapanou PN, Sandros J. *Porphyromonas gingivalis* infection of oral epithelium inhibits neutrophil transepithelial migration. Infect Immun. 1997;65:3983–90.
26. Masunaga H, Tsutae W, Oh H, Shinozuka N, Kishimoto N, Ogata Y. Use of quantitative PCR to evaluate methods of bacteria sampling in periodontal patients. J Oral Sci. 2010;52:615–21.
27. Nanci A, Bosshardt DD. Structure of periodontal tissues in health and disease. Periodontol 2000. 2006;40:11–28.
28. Page RC, Schroeder HE. Pathogenesis of inflammatory periodontal disease. A summary of current work. Lab Investig. 1976;34:235–49.
29. Papapanou PN, Sanz M, et al. Periodontitis: consensus report of workgroup 2 of the 2017 world workshop on the classification of periodontal and Peri-implant diseases and conditions. J Clin Periodontol. 2018;45(Suppl 20):S162–70.
30. Papathanasiou E, Conti P, Carinci F, Lauritano D, Theoharides TC. IL-1 superfamily members and periodontal diseases. J Dent Res. 2020;99(13):1425–34. https://doi.org/10.1177/0022034520945209.
31. Saffar JL, Lasfargues JJ, Cherruau M. Alveolar bone and the alveolar process: the socket that is never stable. Periodontol 2000. 1997;13:76–90.
32. Schroeder HE, Munzel-Pedrazzoli S, Page R. Correlated morphometric and biochemical analysis of gingival tissue in early chronic gingivitis in man. Arch Oral Biol. 1973;18:899–923.
33. Schroeder HE, Listgarten MA. The gingival tissues: the architecture of periodontal protection. Periodontol 2000. 1997;13:91–120.
34. Smith RG, Cakici S, Newcombe RG. Variations in the clinical sulcus depth of healthy human gingiva: a longitudinal study. J Periodontal Res. 1996;31:181–6.
35. Silva BSE, Fagundes NCF, Nogueira BCL, Neto VJ, Normando D, Lima RR. Epithelial rests of Malassez: from latent cells to active participation in orthodontic movement. Dental Press J Orthod. 2017;22:119–25.
36. Taubman MA, Valverde P, Han X, Kawai T. Immune response: the key to bone resorption in periodontal disease. J Periodontol. 2005;76:2033–41.
37. Vacek JS, Gher ME, Assad DA, Richardson AC, Giambarresi LI. The dimensions of the human dentogingival junction. Int J Periodontics Restorative Dent. 1994;14:154–65.
38. Van Dyke TE. Shifting the paradigm from inhibitors of inflammation to resolvers of inflammation in periodontitis. J Periodontol. 2020;91 Suppl 1(Suppl 1):S19–25. https://doi.org/10.1002/JPER.20-0088.
39. Yucel-Lindberg T, Båge T. Inflammatory mediators in the pathogenesis of periodontitis. Expert Rev Mol Med. 2013;15:e7. Published 2013 Aug 5. https://doi.org/10.1017/erm.2013.8.

Periodontal and Gingival Health

2

Contents

Until the 2018 Classification of Periodontal Diseases and Conditions, which codified and defined periodontal and gingival health, articles focused on defining periodontal health were lacking. Having a definition of periodontal health is critical because it provides a benchmark against which to evaluate the status of the periodontium and appraise treatment outcomes.

Definition Clinical gingival health on an intact periodontium is characterized by the absence of bleeding on probing, erythema and edema, patient symptoms, and attachment and bone loss. Physiological bone levels are 1–3 mm apical to the cementoenamel junction. Clinical gingival health is typically associated with a histopathologically evident inflammatory infiltrate and a host response consistent with homeostasis. Periodontal health is assessed and defined at both the patient and the site level.

Clinical Features The features of clinical gingival health *on a site level* vary depending on the integrity of the periodontium.

- On an intact periodontium:
  - Absence of bleeding on probing, erythema and edema, patient symptoms, and attachment and bone loss, with probing depths ≤3 mm (no pseudopockets present).
- On a reduced periodontium, non-periodontitis patient (e.g., patient with gingival recession or patient undergone crown lengthening):
  - Absence of bleeding on probing, erythema, edema, and patient symptoms, in the presence of reduced clinical attachment and bone levels, with probing depths ≤3 mm (no pseudopockets present).
- On a reduced periodontium, successfully treated periodontitis patient:
  - Absence of bleeding on probing, erythema, edema, and patient symptoms, in the presence of reduced clinical attachment and bone levels, with probing depths ≤4 mm (no pseudopockets present).
- The diagnosis is mainly based on clinical and radiographic findings and history.
- When defining health *on a patient level*, as opposed to a specific site, a case of gingival health can be defined based on the above features, with the added qualification that bleeding on probing may be present in less than 10% of available sites (all three categories listed above) and with no site ≥4 mm being positive for bleeding on probing (reduced periodontium in successfully treated periodontitis patient).
- The clinical characteristics of healthy periodontal tissues have been detailed in Chap. 1 of this textbook (Normal Periodontium).

Laboratory Tests There are no specific tests.

G. Laskaris et al., *Periodontal Manifestations of Local and Systemic Diseases*, https://doi.org/10.1007/978-3-031-10828-0_2

References

1. Chapple ILC, Mealey BL, Van Dyke TE, et al. Periodontal health and gingival diseases and conditions on an intact and a reduced periodontium: consensus report of workgroup 1 of the 2017 world workshop on the classification of periodontal and peri-implant diseases and conditions. J Clin Periodontol. 2018;45(Suppl 20):S68–77.
2. Lang NP, Bartold PM. Periodontal health. J Clin Periodontol. 2018;45(Suppl 20):S9–S16.
3. Trombelli L, Farina R, Silva CO, Tatakis DN. Plaque-induced gingivitis: case definition and diagnostic considerations. J Clin Periodontol. 2018;45(Suppl 20):S44–67.

Part II

Local Diseases and Conditions Affecting Periodontal Tissues

Gingival Diseases

3

Contents

Gingivitis: Dental Biofilm-Induced

Definition Inflammatory lesion resulting from the interaction between dental plaque biofilm and host response. Such lesion, which is reversible upon reduction of dental plaque levels, remains contained within the gingiva and does not extend beyond the mucogingival junction or to the remainder of the periodontal attachment apparatus.

Etiology Dental biofilm (plaque) accumulation at the gingival margin area and apical to it. It can be associated with biofilm alone or mediated by various modifying (e.g., smoking, hyperglycemia, sex steroid hormones) or predisposing (e.g., oral dryness, prominent restoration margins) factors.

Gingival Involvement Exclusively; affects majority of population.

Other Sites of Involvement None.

Clinical Features

- One of the most prevalent oral diseases worldwide.
- Clinically, it presents painless, with bleeding upon provocation (i.e., toothbrushing, periodontal probing, biting into hard foods, e.g., apples), gingival redness and edema (Fig. 3.1). Eventually may result in mild gingival enlargement (Figs. 3.2 and 3.3).

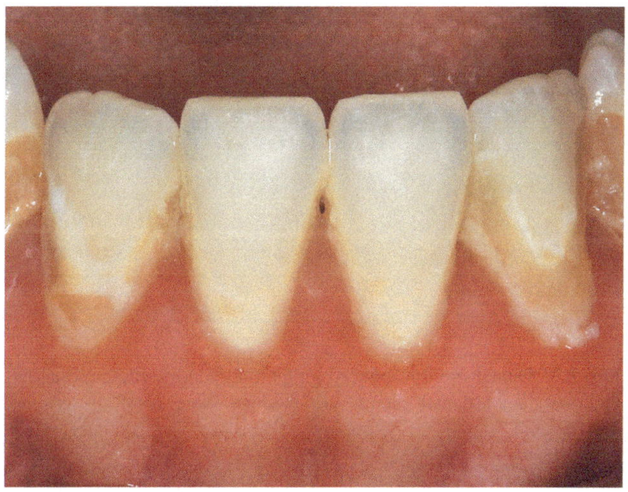

Fig. 3.1 Dental biofilm induced gingivitis, redness and edema. Accumulated dental biofilm evident

- May develop on an intact periodontium (gingivitis on an intact periodontium) or on a reduced periodontium in a non-periodontitis patient (e.g., patient with recession or history of crown lengthening; gingivitis on a reduced periodontium), or on a reduced periodontium in a successfully treated periodontitis patient (in this case, recurrent periodontitis cannot be ruled out).
- The diagnosis is mainly based on the clinical features and dental history.

G. Laskaris et al., *Periodontal Manifestations of Local and Systemic Diseases*, https://doi.org/10.1007/978-3-031-10828-0_3

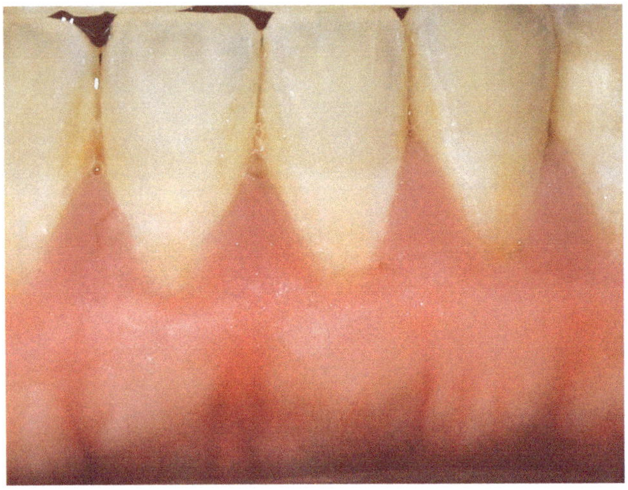

Fig. 3.2 Dental biofilm induced gingivitis, redness and edema, especially in papillary areas

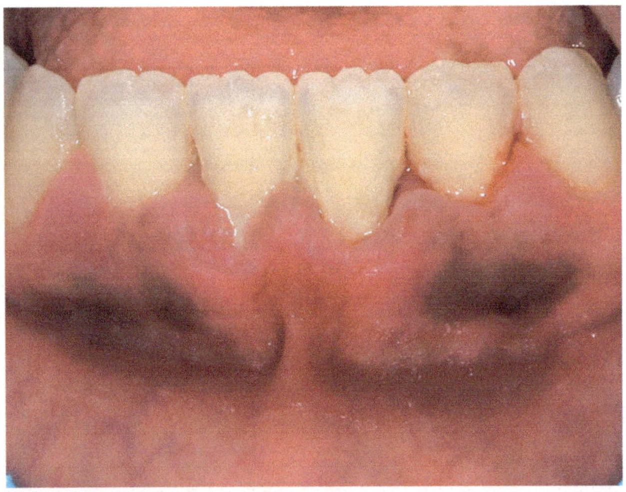

Fig. 3.3 Dental biofilm induced gingivitis, redness, edema, bleeding and associated dental plaque are evident. Note resulting gingival enlargement

Differential Diagnosis

- Periodontitis
- Plasma cell gingivitis
- Desquamative gingivitis
- Localized juvenile spongiotic gingivitis
- Specific bacterial, viral, or fungal infections
- Trauma
- Drug-induced gingival enlargement
- Systemic diseases affecting periodontal tissues (see Part IV)

Laboratory Tests There are no specific tests. Occasionally, radiographic imaging may help support the clinical diagnosis.

Treatment Oral hygiene instruction (plaque control). When needed, nonsurgical periodontal therapy (prophylaxis; calculus removal by scaling and polishing). Occasionally, antimicrobial mouthrinse use, which will aid in plaque control and subsequent resolution of inflammation.

Mouth Breathing Gingivitis

Definition A descriptive term for biofilm-induced gingivitis related to mouth breathing.

Etiology The various factors that can cause a mouth breathing habit, resulting in gingivitis with gingival enlargement, include asthma, allergies, obstruction of the upper airway (e.g., nasal septum deviation), allergic rhinitis, malocclusion. Associated with dental biofilm.

Gingival Involvement Common.

Other Sites of Involvement None.

Clinical Features

- Mouth breathing is observed in mouth breathers (usually due to nasal septum deviation, or hypertrophy of pharyngeal lymphoid tissue-tonsils and adenoids).
- It is common in children and adolescents and mostly affects the maxillary anterior gingiva roughly corresponding to areas lacking lip coverage.
- Mouth breathing is associated with a high level of dental biofilm (or plaque) oral dryness, resulting in gingival inflammation, that can lead to enlarged gingiva, especially labially in the anterior maxilla (Figs. 3.4 and 3.5).

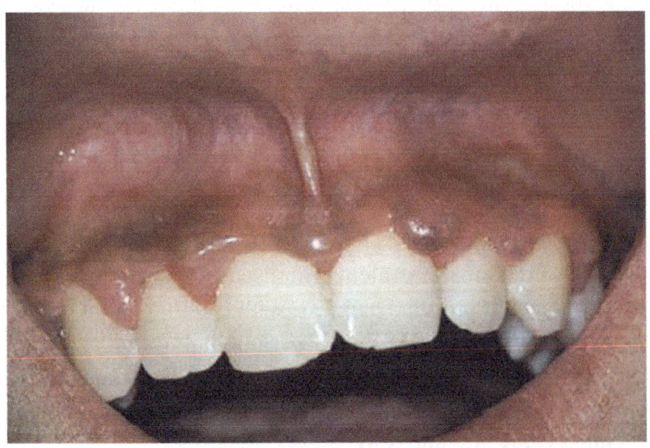

Fig. 3.4 Mouth breathing gingivitis, enlarged gingiva labially on the anterior maxilla

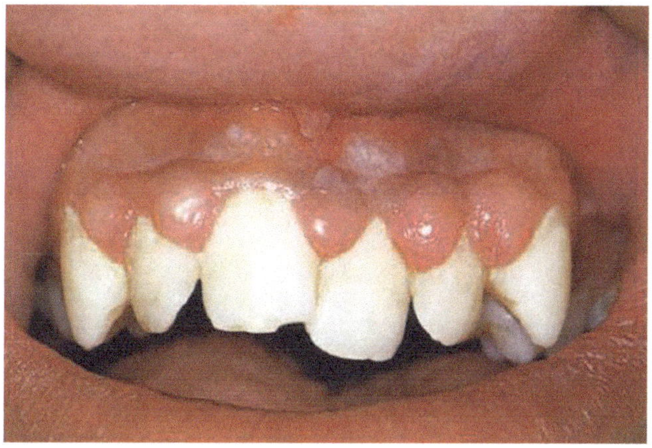

Fig. 3.5 Mouth breathing gingivitis, enlarged gingiva labially at the anterior maxilla

- Clinically, the free gingiva and predominantly the interdental papillae are enlarged, dry, erythematous, and shiny and cover part of the tooth's crown. Pseudopockets are present at sites of enlargement.
- Diagnosis is based on history and clinical features.

Differential Diagnosis
- Chronic gingivitis
- Hereditary gingival fibromatosis
- Drug-induced gingival enlargement
- Pregnancy gingivitis
- Sarcoidosis
- Crohn disease
- Leukemia
- Wegener granulomatosis
- Amyloidosis
- Scurvy
- Mucopolysaccharidoses

Laboratory Tests None.

Treatment Management of the etiology underlying mouth breathing, e.g., examination of the upper respiratory tract by an Otolaryngologist. High level of oral hygiene and occasionally gingivectomy.

Specific Non-dental Biofilm-Induced Gingivitis

Granulomatous Gingivitis

Definition Swelling of gingival tissues in association with histologic evidence of noncaseating granulomatous inflammation.

Etiology Unclear, often idiopathic. Typically, component of orofacial granulomatosis, which itself may be the localized clinical manifestation of diseases such as Melkersson-Rosenthal syndrome, chronic granulomatous cheilitis, Crohn disease, sarcoidosis, and others (e.g., Anderson-Fabry disease). May also represent reaction to food additives (e.g., cinnamic aldehyde) or a foreign body embedded in the gingiva.

Gingival Involvement Rare.

Other Sites of Involvement Lips, oral mucosa, face.

Clinical Features
- Granulomatous red gingival enlargement that maybe be accompanied by mucosal lesions such as cobblestone appearance due to thickening and folding, mucosal tags, linear ulcers in the vestibule, often with adjacent granulomatous masses (Figs. 3.6 and 3.7).

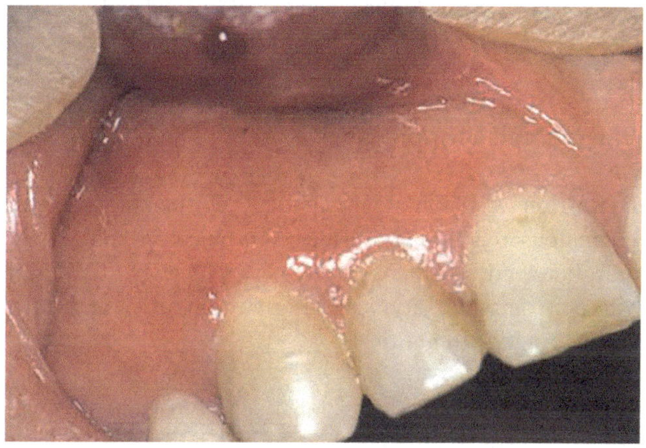

Fig. 3.6 Granulomatous gingivitis, mucosal tags and ulcers

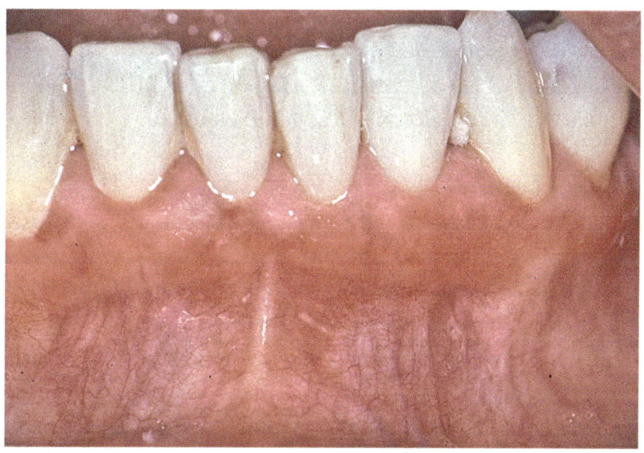

Fig. 3.7 Granulomatous gingivitis, gingival enlargement. Patient with Crohn disease

- Fairly common (20–30%) among patients presenting with orofacial granulomatosis.
- Diagnosis is based on history and clinical features, supplemented by histopathology.

Differential Diagnosis
- Plasma cell gingivitis
- Foreign-body gingivitis
- Crohn disease
- Sarcoidosis
- Kaposi sarcoma
- Wegener granulomatosis
- Tuberculosis
- Leprosy

Laboratory Tests Histopathologic and histochemical examination.

Treatment Management of underlying systemic condition, avoidance of eliciting diet elements. Topical or intralesional or systemic corticosteroids.

Plasma Cell Gingivitis

Definition A non-symptomatic, erythematous, and edematous reaction to various substances, found in the marginal and attached gingiva. Also known as allergic gingivostomatitis, atypical gingivostomatitis, and idiopathic gingivostomatitis.

Etiology Unclear, often idiopathic. Hypersensitivity to components or additives of food, toothpaste, and other orally used products (e.g., lozenges), such as cinnamaldehyde, cinnamon oil, hexylresorcinol, and mint.

Gingival Involvement Rare.

Other Sites of Involvement Rarely, other oral (lips, tongue) or pharyngeal (epiglottis) sites, genital mucosa.

Clinical Features
- Clinically, plasma cell gingivitis presents as a diffuse, sharply demarcated red and edematous area within the attached and marginal gingiva, friable, granular, and readily bleeding upon slight provocation (Figs. 3.8, 3.9 and 3.10). May also rarely present with bullous or verruciform appearance.
- Diagnosis is based on history and clinical features, supplemented by histopathology.

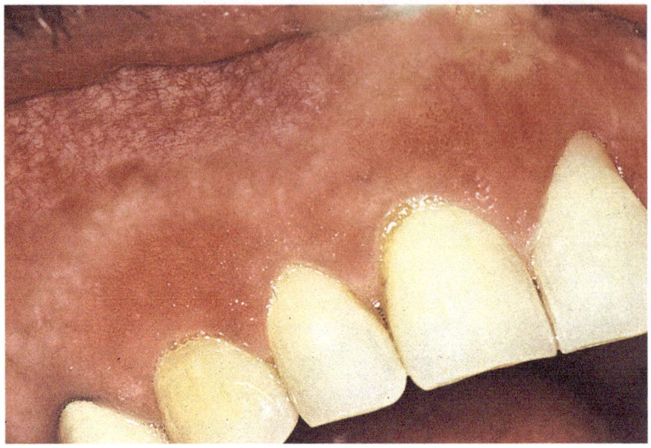

Fig. 3.8 Plasma cell gingivitis, erythematous granular lesions on upper gingiva

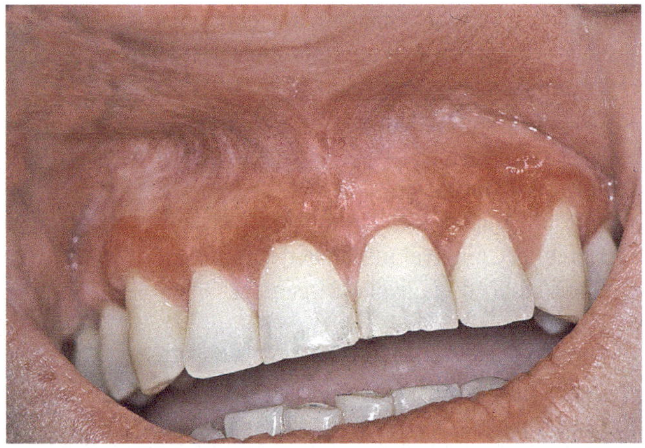

Fig. 3.9 Plasma cell gingivitis, generalized erythematous and edematous lesions on the upper gingiva

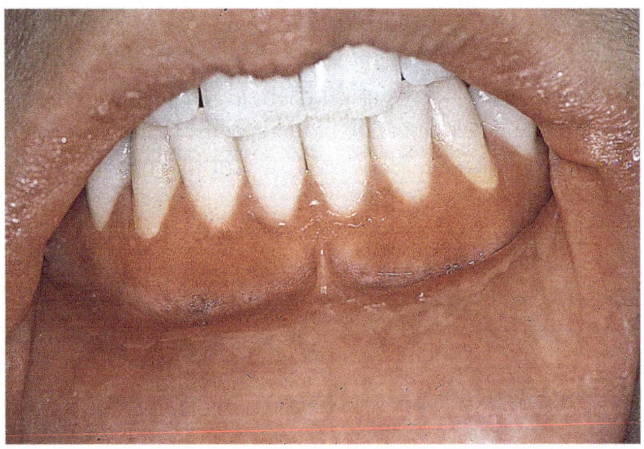

Fig. 3.10 Plasma cell gingivitis, erythematous diffuse lesions on lower gingiva

Differential Diagnosis
- Gingivitis dental biofilm-induced
- Localized juvenile spongiotic gingivitis
- Desquamative gingivitis
- Sarcoidosis
- Crohn disease
- Leukemia
- Wegener granulomatosis
- Amyloidosis
- Scurvy
- Mucopolysaccharidoses
- Mucolipidoses

Laboratory Tests Histopathological and histochemical examination.

Treatment Identification and elimination of eliciting agent. Reinforcement of oral hygiene, antimicrobial rinse and topical corticosteroids, or systemic in severe cases.

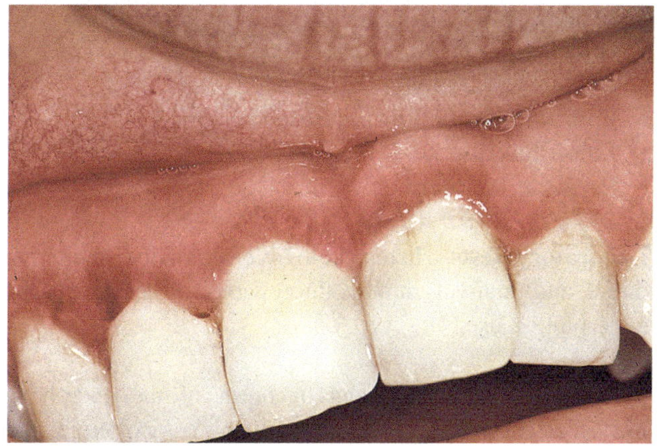

Fig. 3.11 Desquamative gingivitis, typical lesions on the gingiva of mucous membrane pemphigoid

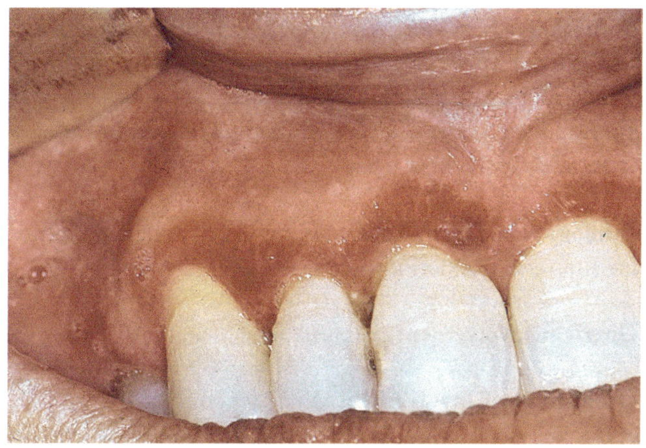

Fig. 3.12 Desquamative gingivitis, clinical manifestation of mucous membrane pemphigoid

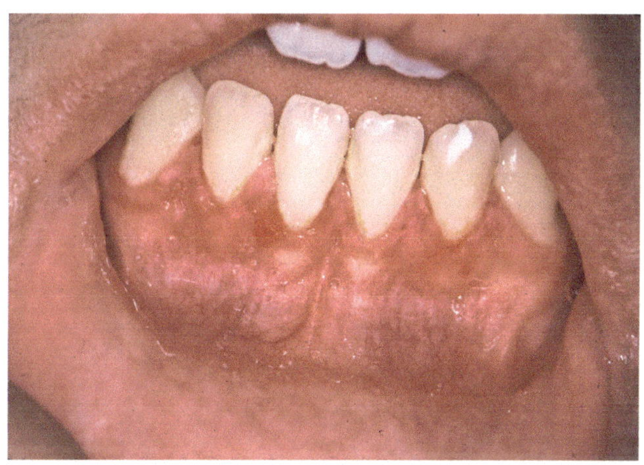

Fig. 3.13 Desquamative gingivitis, lesions of mucous membrane pemphigoid presenting with small hemorrhagic bulla formation at a child

Desquamative Gingivitis

Definition A descriptive term for a gingival inflammatory lesion characterized by erythema, desquamation (shedding) of the epithelium and/or bullous formation after pressure of the gingiva. It is a manifestation of several mucocutaneous diseases.

Etiology Several vesiculobullous diseases may manifest as desquamative gingivitis. Lichen planus, mucous membrane pemphigoid, and pemphigus vulgaris are the most prevalent.

Gingival Involvement Common.

Other Sites of Involvement Oral mucosa (buccal mucosa, lips, tongue, palate) and non-oral (conjunctiva, pharynx, genitalia) mucosa. Skin lesions may also be present, depending on the underlying disease.

Clinical Features
- Clinically, desquamative gingivitis presents with erythematous, edematous, and desquamating areas, often with painful erosions and occasionally ulcerations (Figs. 3.11, 3.12 and 3.13).
- Bullae formation, desquamation, and bleeding upon provocation are characteristic features.
- Clinical diagnosis must be confirmed by laboratory tests.

Differential Diagnosis
- Plasma cell gingivitis
- Lichen planus

- Mucous membrane pemphigoid
- Pemphigus vulgaris
- Bullous pemphigoid
- Epidermolysis bullosa acquisita
- Linear IgA disease
- Erythema multiforme.

Laboratory Tests Histopathologic examination, including direct and indirect immunofluorescence to establish the underlying cause.

Treatment Identification and treatment of the underlying mucocutaneous disease. Topical or systemic corticosteroids and other immunosuppressant drugs. Reinforcement of oral hygiene.

Localized Juvenile Spongiotic Gingivitis

Definition Localized juvenile spongiotic gingivitis or localized juvenile spongiotic gingival hyperplasia is a rare, unique form, from a clinical and histopathological perspective, of gingival hyperplasia affecting primarily children and adolescents, and rarely other ages.

Etiology Unknown. Apparently unrelated to dental biofilm. Possibly due to exteriorized junctional epithelium.

Gingival Involvement Exclusively.

Other Sites of Involvement None reported.

Clinical Features

- Clinically it presents as a bright red, well-demarcated, elevated, and painless, usually sessile gingival lesion, mostly solitary. It demonstrates granular, papillary, or velvety surface appearance and is bleeding upon provocation (Fig. 3.14).

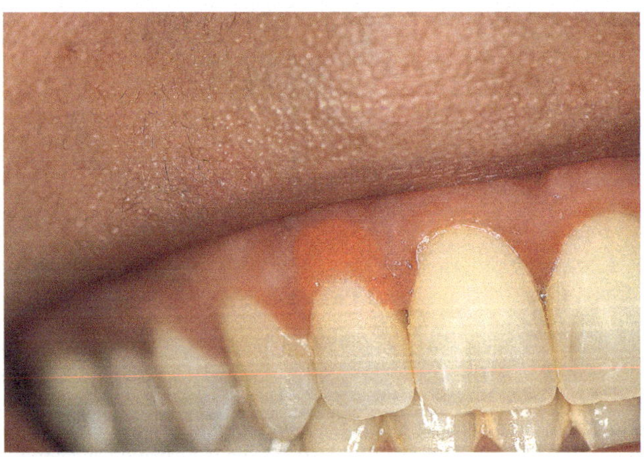

Fig. 3.14 Spongiotic gingival hyperplasia, localized lesion on the upper gingiva

- Often localized in maxillary anterior buccal attached and marginal gingiva.
- Diagnosis is based on history and clinical features, supplemented by the characteristic histopathologic pattern (cellular spongiosis and neutrophils exocytosis).

Differential Diagnosis

- Gingivitis-dental biofilm-induced
- Granulomatous gingivitis
- Plasma cell gingivitis
- Soft tissue plasmacytoma
- Pyogenic granuloma

Laboratory Tests Histopathologic and histochemical examination.

Treatment Conservative surgical excision is the treatment of choice. A slight tendency for recurrence. Spontaneous resolution is possible.

Gingivitis as a Manifestation of Systemic Diseases (see Part IV)

These clinical entities are presented in Part IV.

References

1. Chapple ILC, Mealey BL, Van Dyke TE, et al. Periodontal health and gingival diseases and conditions on an intact and a reduced periodontium: consensus report of workgroup 1 of the 2017 world workshop on the classification of periodontal and peri-implant diseases and conditions. J Clin Periodontol. 2018;45(Suppl 20):S68–77.
2. Trombelli L, Farina R, Silva CO, Tatakis DN. Plaque-induced gingivitis: case definition and diagnostic considerations. J Clin Periodontol. 2018;45(Suppl 20):S44–67.
3. McCartan BE, Healy CM, McCreary CE, et al. Characteristics of patients with orofacial granulomatosis. Oral Dis. 2011;17(7):696–704. https://doi.org/10.1111/j.1601-0825.2011.01826.x.
4. Lourenço SV, Lobo AZ, Boggio P, et al. Gingival manifestations of orofacial granulomatosis. Arch Dermatol. 2008;144(12):1627–30. https://doi.org/10.1001/archderm.144.12.1627.
5. Gordon SC, Daley TD. Foreign body gingivitis: clinical and microscopic features of 61 cases. Oral Surg Oral Med Oral Pathol Oral Radiol Endod. 1997;83(5):562–70. https://doi.org/10.1016/s1079-2104(97)90121-9.
6. Antunes KB, Miranda AM, Carvalho SR, et al. Sarcoidosis presenting as gingival erosion in a patient under long-term clinical control. J Periodontol. 2008;79(3):556–61. https://doi.org/10.1902/jop.2008.070139.
7. Leuci S, Coppola N, Adamo N, et al. Clinico-pathological profile and outcomes of 45 cases of plasma cell gingivitis. J Clin Med. 2021;10(4):830. https://doi.org/10.3390/jcm10040830.
8. Prasanna JS, Mutyap DA, Pantula VR, et al. Plasma cell gingivits–a conflict of diagnosis. J Clin Diagn Res. 2016;10(11):ZD01–3. https://doi.org/10.7860/JCDR/2016/21148.8763.

9. Vishnu V, Ramesh R, Radhakrishnan RP, Sreelakshmi RM. Plasma cell gingivitis mimicking granulomatous disease: a diagnostic dilemma. Clin Adv Periodontics. 2020;11(4):220–4. https://doi.org/10.1002/cap.10108. Epub ahead of print
10. Cabras M, Gambino A, Broccoletti R, Arduino PG. Desquamative gingivitis: a systematic review of possible treatments. J Biol Regul Homeost Agents. 2019;33(2):637–42.
11. Tofan EC, Părlătescu I, Ţovaru Ş, et al. Desquamative gingivitis–a clinicopathological review. Curr Health Sci J. 2018;44(4):331–6. https://doi.org/10.12865/CHSJ.44.04.01.
12. Maderal AD, Lee Salisbury P 3rd, Jorizzo JL. Desquamative gingivitis: clinical findings and diseases. J Am Acad Dermatol. 2018;78(5):839–48. https://doi.org/10.1016/j.jaad.2017.05.056.
13. Yih WY, Maier T, Kratochvil FJ, Zieper MB. Analysis of desquamative gingivitis using direct immunofluorescence in conjunction with histology. J Periodontol. 1998;69(6):678–85. https://doi.org/10.1902/jop.1998.69.6.678.
14. Nisengard RJ, Neiders M. Desquamative lesions of the gingiva. J Periodontol. 1981;52(9):500–10. https://doi.org/10.1902/jop.1981.52.9.500.
15. Laskaris G, Demetriou N, Angelopoulos A. Immunofluorescent studies in desquamative gingivitis. J Oral Pathol. 1981;10(6):398–407. https://doi.org/10.1111/j.1600-0714.1981.tb01291.x.
16. Sklavounou A, Laskaris G. Frequency of desquamative gingivitis in skin diseases. Oral Surg Oral Med Oral Pathol. 1983;56(2):141–4. https://doi.org/10.1016/0030-4220(83)90278-5.
17. McNamara KK, Kalmar JR. Erythematous and vascular oral mucosal lesions: a clinicopathologic review of red entities. Head Neck Pathol. 2019;13(1):4–15. https://doi.org/10.1007/s12105-019-01002-8.
18. Chang JY, Kessler HP, Wright JM. Localized juvenile spongiotic gingival hyperplasia. Oral Surg Oral Med Oral Pathol Oral Radiol Endod. 2008;106(3):411–8. https://doi.org/10.1016/j.tripleo.2008.04.024.
19. Darling MR, Daley TD, Wilson A, Wysocki GP. Juvenile spongiotic gingivitis. J Periodontol. 2007;78(7):1235–40. https://doi.org/10.1902/jop.2007.060502.
20. Eslami A, Sadeghi EM. Mouth breather's gingivitis: a clinicopathologic review. Compendium. 1987;8(1):20–4.
21. Wagaiyu EG, Ashley FP. Mouth breathing, lip seal and upper lip coverage and their relationship with gingival inflammation in 11-14 year-old schoolchildren. J Clin Periodontol. 1991;18(9):698–702. https://doi.org/10.1111/j.1600-051x.1991.tb00112.x.
22. Gulati MS, Grewal N, Kaur A. A comparative study of effects of mouth breathing and normal breathing on gingival health in children. J Indian Soc Pedod Prev Dent. 1998;16(3):72–83.
23. Sharma RK, Bhatia A, Tewari S, Narula SC. Distribution of gingival inflammation in mouth breathing patients: an observational pilot study. J Dent Indones. 2016;23:28–32.

Periodontitis

4

Contents

Periodontitis: Dental Biofilm-Induced

Definition Periodontitis is defined as an inflammatory disease ensuing from the interaction between dysbiotic dental plaque biofilm and host response and resulting in irreversible and progressive destruction of the periodontal apparatus supporting the tooth, affecting the gingiva, alveolar bone, periodontal ligament, and cementum.

Etiology The etiology is dental plaque biofilm accumulation and dysbiosis in a susceptible host. Established risk factors include smoking and diabetes.

Periodontal Involvement Common.

Other Sites of Involvement Periodontitis has been linked to and investigated as a possible risk factor for several systemic diseases (See Chap. 24), with the associations explained by the distant effects of the dysbiotic biofilm originating from the diseased periodontium and/or the systemic effects of the intensified local inflammatory and immune response.

Clinical Features

- Clinically it presents with gingival redness, edema, and bleeding upon provocation, deep periodontal pockets (deepened gingival sulci), and gingival recession, especially with advancing disease. Exudate, debris, and purulence (pyorrhea) may be elicited from the pockets. Supra- and subgingival calculus is typically present (Figs. 4.1 and 4.2).
- Primarily painless, often associated with halitosis (oral malodor) and taste alteration (foul taste).
- Alveolar bone (alveolar bone loss) and periodontal ligament destruction, whose progressive nature leads to diminished tooth support and ensuing increase in tooth mobility. Root resorption may also be present.
- Often presenting with tooth mobility and pathologic tooth migration, signs noticed by the patients and driving them to seek care (Fig. 4.3). In severely advanced cases teeth may exfoliate (Fig. 4.4).

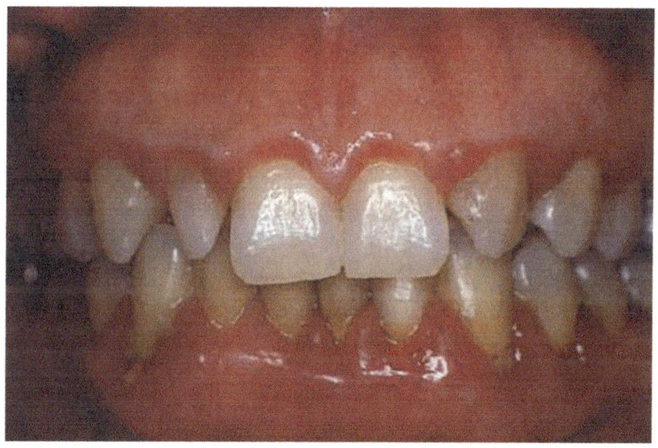

Fig. 4.1 Dental biofilm-induced periodontitis, incipient disease; inflamed gingiva and local factors (plaque and calculus) are evident

G. Laskaris et al., *Periodontal Manifestations of Local and Systemic Diseases*, https://doi.org/10.1007/978-3-031-10828-0_4

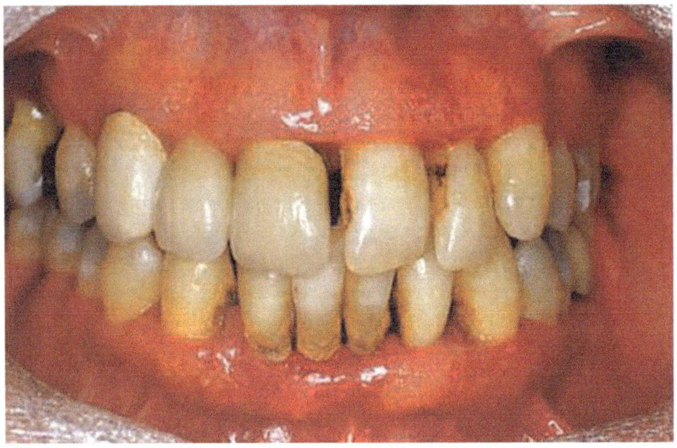

Fig. 4.2 Dental biofilm-induced periodontitis, severe disease with evident loss of attachment, gingival inflammation, and local factors (plaque and calculus)

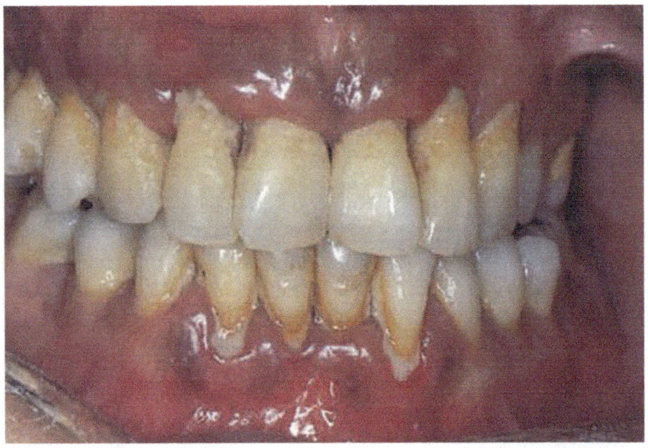

Fig. 4.3 Dental biofilm-induced periodontitis, severe disease with evident loss of attachment, gingival inflammation, local factors, and pathologic tooth migration

- Typically presenting in adults, more prevalent with increasing age, but may also manifest in children and adolescents. Preceded by gingivitis. Worldwide, one of the most prevalent diseases, both among oral diseases and in general.
- The diagnosis is based on the clinical features, including the results of periodontal examination (probing), and dental history and is supported by radiographic imaging. The 2018 Classification of Periodontal Diseases and Conditions introduced a Staging and Grading diagnostic scheme for periodontitis, briefly summarized below.
  - *Stages I, II, III, and IV*: Stages reflect disease severity at presentation and anticipated complexity of disease management; they include description of disease extent and distribution throughout the dentition.
  - *Stage I*: initial or incipient disease, limited clinical attachment loss. No tooth loss due to periodontitis.

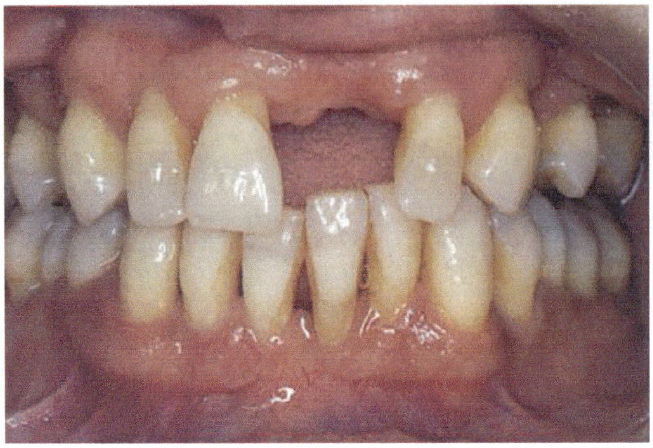

Fig. 4.4 Dental biofilm-induced periodontitis, advanced disease with evident loss of attachment, gingival inflammation, and tooth loss

  - *Stage II*: established disease with periodontal tissue destruction affecting the coronal third of the root; no tooth loss due to periodontitis.
  - *Stage III*: severe disease with periodontal destruction extending to or beyond half of the root length. Limited tooth loss due to the disease and potential for additional tooth loss.
  - *Stage IV*: advanced disease with destruction extending to or beyond half of the root length. Extensive tooth loss and potential loss of the entire dentition.
- For each stage, extent, and distribution may be localized (<30% of teeth involved), generalized (≥30% of teeth), or molar/incisor pattern. Complexity, especially in terms of management/rehabilitation, differentiates primarily Stage III from Stage IV (greatest complexity).
- *Grades A, B, C*: Grades reflect information about biological features, including the rate of disease progression, risk assessment for further progression, possible poor treatment outcomes, and risk assessment for systemic effects of the disease.
  - *Grade A*: slow progression rate.
  - *Grade B*: moderate rate of progression.
  - *Grade C*: rapid progression rate.
  - *Grade modifiers*: presence/absence of risk factors (smoking and diabetes).

Differential Diagnosis

- Gingivitis
- Periodontitis as manifestation of systemic disease (see Part IV)
- Other causes (localized or systemic) of tooth mobility and/or periodontal tissue destruction are trauma (including factitious injury), root fracture, endodontic lesions, and neoplastic diseases

Laboratory Tests There are no specific tests. Current research is focused on potential noninvasive salivary molecular diagnostics.

Treatment The treatment should address the etiology, control the disease process, correct any disease-induced deformities (e.g., deep pockets, craters) that complicate plaque control, and, if possible, reconstruct lost tissues, to provide the patient with optimal function and esthetics. Removal of etiologic factors and elimination of risk factors through oral hygiene instruction (improvement of plaque control), smoking cessation, and improved diabetic control, where indicated. The arrest of the disease process through nonsurgical periodontal therapy, which includes mechanical removal of plaque and calculus through scaling and root planing, using hand and ultrasonic instruments, and extraction of hopeless teeth. Use of adjunctive systemic antibiotic therapy may be indicated in severe cases or severely compromised/highly susceptible patients (evidence of rapid destruction). Pocket elimination through surgical periodontal therapy may be necessary after reevaluation of the outcomes of nonsurgical therapy. Surgical treatment to reconstruct and regenerate lost tissues may also be indicated. Long-term maintenance therapy is essential to prevent or minimize recurrence.

Periodontitis as Manifestation of Systemic Diseases (see Part IV)

These clinical entities are presented in Part IV.

References

1. Sanz M, Papapanou PN, Tonetti MS, et al. Guest editorial: clarifications on the use of the new classification of periodontitis. J Clin Periodontol. 2020;47(6):658–9. https://doi.org/10.1111/jcpe.13286.
2. Chapple ILC, Mealey BL, Van Dyke TE, et al. Periodontal health and gingival diseases and conditions on an intact and a reduced periodontium: consensus report of workgroup 1 of the 2017 world workshop on the classification of periodontal and peri-implant diseases and conditions. J Clin Periodontol. 2018;45(Suppl 20):S68–77.
3. Tonetti MS, Greenwell H, Kornman KS. Staging and grading of periodontitis: framework and proposal of a new classification and case definition. J Clin Periodontol. 2018;89(Suppl 1):S159–72. https://doi.org/10.1111/jcpe.12945.
4. Papapanou PN, Sanz M, Buduneli N, et al. Periodontitis: consensus report of workgroup 2 of the 2017 world workshop on the classification of periodontal and peri-implant diseases and conditions. J Clin Periodontol. 2018;45(Suppl 20):S162–70. https://doi.org/10.1111/jcpe.12946.

5 Necrotizing Periodontal Diseases

Contents

Necrotizing Gingivitis

Definition A rapidly destructive, noncontagious, microbial infection of the gingiva, usually in persons with immune system impairment. Previously known as acute necrotizing ulcerative gingivitis (ANUG).

Etiology The etiology is microbial, in association with impaired antibacterial defenses. Implicated bacteria include Spirochetes (*Treponema* spp.) and other Gram-negative anaerobic bacteria, such as *Prevotella intermedia*, *Selenomonas* spp. and *Fusobacterium* spp. Existing gingivitis, smoking, immunosuppression, diminished coping with psychological stress, and malnutrition are strongly associated predisposing factors.

Gingival Involvement Uncommon, with prevalence higher in susceptible populations.

Other Sites of Involvement Is considered part of a disease spectrum that includes necrotizing periodontitis, necrotizing stomatitis, and noma (cancrum oris), suggestive of potential spread of the infection to nearby tissues. Considered possible precursor of necrotizing periodontitis.

Clinical Features

- Clinically, necrotizing gingivitis is characterized by an acute presentation with pain (from dull ache to severe, sharp pain), gingival bleeding, and interdental papillae ulceration ("punched out" papillae). Tissue necrosis and ulceration usually start at papilla tip (Figs. 5.1 and 5.2)

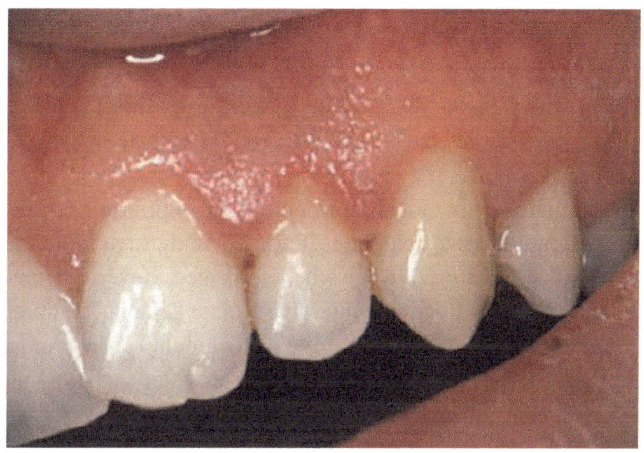

Fig. 5.1 Early stage of necrotizing gingivitis involving only the tips of the papillae

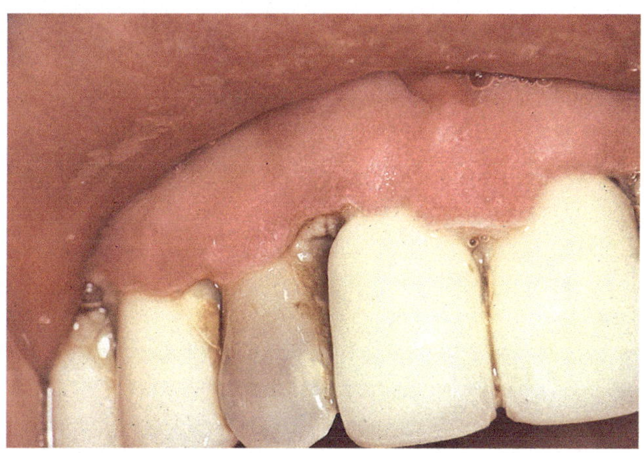

Fig. 5.2 Necrotizing gingivitis, crater formation on upper gingiva

G. Laskaris et al., *Periodontal Manifestations of Local and Systemic Diseases*, https://doi.org/10.1007/978-3-031-10828-0_5

and may spread to entire papilla, marginal gingiva, and attached gingiva with increasing severity (Fig. 5.3). No evidence of attachment loss or alveolar bone involvement.
- Characteristically associated with halitosis (oral malodor) and presence of pseudomembrane over the necrotic tissue. Less commonly, presents with lymphadenopathy and fever.
- Typically presenting in malnourished children and in young adults. Affected young adults are usually immunocompromised (e.g., HIV patients) or under stress (students, soldiers), and mostly smokers. Recurrence is frequent.
- The diagnosis is based on the history and the essential clinical features.

Differential Diagnosis
- Herpetic gingivitis and stomatitis
- Desquamative gingivitis
- Specific bacterial or viral infections of the gingiva
- Acute leukemia
- Necrotizing periodontitis

Laboratory Tests There are no specific tests. Gram-staining of plaque sample smear may support clinical diagnosis.

Treatment Gentle local debridement, antiseptic and antimicrobial mouthrinse, analgesics if needed, and use of systemic antibiotics (metronidazole) when indicated (fever, lymphadenopathy). Following acute phase management, comprehensive periodontal assessment and treatment (prophylaxis, oral hygiene instruction) should be provided and should include management of predisposing factors (e.g., smoking cessation) and institution of regular periodontal maintenance to prevent recurrence.

Necrotizing Periodontitis

Definition A rapidly destructive, noncommunicable, inflammatory disease process of microbial origin, resulting in the destruction of the periodontal apparatus, usually in immunosuppressed individuals.

Etiology The etiology is microbial, with several commonly encountered Gram-negative periodontal pathogens (e.g., Spirochetes (*Treponema* spp.), *Tannerella forsythia*, *Prevotella intermedia*, *Fusobacterium* spp.), and other bacterial species rarely encountered in periodontitis (e.g., *Staphylococcus aureus, Pseudomonas aeruginosa, Enterococcus faecalis*), and *Candida albicans* being implicated, in combination with diminished defenses to bacterial infections. The primary predisposing factor is immunosuppression (especially HIV), with malnutrition, psychological stress, and tobacco smoking, along with preexisting periodontitis or necrotizing gingivitis, considered associated predisposing factors.

Periodontal Involvement Overall rare, with prevalence varying by predisposing condition.

Other Sites of Involvement Is considered part of a disease spectrum that includes necrotizing gingivitis, necrotizing stomatitis, and noma (cancrum oris), suggestive of potential spread of the infection to nearby tissues.

Clinical Features
- Clinically it presents with acutely developing pain (usually severe), with gingival bleeding (often spontaneous), necrosis of the gingiva (ulceration), and attachment loss (Fig. 5.4). As the necrotizing disease process progresses, visible craters develop interproximally (Figs. 5.5 and

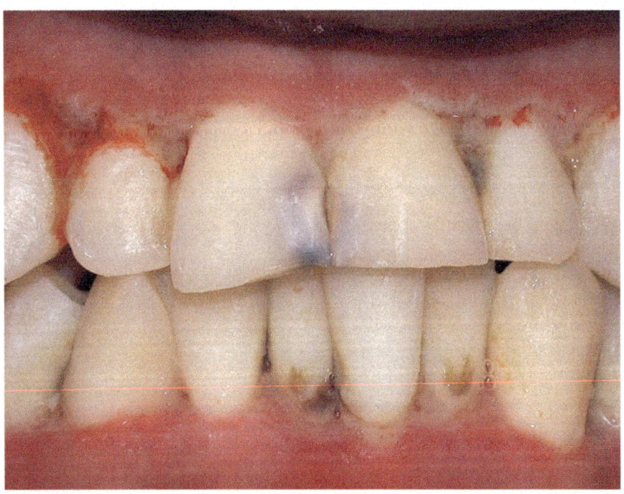

Fig. 5.3 Advanced necrotizing gingivitis

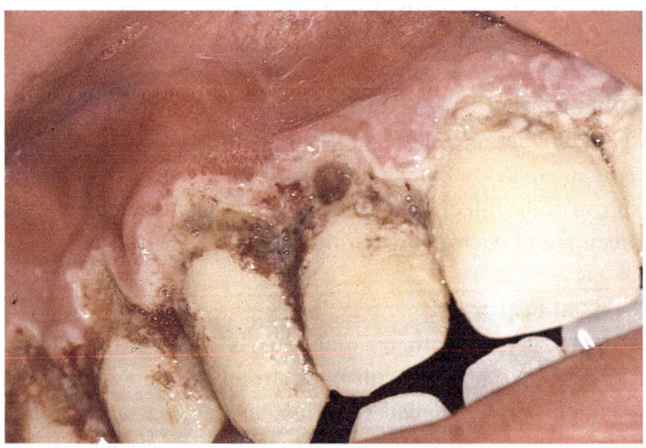

Fig. 5.4 Necrotizing periodontitis, extensive lesions on the gingiva and alveolar bone of an immunosuppressed patient

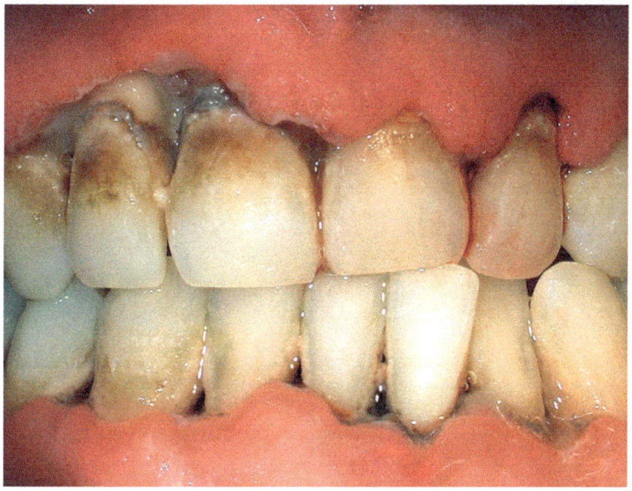

Fig. 5.5 Necrotizing periodontitis with interdental craters

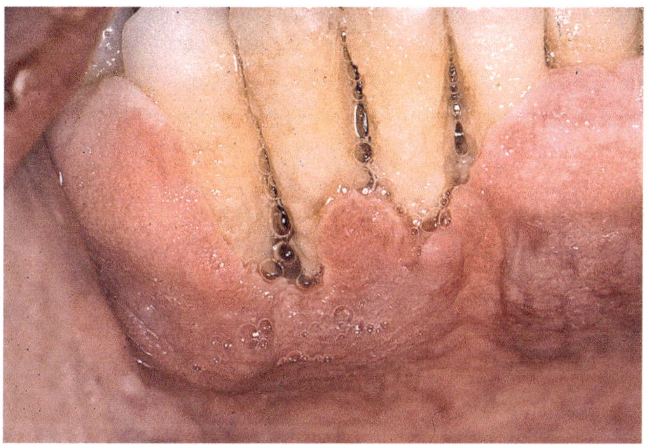

Fig. 5.6 Severe necrotizing periodontitis of an AIDS patient

5.6). Alveolar bone exposure and bone sequestration, due to overlying gingival tissue loss, may also be present. Tooth loss may occur due to severe attachment loss.

- It is associated with halitosis (oral malodor) and the presence of pseudomembrane over the necrotic tissue. May present with lymphadenopathy, fever, and malaise.
- Typically presenting in malnourished children and in young adults. Affected young adults are usually immunocompromised (e.g., HIV patients) or under stress (students, soldiers), and often smokers. Recurrence is frequent.
- The diagnosis is based on the essential clinical features and supported by radiographic evidence of alveolar bone loss.

Differential Diagnosis
- Necrotizing gingivitis
- Acute leukemia
- Neutropenia
- Agranulocytosis
- Scurvy
- Invasive fungal infections

Laboratory Tests There are no specific tests.

Treatment Gentle local debridement, antiseptic and antimicrobial mouthrinse, and, when indicated (fever, lymphadenopathy), use of systemic antibiotics (metronidazole). Following acute phase management, comprehensive periodontal assessment and treatment (prophylaxis, oral hygiene instruction, extraction of hopeless teeth, corrective surgical periodontal therapy) should be provided and should include diagnosis and management of predisposing conditions and factors (e.g., immunosuppression), through medical consultation, and institution of regular periodontal maintenance to prevent recurrence.

References

1. Herrera D, Retamal-Valdes B, Alonso B, Feres M. Acute periodontal lesions (periodontal abscesses and necrotizing periodontal diseases) and endo-periodontal lesions. J Clin Periodontol. 2018;45(Suppl 20):S78–94. https://doi.org/10.1111/jcpe.12941.
2. Dufty J, Gkranias N, Donos N. Necrotising ulcerative gingivitis: a literature review. Oral Health Prev Dent. 2017;15(4):321–7. https://doi.org/10.3290/j.ohpd.a38766.
3. Jia J, Zhou Y, Wang X, Liu Y. Subgingival microbiome dynamic alteration associated with necrotizing periodontal disease: a case report. Medicine (Baltimore). 2021;100(8):e24311. https://doi.org/10.1097/MD.0000000000024311.
4. Nakou M, Kamma J, Gargalianos P, Laskaris G, et al. Periodontal microflora of HIV infected patients with periodontitis. Anaerobe. 1997;3(2–3):97–102. https://doi.org/10.1006/anae.1997.0081.

6 Peri-Implant Diseases

Contents

Peri-Implant Health

Peri-implant health is characterized by the absence of clinical signs of inflammation or infection (bleeding on probing, erythema, edema, suppuration). The range of probing depths compatible with peri-implant health has not been possible to define. It is possible, after successful treatment, to have peri-implant health around endosseous dental implants that have previously experienced bone loss, i.e., that exhibit reduced bone support.

When the periodontal tissues under normal healthy conditions (see Chap. 1) are compared to normal healthy peri-implant tissues, there are not readily, visibly distinguishable, clinical differences. However, there are possible differences, which may include shorter papillae (interproximally) at implant sites compared to papillae around teeth (Fig. 6.1), and generally deeper probing depths around implants than around teeth. As stated above, it has not been possible to define a range of probing depths compatible with health around a dental implant.

Healthy peri-implant soft tissues typically consist of mucosa, 3–4 mm in height, which is either masticatory mucosa (keratinized epithelium) or lining mucosa (non-keratinized epithelium). The implant/abutment-facing aspect of the peri-implant mucosa includes a coronal part, lined by sulcular epithelium, followed apically by a thin junctional epithelium. Apical to the junctional epithelium is the supracrestal connective tissue, which is in direct contact with the surface of the implant. As with the periodontal tissues in clinical health (see Chap. 1), an inflammatory cell infiltrate is present in the clinically healthy peri-implant supracrestal connective tissue, mainly lateral to the sulcular epithelium.

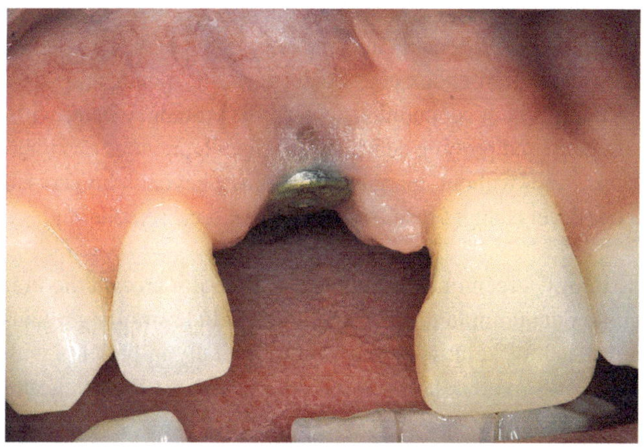

Fig. 6.1 Dental implant with healthy peri-implant tissues, compare interproximal papilla height between teeth and implant

There are several histological differences between healthy periodontal and peri-implant tissues. A main difference between the two organized structures is the lack of cementum and periodontal ligament around implants. The lack of periodontal ligament precludes any implant mobility, in

G. Laskaris et al., *Periodontal Manifestations of Local and Systemic Diseases*, https://doi.org/10.1007/978-3-031-10828-0_6

health, and results in reduced vascularization of the supracrestal connective tissue around implants, due to the absence of the periodontal ligament-originating vascular network. Another difference with respect to the supracrestal connective tissue is the lack of inserting fibers into the implant. The peri-implant epithelium is often longer than the corresponding epithelium around teeth. The aforementioned differences may explain the presence of usually deeper probing depths around implants, compared to teeth, in health.

Osseointegration, which is defined as the direct attachment or connection of vital osseous tissue to the surface of an implant, without intervening connective tissue, results in rigid fixation of the implant in the alveolar or basal bone. Under function, 100% bone-to-implant contact does not exist; the average bone-to-implant contact has been reported to be approximately 60%. Therefore, the portion of the dental implant that is in bone (endosseous) is mostly in direct contact with mineralized bone, with the remaining implant surface facing bone lacunae, bone marrow, osseous vascular channels, or fibrous tissue.

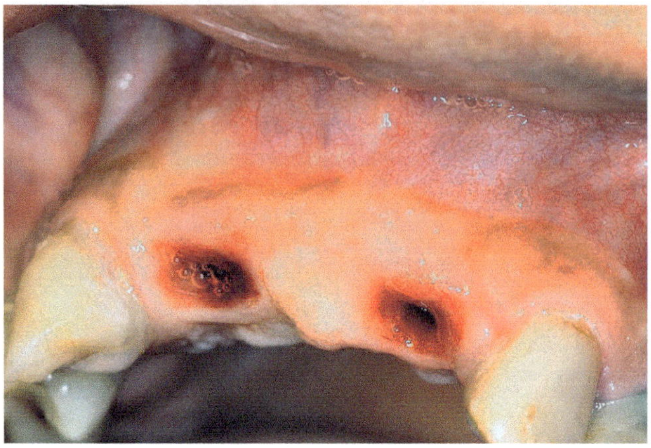

Fig. 6.2 Peri-implant mucositis around two maxillary anterior implants; mucosal redness and slight edema are present

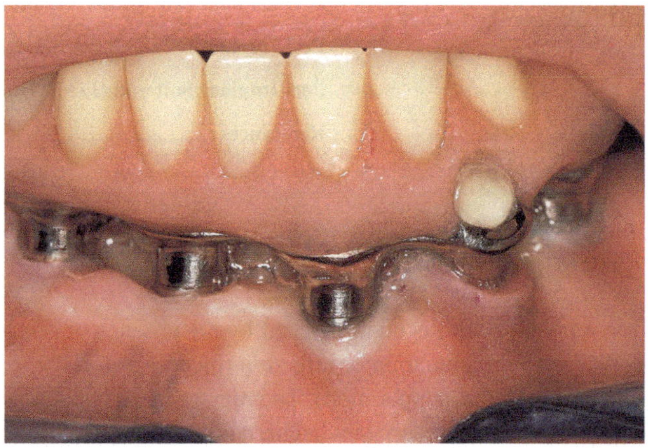

Fig. 6.3 Implant (fourth from left) presenting with peri-implant mucositis; redness and edema are evident

Peri-Implant Mucositis

Definition A reversible inflammatory lesion of the soft tissues surrounding an endosseous dental implant, manifesting with bleeding and/or suppuration upon gentle probing, with or without increased probing depth compared with previous examinations, and without marginal bone loss beyond any crestal bone-level changes resulting from initial bone remodeling.

Etiology Accumulation of bacterial biofilm around the titanium dental implant. Risk indicators include smoking, radiation, lack of keratinized mucosa (especially in patients with poor oral hygiene), excess prosthetic cement material, and diabetes.

Peri-Implant Involvement Common.

Other Sites of Involvement May affect all types of dental implants (endosseous and non-endosseous).

Clinical Features
- Mucosal redness, edema and/or mild tissue enlargement, and bleeding upon provocation (i.e., toothbrushing, periodontal probing, biting into hard foods, e.g., apples); associated biofilm and calculus often present; painless or mild discomfort, often associated with mechanical stimulation (e.g., brushing) (Figs. 6.2 and 6.3).
- Absence of marginal bone loss beyond crestal bone-level changes resulting from initial bone remodeling.
- Highly prevalent worldwide. Considered precursor of peri-implantitis.
- The diagnosis is mainly based on the clinical features and dental history, and supported by radiographic evidence of lack of continuing alveolar bone loss.

Differential Diagnosis
- Peri-implantitis
- Peripheral giant cell granuloma
- Pyogenic granuloma
- Rarely, primary and metastatic malignancies

Laboratory Tests There are no specific tests.

Treatment Control of biofilm results in reversal of inflammation. Mechanical debridement (biofilm and calculus removal) and oral hygiene instruction are essential and may be aided by antimicrobial mouthrinse or gel use. Evaluation of implant-supported restoration and, when indicated, removal of excess cement and/or fabrication of improved restoration. Establishment of regular periodontal maintenance is necessary to prevent recurrence and/or progression to peri-implantitis.

Peri-Implantitis

Definition A destructive inflammatory lesion of the soft and hard tissues surrounding an endosseous dental implant, defined by bleeding and/or suppuration upon gentle probing, increased probing depth compared with previous examinations, and accompanied by progressive peri-implant bone loss beyond any crestal bone-level changes resulting from initial bone remodeling.

Etiology Accumulation and dysbiosis of bacterial biofilm around the titanium dental implant, with disease severity being commensurate with the level of biofilm dysbiosis. Risk indicators are periodontitis or history thereof, biofilm accumulation, lack of regular maintenance therapy, improper implant placement/positioning, plaque retentive factors (excess prosthetic cement material, poorly designed prosthesis), lack of keratinized mucosa (especially in patients whose oral hygiene is lacking), smoking, and hyperglycemia. Potential contributing factors include occlusal overload and release/presence of titanium particles.

Peri-Implant Involvement Common.

Other Sites of Involvement May affect all types of dental implants (endosseous and non-endosseous).

Clinical Features
- Bleeding and/or suppuration upon gentle provocation (e.g., periodontal probing, toothbrushing, biting into hard foods); mucosal redness, edema and/or mild tissue enlargement; associated biofilm and calculus usually present; increased periodontal probing relative to prior examinations (painless or mild discomfort); may be accompanied by mucosal deficiency (soft tissue recession) around the implant and exposure of implant threads (Fig. 6.4).
- Evidence of continuing marginal bone loss, beyond any crestal bone-level changes associated with the initial bone remodeling; progress in accelerating manner.
- In the absence of prior examination data, probing depths ≥6 mm and bone level ≥ 3 mm apical of the most coronal portion of the intraosseous part of the implant.
- Increased severity may lead to implant failure, complete loss of osseointegration, implant mobility, and exfoliation.
- Highly prevalent worldwide. Preceded by peri-implant mucositis.
- The diagnosis is mainly based on the clinical features and dental history, and supported by radiographic evidence of progressive alveolar bone loss.

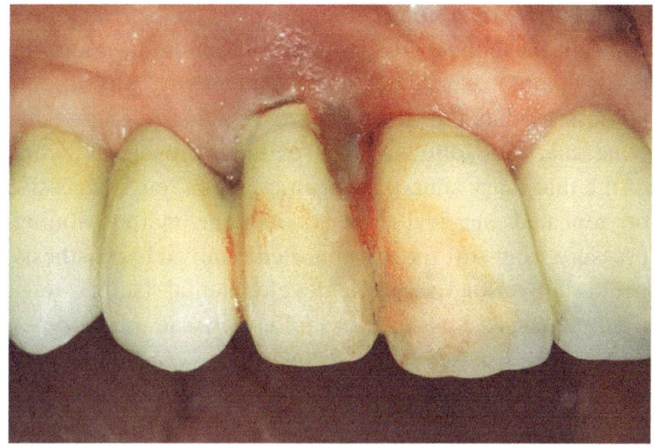

Fig. 6.4 Maxillary implant presenting with peri-implantitis, note inflammation and suppuration; deep probing depths are also present

Differential Diagnosis
- Peri-implant mucositis
- Common benign oral mucosal lesions
- Rarely, primary and metastatic malignancies

Laboratory Tests There are no specific tests.

Treatment Therapeutic aims include arresting the disease process (resolve inflammation, remove biofilm and plaque retentive factors, improve oral hygiene), correcting soft tissue morphology (pocket elimination, through flap surgery or gingivectomy), regenerating lost bone to increase support (surface decontamination, guided bone regeneration; re-osseointegration of the exposed part may be possible), eliminating or reducing contributing factors (smoking cessation, soft tissue grafting to increase keratinized mucosa), and establishing proper maintenance regimen.

Peri-Implant Soft and Hard Tissue Deficiencies

Definition Soft tissue defects around implants include both quantitative (e.g., reduced volume, presence of soft tissue dehiscence or recession) and qualitative (lack of keratinized tissue) deficiencies. Hard tissue defects include horizontal and/or vertical ridge defects, bone dehiscence, and fenestration.

Etiology The etiology can be multifactorial for both soft and hard tissue deficiencies. The identified etiologic factors include orofacial trauma (e.g., automobile accidents); local diseases affecting adjacent teeth (e.g., endodontic infections, longitudinal root fractures), adjacent periodontal tissues (e.g., periodontitis), and the peri-implant tissues (e.g., peri-implantitis); physiologic processes related to tissue healing or aging (e.g., alveolar bone resorption following tooth extraction, pneumatization of the maxillary sinus); iatrogenic factors (e.g., excessive or repeated surgical trauma, implant malpositioning, pressure from soft tissue-supported removable prosthesis, occlusal overload); genetic/developmental factors (e.g., tooth agenesis, tissue morphology, tissue phenotype); systemic diseases and conditions and systemic medications. The severity of the resulting soft or hard tissue defect may increase when multiple etiologic factors are present concurrently.

Peri-Implant Involvement Common.

Other Sites of Involvement May affect all types of dental implants (endosseous and non-endosseous).

Clinical Features

- The clinical features vary depending on the nature of the defect. These defects may lead to soft tissue inflammation, soft tissue recession, and increase in marginal bone loss (Fig. 6.5). These in turn may compromise implant function and survival.
- Lack of keratinized mucosa may impair plaque removal and increase patient discomfort. Any associated discomfort and/or aesthetic complications may also negatively impact the patient's quality of life.
- Compromised marginal bone levels (reduced alveolar crest height) may manifest with reduced interproximal papilla height.

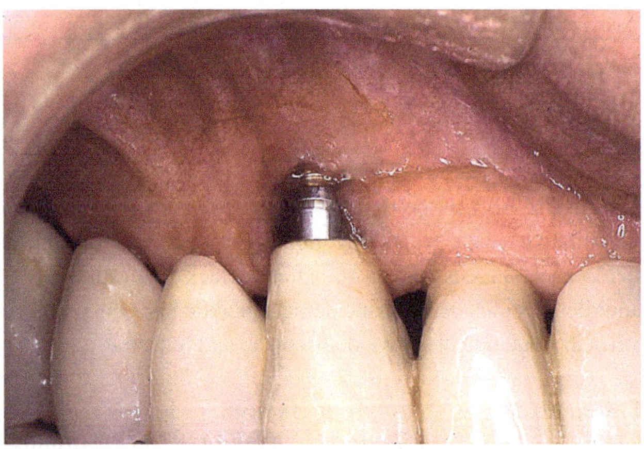

Fig. 6.5 Soft and hard tissue defects on the buccal aspect of a maxillary implant, likely due to malpositioning

- The diagnosis is primarily based on the clinical features and dental history, and is supported by radiographic findings.

Differential Diagnosis

- Primarily concerns differentiation/identification of the underlying etiologic factor(s).

Laboratory Tests There are no specific tests.

Treatment Therapeutic interventions are typically surgical, aiming to reconstruct the presenting soft and hard tissue defects, and preventative, aiming to eliminate or control the identified etiologies.

References

1. Renvert S, Persson GR, Pirih FQ, Camargo PM. Peri-implant health, peri-implant mucositis, and peri-implantitis: case definitions and diagnostic considerations. J Clin Periodontol. 2018;45(Suppl 20):S278–85. https://doi.org/10.1111/jcpe.12956.
2. Berglundh T, Armitage G, Araujo MG, et al. Peri-implant diseases and conditions: consensus report of workgroup 4 of the 2017 world workshop on the classification of periodontal and Peri-implant diseases and conditions. J Clin Periodontol. 2018;45(Suppl 20):S286–91. https://doi.org/10.1111/jcpe.12957.
3. Heitz-Mayfield LJA, Salvi GE. Peri-implant mucositis. J Clin Periodontol. 2018;45(Suppl 20):S237–45. https://doi.org/10.1111/jcpe.12953.
4. Román-Quesada N, González-Navarro B, Izquierdo-Gómez K, et al. An analysis of the prevalence of peripheral giant cell granuloma and pyogenic granuloma in relation to a dental implant. BMC Oral Health. 2021;21(1):204. Published 2021 Apr 23. https://doi.org/10.1186/s12903-021-01566-4.
5. Miranda Galvis M, Schausltz Pereira Faustino I, Cabral Ramos J, et al. Oral cancer adjacent to dental implants mimicking benign lesions: a case series study. Aust Dent J. 2021;66(1):112–8. https://doi.org/10.1111/adj.12793.
6. Schwarz F, Derks J, Monje A, Wang HL. Peri-implantitis. J Clin Periodontol. 2018;45(Suppl 20):S246–66. https://doi.org/10.1111/jcpe.12954.
7. Kröger A, Hülsmann C, Fickl S, et al. The severity of human peri-implantitis lesions correlates with the level of submucosal microbial dysbiosis. J Clin Periodontol. 2018;45(12):1498–509. https://doi.org/10.1111/jcpe.13023.
8. Kumar PS, Dabdoub SM, Hegde R, et al. Site-level risk predictors of peri-implantitis: a retrospective analysis. J Clin Periodontol. 2018;45(5):597–604. https://doi.org/10.1111/jcpe.12892.
9. Raiser V, Abu-El Naaj I, Shlomi B, et al. Primary oral malignancy imitating peri-implantitis. J Oral Maxillofac Surg. 2016;74(7):1383–90. https://doi.org/10.1016/j.joms.2016.02.008.
10. Hämmerle CHF, Tarnow D. The etiology of hard- and soft-tissue deficiencies at dental implants: a narrative review. J Clin Periodontol. 2018;45(Suppl 20):S267–77. https://doi.org/10.1111/jcpe.12955.

Part III

Other Local Non-Dental Biofilm Induced Conditions Affecting Periodontal Tissues

7 Periodontal Abscesses

Contents

Periodontal Abscesses

Definition A destructive inflammatory lesion, defined as an abscess (pus accumulation), localized within the gingival wall of the periodontal pocket.

Etiology Invasion of bacteria into the soft tissues around a periodontal pocket, resulting in acute inflammatory infiltrate and subsequent pus formation and, ultimately, localized pus accumulation if conditions prevent drainage. May ensue following foreign body impaction in the periodontal pocket. Rarely, may be associated with lateral root canal of non-vital tooth draining into a periodontal pocket (endodontic-periodontal lesion).

Periodontal Involvement Common.

Other Sites of Involvement Periodontal abscesses have the potential to cause severe infections in distant tissues and organs, with dissemination associated with untreated abscesses or occurring during therapy.

Clinical Features

- Typically presenting with gingival swelling, bleeding and/or suppuration upon periodontal probing, and often pain. Deep periodontal pockets and tooth mobility may also be present. Patients may report tooth feeling "high" (Figs. 7.1, 7.2, and 7.3).
- Rarely, signs of systemic involvement (fever, lymphadenopathy) may develop.
- Often develops in untreated periodontitis patients, i.e., in an existing periodontal pocket. May also develop in patients who have received nonsurgical or maintenance therapy for periodontitis, or in patients having received systemic antibiotics. Prevalence may be increased in systemically compromised patients susceptible to bacterial infections (e.g., diabetics).
- The diagnosis is based on the clinical features and dental history and supported by vitality testing (tooth found vital) and radiographic evidence that can help with differential diagnosis.

Differential Diagnosis

- Gingival abscess
- Periapical abscess
- Other localized swellings (e.g., pyogenic granuloma, lateral periodontal cyst)
- Rarely, primary and metastatic malignancies

Laboratory Tests There are no specific tests.

Treatment Establishment of drainage, usually by means of mechanical instrumentation of the periodontal pocket, and irrigation, along with the removal of local debris and contributing factors (e.g., calculus, foreign body). Systemic antibiotics may be indicated when systemic involvement is present. Analgesics may ease patient discomfort. After resolution, comprehensive periodontal assessment and treatment is necessary to prevent recurrence.

G. Laskaris et al., *Periodontal Manifestations of Local and Systemic Diseases*, https://doi.org/10.1007/978-3-031-10828-0_7

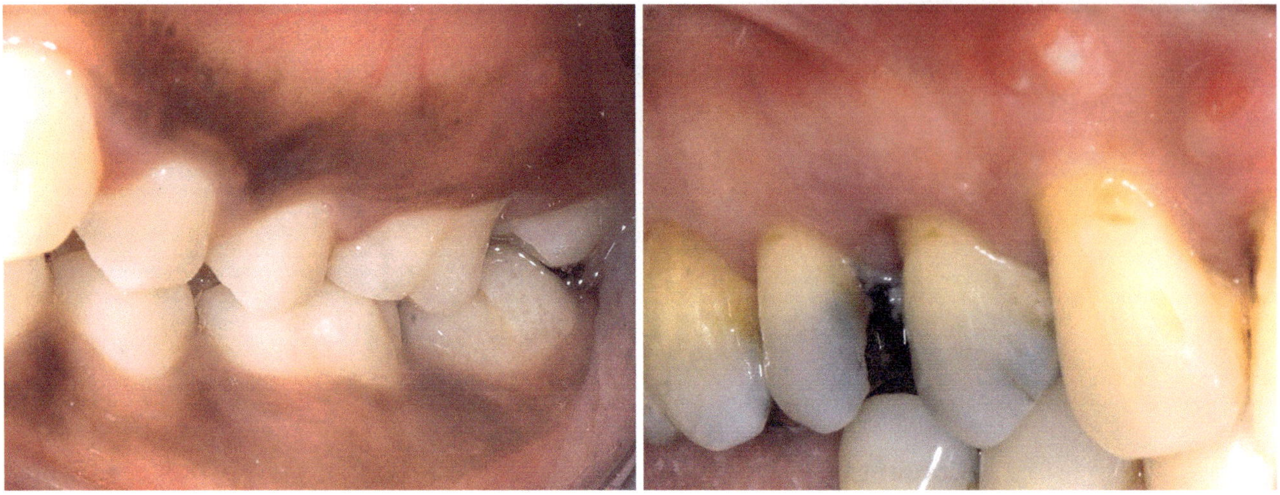

Figs. 7.1 and 7.2 Periodontal abscesses; note associated gingival swelling

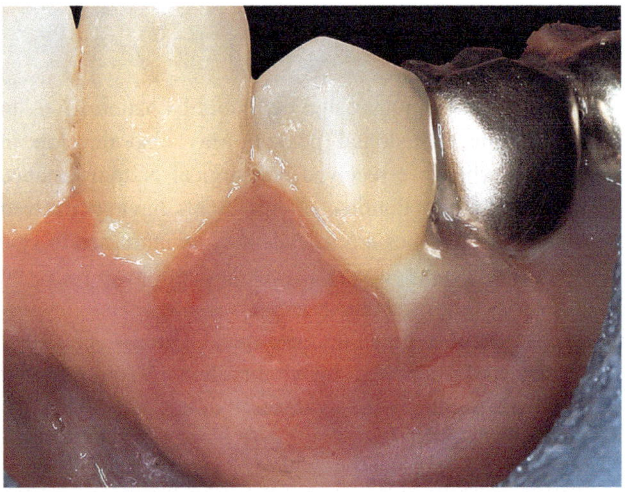

Fig. 7.3 Periodontal abscess; note marked suppuration

References

1. Meng HX. Periodontal abscess. Ann Periodontol. 1999;4(1):79–83. https://doi.org/10.1902/annals.1999.4.1.79.
2. Wadia R, Ide M. Periodontal emergencies in general practice. Prim Dent J. 2017;6(2):46–51. https://doi.org/10.1308/205016817821281774.
3. Herrera D, Retamal-Valdes B, Alonso B, Feres M. Acute periodontal lesions (periodontal abscesses and necrotizing periodontal diseases) and endo-periodontal lesions. J Clin Periodontol. 2018;45(Suppl 20):S78–94. https://doi.org/10.1111/jcpe.12941.
4. Papapanou PN, Sanz M, Buduneli N, et al. Periodontitis: consensus report of workgroup 2 of the 2017 world workshop on the classification of periodontal and Peri-implant diseases and conditions. J Clin Periodontol. 2018;45(Suppl 20):S162–70. https://doi.org/10.1111/jcpe.12946.

8 Mucogingival Deformities and Conditions Around Teeth

Contents

Gingival/Soft Tissue Recession

Definition The shift of the gingival/soft tissue margin apical to the cementoenamel junction. Typically confined to buccal or lingual aspects of the teeth.

Etiology Typically multifactorial. Commonly attributed to chronic mechanical trauma to the tissues (e.g., aggressive toothbrushing, self-inflicted injuries). Several predisposing factors have been suggested, including anatomical (e.g., aberrant tooth position, thin periodontal phenotype, lack of attached gingiva, aberrant frenum), behavioral (e.g., smoking), and iatrogenic factors (e.g., orthodontic tooth movement, cervical restorations, removable appliances). Rarely, may result from local disease (e.g., herpetic lesions).

Gingival Involvement Common on facial aspect of teeth.

Other Sites of Involvement Lingual/palatal aspect of teeth.

Clinical Features

- Gingival/soft tissue margin located apical to the cementoenamel junction, with concomitant exposure of the tooth root and evident loss of attachment (Fig. 8.1).

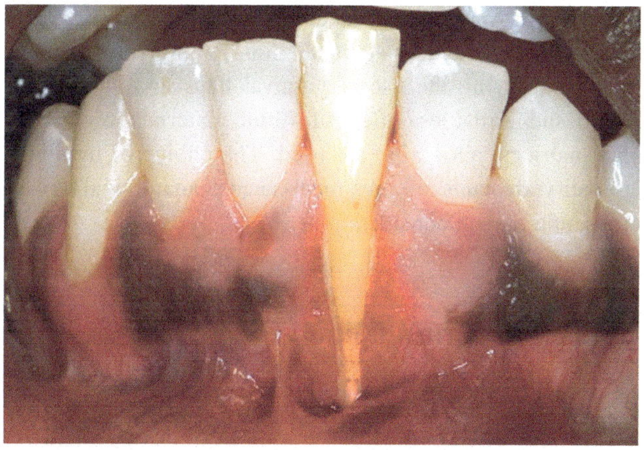

Fig. 8.1 Deep recession defect on mandibular central incisor, with associated lack of keratinized gingiva

- May be associated with dentin hypersensitivity and with carious and non-carious cervical lesions (e.g., abrasions) (Fig. 8.2) and may be associated with lack of keratinized gingiva (Fig. 8.1).
- Patients may present complaining of associated esthetic concerns.
- Highly prevalent in adults; common in persons with both excellent and poor oral hygiene. Prevalence, severity, and extent increase with age.
- Diagnosis is based on clinical features.

G. Laskaris et al., *Periodontal Manifestations of Local and Systemic Diseases*, https://doi.org/10.1007/978-3-031-10828-0_8

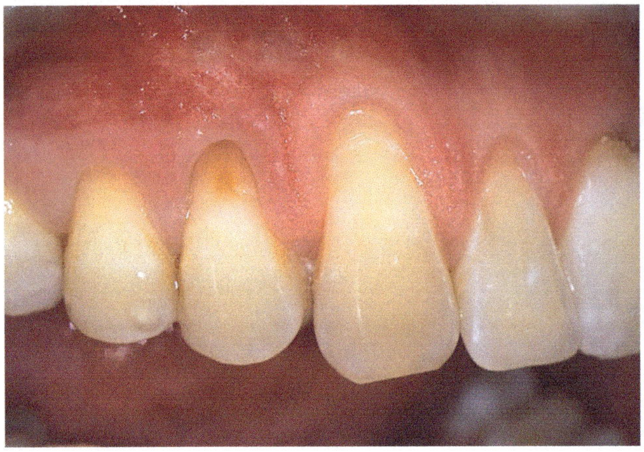

Fig. 8.2 Recession defect on maxillary canine, with associated noncarious cervical lesion, and recession with associated carious lesion on first premolar

Differential Diagnosis
- Uneven gingival margins (pseudo-recession).
- Enamel structure loss at cementoenamel junction.

Laboratory Tests There are no specific tests.

Treatment Various surgical approaches are used to accomplish root coverage or augmentation of gingival thickness, often employing the use of gingival flaps and autogenous soft tissue grafts; less often, substitute materials (e.g., collagen matrices, allografts) are used. The choice of treatment modality depends on treatment needs, anatomical conditions, and patient considerations.

Lack of Keratinized Gingiva

Definition The absence of keratinized gingiva around the tooth.

Etiology Typically multifactorial. Commonly attributed to chronic mechanical trauma to the tissues (e.g., aggressive toothbrushing, self-inflicted injuries) and associated with gingival recession. Occasionally iatrogenic (postsurgical). Several predisposing factors have been suggested, including anatomical (e.g., aberrant tooth position, thin periodontal phenotype, aberrant frenum), and iatrogenic factors (e.g., orthodontic tooth movement, cervical restorations).

Gingival Involvement Common on facial aspect of teeth.

Other Sites of Involvement Lingual aspect of mandibular anterior teeth. It may also commonly occur around dental implants.

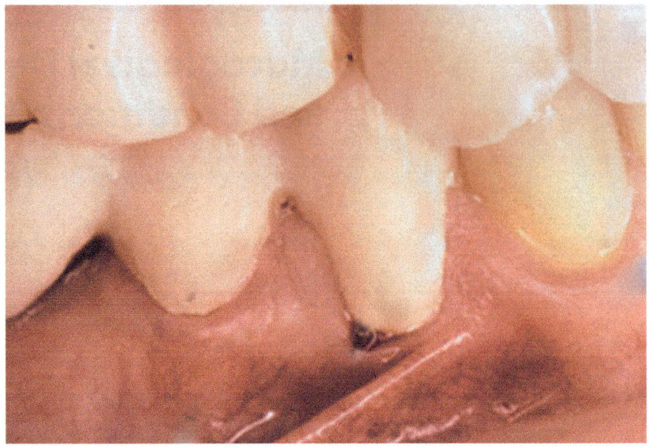

Fig. 8.3 Lack of keratinized gingiva on the buccal aspect of first premolar; note an associated aberrant frenum

Clinical Features
- The clinical presentation is that of soft tissue margin consisting of alveolar mucosa, that may be associated with soft tissue recession (Fig. 8.3).
- Patients may present complaining of tenderness during toothbrushing or eating.
- Diagnosis is based on clinical features.

Differential Diagnosis
- Uneven gingival margins (pseudo-recession).

Laboratory Tests There are no specific tests.

Treatment Various surgical approaches are used to accomplish gingival augmentation, often including use of autogenous soft tissue grafts, and less often including use of substitute materials (e.g., collagen matrices, allografts). The choice of treatment procedure depends on anatomical conditions and patient considerations.

Aberrant Frenum

Definition Atypical/abnormal insertion of labial, buccal, or lingual frenula capable of retracting gingival margins, creating diastemas, and limiting lip and tongue movements (ankyloglossia).

Etiology Developmental. Rarely may be a sequela of periodontal disease or surgical treatment. Also associated with rare genetic conditions (e.g., Ellis-van Creveld syndrome).

Gingival Involvement Fairly common in maxillary and mandibular central incisor areas (facial aspect).

Other Sites of Involvement Facial aspect of other teeth. Rarely, lingual aspect of mandibular central incisors (lingual frenum).

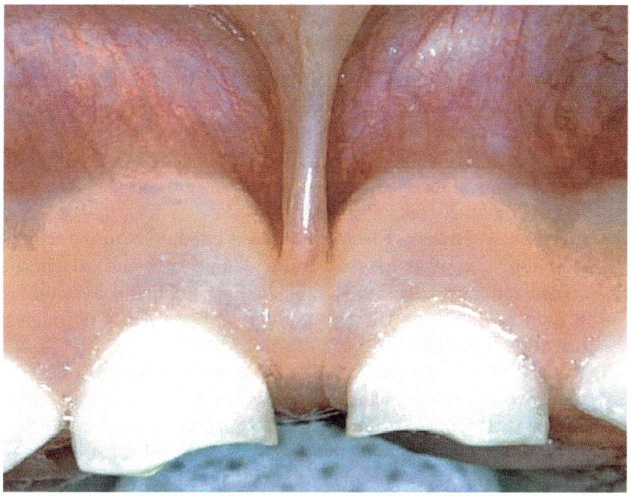

Fig. 8.4 Aberrant maxillary labial frenum in a child, with associated midline diastema

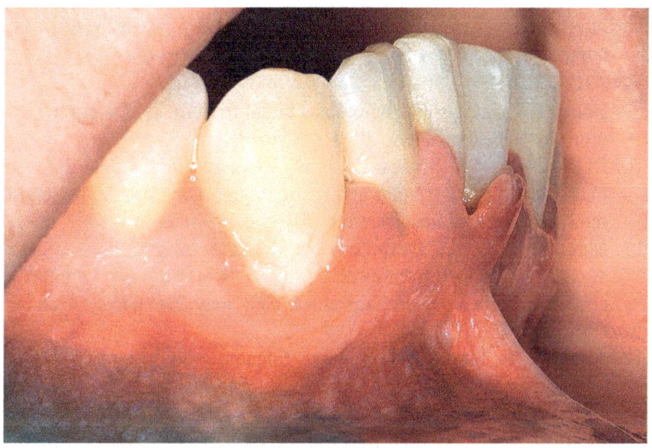

Fig. 8.5 Aberrant mandibular labial frenum; note how the pull from the frenum moves the buccal gingiva away from the central incisor teeth

Clinical Features

- Clinically it may be associated with midline diastema, especially in maxilla (Fig. 8.4).
- High frenum attachment that may cause mobility of gingiva by encroaching on the marginal gingival usually associated with increased local plaque accumulation, gingival inflammation, and gingival recession, especially in mandible (Figs. 8.3 and 8.5).
- Patients may present with complaints of difficulty brushing in the area.
- Diagnosis is based on clinical features.

Differential Diagnosis

- Injured/torn frenum in addition to other traumas and questionable history may be indicative of child or elder abuse.

Laboratory Tests There are no specific tests.

Treatment Surgical excision (frenectomy), either alone or in combination with root coverage procedures when indicated.

Gingival Excess—Gingival Enlargement

Definition The presence of excessive gingival tissue, resulting in greater than normal coverage of the anatomical crown of the tooth. It may manifest as pseudo pocketing (increased probing depths in the absence of attachment loss), inconsistent gingival margins, gingival enlargement, or combinations thereof. The term "gingival excess" may also refer to excessive gingival display (typically greater than 2 mm) during smiling, often referred to as "gummy smile," which may or may not be accompanied by greater than normal coverage of the anatomical crown.

Etiology Multifactorial. It may be of developmental (e.g., altered passive eruption), genetic (e.g., hereditary gingival fibromatosis), inflammatory (e.g., mouth breathing, orthodontic treatment), drug-related (e.g., drug-induced gingival enlargement), or disease-related (e.g., leukemia) origin. Multiple etiologies may be present concurrently.

Gingival Involvement Fairly common, especially in maxillary anterior dentition.

Other Sites of Involvement Posterior dentition, retromolar areas.

Clinical Features

- Clinically gingival excess presents as increased amount (often volume) of gingival tissue, which may have normal, fibrotic, or inflamed appearance, depending on the underlying etiology and local plaque levels. (Fig. 8.6).
- Teeth may appear short and/or square, with gingiva covering more than 20% of the anatomical crown length. (Fig. 8.7).
- Diagnosis is based on clinical features and history and is supported by radiographic documentation.

Differential Diagnosis

- Differentiation between the various etiologies is the main concern.

Laboratory Tests There are no specific tests.

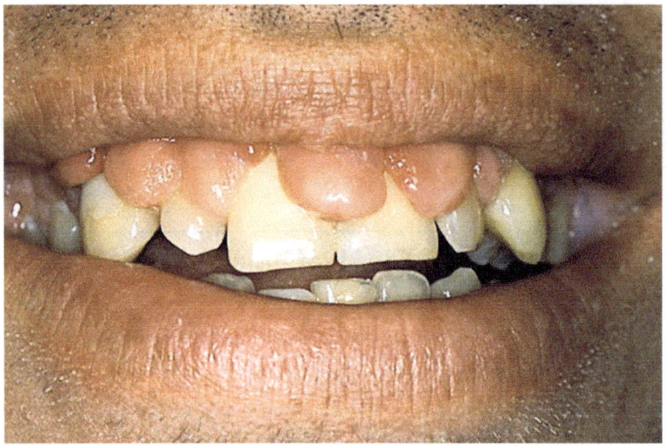

Fig. 8.6 Gingival excess in a case of drug-induced gingival enlargement

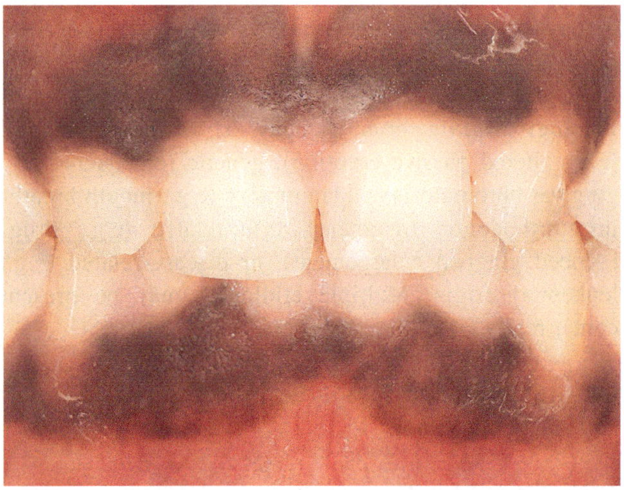

Fig. 8.7 Gingival excess in a case of altered passive eruption; several teeth appear short and square

Treatment Surgical excision in most cases. Recurrence may be common for certain etiologies (e.g., genetic and drug-induced enlargements, persistent mouth breathing). Whenever possible, addressing the underlying etiology (e.g., change of medications, debonding after completion of orthodontic treatment) may lead to partial or complete resolution. For gummy smile, treatment is dictated by the underlying etiology and may vary from orthognathic surgery and lip repositioning surgery to periodontal surgery and restorative treatment.

References

1. Chambrone L, Tatakis DN. Periodontal soft tissue root coverage procedures: a systematic review from the AAP regeneration workshop. J Periodontol. 2015;86(2 Suppl):S8–S51.
2. Chambrone L, Tatakis DN. Long-term outcomes of untreated buccal gingival recessions: a systematic review and meta-analysis. J Periodontol. 2016;87:796–808.
3. Cortellini P, Bissada NF. Mucogingival conditions in the natural dentition: narrative review, case definitions, and diagnostic considerations. J Clin Periodontol. 2018;45(Suppl 20):S190–8.
4. Kassab MM, Cohen RE. The etiology and prevalence of gingival recession. J Am Dent Assoc. 2003;134:220–5.
5. Tatakis DN, Chambrone L, Allen EP, et al. Periodontal soft tissue root coverage procedures: a consensus report from the AAP regeneration workshop. J Periodontol. 2015;86(2 Suppl):S52–5.
6. Scheyer ET, Sanz M, Dibart S, et al. Periodontal soft tissue non-root coverage procedures: a consensus report from the AAP regeneration workshop. J Periodontol. 2015;86(2 Suppl):S73–6.
7. Bertl K, Melchard M, Pandis N, et al. Soft tissue substitutes in non-root coverage procedures: a systematic review and meta-analysis. Clin Oral Investig. 2017;21(2):505–18.
8. Dragan IF, Hotlzman LP, Karimbux NY, et al. Clinical outcomes of comparing soft tissue alternatives to free gingival graft: a systematic review and meta-analysis. J Evid Based Dent Pract. 2017;17(4):370–380.e3.
9. Boutsi EA, Tatakis DN. Maxillary labial frenum attachment in children. Int J Paediatr Dent. 2011;21:284–8.
10. Delli K, Livas C, Sculean A, et al. Facts and myths regarding the maxillary midline frenum and its treatment: a systematic review of the literature. Quintessence Int. 2013;44:177–87.
11. Maguire S, Hunter B, Hunter L, et al. Diagnosing abuse: a systematic review of torn frenum and other intra-oral injuries [published correction appears in arch dis child. 2008 may;93(5):453]. Arch Dis Child. 2007;92:1113–7.
12. Andijani RI, Tatakis DN. Hypermobile upper lip is highly prevalent among patients seeking treatment for gummy smile. J Periodontol. 2019;90(3):256–62. https://doi.org/10.1002/JPER.18-0468.
13. Mele M, Felice P, Sharma P, et al. Esthetic treatment of altered passive eruption. Periodontol. 2018;77(1):65–83. https://doi.org/10.1111/prd.12206.
14. Kalsi HJ, Hussain Z, Darbar U. An update on crown lengthening. Part 1: gingival tissue excess. Dent Update. 2015;42(2):144–53. https://doi.org/10.12968/denu.2015.42.2.144.
15. Silva CO, Ribeiro-Júnior NV, Campos TV, et al. Excessive gingival display: treatment by a modified lip repositioning technique. J Clin Periodontol. 2013;40(3):260–5. https://doi.org/10.1111/jcpe.12046.
16. Silberberg N, Goldstein M, Smidt A. Excessive gingival display–etiology, diagnosis, and treatment modalities. Quintessence Int. 2009;40(10):809–18.
17. Dahllöf G, Axiö E, Modéer T. Regression of phenytoin-induced gingival overgrowth after withdrawal of medication. Swed Dent J. 1991;15(3):139–43.

9 Endodontic and Periodontal Lesions

Contents

Definition Endodontic-periodontal lesions, often referred to as "Endo-Perio" or "Perio-Endo" lesions, are defined as acute or chronic pathologic communications between the periodontal and pulpal tissues of a tooth.

Etiology The etiology is the respective etiologies of periodontitis and endodontic involvement, i.e., dysbiotic biofilm in a susceptible host and the infectious (e.g., caries) or non-infectious (e.g., trauma, restorative procedures, tooth fracture) causes of pulpal disease/necrosis. Contributing factors are anatomical deformities of the root, e.g., accessory canals and deep developmental grooves, and loss of cementum resulting in exposure of open dentinal tubules, all of which can develop into patent direct anatomical communication between the pulp and the periodontal ligament or periodontal pocket space.

Periodontal Involvement Fairly common.

Clinical Features

- The typical signs of these lesions include a deep periodontal pocket, usually localized and often extending to the apex of the root, and/or negative or altered pulpal response to vitality testing.
- Clinically endodontic-periodontal lesions have been classified into the following categories:
  - *Primary endodontic lesion.* This is an acute inflammatory lesion, usually developing from a chronic periapical lesion, on a tooth with a necrotic pulp, which may drain through the periodontal ligament into the gingival sulcus. This represents a sinus tract (from the pulp to the periodontal ligament and sulcus) that clinically may present as a periodontal abscess.
  - *Primary periodontal lesion.* In this lesion, bacteria from a deep periodontal pocket gain access to the pulp, typically from the apical foramen, and cause localized changes, although the tooth will mostly provide a normal response to pulpal testing.
  - *Primary endodontic lesion with secondary periodontal involvement.* If a primary endodontic lesion does not receive treatment, it will become chronic and can lead to extensive periodontal tissue damage and loss of periodontal support (retrograde periodontitis). Such lesions may also be the result of endodontic or restorative treatment complications (e.g., root perforation occurring during root canal therapy or post and pin placement during tooth buildup), or the manifestation of a root fracture, especially in endodontically treated teeth with posts and cores. The clinical signs may vary, from an acute, painful, periodontal abscess to a painless, localized, deep periodontal pocket with associated typical inflammatory characteristics (e.g., redness, bleeding on probing).
  - *Primary periodontal lesion with secondary endodontic involvement.* A long-standing periodontitis lesion that has reached the apical foramen may lead to pulpal necrosis, due to the bacterial biofilm and the elevated levels of host pro-inflammatory molecules gaining access to the pulp. Such lesions may also develop following periodontal therapy, because the necessary root instrumentation may create access to the pulp through dentinal tubules and accessory canals or possibly through severed pulpal blood vessels (e.g., in an exposed accessory canal).
  - *True combined lesion.* A lesion where periodontal and pulpal disease develop independently and even-

G. Laskaris et al., *Periodontal Manifestations of Local and Systemic Diseases*, https://doi.org/10.1007/978-3-031-10828-0_9

tually communicate. This is the least common category.
- The diagnosis is based on the clinical features and history, supported by radiographic evidence and pulp testing.

Differential Diagnosis
- Ascertainment of the primary lesion.
- Periapical abscess.

Laboratory Tests There are no specific tests.

Treatment The treatment options and sequence of treatment are dictated by the type of lesion and tooth prognosis. Extraction is the only option for hopeless teeth (e.g., teeth with a vertical root fracture). In cases where endodontic involvement is confirmed, endodontic treatment should be completed first. For primary endodontic lesions, endodontic therapy alone is expected to provide complete resolution in most cases. For primary periodontal lesions, periodontal therapy alone should be sufficient. In cases of primary endodontic-secondary periodontal lesion, periodontal therapy should follow endodontic treatment, typically 3 months later and provided that acute symptoms have subsided. In cases of primary periodontal-secondary endodontic lesions and true combined lesions, periodontal treatment should follow immediately after the successful completion of endodontic therapy.

References

1. Solomon C, Chalfin H, Kellert M, Weseley P. The endodontic-periodontal lesion: a rational approach to treatment. J Am Dent Assoc. 1995;126(4):473–9. https://doi.org/10.14219/jada.archive.1995.0210.
2. Herrera D, Retamal-Valdes B, Alonso B, Feres M. Acute periodontal lesions (periodontal abscesses and necrotizing periodontal diseases) and endo-periodontal lesions. J Clin Periodontol. 2018;45(Suppl 20):S78–94. https://doi.org/10.1111/jcpe.12941.
3. Papapanou PN, Sanz M, Buduneli N, et al. Periodontitis: consensus report of workgroup 2 of the 2017 world workshop on the classification of periodontal and Peri-implant diseases and conditions. J Clin Periodontol. 2018;45(Suppl 20):S162–70. https://doi.org/10.1111/jcpe.12946.

Traumatic Occlusal Forces and Occlusal Trauma

10

Contents

Definitions Traumatic occlusal forces are defined as occlusal forces that exceed the reparative capacity of the periodontal attachment apparatus, resulting in occlusal trauma and/or causing excessive tooth wear. Occlusal trauma is defined as injury which results in histologic alterations in the attachment apparatus, i.e., the periodontal ligament, alveolar bone, and cementum, as a result of occlusal forces. Occlusal trauma may be *primary* (injury from excessive occlusal forces applied to a tooth or teeth with normal periodontal support) or *secondary* (normal or excessive occlusal forces applied to a tooth or teeth with reduced periodontal support).

Etiology Physiological occlusal forces may become traumatic when improper, irregular, and/or unbalanced tooth contact relationships (occlusal discrepancies) are established due to developmental (e.g., malocclusion, tooth malposition, tooth malformation) or other reasons (e.g., wrongly designed or poorly fabricated restorations, partial edentulism), or when the periodontal attachment apparatus is significantly reduced (e.g., loss of periodontal support due to periodontitis). Parafunctional habits may also result in traumatic occlusal forces.

Periodontal Involvement Common.

Other Sites of Involvement Traumatic occlusal forces, often referred to as occlusal overload, may also affect dental implants.

Clinical Features

- May typically present with fremitus, progressive tooth mobility, wear facets, occlusal discrepancies, widened periodontal ligament space (Fig. 10.1), discomfort or pain on chewing, and thermal sensitivity.
- In increasingly severe and long-standing cases, it may present with tooth migration, tooth fracture, root resorption, and cemental tear.
- Occlusal trauma does not initiate periodontal attachment loss; however, it may contribute to the progression of established disease.
- The clinical diagnosis is mainly based on the clinical features and dental history and supported by radiographic evidence. Occlusal trauma can only be definitively confirmed through histological examination.

Differential Diagnosis

- Other causes (localized or systemic) of tooth mobility
- Periodontitis
- Endodontic lesions
- Neoplastic diseases
- Other causes of tooth wear, such as coarse, abrasive, or attritive diet, parafunctional habits, e.g., bruxism.

Laboratory Tests There are no specific tests.

Treatment In the presence of clinical signs of occlusal trauma, occlusal therapy, consisting of occlusal adjustment,

G. Laskaris et al., *Periodontal Manifestations of Local and Systemic Diseases*, https://doi.org/10.1007/978-3-031-10828-0_10

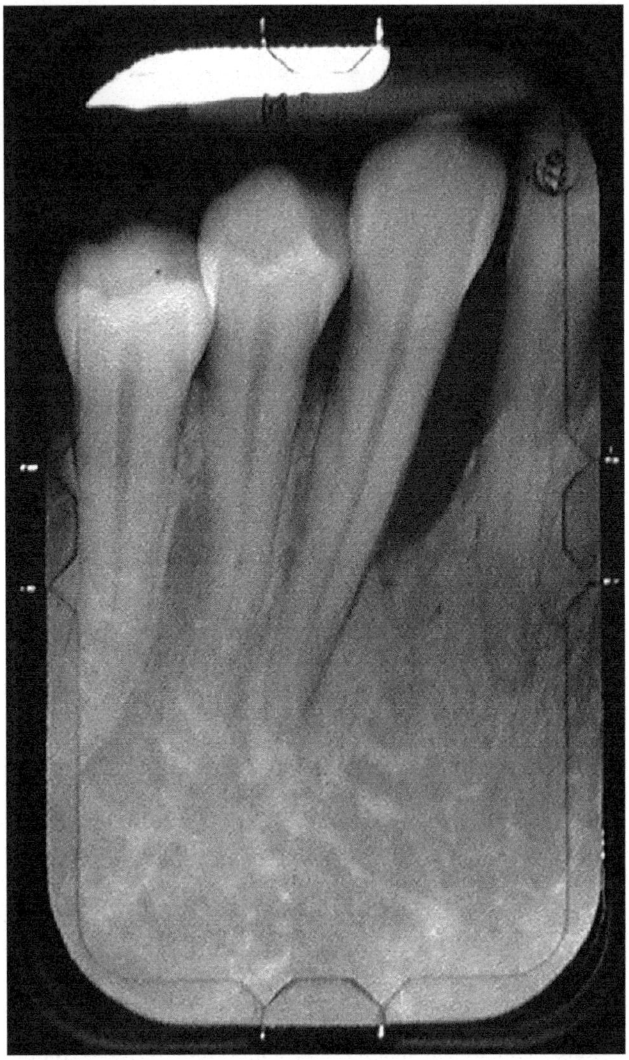

Fig. 10.1 Mandibular canine with widened periodontal ligament, suggestive of secondary occlusal trauma (note severe bone loss on mesial aspect)

i.e., reshaping of the occluding surfaces of opposing teeth to establish appropriate and balanced tooth contacts and reduce the resulting forces, will help improve the masticatory function of the dentition and the comfort of the patient. Occlusal therapy may also include the use of bite guards, especially in cases of secondary occlusal trauma. For patients with periodontitis and clinical signs of occlusal trauma, reduction of inflammation through routine nonsurgical periodontal therapy remains the primary therapeutic goal and should precede any definitive occlusal therapy.

References

1. Reinhardt RA, Killeen AC. Do mobility and occlusal trauma impact periodontal longevity? Dent Clin N Am. 2015;59(4):873–83. https://doi.org/10.1016/j.cden.2015.06.003.
2. Fan J, Caton JG. Occlusal trauma and excessive occlusal forces: narrative review, case definitions, and diagnostic considerations. J Clin Periodontol. 2018;45(Suppl 20):S199–206. https://doi.org/10.1111/jcpe.12949.
3. Jepsen S, Caton JG, Albandar JM, et al. Periodontal manifestations of systemic diseases and developmental and acquired conditions: consensus report of workgroup 3 of the 2017 world workshop on the classification of periodontal and Peri-implant diseases and conditions. J Clin Periodontol. 2018;45(Suppl 20):S219–29. https://doi.org/10.1111/jcpe.12951.
4. Campiño JI, Ríos CC, Rodriguez-Medina C, Botero JE. Association between traumatic occlusal forces and periodontitis: a systematic review. J Int Acad Periodontol. 2019;21(4):148–58. Published 2019 Oct 1

Tooth- and Prosthesis-Related Factors

11

Contents

Cervical Enamel Projection

Definition An anatomical tooth variation where there is an ectopic enamel deposit, continuous with and apical to the typical cementoenamel junction level, which has a tapering form extending toward the root furcation area.

Etiology Cervical enamel projections are a developmental irregularity. The presence of enamel apical to the normal cementoenamel junction position prevents connective tissue attachment, which is thought to make the involved areas more susceptible to biofilm accumulation and periodontal breakdown. The presence of cervical enamel projections is significantly associated with furcation involvement (periodontal attachment loss).

Periodontal Involvement Common in molar furcation areas, especially the buccal aspect of mandibular molars.

Other Sites of Involvement Extremely rare in other tooth types, including single rooted and anterior teeth.

Clinical Features

- Cervical enamel projections are typically flat and have a triangular form (Fig. 11.1). They have been classified on the basis of the extent to which they deviate from the normal cementoenamel junction level and the proximity of their most apical part to the furcation opening. The more a cervical enamel projection extends toward the furcation, the more likely it is to contribute to furcation involvement; also, the more likely that a major portion of the projection will be located subgingivally.
- Cervical enamel projection classification:
  - Grade I. Distinct change in cementoenamel junction course with enamel projecting toward the furcation (Fig. 11.1).
  - Grade II. Enamel projection approaching the furcation, but not actually making contact with it.
  - Grade III. Enamel projection extending into the furcation proper (Fig. 11.2).

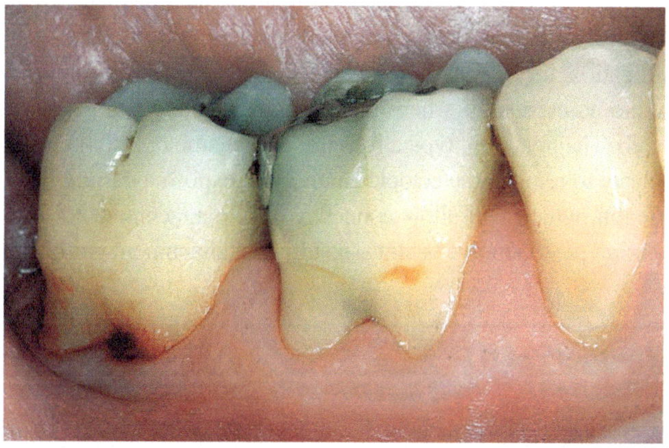

Fig. 11.1 Cervical enamel projection (Grade I) on first molar

G. Laskaris et al., *Periodontal Manifestations of Local and Systemic Diseases*, https://doi.org/10.1007/978-3-031-10828-0_11

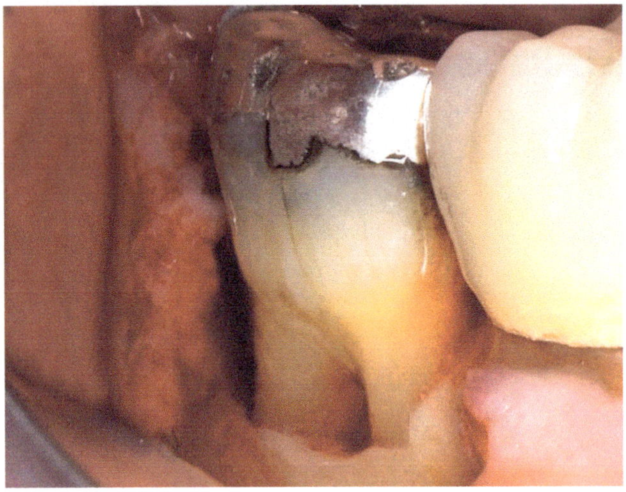

Fig. 11.2 Cervical enamel projection (Grade III) on second molar

- Clinically, the only sign may be the presence of a localized deep pocket, associated with furcation involvement. If the associated furcation area has experienced gingival recession, then the cervical enamel projection will be readily visible (Fig. 11.1).
- The diagnosis is based on the clinical features with, rarely, supportive evidence from radiographic imaging. Elevation of a full-thickness flap and exposure of the furcation area may be necessary to properly assess the extent of a cervical enamel projection (Fig. 11.2) in cases where soft tissue levels are normal (i.e., at the level of the cementoenamel junction).

Differential Diagnosis
- Enamel pearl
- Other localized developmental or iatrogenic factors

Laboratory Tests There are no specific tests.

Treatment Cervical enamel projections located supragingivally, or ones that will become/remain supragingival after periodontal therapy in the involved furcation area, do not require any intervention. Cervical enamel projections associated with furcation involvement should be treated as part of furcation therapy, especially when regenerative procedures are considered. The treatment typically consists of enameloplasty/odontoplasty to remove the ectopic enamel and expose the underlying dentin, which will allow connective tissue attachment to form during postoperative healing (resulting in attachment gain).

Enamel Pearl

Definition An anatomical tooth variant where there is an ectopic globular enamel deposit, firmly attached to the tooth surface.

Etiology These formations are of developmental origin. The presence of an enamel pearl, whose contour and location may result in inevitable biofilm retention and accumulation, impedes connective tissue attachment; together, these are considered the factors that allow enamel pearls to predispose an area to localized periodontal attachment loss.

Periodontal Involvement Uncommon. Usually found on the distal proximal surfaces of maxillary molars, particularly third and second molars, and on the buccal/lingual surfaces of mandibular molars.

Other Sites of Involvement Extremely rare in other tooth types, including anterior teeth, or on the apical root portion of molar teeth.

Clinical Features
- Enamel pearls are small round or ovoid globules (Fig. 11.3), with a sessile base, that are typically found in the furcation area. Histologically they may contain only enamel (real enamel pearl) or include a dentin core (composite enamel pearl) and, occasionally, even a pulp tissue center (enamel-dentin-pulp pearl).
- Clinically, the only sign may be the presence of a localized deep pocket in a furcation or interproximal area. Depending on the position of the pearl and the location of the soft tissue margin, an enamel pearl may be readily visible.
- The diagnosis is based on the clinical features with, occasionally, supportive evidence from radiographic imaging. Elevation of a mucoperiosteal flap and exposure of the affected area may be necessary to confirm the diagnosis and properly evaluate a suspected enamel pearl.

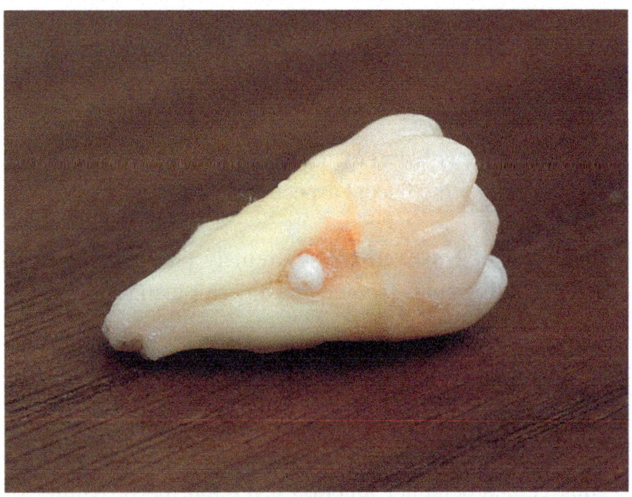

Fig. 11.3 Enamel pearl on extracted third molar

Differential Diagnosis

- Cervical enamel projection
- Other localized developmental or iatrogenic factors

Laboratory Tests There are no specific tests.

Treatment The location, size, and type of the enamel pearl, along with the associated periodontal tissue destruction, will dictate the treatment. Often, given the interproximal location of the pearl, the associated periodontal attachment loss, and the technical difficulties inherent in any attempt to remove a pearl from the distal aspect of a posterior tooth, the sensible treatment is tooth extraction.

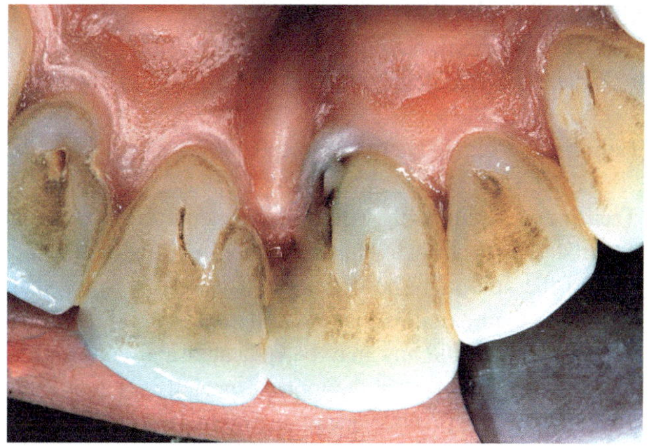

Fig. 11.4 Palatogingival grooves on maxillary central incisors; there is associated localized deep probing depth on the right side

Developmental Groove

Definition An anatomical abnormality where a groove or concavity is present, either on the crown and maybe extending to the root or just on the tooth root, with variable depth, width, length, direction and location (tooth aspect). The *palatogingival groove*, which is found on maxillary incisors, is typically starting in the central fossa and, after crossing the cingulum, extends apically on the palatal aspect of the root, with varying course. *Proximal root grooves* and *concavities*, usually found on mandibular anterior and maxillary premolar teeth, are another form of developmental groove.

Etiology As their name implies, these are developmental deformities. The presence of grooves leads to localized biofilm accumulation, subsequent gingival inflammation, deepening localized and narrow probing depths, and often relatively rapid attachment loss.

Periodontal Involvement Fairly common for the specific tooth types.

Other Sites of Involvement Rare in other tooth types.

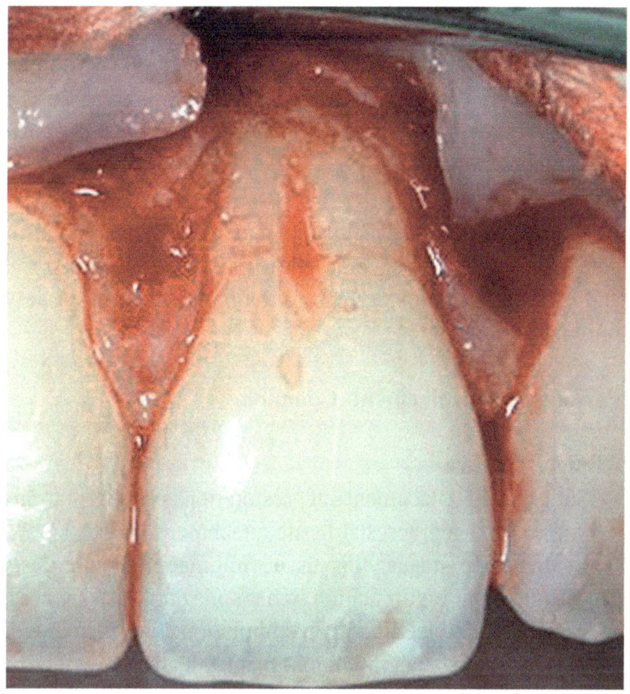

Fig. 11.5 Buccal developmental groove on maxillary central incisor, evident during exploratory surgery

Clinical Features

- Palatogingival grooves are most commonly found on maxillary lateral incisor teeth while proximal grooves are most likely to be present on mandibular incisor teeth and maxillary premolars. Proximal grooves on maxillary premolars tend to be more v-shaped, wider closer to the cementoenamel junction, mostly located on the mesial, and they extend further toward the apical part of the root; those on mandibular incisors tend to be more u-shaped and can fade toward the apical part.
- Clinically, the typical palatogingival groove is visible in the cingulum and cementoenamel junction area and, when it extends apically, a localized narrow and deep pocket may be present (Fig. 11.4). Proximal grooves may or may not be visible, depending on the presence or absence of interproximal tissue loss, but are often detectable by probing.
- Deeper grooves may also be associated with altered root canal morphology, which can complicate endodontic therapy and/or lead to the development of endodontic-periodontal lesions.
- The diagnosis is based on the clinical features with, rarely, supportive evidence from routine radiographic imaging. However, cone-beam computed tomography, i.e., three-dimensional imaging, can provide detailed morphologic and diagnostic information. Surgical access can facilitate identification (Fig. 11.5).

Differential Diagnosis

- Enamel projection
- Other localized developmental or iatrogenic factors

Laboratory Tests There are no specific tests.

Treatment Teeth with localized periodontal involvement associated with grooves that are deeper and extend farther toward the apex may be hopeless. When grooves are shallower and their extent is limited, odontoplasty and regenerative periodontal therapy may be indicated and could allow for long-term survival of the tooth, especially for motivated patients who can practice adequate oral hygiene.

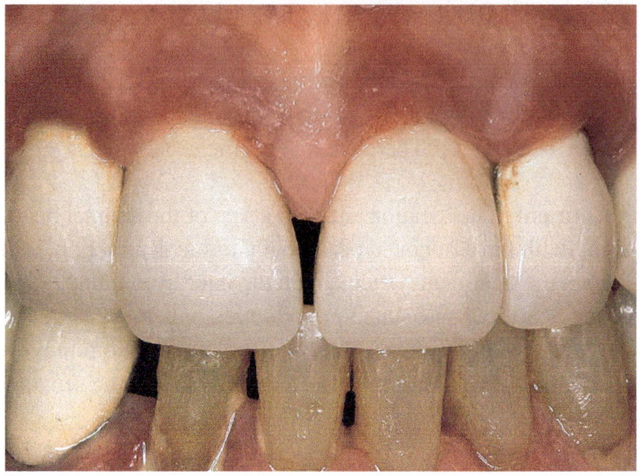

Fig. 11.6 Prosthesis related factors; subgingival placement of crown margins impinging on the supracrestal tissue attachment and resulting in gingival inflammation (redness, swelling, and bleeding upon stimulation)

Prosthesis-Related Factors

Definition Restorative aspects, related to fixed prostheses, dental restorations, removable prostheses, and/or dental materials, that can contribute to plaque accumulation and/or tissue trauma, inflammation, and ultimately lead to periodontal attachment loss.

Etiology Most of these factors may be considered iatrogenic. However, the specific etiology can be multifactorial and is often inflammatory and/or traumatic, and more rarely immunologic in nature.

Periodontal Involvement Common.

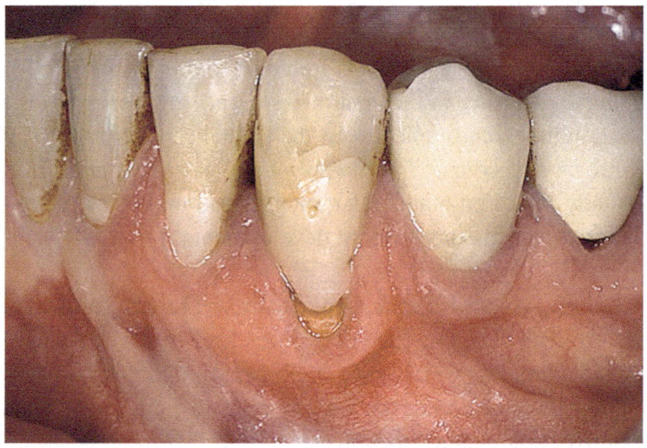

Fig. 11.7 Prosthesis related factors; deteriorating marginal quality of restoration likely contributing to associated gingival inflammation and gingival recession on mandibular canine

Clinical Features

- Subgingival placement of restorations/crown margins impacts the supracrestal tissue attachment (see Chap. 1). In the early stages, this tissue impingement manifests with gingival inflammation, which presents with redness, swelling, and bleeding upon stimulation (Fig. 11.6). With time, this persistent inflammation may lead to loss of periodontal support, either in the form of gingival recession (sites with thin phenotype; (Fig. 11.7)) or increased probing depths and alveolar bone loss (sites with thick phenotype), or both.
- Direct and indirect restoration overhangs hamper oral hygiene efforts, promote biofilm accumulation, and are associated with increased gingival inflammation, deepening periodontal pockets, and loss of crestal bone. These detrimental effects are proportional to the dimensions of the overhang.
- The inevitable intraoral procedural aspects of dental restoration and fixed prosthesis fabrication, such as tooth preparation (especially subgingivally), gingival displacement for impression taking, impression taking, and placement of provisional restorations, may contribute to the development of gingival inflammation, gingival recession, and periodontal tissue loss, especially in cases of thin phenotype. Also associated with these procedures are the potential detrimental direct effects of required materials, such as restorative cements and resins.
- Removable dental prostheses may also contribute, indirectly, through increased plaque retention, to the development of gingivitis and periodontal attachment loss. Distal extension removable prostheses may cause increased mobility to the abutment teeth, due to possible increased applied torque and forces.
- Dental materials used to fabricate dental restorations and prostheses may have direct effects, irrespective of restoration type or design. For example, surface roughness may contribute to increased plaque accumulation and lead to gingival inflammation. Release of specific metal ions and particles has been associated with hypersensitivity reac-

tions, which also result in the development of localized gingival inflammation and gingival pigmentation.

- The diagnosis is based on the clinical features with, occasionally, supportive evidence from radiographic imaging (e.g., interproximal overhangs).

Differential Diagnosis

- Other localized developmental or iatrogenic factors.

Laboratory Tests There are no specific tests, except in cases where hypersensitivity to dental materials is suspected; hypersensitivity testing can then be used to identify the allergen.

Treatment Proper oral hygiene and periodontal maintenance are essential to minimize the potentially damaging effects of prosthesis-related factors. Poorly designed or made restorations should be corrected, e.g., by recontouring or removal of overhangs, or replaced. Removable prostheses, especially distal extension ones, must be regularly examined and, if indicated, relined. Metal restorations associated with metal hypersensitivity should be replaced by nonmetal restorations.

References

1. Machtei EE, Wasenstein SM, Peretz B, Laufer D. The relationship between cervical enamel projection and class II furcation defects in humans. Quintessence Int. 1997;28(5):315–20.
2. Ercoli C, Caton JG. Dental prostheses and tooth-related factors. J Clin Periodontol. 2018;45(Suppl 20):S207–18. https://doi.org/10.1111/jcpe.12950.
3. Jepsen S, Caton JG, Albandar JM, et al. Periodontal manifestations of systemic diseases and developmental and acquired conditions: consensus report of workgroup 3 of the 2017 world workshop on the classification of periodontal and Peri-implant diseases and conditions. J Clin Periodontol. 2018;45(Suppl 20):S219–29. https://doi.org/10.1111/jcpe.12951.
4. Moskow BS, Canut PM. Studies on root enamel (2). Enamel pearls. A review of their morphology, localization, nomenclature, occurrence, classification, histogenesis and incidence. J Clin Periodontol. 1990;17(5):275–81. https://doi.org/10.1111/j.1600-051x.1990.tb01089.x.
5. Versiani MA, Cristescu RC, Saquy PC, et al. Enamel pearls in permanent dentition: case report and micro-CT evaluation. Dentomaxillofac Radiol. 2013;42(6):20120332. https://doi.org/10.1259/dmfr.20120332.
6. Hou GL, Tsai CC. Relationship between palato-radicular grooves and localized periodontitis. J Clin Periodontol. 1993;20(9):678–82. https://doi.org/10.1111/j.1600-051x.1993.tb00715.x.
7. Leknes KN, Lie T, Selvig KA. Root grooves: a risk factor in periodontal attachment loss. J Periodontol. 1994;65(9):859–63. https://doi.org/10.1902/jop.1994.65.9.859.
8. Zhao H, Wang H, Pan Y, et al. The relationship between root concavities in first premolars and chronic periodontitis. J Periodontal Res. 2014;49(2):213–9. https://doi.org/10.1111/jre.12097.
9. Tan X, Zhang L, Zhou W, et al. Palatal radicular groove morphology of the maxillary incisors: acase series report. J Endod. 2017;43(5):827–33. https://doi.org/10.1016/j.joen.2016.12.025.
10. Schätzle M, Land NP, Anerud A, et al. The influence of margins of restorations of the periodontal tissues over 26 years. J Clin Periodontol. 2001;28(1):57–64. https://doi.org/10.1034/j.1600-051x.2001.280109.x.
11. Mittermüller P, Hiller KA, Schmalz G, Buchalla W. Five hundred patients reporting on adverse effects from dental materials: frequencies, complaints, symptoms, allergies. Dent Mater. 2018;34(12):1756–68. https://doi.org/10.1016/j.dental.2018.09.012.
12. Moldovan O, Rudolph H, Luthardt RG. Biological complications of removable dental prostheses in the moderately reduced dentition: a systematic literature review. Clin Oral Investig. 2018;22(7):2439–61. https://doi.org/10.1007/s00784-018-2522-y.

12 Developmental Disorders

Contents

Torus Mandibularis

Definition A bony exophytic growth on the mandible that is benign, asymptomatic, and usually occurs bilaterally on the lingual side near the premolars.

Etiology Developmental. Possibly they are inherited in an autosomal dominant trait; however, environmental and functional factors may have been associated.

Gingival Involvement Relatively rare on the gingiva.

Other Sites of Involvement Often associated with torus palatinus and multiple exostoses of the jaw.

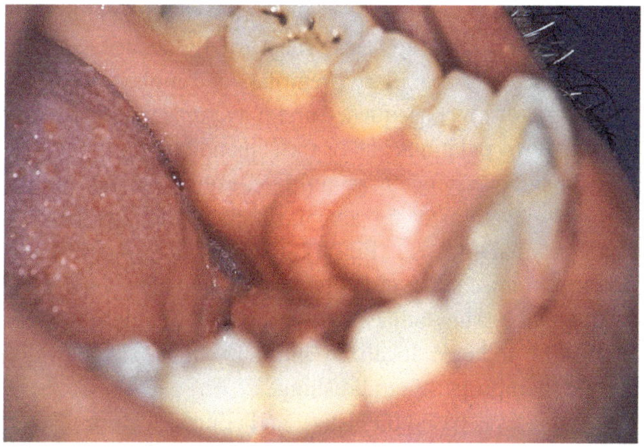

Fig. 12.1 Torus mandibularis

Clinical Features
- Seen most frequently in Asian and Black races and rarely in Turner's syndrome (45, X). Prevalence ranges from 6% to 40% with both sexes being affected roughly equally.
- Secondary gingival lesions are a result of mechanical irritation. Biofilm-induced gingivitis can develop due to inappropriate tooth brushing of the area.
- Clinically, they present as hard, asymptomatic, slow-growing bony lumps, with normal overlying mucosa. The malformations appear during adolescence and usually cease growing in late teens (Fig. 12.1). The size varies from 0.5 to several centimeters and may be single or multiple. Patients are usually not aware of the lesion unless secondary erosion or ulcer develops following mechanical trauma.
- Diagnosis is based on history and clinical features.

Differential Diagnosis
- Osteoma
- Gardner syndrome
- Chronic tooth abscess
- Unerupted teeth
- Osteosarcoma
- Other neoplasms

G. Laskaris et al., *Periodontal Manifestations of Local and Systemic Diseases*, https://doi.org/10.1007/978-3-031-10828-0_12

Laboratory Tests Radiographic examination may be performed.

Treatment No treatment is needed unless the fabrication of dentures is complicated.

Multiple Exostoses

Definition Buccal exostoses occur as multiple bony hard masses along the facial aspect of the maxillary and/or mandibular alveolar ridge.

Etiology Etiology is multifactorial and involves interplay of genetic and environmental factors.

Gingival Involvement Relatively rare.

Other Sites of Involvement Occasionally arise beneath a bridge pontic.

Clinical Features
- Aging-associated disorders that grow slowly and usually cease growth in late teens. They usually occur bilaterally and buccal to maxillary premolars and molars. They are benign, of no consequence and may present concurrently with torus palatinus and/or torus mandibularis.
- Clinically, they occur as multiple, asymptomatic nodular bony elevations of the alveolar bone of the jaws covered by normal mucosa (Fig. 12.2 and 12.3). Occasionally, ulcerations can develop due to mechanical trauma to the gingival tissues adjacent to exostoses, leading to pain. Biofilm-induced localized gingivitis may also develop due to improper tooth brushing.
- Diagnosis is based on history and clinical features.

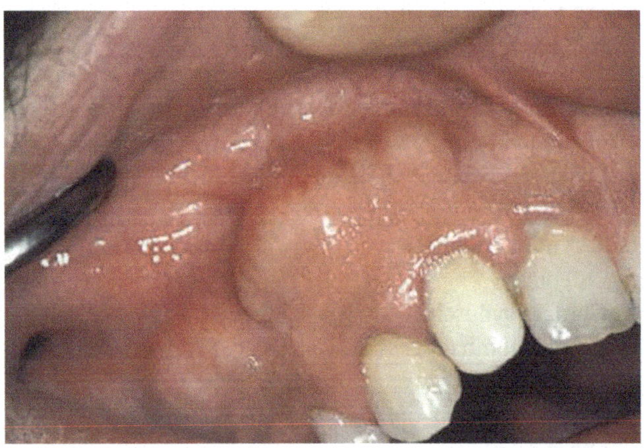

Fig. 12.2 Multiple exostoses

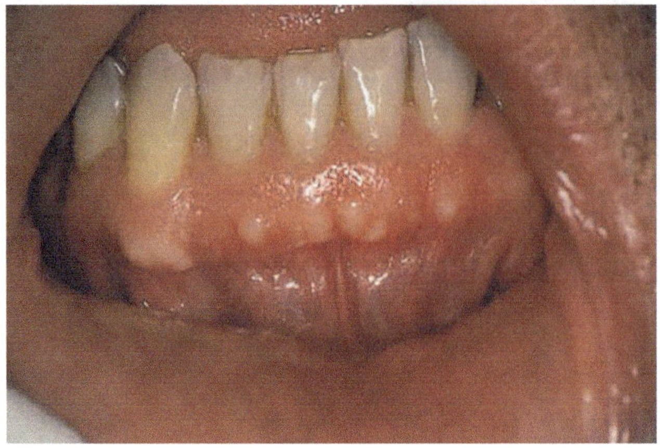

Fig. 12.3 Multiple exostoses

Differential Diagnosis
- Multiple osteomas
- Gardner syndrome
- Paget disease of bone
- Fibrous dysplasia

Laboratory Tests Radiography may be useful.
Treatment No treatment is required. Patient reassurance. Excise or reduce only if causing difficulties with prostheses or other complications. May serve as a source of autogenous bone graft.

Fibrous Tuberosity Enlargement

Definition Rare developmental benign malformation of fibrous tissue.

Etiology Idiopathic.

Gingival Involvement Common.

Other Sites of Involvement None.

Clinical Features
- Most frequently they begin during childhood or puberty and may exhibit rapid or insidious growth. The size extends to several centimeters and occasionally can touch both sides creating speech, chewing, and swallowing problems. Lesions usually remain stable after the third decade of life.
- The malformation most commonly appears as bilaterally symmetrical on the maxillary alveolar tuberosity regions, mainly palatally and less frequently on the retromolar region of the mandible.

- Clinically, they appear as painless fibrous overgrowths with smooth surface and firm on palpation, that are covered by normal mucosa with pale color (Figs. 12.4 and 12.5). The fibrous mass is firmly attached to the underlying bone, but occasionally may be movable. The gingiva is hard in consistency and is covered by normal mucosa.
- Diagnosis is based on history and clinical features.

Differential Diagnosis
- Hereditary gingival fibromatosis
- Fibroma
- Neurofibroma
- Oral focal mucinosis
- Drug-related enlargement
- Neoplasms

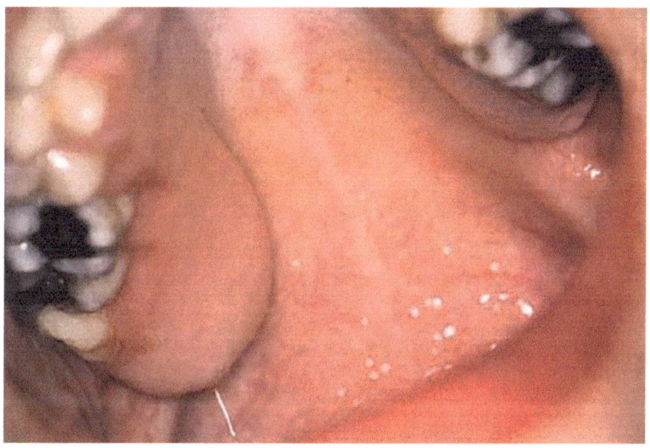

Fig. 12.4 Maxillary fibrous tuberosity, unilateral

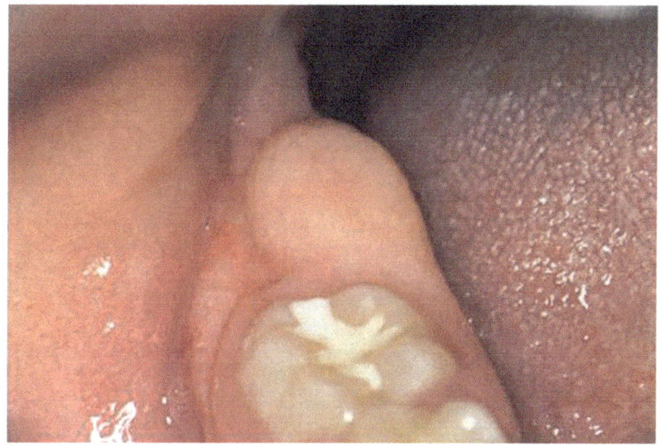

Fig. 12.5 Mandibular fibrous tuberosity

Laboratory Tests Rarely histopathlogic examination.

Treatment Occasionally conservative surgical excision is performed.

References

1. Ahn SH, Ha JG, Kim JW, et al. Torus mandibularis affects the severity and position-dependent sleep apnoea in non-obese patients. Clin Otolaryngol. 2019;44(3):279–85.
2. Loukas M, Hulsberg P, Tubbs RS, et al. The Tori of the mouth and ear: a review. Clin Anat. 2013;26(8):953–60.
3. Kannan S, Muthusamy S, Muthu K, Sidhu P. Multiple bony overgrowths in the mouth–report of two cases. Clin Cases Miner Bone Metab. 2015;12(3):260–1.
4. Gomes GH, Pegoraro GO, Mazzetti T, Martos J. Esthetic treatment of buccal exostoses: a case report. Gen Dent. 2020;68(6):75–7. PMID: 33136051
5. Currie WJ, Hill R, Keshani DK. An unusual cause of maxillary tuberosity enlargement. Br Dent J. 1994;177(2):60–2. (ISSN:0007-0610)

Heavy Metal and Foreign Bodies Depositions

13

Contents

Amalgam Tattoo

Definition Amalgam tattoo is the most frequent cause of exogenous pigmentation in the oral mucosa.

Etiology Usually, it is due to incorporation of dental amalgam particles or salts into the tissues during restorative or endodontic procedures.

Gingival Involvement Common.

Other Sites of Involvement Oral mucosa (e.g., floor of the mouth, buccal mucosa, alveolar mucosa, hard palate).

Clinical Features

- Clinically, amalgam tattoo presents as a bluish-black discoloration that is well-defined and asymptomatic. It is usually flat, irregular, and can vary in size (Figs. 13.1, 13.2, and 13.3). Lesions can occur as solitary or multiple, associated with history of amalgam restorations near the area.
- Diagnosis is usually based on history and clinical features. Sometimes, laboratory tests are needed to confirm diagnosis.

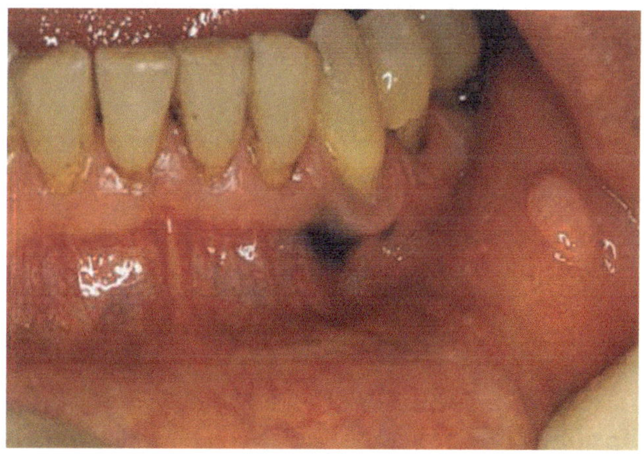

Fig. 13.1 Gingival pigmentation, amalgam deposition

Differential Diagnosis

- Racial pigmentation
- Smoking melanosis
- Drug-related discoloration
- Pigmented nevi
- Ephelides
- Lentigo simplex
- Melanoacanthoma
- Lentigo maligna

G. Laskaris et al., *Periodontal Manifestations of Local and Systemic Diseases*, https://doi.org/10.1007/978-3-031-10828-0_13

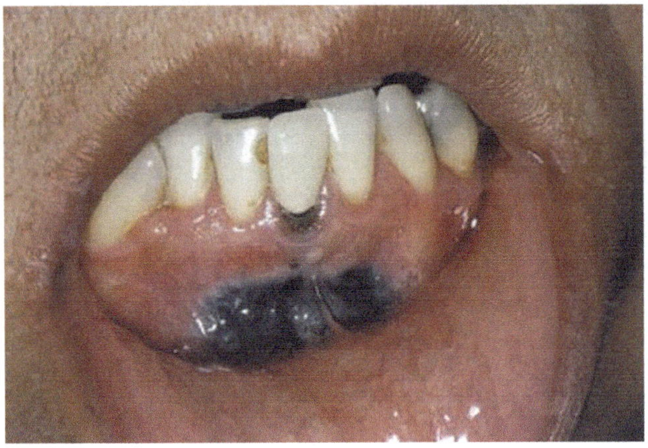

Fig. 13.2 Gingival pigmentation, amalgam deposition

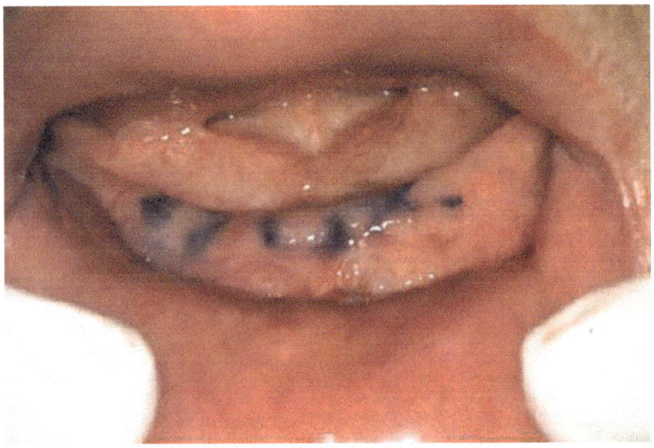

Fig. 13.3 Alveolar pigmentation, amalgam deposition

- Malignant melanoma
- Kaposi sarcoma
- Silver and graphite implantation

Laboratory Tests Histopathologic examination and radiographs.

Treatment No treatment is necessary when diagnosis is accurate or the metallic fragments are evident radiographically. Conservative surgical excision is the treatment of choice in diagnostically uncertain cases.

Silver and Graphite Deposits

Definition Discoloration of the tissue due to exogenous deposition of silver or graphite.

Etiology Silver deposition may be the result of migration and deposition within the oral soft tissues after an endodontic procedure. Graphite deposition is usually the result of repeated trauma-related implantation of pencil tip material, by the patient.

Gingival Involvement Relatively rare. Non-dental biofilm-induced lesions.

Other Sites of Involvement Alveolar mucosa and hard palate.

Clinical Features
- Clinically, gingival lesions present as brownish, gray, or black asymptomatic macules or small plaques, close to the apex of endodontically treated teeth (Fig. 13.4). Graphite material is usually implanted after self-induced trauma with pencils (Fig. 13.5).
- Diagnosis is usually based on history and clinical features, but it should be confirmed by laboratory tests.

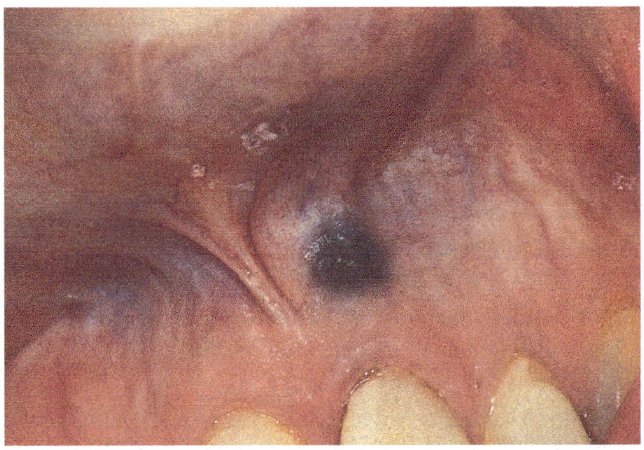

Fig. 13.4 Tatoo from endodontic treatment with silver cone

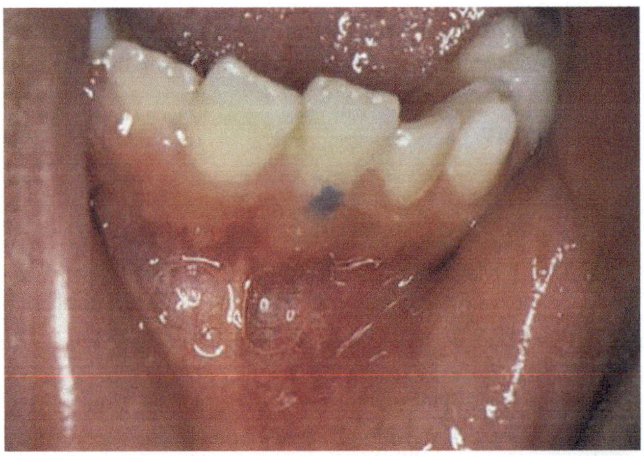

Fig. 13.5 Gingival pigmentation, graphite deposition

Differential Diagnosis
- Amalgam tattoo
- Pigmented nevi
- Ephilides
- Lentigo simplex
- Melanoacanthoma
- Malignant melanoma

Laboratory Tests Usually are not required. Histopathologic examination in some cases.

Treatment Treatment is usually not recommended. Conservative surgical excision is the treatment of choice mainly for cosmetic reasons or when a diagnostic dilemma exists.

Bismuth Deposition

Definition Tissue discoloration due to bismuth pigmentation.

Etiology Deposition of bismuth due to systemic administration as treatment of syphilis and other skin diseases in the past, or by occupational exposure.

Gingival Involvement Rare.Non-biofilm-related lesions.

Other Sites of Involvement Tongue, borders of oral ulcers, skin.

Clinical Features
- Clinically it appears as a bluish-gray line along the marginal and interdental gingiva forming a characteristic pattern, known as *"bismuth line"* (Fig. 13.6). Patients complain of burning mouth sensation and increased salivation. In rare cases, ulcerations may occur.

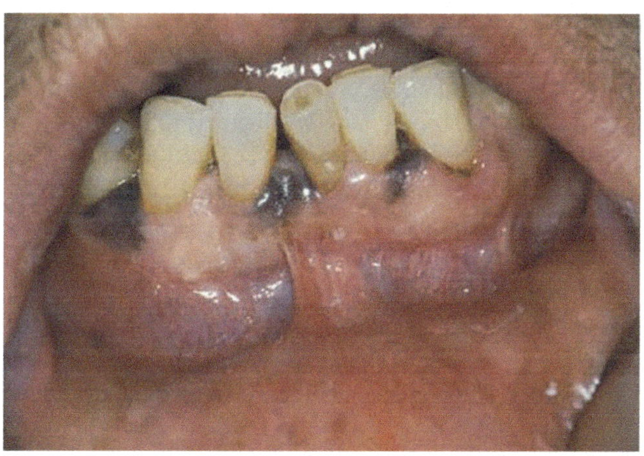

Fig. 13.6 Gingival pigmentation due to bismuth (bismuth line)

- Poor oral hygiene is a risk factor for developing oral lesions.
- Diagnosis is based on history and clinical features.

Differential Diagnosis
- Lead deposition
- Silver deposition
- Amalgam tattoo
- Drug-related discoloration
- Addison disease
- Racial pigmentation

Laboratory Tests Usually not required. Histopathologic examination can be performed.

Treatment Discontinuation of further exposure to the bismuth is suggested. The oral discoloration does not need any treatment.

Lead Deposition

Definition Tissue staining caused by lead.

Etiology It is caused by contact with lead-contaminated food and water. Exposure at work is a common cause of lead poisoning in adults. It is a black precipitate of lead sulfide resulting from the reaction of bacterial hydrogen sulfide and lead salt.

Gingival Involvement Relatively rare. Non-biofilm-related lesions. Severe periodontal disease can occur.

Other Sites of Involvement Tongue, buccal mucosa, several organs (kidneys, bone marrow, bone, joints, nervous system, and gastrointestinal tract).

Clinical Features
- Clinically, a characteristic bluish-black line is observed along the marginal gingiva which is called *"lead line"* (Fig. 13.7).
- Less frequently, nonspecific ulcerations and bluish-gray spots may be observed on the tongue and buccal mucosa. Excessive salivation, metallic taste, severe periodontal disease, and tremor of the tongue may also occur.
- Diagnosis is mainly based on history and clinical features.

Differential Diagnosis
- Bismuth deposition
- Other heavy metal deposition
- Amalgam tattoo

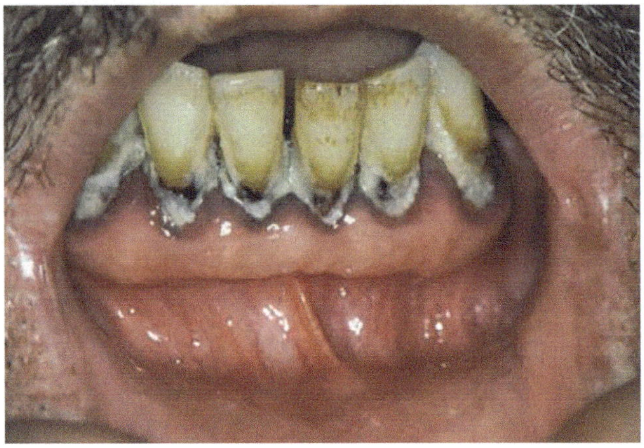

Fig. 13.7 Gingival pigmentation due to lead (lead line)

Laboratory Tests Histopathologic examination and/or measurement of lead levels in the blood may be useful in diagnosis.

Treatment Discontinuation of exposure to lead, supportive care, and administration of chelating agents. In cases of severe lead poisoning 2,3-dimercaptosuccinic acid (DMSA) and 2,3-dimercaptopropane-1-sulfonate (DMPS) or D-penicillamine are the drugs of choice. Patients should be treated by Specialists.

Materia Alba

Definition Materia alba is a soft whitish deposit found on teeth at the gum line consisting of bacteria, dead epithelial cells, and food debris.

Etiology Poor oral hygiene.

Gingival Involvement Common along the gingival margins. Dental biofilm-induced condition.

Other Sites of Involvement Alveolar mucosa.

Clinical Features
- Clinically, material alba presents as whitish or white-gray soft plaques that can easily be removed with gauze leaving a reddish surface (Fig. 13.8.)
- Diagnosis is based on history and clinical features.

Differential Diagnosis
- Candidiasis
- Lichen planus
- Mechanical keratosis
- Chemical burn
- Cinnamon contact stomatitis
- Leukoplakia

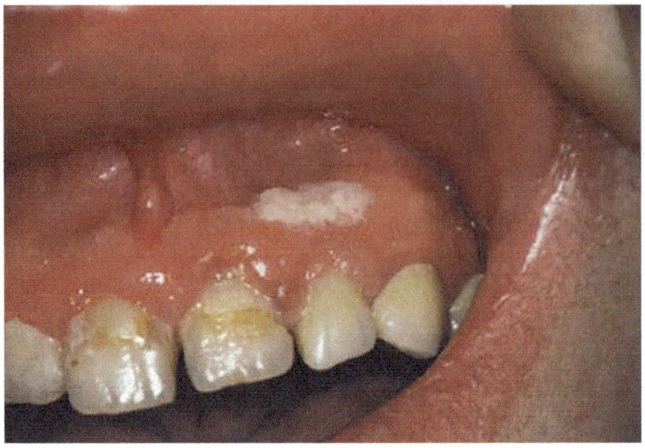

Fig. 13.8 Materia alba on the gingiva and alveolar mucosa

Laboratory Tests No laboratory tests are needed.

Treatment Good oral hygiene.

Various Foreign Body Depositions

Definition Foreign body impaction in the oral cavity.

Etiology Traumatic or iatrogenic injury. It may be the result of an accident, hard food stuffs, or dental and medical procedures in the oral cavity.

Gingival Involvement Relatively common. Non-biofilm-induced lesions.

Other Sites of Involvement Buccal mucosa, palate.

Clinical Features
- Gingival inflammation associated with foreign bodies is termed *foreign body gingivitis*.
- Clinically, the most common features induce a nonspecific red or brown-red, painful, reaction associated with intense gingival inflammation (Fig. 13.9). Discoloration of the surrounding tissues may occur, depending on the color and the size of the foreign body (Fig. 13.10).
- Diagnosis is based on history and clinical features.

Differential Diagnosis
- Traumatic lesions
- Metallic deposits
- Benign and malignant tumors

Laboratory Tests Histopathologic examination, imaging.

Treatment If easy removal of the foreign body is not possible surgical excision will be the treatment of choice.

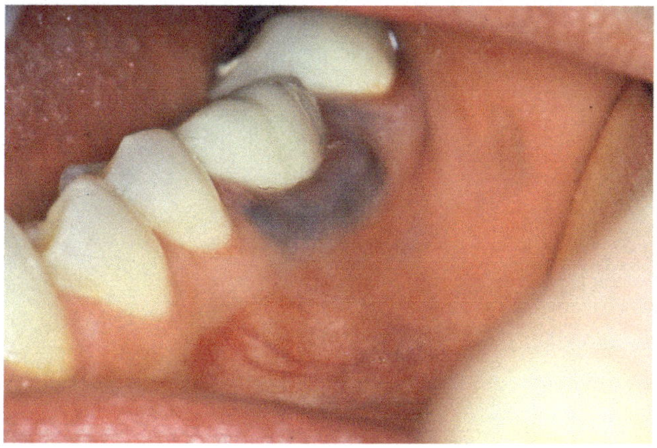

Fig. 13.9 Pigmentation of the gingiva as a reaction to the metal crown

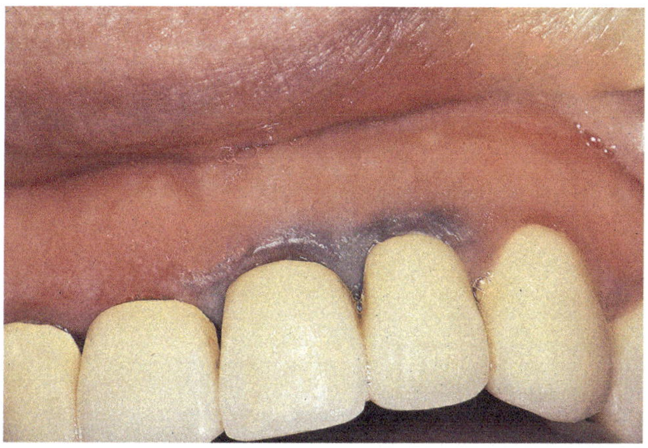

Fig. 13.10 Pigmentation of the gingiva as a reaction to the metal crown

References

1. Rosebush MS, Briody AN, Cordell KG. Black and Brown: non-neoplastic pigmentation of the oral mucosa. Head Neck Pathol. 2019;13(1):47–55. https://doi.org/10.1007/s12105-018-0980-9. Epub 2019 Jan 22. PMID: 30671761; PMCID: PMC6405786
2. Tran HT, Anandasabapathy N, Soldano AC. Amalgam tattoo. Dermatol Online J. 2008;14:19.
3. Anderegg CR Jr, Lyles MB. Graphite tattoo: report of a case and differential diagnosis. Mil Med. 1992;157:323–4.
4. Galletta VC, Artico G, Dal Vechio AM, et al. Extensive amalgam tattoo on the alveolar-gingival mucosa. An Bras Dermatol. 2011;86(5):1019–21. https://doi.org/10.1590/s0365-05962011000500026. PMID: 22147048
5. Khalil A. Lead poisoning. Br Dent J. 2009;206:608.
6. Lai Y, Xu Z, Chen J, et al. Biofunctionalization of microgroove surfaces with antibacterial nanocoatings. Biomed Res Int. 2020;2020:8387574. https://doi.org/10.1155/2020/8387574. PMID: 32626766; PMCID: PMC7317309
7. Gravitis K, Perio C, Daley TD, Marie A. Lochhead management of patients with foreign body gingivitis: report of 2 cases with histologic findings. J Can Dent Assoc. 2005;71(2):105–9.
8. Tatakis DN, Trombelli L. Adverse effects associated with a bioabsorbable guided tissue regeneration device in the treatment of human gingival recession defects: a clinicopathologic case report. J Periodontol. 1999;70(5):542–7. https://doi.org/10.1902/jop.1999.70.5.542. PMID: 10368059

14 Mechanical Gingival Lesions

Contents

Traumatic Ulcer

Definition Traumatic ulcer is one of the most common gingival lesions, caused by acute or chronic injury.

Etiology Abrasive tooth brushing, chewing on sticks, a sharp or broken tooth, rough fillings, sharp full or partial dentures, hard food and other foreign bodies, biting of the mucosa, misuse of dental instruments, mental impairment, and self-induced wounds are the most common causes.

Gingival Involvement Common. Non-biofilm-related lesions.

Other Sites of Involvement Most commonly on the lateral borders of the tongue, buccal mucosa, lips, buccal alveolar, and labio-alveolar grooves.

Clinical Features

- Clinically, traumatic ulcer on the gingiva presents as a single and painful lesion, soft on palpation, with a smooth red or white-yellow surface and occasionally thin erythematous or whitish halo due to reactive hyperkeratosis. Erosive lesions by toothbrushing appear as small, oval, round, or band-like superficial epithelial loss that is covered by a whitish pseudomembrane. (Figs. 14.1, 14.2, and 14.3).
- Traumatic ulcers occurring in other mucosal sites exhibit a similar presentation pattern.

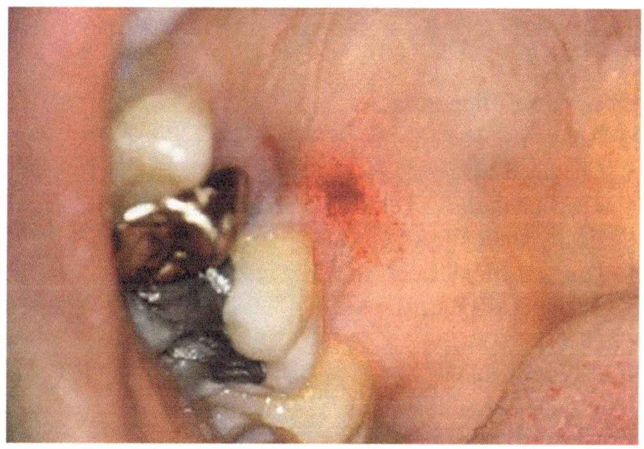

Fig. 14.1 Gingival trauma from tooth brushing

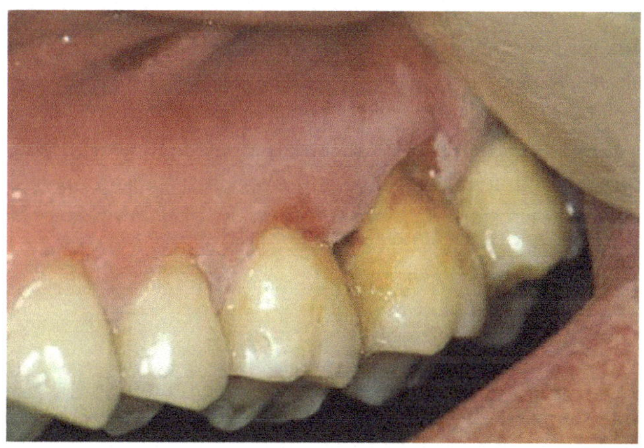

Fig. 14.2 Gingival trauma from tooth brushing

G. Laskaris et al., *Periodontal Manifestations of Local and Systemic Diseases*, https://doi.org/10.1007/978-3-031-10828-0_14

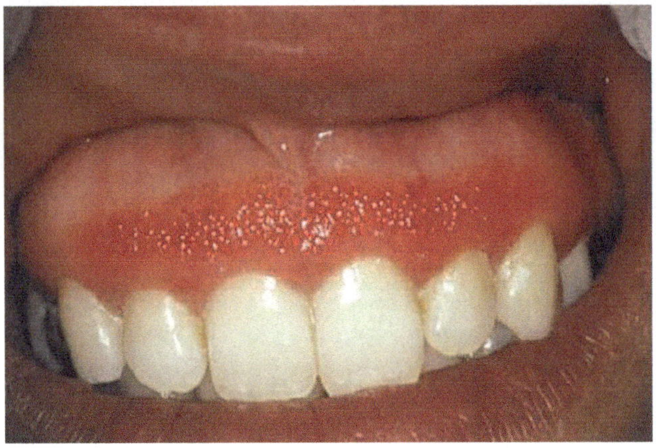

Fig. 14.3 Gingival inflammation and hyperplasia due to tooth brushing

- The ulcers usually heal spontaneously, without scarring within 6–10 days following elimination of the causative factor. Occasionally, the traumatic ulcer may clinically mimic oral squamous cell carcinoma.
- Diagnosis is mainly based on history and clinical features. Sometimes, diagnosis should be confirmed by laboratory tests.

Differential Diagnosis

- Aphthous ulcer
- Chemical burn
- Thermal burn
- Eosinophilic ulcer
- Drug reaction ulcers
- Tuberculosis ulcer
- Chancre
- Other infections
- Wegener granulomatosis
- Squamous cell carcinoma
- Non-Hodgkin lymphoma

Laboratory Tests Histological examination is recommended to rule out malignancy when an ulcer persists longer than 10 days.

Treatment Removal of the causative agent. Topical corticosteroid ointments in Orabase. Low doses, short-term systemic corticosteroids, and short-term use of mouthwashes.

Factitious Trauma

Definition Self-inflicted oral trauma is common in people with intellectual disabilities or severe emotional distress.

Etiology The trauma is usually caused by fingernails or sharp objects.

Gingival Involvement Common. Non-biofilm-related lesions.

Other Sites of Involvement Buccal mucosa, tongue, lips, skin.

Clinical Features

- Clinically, factitious trauma usually appears as a mild or severe, small or large painful ulceration on the gingiva, or other sites of oral mucosa that can be reached by fingers and instruments (Figs. 14.4 and 14.5).
- Due to chronic inflammation ulcers may become irregular with vegetations, raised border, and indurated base.
- The diagnosis depends on a strong clinical suspicion, detailed history, and a thorough examination. Occasionally, it should be confirmed by laboratory tests.

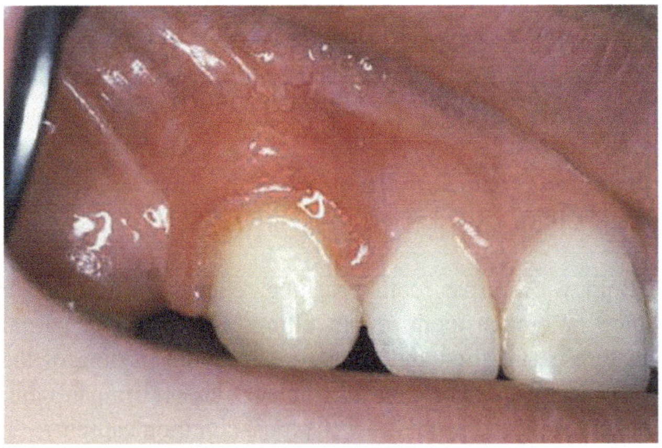

Fig. 14.4 Gingival factitious trauma from fingernail

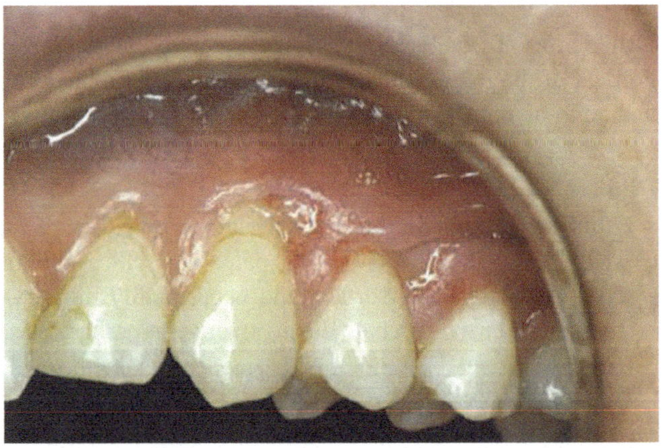

Fig. 14.5 Gingival factitious trauma from fingernail

Differential Diagnosis
- Mechanical ulcerations
- Aphthous ulcer
- Squamous cell carcinoma
- Tuberculosis
- Syphilis
- Eosinophilic ulcer
- Other nonspecific ulcerations

Laboratory Tests Usually not required. If ulceration persists longer than 10 days, biopsy for histopathological examination is suggested.

Treatment The treatment of factitious oral ulcers should be individually tailored for each patient with periodic clinical control and psychotherapy. Topical corticosteroid ointment in Orabase and short-term use of antibacterial mouthwashes are suggested measures.

Frictional Keratosis

Definition Frictional hyperkeratosis is a benign white lesion of the gingiva or the oral mucosa.

Etiology The distinctive lesion is caused by mild chronic trauma (e.g., impaction of food, inappropriate toothbrushing or dental floss use, chronic movement of an ill-fitting denture on the gingiva or alveolar mucosa), or direct trauma from a hyper-erupted tooth.

Gingival Involvement Common. Non-biofilm-induced lesion.

Other Sites of Involvement Oral mucosa, alveolar mucosa, retromolar pad.

Clinical Features
- Clinically, it presents as a poorly demarcated white papule or plaque on the keratinized mucosa of the retromolar pad or alveolar ridge mucosa (often edentulous). The surface of the lesion appears whitish-gray in color, can be rough, and may rarely be associated with erosions (Figs. 14.6, 14.7, and 14.8).
- When lesions are related to inappropriate tooth brushing, they present as a superficial, horizontal gingival laceration to major loss of tissue often resulting in gingiva recession. Characteristic findings in these patients include extremely good oral hygiene, cervical tooth abrasion, and unaffected tips of the interdental papillae at the site of injury.

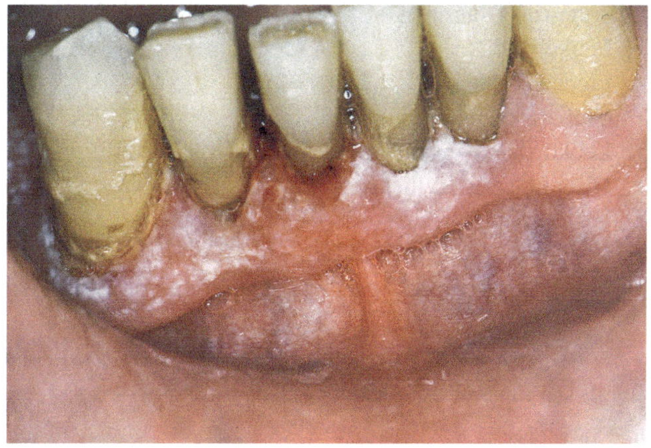

Fig. 14.6 Friction keratosis related to hard brushing

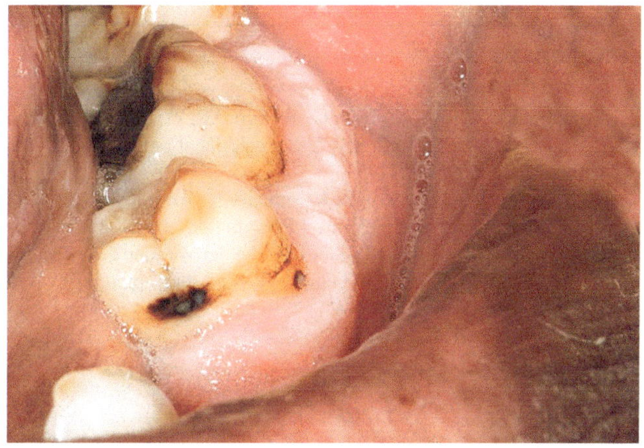

Fig. 14.7 Frictional keratosis on the gingiva

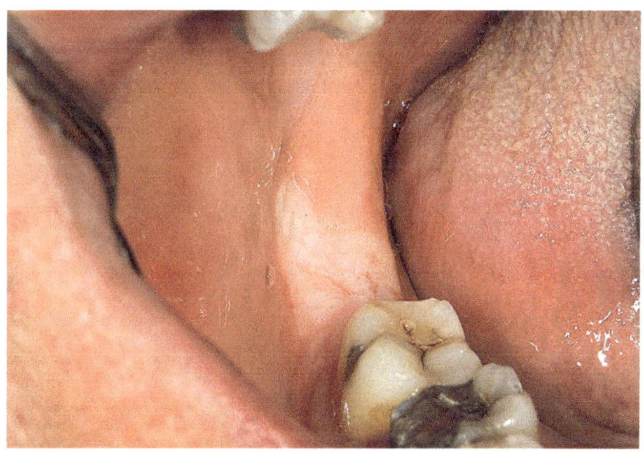

Fig. 14.8 Frictional keratosis on the retromolar area

- It should be clearly distinguished from true leukoplakia, a potentially malignant disorder.
- Diagnosis is mainly based on clinical criteria. Sometimes, laboratory tests are needed.

Differential Diagnosis

- Leukoplakia
- Lichen planus
- Cinnamon contact stomatitis
- Leukoedema
- Discoid lupus erythematosus
- White sponge nevus
- Dyskeratosis congenital
- Pachyonychia congenital

Laboratory Tests Histopathologic examination will be helpful, if the exact clinical diagnosis is not possible.

Treatment Follow-up. Elimination of the causative factor contributing to friction.

References

1. Compilato D, Cirillo N, Termine N, Kerr AR, et al. Longstanding oral ulcers: proposal for a new 's-c-d classification system'. J Oral Pathol Med. 2009;38:241–53.
2. Er N, Ozkavaf A, Berberoglu A, Yamalik N. An unusual cause of gingival recession: oral piercing. J Periodontol. 2000;171:1767–9.
3. Hennequin-Hoenderdos NL, Slot DE, van der Weijden GA. Trauma to the gingiva by oral hygiene aids and oral piercings. Ned Tijdschr Tandheelkd. 2017;124(12):653–6. https://doi.org/10.5177/ntvt.2017.12.17187.
4. Kofina V, An H, Rawal SY. Iatrogenic acid-induced gingival recession during crown cementation: a case report. Aust Dent J. 2021;66(3):332–6. https://doi.org/10.1111/adj.12820. Epub ahead of print. PMID: 33438220
5. Rajiv S, Biju T, Maithreyi VP. Self-inflicted traumatic injuries of the gingiva–a case series. J Int Oral Health. 2010;2(2):43.
6. Krejci CB. Self-inflicted gingival injury due to habitual fingernail biting. J Periodontol. 2000;71:1029–31.
7. Müller S. Frictional keratosis, contact keratosis and smokeless tobacco keratosis: features of reactive white lesions of the oral mucosa. Head Neck Pathol. 2019;13(1):16–24.
8. Suwasini S, Chatterjee K, Purkait SK, et al. Expression of P53 protein and Ki-67 antigen in oral leukoplakia with different histopathological grades of epithelial dysplasia. J Int Soc Prev Community Dent. 2018;8(6):513–22.

Chemical and Thermal Lesions of the Gingiva

15

Contents

Chemical Lesions

Definition Chemically induced lesions often present as mucosal burns, erosions, or white lesions.

Etiology Lesions are caused by a large number of caustic chemical agents that are improperly applied topically. These agents include analgesic tablets, such as aspirin, cocaine deliberately rubbed into the gingiva or vestibule, mouthwashes, chemical agents used in dental practice, tobacco products, including smokeless tobacco, sanguinaria, areca nut, and alcoholic products. Accidental ingestion of household chemicals or dental chemicals (e.g., kitchen cleansers, eugenol, hydrogen peroxide, root canal cleansers) may also cause chemical lesions on the gingiva.

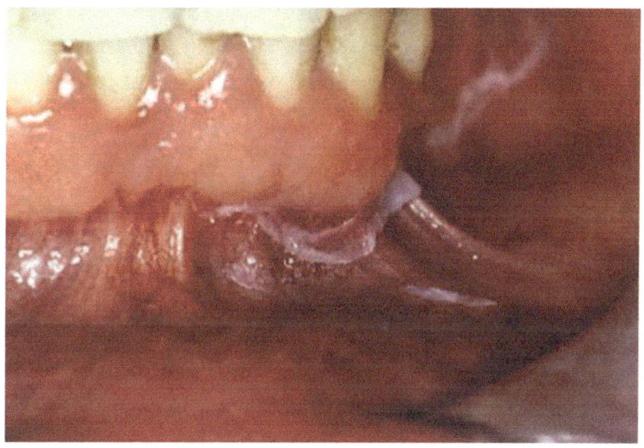

Fig. 15.1 Mucosal chemical burn from mouthwash

Gingival Involvement Relatively common.

Other Sites of Involvement Tongue, palate, floor of the mouth, buccal mucosa, lips.

Clinical Features

- Clinically, chemical lesions on the gingiva present as erythematous lesions that may slough a coagulated surface. Vesicles and sometimes ulceration, petechiae, or erosion, are observed. (Figs. 15.1, 15.2, 15.3, 15.4, 15.5 and 15.6).
- On other oral mucosa sites, chemically induced lesions initially present as an irregular whitish and wrinkled area. Later, the necrotic epithelium desquamates exposing an underlying painful erosion.
- The severity of the lesion depends on the causative agent, its concentration, and the duration of tissue contact.
- Lesions usually heal within 4–6 days after discontinuing the agent.
- Diagnosis is based on history and clinical features.

Differential Diagnosis

- Thermal burns
- Traumatic lesions
- Friction keratoses
- Leukoplakia
- Materia alba
- Squamous cell carcinoma
- Candidiasis

G. Laskaris et al., *Periodontal Manifestations of Local and Systemic Diseases*, https://doi.org/10.1007/978-3-031-10828-0_15

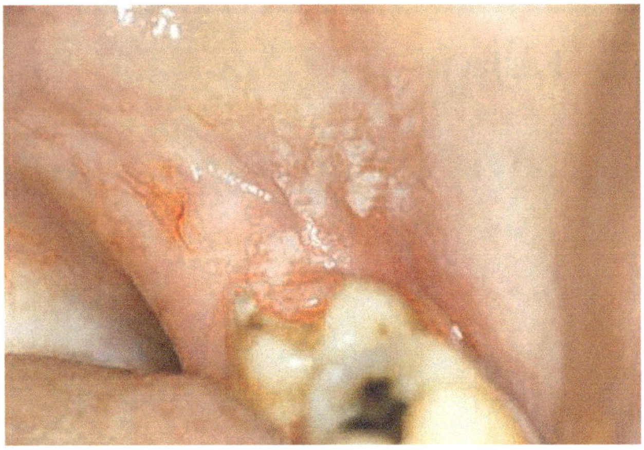

Fig. 15.2 Mucosal chemical burn from topical application of aspirin

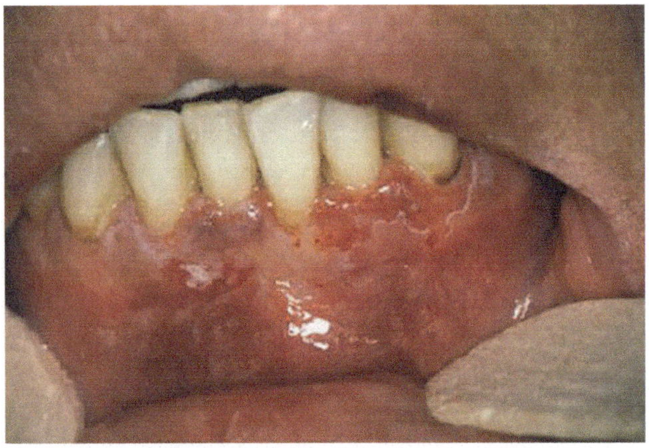

Fig. 15.3 Mucosal chemical burn from hydrogen peroxide

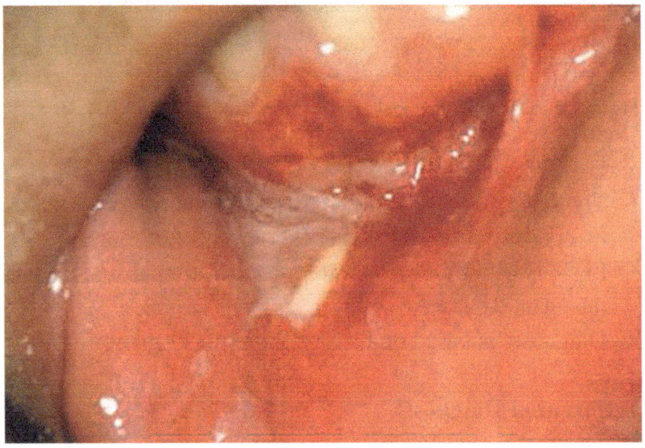

Fig. 15.4 Mucosal chemical burn from trichloracetic acid

- Syphilis
- Lichen planus
- Drug reaction
- Cinammon contact stomatitis
- Desquamative gingivitis

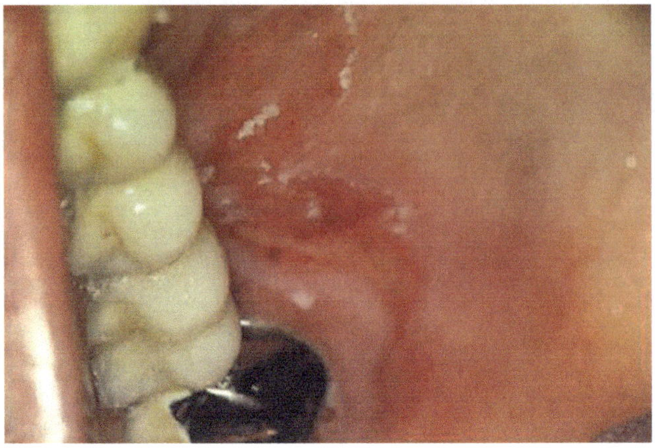

Fig. 15.5 Mucosal chemical burn from alcohol

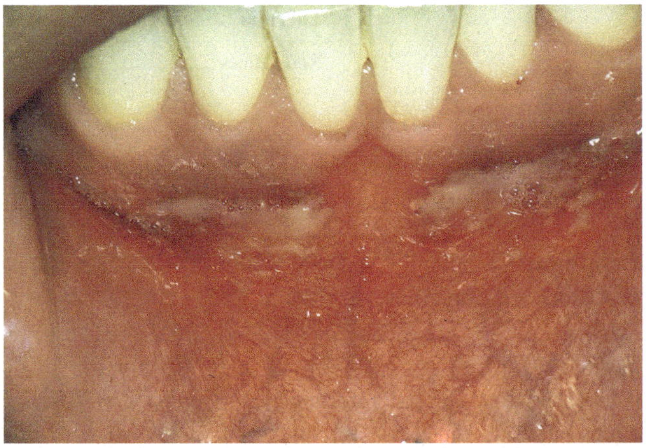

Fig. 15.6 Erythema due to chemical burn from mouthwash

Laboratory Tests No laboratory tests are required.

Treatment Removal of the offending agent and use of a chamomile mouthwash. In severe cases, low dose, short-term systemic corticosteroids.

Thermal Lesions

Definition Thermal is a frequent cause that can produce mild or severe tissue damage.

Etiology Thermally induced lesions may be caused by hot foods or beverages, (e.g., pizza, melted cheese, tea), accidental contact with hot dental instruments, electrosurgery, cryosurgery, laser surgery, and long-term heavy smoking.

Gingival Involvement Relatively common.

Other Sites of Involvement Tongue, palate, floor of the mouth, buccal mucosa, lips.

Clinical Features

- Most commonly, thermal lesions on the gingiva appear as erythematous lesions that may undergo epithelial desquamation. Vesicles, ulcerations, petechiae, or erosions are observed. (Figs. 15.7, 15.8, and 15.9). Multifocal pigmentation may also be seen when the patient is a heavy smoker (*Smoker's melanosis*). Melanosis is due to increased melanin production because of the elevated temperature in the mouth for a long period.
- On other oral mucosa sites, thermal lesions appear as irregular, whitish, and wrinkled areas whose superficial necrotic epithelial cells normally desquamate exposing an underlying painful erosion.
- The severity of the lesion depends on the causative agent, its temperature, and the duration of tissue contact.
- Lesions usually heal within 4–6 days after discontinuation of the causative agent.
- Diagnosis is based on history and clinical features.

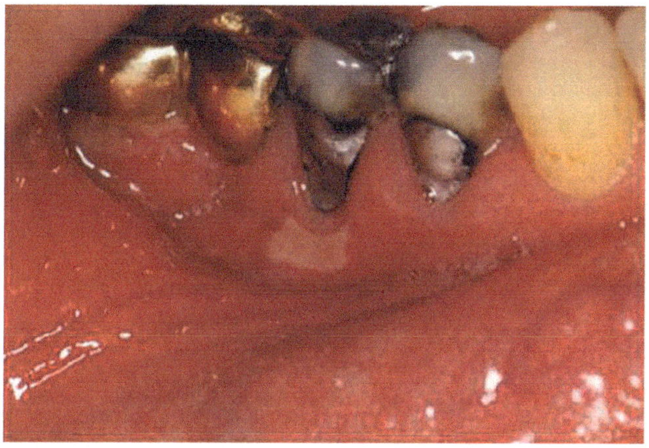

Fig. 15.7 Mucosal thermal burn from hot beverage

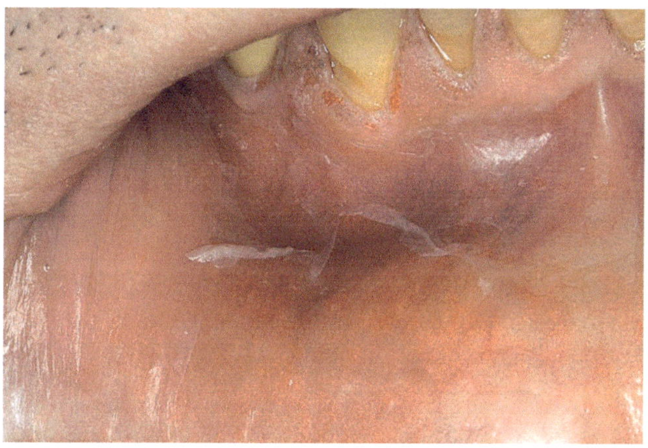

Fig. 15.8 Mucosal thermal burn from hot beverage

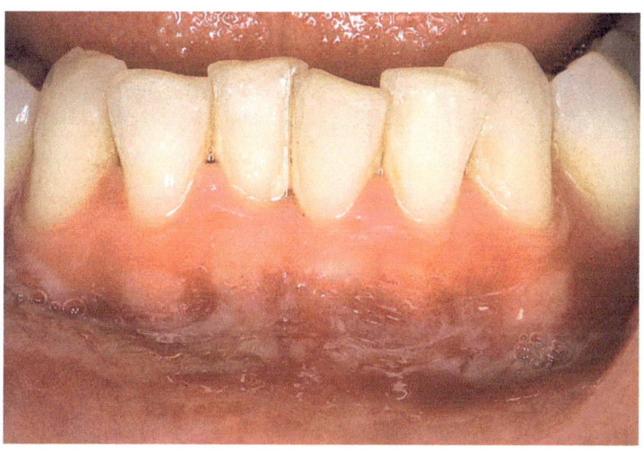

Fig. 15.9 Mucosal thermal burn from hot beverage

Differential Diagnosis

- Traumatic erosions
- Chemical burns
- Drug reaction
- Cinnamon contact stomatitis
- Desquamative gingivitis
- Vesiculobullous diseases
- Squamous cell carcinoma
- Candidiasis

Laboratory Tests No laboratory tests are required.

Treatment Removal of the offending agent and use of chamomile mouthwash. Low dose, short-term systemic corticosteroids in severe cases.

References

1. Taybos G. Oral changes associated with tobacco use. Am J Med Sci. 2003;326:179–82.
2. Ahmadzadeh A, Majd NE, Chasteen J, et al. Inflammatory response of canine gingiva to a chemical retraction agent placed at different time intervals. Dent Res J (Isfahan). 2014;11(1):81–6. PMID: 24688565; PMCID: PMC3955320
3. Rawal SY, Claman LJ, Kalmar JR, Tatakis DN. Traumatic lesions of the gingiva: a case series. J Periodontol. 2004;75:762–9. https://doi.org/10.1902/jop.2004.75.5.762
4. Angiero F, Parma L, Crippa R, Benedicenti S. Diode laser (808 nm) applied to oral soft tissue lesions: a retrospective study to assess histopathological diagnosis and evaluate physical damage. Lasers Med Sci. 2012;27(2):383–8. https://doi.org/10.1007/s10103-011-0900-7. Epub 2011 Mar 9

Drug-Influenced Gingival Lesions

16

Contents

Gingival Enlargement Due to Phenytoin, Cyclosporine, and Calcium Channel Blockers

Definition Gingival overgrowth in response to the use of these drugs.

Etiology The exact mechanism is unknown. There is a positive correlation between the severity of gingival overgrowth and inflammation, plaque biofilm score, calculus accumulation, and pocket depths. These particular drugs possibly effect various molecular pathways and get implicated in increased expression of markers of gingival fibrosis and gingival fibroblasts.

Gingival Involvement Common. Associated with dental biofilm, when poor oral hygiene exists.

Other Sites of Involvement Skin, hair.

Clinical Features

- Clinically, gingival overgrowth presents as a characteristically firm, lobulated, or smooth and painless tissue mass with normal or red color. It is tough with coarse stippling and relatively little bleeding tendency, which often occurs in the interdental papillae, that enlarge to form false vertical clefts. The enlargement gradually involves both the free and attached gingiva and is found more on buccal and labial gingiva opposed to palatal and lingual (Figs. 16.1, 16.2, 16.3, 16.4, 16.5, 16.6, 16.7 and 16.8). It is absent in edentulous areas.

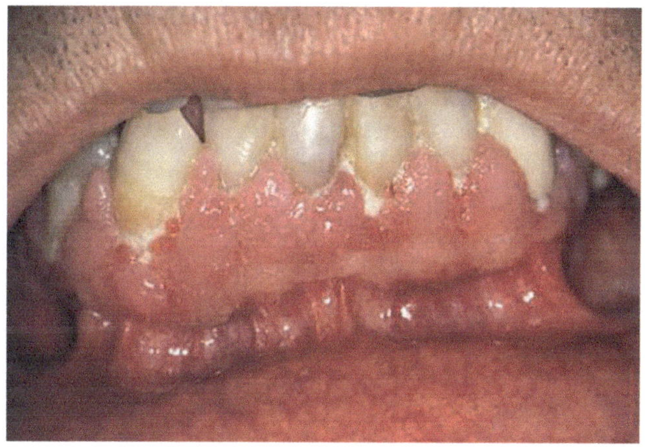

Fig. 16.1 Drug induced gingival enlargement due to phenytoin

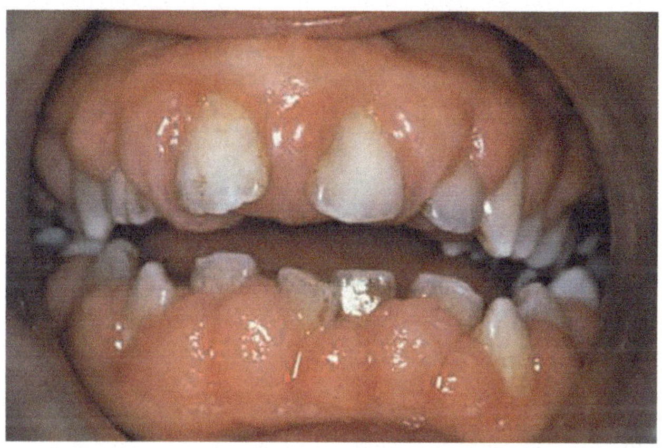

Fig. 16.2 Drug induced gingival enlargement due to phenytoin

G. Laskaris et al., *Periodontal Manifestations of Local and Systemic Diseases*, https://doi.org/10.1007/978-3-031-10828-0_16

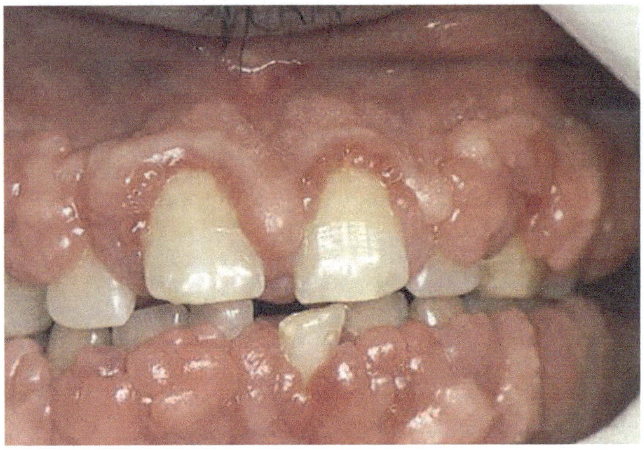

Fig. 16.3 Drug induced gingival enlargement due to cyclosporine

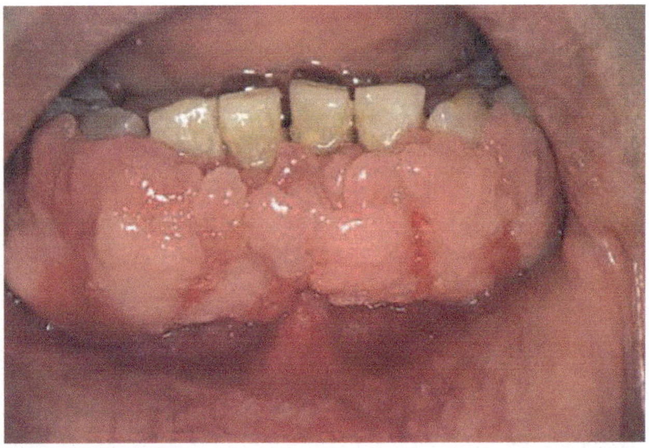

Fig. 16.4 Drug induced gingival enlargement due to cyclosporine

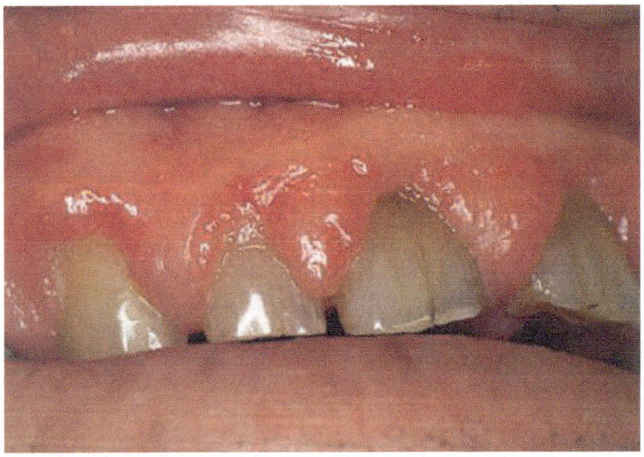

Fig. 16.5 Drug induced gingival enlargement due to cyclosporine

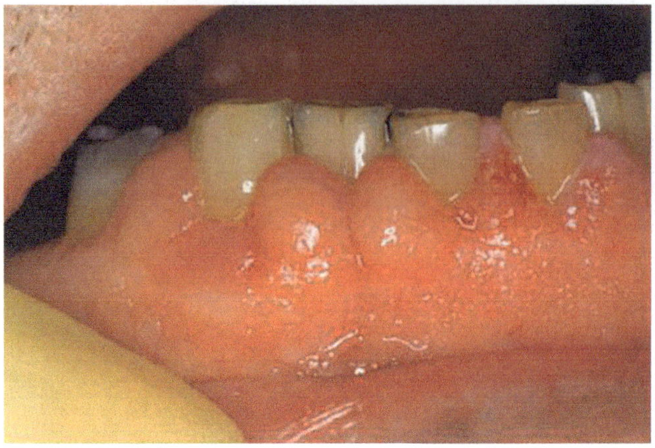

Fig. 16.6 Drug induced gingival enlargement due to nifedipine

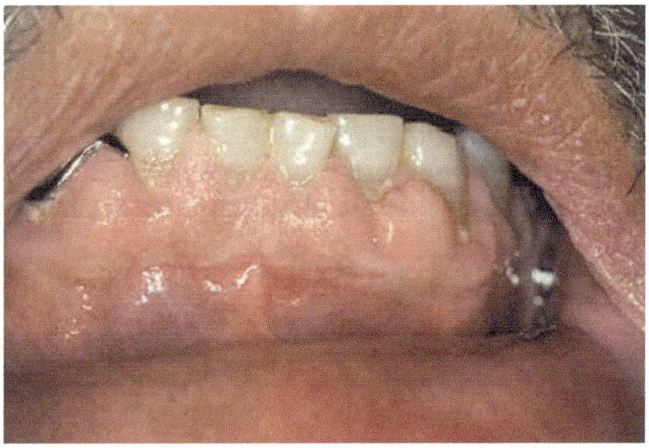

Fig. 16.7 Drug induced gingival enlargement due to nifedipine

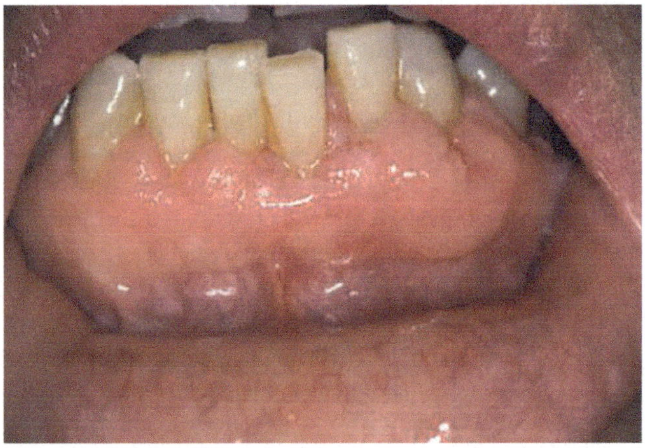

Fig. 16.8 Drug induced gingival enlargement due to nifedipine

- The enlargement develops slowly over weeks and is usually *generalized*, but it *can be limited* to a few teeth and it is more commonly noted in the anterior areas.
- The frequency and degree of gingival enlargement depends usually on the treatment regime and its duration. The gingiva may partially or entirely cover the crowns of the teeth. The enlargement develops within the first 2–3 months of starting treatment and is peaking at around 1 year of drug use. It is aggravated by poor oral hygiene.
- Diagnosis is based on history and clinical features.

Differential Diagnosis
- Dental biofilm-induced gingivitis
- Hereditary gingival fibromatosis
- Pregnancy gingivitis
- Sarcoidosis
- Crohn disease
- A-aminosidosis
- Acanthosis nigricans
- Leukemia
- Wegener granulomatosis
- Amyloidosis
- Hurler syndrome
- Zimmermann-Laband syndrome

Laboratory Tests Usually not required.

Treatment Following consultation with physician, change in the drug regime or dose reduction. Improvement of oral hygiene. Gingival surgery may be needed. Adjunctive use of azithromycin may reduce lesion size. With continuous medication use, recurrence is common.

Lesions Induced by Bisphosphonates and RANKL Inhibitors

Definition Osteonecrosis of the jaw, caused by bisphosphonates and Rank ligand (RANKL) inhibitors.

Etiology The exact mechanism of the disease remains unclear. Bisphosphonates are agents that inhibit bone resorption and bone remodeling leading to jaw necrosis, while RANKL inhibitors prohibit angiogenesis.

Gingival Involvement Relatively rare. Non-dental biofilm-related lesions.

Other Sites of Involvement Alveolar mucosa, oral mucosa (rare).

Clinical Features
- Clinically, the periodontal attachment apparatus appears inflamed, edematous, ulcerated, and necrotic.

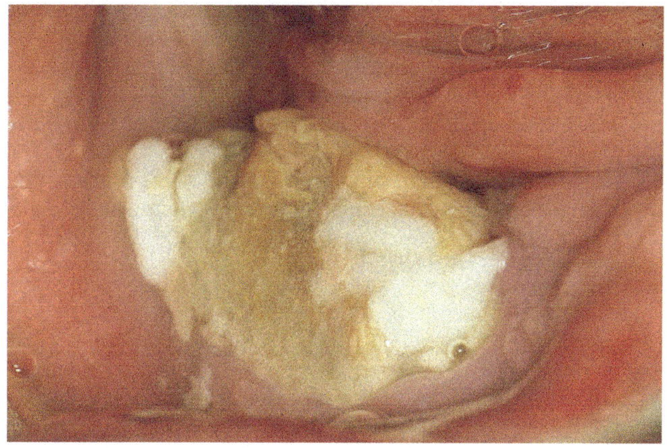

Fig. 16.9 Osteonecrosis of the mandible due to biphosphonates of a patient with multiple myeloma

- There is painful bone exposure with inflammation and edema that may lead to osteomyelitis, necrosis, and sequestration (Fig. 16.9). The mandible is affected more commonly.
- An irregular, painful ulceration may be observed in adjacent oral mucosa sites.
- Diagnosis is based on history as well as on clinical and laboratory tests.

Differential Diagnosis
- Radiotherapy-induced osteonecrosis
- Osteomyelitis
- Actinomycosis
- Ulcerations due to other medications

Laboratory Tests Histopathologic examination, panoramic radiograph, CT scan.

Treatment High level of oral hygiene, systemic antibiotics, conservative surgical debridement.

References

1. Trackman PC, Kantarci A. Molecular and clinical aspects of drug-induced gingival overgrowth. J Dent Res. 2015;94(4):540–6. https://doi.org/10.1177/0022034515571265. Epub 2015 Feb 13
2. Alshargabi R, Sano T, Yamashita A, et al. SPOCK1 is a novel inducer of epithelial to mesenchymal transition in drug-induced gingival overgrowth. Sci Rep. 2020;10(1):9785. https://doi.org/10.1038/s41598-020-66660-z.
3. Kim SS, Jackson-Boeters L, Darling MR, et al. Nifedipine induces periostin expression in gingival fibroblasts through TGF-beta. J Dent Res. 2013;92(11):1022–8. https://doi.org/10.1177/0022034513503659. Epub 2013 Sep 4
4. Rapone B, Ferrara E, Santacroce L, et al. Periodontal microbiological status influences the occurrence of cyclosporine-a and tacrolimus-induced gingival overgrowth. Antibiotics (Basel). 2019;8(3):124. https://doi.org/10.3390/antibiotics8030124.
5. Kim SS, Nikoloudaki G, Darling M, et al. Phenytoin activates Smad3 phosphorylation and periostin expression in drug-induced

gingival enlargement. Histol Histopathol. 2018;33(12):1287–98. https://doi.org/10.14670/HH-18-015. Epub 2018 Jun 19
6. Asif SM, Shaik N, Barthunia B, et al. Nifedipine induced gingival enlargement in an edentulous patient: a case report with one year follow up. BMC Oral Health. 2018;18(1):227. https://doi.org/10.1186/s12903-018-0690-4.
7. Ramírez-Rámiz A, Brunet-LLobet L, Lahor-Soler E, Miranda-Rius J. On the cellular and molecular mechanisms of drug-induced gingival overgrowth. Open Dent J. 2017;31(11):420–35. https://doi.org/10.2174/1874210601711010420.
8. Sven O, et al. Medication-related osteonecrosis of the jaw: prevention, diagnosis and management in patients with cancer and bone metastases. Cancer Treat Rev. 2018;69:177–87.
9. O'Sullivan EM. Nicorandil-induced severe oral ulceration. J Ir Dent Assoc. 2004;50:157–9.
10. Horie N, Kawano R, Kaneko T, Shimoyama T. Methotrexate-related lymphoproliferative disorder arising in the gingiva of a patient with rheumatoid arthritis. Aust Dent J. 2015;60(3):408–11. https://doi.org/10.1111/adj.12235. Epub 2015 Jul 24

Radiation and Chemotherapy-Induced Gingival Lesions

17

Contents

Radiation Mucositis

Definition Radiation-induced oral mucositis is the most common complication of radiotherapy and affects the quality of life of individuals diagnosed with oral cancer.

Etiology Ionizing radiation.

Gingival Involvement Relatively common. Non-dental biofilm-induced lesions.

Other Sites of Involvement Tongue, buccal mucosa, palate, floor of the mouth, salivary glands.

Clinical Features

- Radiation-induced oral mucositis results from direct and indirect effects of radiation on the rapidly proliferating basal epithelial cells of the oral mucosa causing the loss of ability to self-renew and ulceration. Its severity depends on the dose and duration of treatment, the volume of radiated tissue, the type of ionizing radiation, and the preventive care of the mouth before cancer treatment. Mucosal changes can be *acute* (*early*) and *chronic* (*late*).
- Clinically, acute oral mucositis presents with a diffuse erythematous and edematous gingiva associated with burning sensation or pain and erosions (Figs. 17.1, 17.2 and 17.3).
- Gingival bleeding index, plaque index, and gingival recession are all increased after radiotherapy.

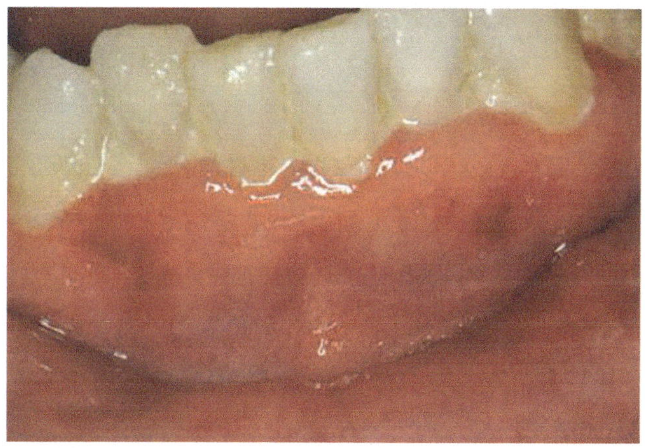

Fig. 17.1 Radiation mucositis on the gingiva and oral mucosa

- Oral mucosal lesions are characterized by thin mucosal lining, vascular fibrosis, erythema, and painful ulcerations. Xerostomia, telangiectasia, dental decay, taste changes, osteoradionecrosis, candidiasis, are also common.
- Diagnosis is mainly based on history and clinical features.

Differential Diagnosis

- Mucositis due to chemotherapy
- Chemical burns
- Thermal burns
- Lichen planus

G. Laskaris et al., *Periodontal Manifestations of Local and Systemic Diseases*, https://doi.org/10.1007/978-3-031-10828-0_17

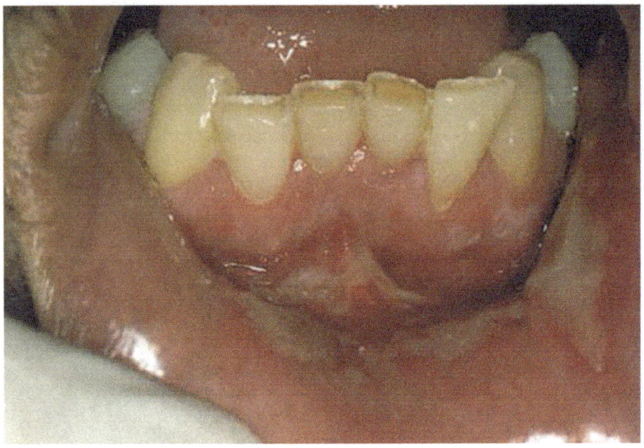

Fig. 17.2 Radiation mucositis on the gingiva and oral mucosa

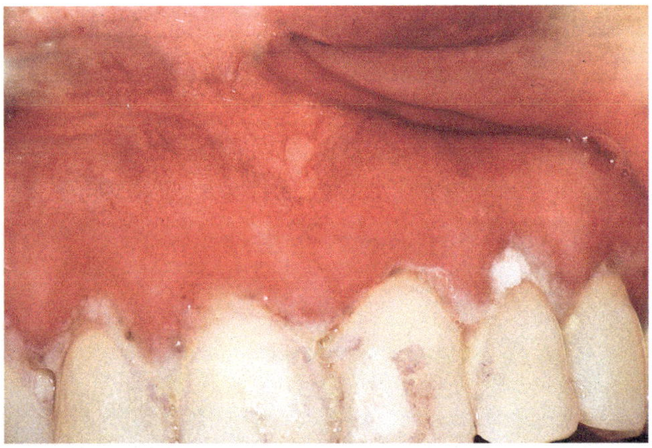

Fig. 17.3 Radiation mucositis of the upper gingiva and alveolar mucosa

- Desquamative gingivitis
- Mucositis from stem cell transplant
- Drug reactions
- Allergic contact stomatitis
- Leukemias

Laboratory Tests Usually not required. Histopathologic examination may be helpful.

Treatment There is no specific treatment.Oral complications can be prevented by healthy diet, high level of oral hygiene, dental and periodontal care, smoking cessation, and alcohol abstinence. Palliative care *locally* and *systemic* treatment of oral mucositis are critical during and after radiation therapy. Aggressive oral care is very important and should be performed before, during, and after therapy.

Osteoradionecrosis

Definition Bone necrosis and infection arising in a previously irradiated jaw.

Etiology The etiology is linked to radiation-induced hypoxic, hypocellular, and hypovascular tissue followed by a defective or delayed wound healing affecting mostly the mandible. The initiating factor is often trauma, such as tooth extraction or infection.

Gingival Involvement Rare. Non-dental biofilm-related lesions.

Other Sites of Involvement Muscle, teeth, salivary glands.

Clinical Features

- Gingival lesions follow bone lesions. Their clinical features include inflammation, erythema, edema, erosions, and ulcerations. They are accompanied by localized infections.
- Clinically, patients with jaw osteonecrosis present with exposed bone and pain with or without external sinuses and/or pathological fracture (Fig. 17.4). Extensive osteonecrosis may cause anesthesia or paresthesia.
- Once established, osteonecrosis may spread to the entire jaw, usually the mandible. Osteonecrosis usually occurs 2–6 months after radiotherapy.
- Diagnosis is mainly based on history and clinical features.

Differential Diagnosis

- Osteomyelitis
- Biphosphonate-induced osteonecrosis
- Monoclonal antibodies-induced osteonecrosis
- Metastatic carcinoma

Laboratory Tests Microbiology, imaging, and histopathologic examination may be helpful.

Treatment Long-term antibiotics, especially tetracycline. Topical use of 0.2% aqueous chlorhexidine is recommended. Minor surgical procedures (sequestration or removal of dead bone).

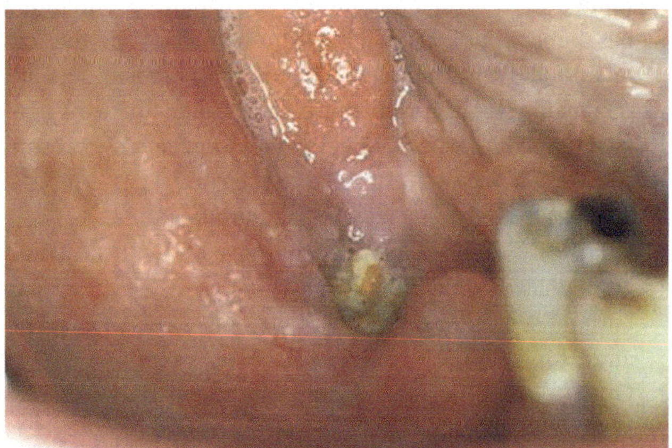

Fig. 17.4 Osteoradionecrosis of the alveolar mucosa

Chemotherapy-Induced Mucositis

Definition Oral mucositis is the outcome of acute direct toxicity related to chemotherapy and occurs in 40–50% of all patients.

Etiology Chemotherapy causes neutropenia, neutrophil dysfunction, and impaired inflammatory response, which may delay tissue healing and damage oral and periodontal tissues.

Gingival Involvement Common. Non-dental biofilm-related lesions. Dental biofilm may modify gingival lesions.

Other Sites of Involvement Oral mucosa, gastric mucosa, others.

Clinical Features

- Chemotherapy-induced oral mucositis depends on the patient's age, the degree of toxicity of the chemotherapeutic agent, treatment dose and duration, concomitant medications, previous treatment, and preexisting oral conditions. The risk of developing oral mucositis increases with the number of chemotherapeutic cycles. It may be *localized* or *diffuse.*
- Clinically, gingival lesions present as erythema associated with extremely painful bleeding and erosions or ulcerations covered with sloughing pseudomembranes. Occasionally osteonecrosis occurs. (Fig. 17.5).
- Similarly, the oral mucosa appears erythematous, atrophic, and usually with multiple painful erosions and ulcerations covered by white-yellowish pseudomembranes.
- Burning sensation, dry mouth and taste changes, candidiasis, herpetic and bacterial infections are common.

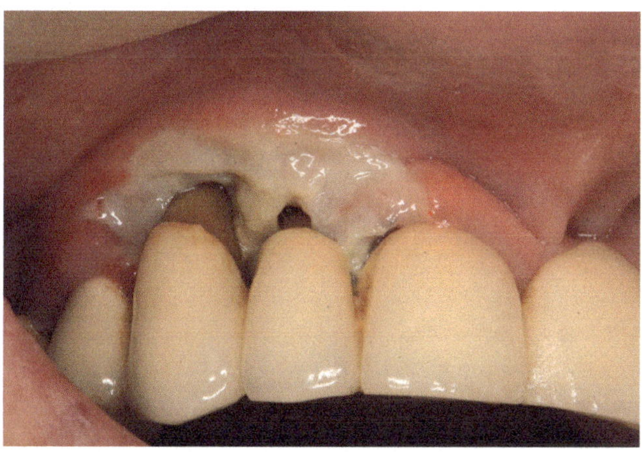

Fig. 17.5 Severe gingival ulceration covered by necrotic pseudomembrane due to methotrexate

- Oral mucositis from chemotherapy gradually resolves within 3–6 weeks following the discontinuation of treatment.
- Diagnosis is based on history and clinical features.

Differential Diagnosis

- Oral mucositis due to radiation
- Drug-induced oral lesions
- Erythema multiforme
- Herpetic stomatitis
- Graft-Versus-Host disease

Laboratory Tests Usually not required. Histopathologic examination.

Treatment There is no universally accepted standard treatment. Numerous local and systemic medicines have been used. High level of oral hygiene before, during, and after chemotherapy is necessary. Topical application of lidocaine, benzocaine, mouthwashes with diphenhydramine, benzydamine hydrochloride or ketoprofen lysine salt 1.6%, and oxygen-releasing mouthwashes is important. Systemic administration of low doses of corticosteroids for 10–15 days is effective, usually in association with high doses of vitamin B complex. Several other treatments have been recommended.

References

1. Alterio D, Jereczek-Fossa BA, Fiore MR, Piperno G, et al. Cancer treatment-induced oral mucositis. Anticancer Res. 2007;27:1105–25.
2. Sven O, et al. Medication-related osteonecrosis of the jaw: prevention, diagnosis and management in patients with cancer and bone metastases. Cancer Treat Rev. 2018;69:177–87.
3. Barasch A, Peterson DE. Risk factors for ulcerative oral mucositis in cancer patients: unanswered questions. Oral Oncol. 2003;39:91–100.
4. Madrid C, Abarca M, Bouferrache K. Osteoradionecrosis: an update. Oral Oncol. 2010;46:471–4.
5. Otmani N, Alami R, Hessissen L, Mokhtari A, et al. Determinants of severe oral mucositis in paediatric cancer patients: a prospective study. Int J Paediatr Dent. 2011;21:210–6.
6. Singh N, Scully C, Joyston-Bechal S. Oral complications of cancer therapies: prevention and management. Clin Oncol. 1996;8:15–24.
7. de Oliveira Lula EC, de Oliveira Lula CE, Alves CM, et al. Chemotherapy-induced oral complications in leukemic patients. Int J Pediatr Otorhinolaryngol. 2007;71(11):1681–5. https://doi.org/10.1016/j.ijporl.2007.07.006. Epub 2007 Sep 11. PMID: 17850887
8. Morais MO, Martins AFL, de Jesus APG, et al. A prospective study on oral adverse effects in head and neck cancer patients submitted to a preventive oral care protocol. Support Care Cancer. 2020;28(9):4263–73. https://doi.org/10.1007/s00520-019-05283-1. Epub 2020 Jan 3. PMID: 31900618

Allergic and Inflammatory Reactions

18

Contents

Allergic Gingivitis

Definition An uncommon erythematous and edematous reaction to various substances.

Etiology Type IV hypersensitivity allergic reaction triggered by oral health care products, specific foods, or constituents found in perfumes, sprays, creams, mouthwashes, dentifrices, breath fresheners, dental materials, and drugs.

Gingival Involvement Rare. Non-dental biofilm-induced lesion.

Other Sites of Involvement Oral mucosa, lips, skin.

Clinical Features
- Clinically, allergic gingivitis presents with inflammation, gingival swelling and redness, vesicles and erosions, whitish areas of necrotic epithelium, and sometimes, without intense features (Fig. 18.1 and 18.2). The most common symptom is a burning sensation or pain.
- Similar signs and symptoms can occur in other oral mucosal sites.
- The diagnosis is determined by the history and clinical features.

Differential Diagnosis
- Dental biofilm-induced gingivitis
- Desquamative gingivitis

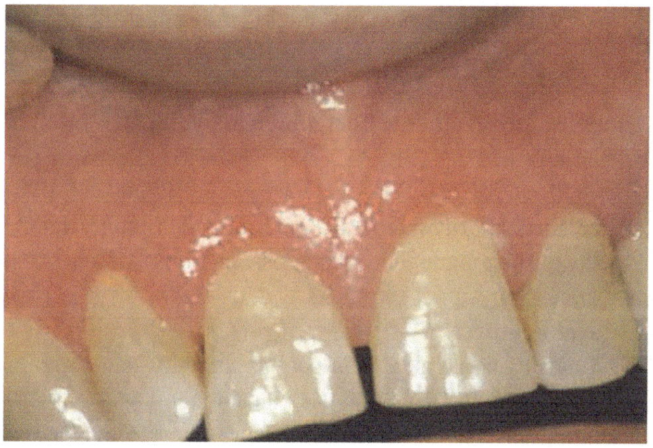

Fig. 18.1 Contact gingivitis from chlorexidine

- Plasma cell gingivitis
- Granular cell gingivitis
- Cinnamon contact stomatitis
- Trauma
- Drugs
- Erythroplakia

Laboratory Tests Usually not required. Histopathologic examination, skin patch tests.

Treatment Withdrawal of the offending agent will usually result in rapid improvement. Systemic corticosteroids in severe cases.

G. Laskaris et al., *Periodontal Manifestations of Local and Systemic Diseases*, https://doi.org/10.1007/978-3-031-10828-0_18

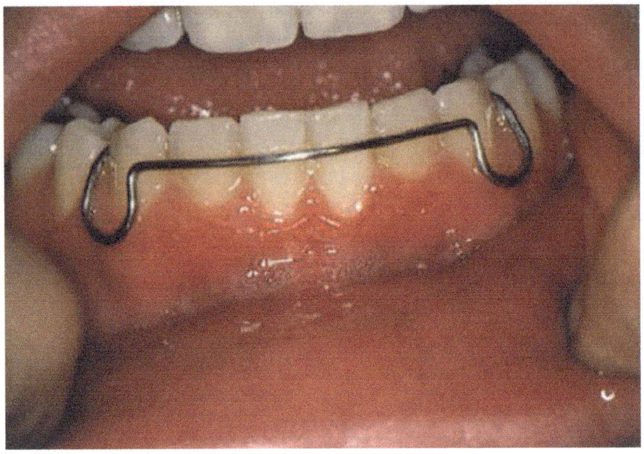

Fig. 18.2 Contact gingivitis from mouthwash containing ethanol

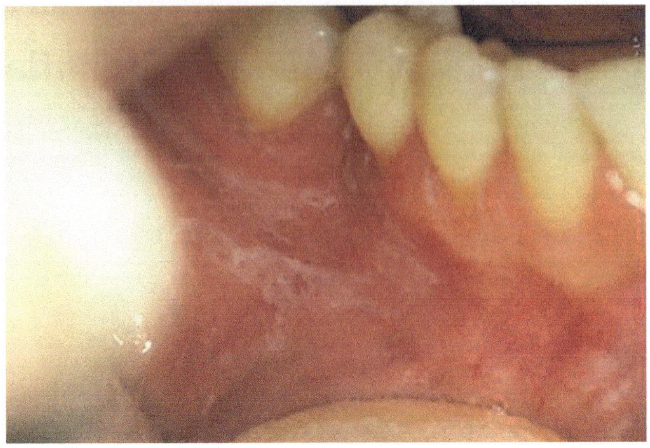

Fig. 18.3 Contact gingivitis from cinnamon

Cinnamon Contact Gingivitis

Definition Hypersensitivity type of allergic reaction of the gingivae to cinnamon.

Etiology Consumption of products containing artificial cinnamon flavor.

Gingival Involvement Uncommon. Non dental biofilm-related lesion.

Other Sites of Involvement Oral mucosa (mainly lateral aspects of the tongue, buccal mucosa, and lips).

Clinical Features
- Clinically, an atypical, nonspecific gingivitis is a common finding in individuals who use cinnamon toothpaste or cinnamon-flavored dental floss. Gingiva can present as red, slightly inflamed, or erosive with whitish lines (striae) (Fig. 18.3).
- Erythematous lesions of the oral mucosa with white hyperkeratotic striations or plaques, and erosions are common (Fig. 18.4).
- A burning sensation and pain are common symptoms.
- Diagnosis is mainly based on history and clinical features.

Differential Diagnosis
- Candidiasis
- Leukoplakia
- Lichen planus
- Plasma cell gingivitis
- Granular cell gingivitis
- Uremic stomatitis
- Chronic biting

Laboratory Tests Histopathologic examination, skin patch test.

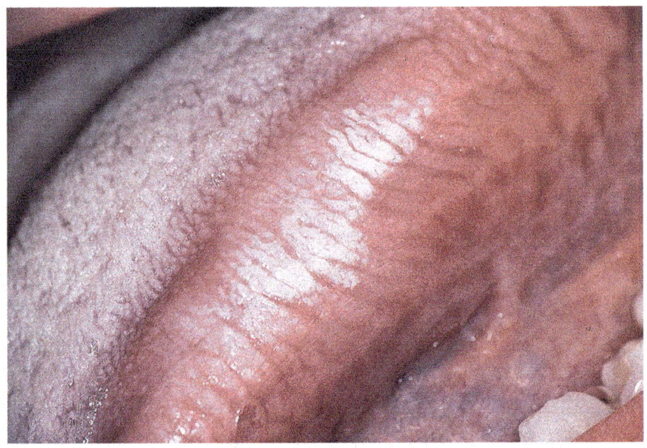

Fig. 18.4 Contact stomatitis from cinnamon on the lateral border of the tongue

Treatment Discontinuing the use of substances containing cinnamon. Topical rinses with chamomile 4–5 times daily. In cases of persistent and severe erosions, short-term and low-dose systemic corticosteroids can be helpful.

References

1. Gawkrodger DJ. Investigation of reactions to dental materials. Br J Dermatol. 2005;153:479–85.
2. Georgakopoulou EA. Cinnamon contact stomatitis. J Dermatol Case Rep. 2010;4:28–9.
3. de Groot A. Contact allergy to (ingredients of) toothpastes. Dermatitis. 2017;28(2):95–114. https://doi.org/10.1097/DER.0000000000000255.
4. Nelwan SC, Nugraha RA, Endaryanto A, et al. Effect of scaling and root planing on level of immunoglobulin E and immunoglobulin G_4 in children with gingivitis and house-dust mite allergy: a pilot randomised controlled trial. Singap Dent J. 2019;39(1):21–31. https://doi.org/10.1142/S2214607519500020. Epub 2020 Feb 14
5. Silvestre JF, Albares MP, Blanes M, et al. Allergic contact gingivitis due to eugenol present in a restorative dental material. Contact Dermatitis. 2005;52(6):341. https://doi.org/10.1111/j.0105-1873.2005.0612c.x.

19 Pigmentary Disorders

Contents

Racial Pigmentation

Definition Physiologic gingival pigmentation related to race.

Etiology It is caused by increased melanin production.

Gingival Involvement Common. Non-dental biofilm-induced lesions.

Other Sites of Involvement Other oral sites may be affected, including buccal mucosa, lips, palate, and tongue.

Clinical Features

- Clinically, it appears as asymptomatic, black-brown, diffusely pigmented areas of varying size and distribution. The most common site of such pigmentation is the anterior labial attached gingiva (Fig. 19.1).
- The pigmentation is more prominent in areas of pressure or friction and becomes more intense with aging.
- Diagnosis is based on clinical criteria.

Differential Diagnosis

- Ephelis
- Lentigo simplex
- Nevus

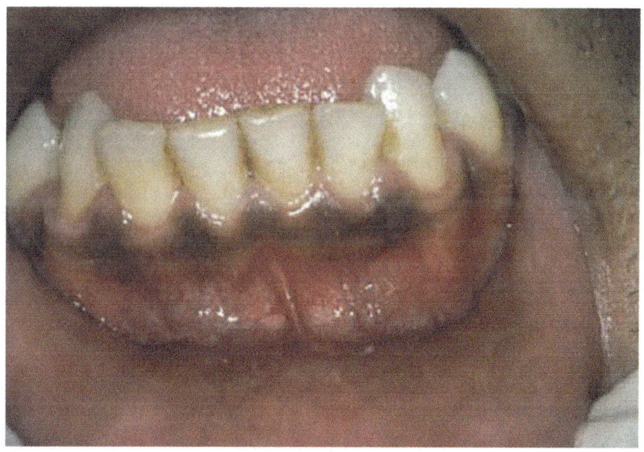

Fig. 19.1 Racial gingival pigmentation

- Melanoacanthoma
- Drug-induced pigmentation
- Addison disease
- Malignant melanoma

Laboratory Tests Usually not required. Histopathologic examination only in doubtful cases. Photographs may be useful for future comparison.

Treatment Reassurance of the patient. No treatment is required.

G. Laskaris et al., *Periodontal Manifestations of Local and Systemic Diseases*, https://doi.org/10.1007/978-3-031-10828-0_19

Ephelides

Definition Benign pigmented lesions of the oral cavity.

Etiology Ephelides (freckles) are caused by increased melanocytic activity and deposition of melanin (melanosomes) into epithelial cells.

Gingival Involvement Rare. Non-dental biofilm-induced lesion.

Other Sites of Involvement Lips, skin.

Clinical Features
- Clinically, ephelides affecting the gingival tissues are rare and they present as nonspecific, round, and solitary brown macules (Fig. 19.2).
- Ephelides may appear on the vermilion border of the lower lip and rarely at other sites intraorally.
- On sun-exposed skin, ephelides appear as multiple, usually brown or red-brown, discrete round/oval lesions, generally less than 5 mm in diameter.
- The clinical diagnosis should be confirmed with laboratory tests.

Differential Diagnosis
- Amalgam tattoo
- Lentigo simplex
- Melanocytic nevi
- Oral melanoacanthoma
- Peutz-Jegher syndrome
- Albright syndrome
- Malignant melanoma

Laboratory Tests Histopathologic and histochemical examination.

Treatment Treatment is usually not required.

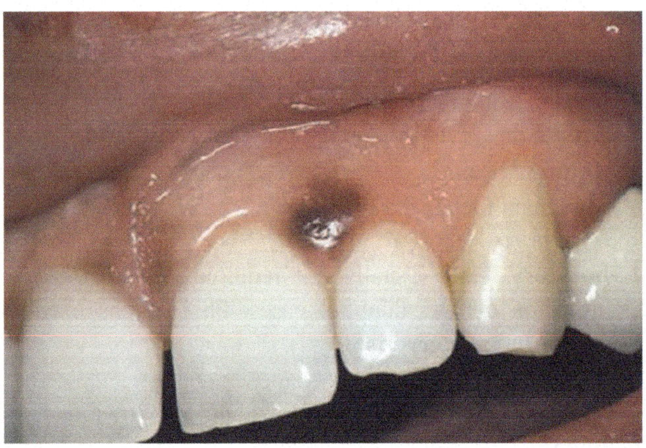

Fig. 19.2 Ephelis on the gingiva

Lentigo Simplex

Definition A benign pigmented lesion.

Etiology Lentigo simplex is caused by increased melanocytes and melanin pigment in the basal layer.

Gingival Involvement Rare. Non-dental biofilm-induced lesion.

Other Sites of Involvement The oral mucosa is rarely affected. The skin is the most commonly involved.

Clinical Features
- Clinically, the gingival lentigines occur in a sharply demarcated distribution. They are flat, round macules or plaques with brown or black-brown color (Fig. 19.3). The most commonly affected oral sites are the lower lip and buccal mucosa.
- Lesions can also arise in the genital mucosa. They are more common on the skin and are not related to sun exposure.
- The clinical diagnosis should be confirmed by laboratory tests.

Differential Diagnosis
- Amalgam tattoo
- Ephelides
- Melanocytic nevi
- Oral melanoacanthoma
- Peutz-Jegher syndrome
- Albright syndrome
- LEOPARD syndrome
- Malignant melanoma

Laboratory Tests Histopathologic and histochemical examination.

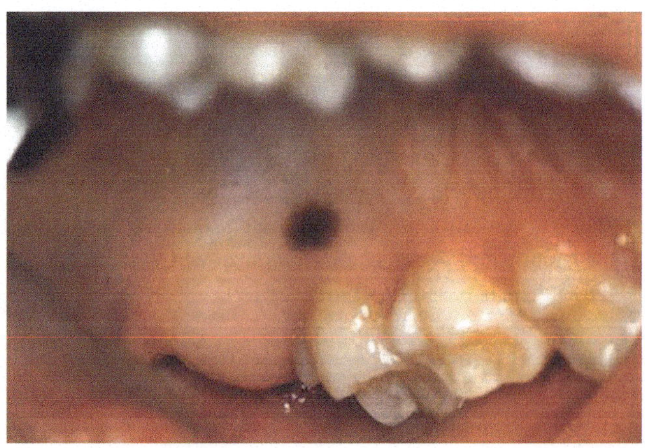

Fig. 19.3 Melanotic macule on the gingiva

Treatment No treatment is required, except for esthetic reasons. However, if lentigo simplex occurs in an area of the mouth that is constantly subjected to mechanical friction, conservative surgical excision should be advised.

Nevi

Definition Nevi are well-circumscribed developmental malformations, usually brown, blue, or black in color.

Etiology They result from the proliferation of modified melanocytes or nevus cells. Genetic factors seem to play a role in the development of nevi. Other factors, such as environmental, hormonal, and immunologic, are also involved in the development of nevi.

Classification There are two main types of melanocytic nevi: a. *congenital nevus* and b. *acquired nevus*. Intraoral acquired nevi are histologically classified into four types depending on the location of nevus cells and the presence or absence of junctional activity: a. *intradermal (intramucosal)*, b. *junctional*, c. *compound,* and d. *blue. Nevus of Ota* is a rare congenital hamartoma (variation of blue nevus) of dermal melanocytes that causes blue-gray hyperpigmentation of the eye and surrounding structures. It mainly affects the ophthalmic and maxillary divisions of the trigeminal nerve.

Gingival Involvement Rare. Non-dental biofilm-induced lesion.

Other Sites of Involvement Oral mucosa, most commonly on the hard palate and buccal mucosa, genitalia, skin, and other mucosae.

Clinical Features

- Clinically, the gingival lesions are typically asymptomatic and may present as black or brown, flat or slightly elevated macules or plaques (Fig. 19.4).
- Melanocytic nevi tend to increase in size and change in color with age, during pregnancy or after the administration of ACTH.
- Intraoral involvement of nevus of Ota is relatively rare. Most commonly, it presents unilaterally on the hard palate Figs. 19.5, 19.6 and 19.7).
- Junctional and compound nevi are associated with an increased risk of transformation to a malignant melanoma due to *junctional activity.*
- The clinical diagnosis should be confirmed by laboratory tests.

Differential Diagnosis

- Racial pigmentation
- Smoker's melanosis
- Amalgam tattoo
- Lentigo simplex
- Ephilides
- Melanoacanthoma
- Lentigo maligna
- Malignant melanoma

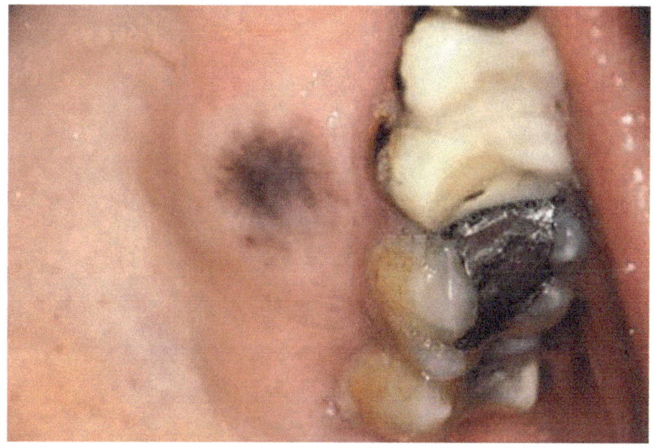

Fig. 19.4 Compound nevus on the gingiva

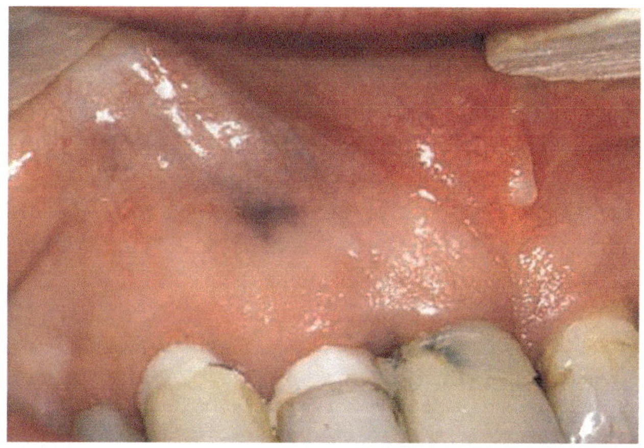

Fig. 19.5 Nevus of Ota on the gingival and alveolar mucosa

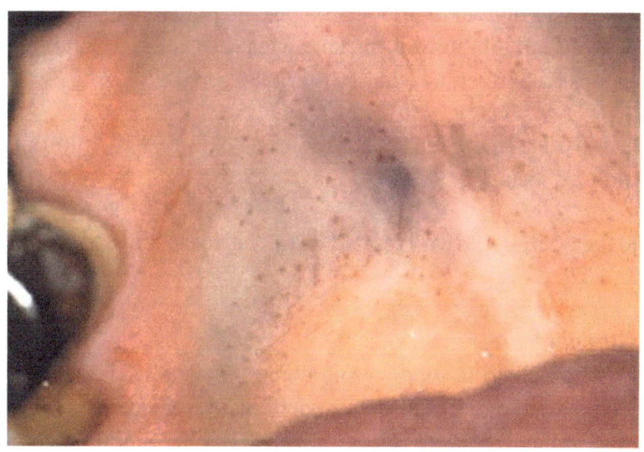

Fig. 19.6 Nevus of Ota on the palatal mucosa

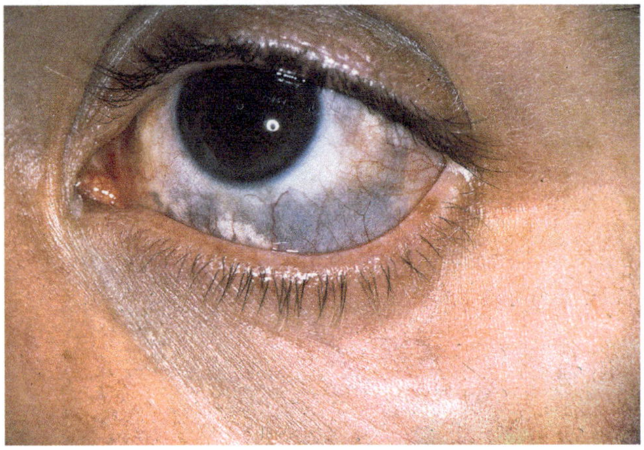

Fig. 19.7 Nevus of Ota, eye involvement

- Kaposi sarcoma
- Addison disease

Laboratory Tests Histopathologic and histochemical examination.

Treatment Conservative surgical excision is recommended primarily for cosmetic reasons and diagnostic purposes, and also to reduce malignant melanoma risk.

Smoker's Melanosis

Definition Benign hyperpigmentation of the oral mucosa caused by tobacco smoking.

Etiology Increased production and deposition of melanin due to stimulation of melanocytes by nicotine and the increased temperature during smoking.

Gingival Involvement Common. Non-dental biofilm-induced lesion.

Other Sites of Involvement Oral mucosa, tongue, palate, and lips.

Clinical Features

- Clinically, the gingival pigmentation usually presents as asymptomatic, multiple, and brown-pigmented macules or plaques. They are localized most frequently at the attached labial anterior gingiva and the interdental papillae of the mandible (Figs. 19.8 and 19.9).
- Melanosis may gradually diminish or disappear after quitting smoking.
- Diagnosis is usually based on history and clinical features.

Differential Diagnosis

- Racial pigmentation
- Amalgam tattoo

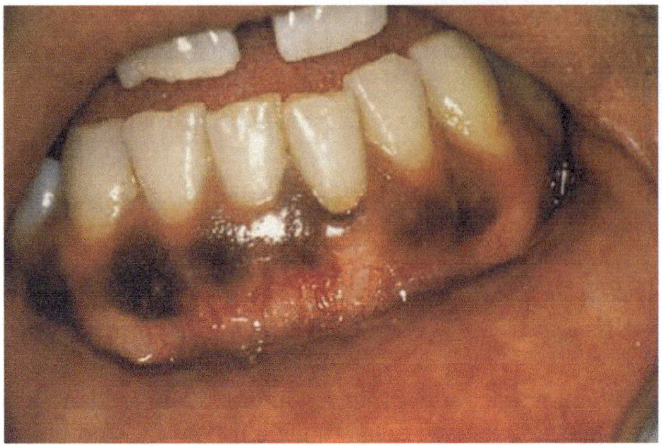

Fig. 19.8 Smoker's melanosis on the gingiva

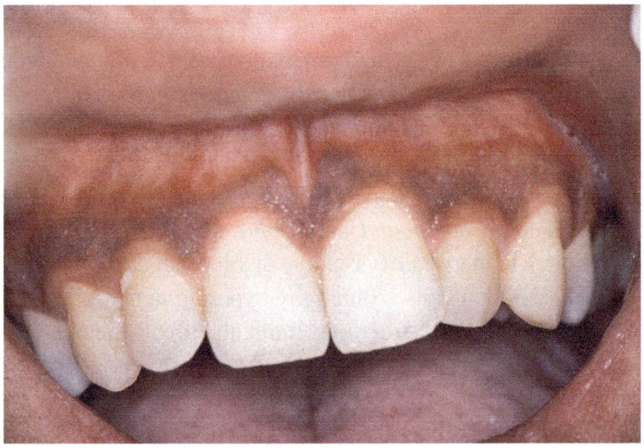

Fig. 19.9 Smoker's melanosis on the gingiva

- Traumatic pigmentation
- Drug-induced pigmentation
- Pigmented nevi
- Lentigo simplex
- Freckles
- Malignant melanoma
- Peutz-Jeghers syndrome
- Albright syndrome

Laboratory Tests Histopathologic examination may be needed to rule out other pigmented disorders.

Treatment No treatment is required**.** Strict smoking secession is urgently required.

References

1. Rawal SY, Burrell R, Hamidi CS, et al. Diffuse pigmentation of maxillary attached gingiva: four cases of the cultural practice of gingival tattoo. J Periodontol. 2007;78:170–6.
2. Rosebush MS, Briody AN, Cordell KG. Black and Brown: non-neoplastic pigmentation of the oral mucosa. Head Neck Pathol.

2019;13(1):47–55. https://doi.org/10.1007/s12105-018-0980-9. Epub 2019 Jan 22

3. Rehab A, Moneim A, El Deeb M, Rabea AA. Gingival pigmentation (cause, treatment and histological preview). Future Dental Journal. 2017;3:1–7.
4. Tavares TS, Meirelles DP, de Aguiar MCF, Caldeira PC. Pigmented lesions of the oral mucosa: a cross-sectional study of 458 histopathological specimens. Oral Dis. 2018;24(8):1484–91. https://doi.org/10.1111/odi.12924. Epub 2018 Jul 10
5. Buchner A, Hansen LS. Pigmented nevi of the oral mucosa: a clinicopathologic study of 36 new cases and review of 155 cases from the literature. Part II: analysis of 191 cases. Oral Surg Oral Med Oral Pathol. 1987;63:676–82.
6. Amérigo-Góngora M, Machuca-Portillo G, Torres-Lagares D, et al. Clinicopathological and immunohistochemical analysis of oral melanocytic nevi and review of the literature. J Stomatol Oral Maxillofac Surg. 2017;118(3):151–5. https://doi.org/10.1016/j.jormas.2017.03.003. Epub 2017 Mar 29
7. Hassona Y, Sawair F, Al-Karadsheh O, Scully C. Prevalence and clinical features of pigmented oral lesions. Int J Dermatol. 2016;55(9):1005–13. https://doi.org/10.1111/ijd.13133. Epub 2015 Dec 28
8. Pennacchiotti G, Oviedo C, Ortega-Pinto A. Solitary pigmented lesions in oral mucosa in Latin American children: a case series. Pediatr Dermatol. 2018;35(3):374–7. https://doi.org/10.1111/pde.13465. Epub 2018 Mar 24
9. Nwhator SO, Winfunke-Savage K, Ayanbadejo P, Jeboda SO. Smokers' melanosis in a Nigerian population: a preliminary study. J Contemp Dent Pract. 2007;8(5):68–75.
10. Treister NS, Magalnick D, Woo SB. Oral mucosal pigmentation secondary to minocycline therapy: report of two cases and a review of the literature. Oral Surg Oral Med Oral Pathol Oral Radiol Endod. 2004;97(6):718–25. https://doi.org/10.1016/j.tripleo.2003.11.006.

20 Bacterial Gingival Infections

Contents

Necrotizing Gingivitis (see p. 33)

Necrotizing Periodontitis (see p. 34)

Pericoronitis

Definition Inflammation of the operculum around a partially erupted or impacted tooth.

Etiology Mechanical trauma and dental plaque accumulation are the etiological factors.

Gingival Involvement Common in adolescents and teenagers.

Other Sites of Involvement None.

Clinical Features

- Clinically, there is redness and swelling of the gingiva and the mucosal flap overlying and surrounding the crown of an unerupted tooth. Frequently, ulceration and abscess formation may occur (Fig. 20.1).
- Patients complain of pain, trismus, swelling of operculum, halitosis, facial swelling, fever, regional lymphadenitis, and malaise.

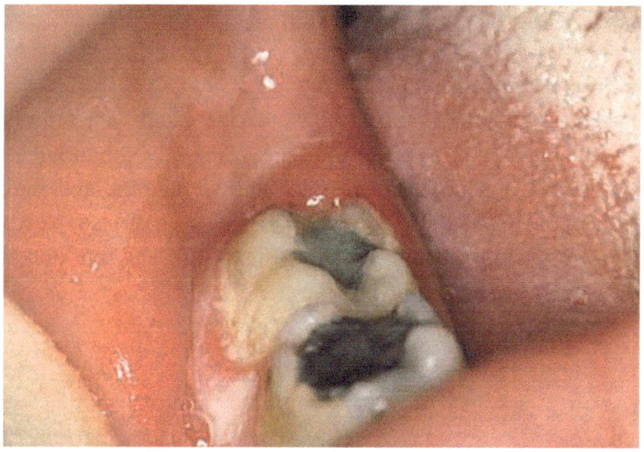

Fig. 20.1 Pericoronitis of mandibular third molar

- Pericoronitis is often associated with impacted mandibular third molars, but it is occasionally seen in relation to lower second molars.
- The diagnosis is usually based on clinical criteria.

Differential Diagnosis

- Necrotizing gingivitis
- Necrotizing periodontitis
- Tooth abscess
- Infectious mononucleosis

G. Laskaris et al., *Periodontal Manifestations of Local and Systemic Diseases*, https://doi.org/10.1007/978-3-031-10828-0_20

- Herpetic gingivitis
- Leukemia
- Non-Hodgkin lymphoma
- Mucoepidermoid carcinoma

Laboratory Tests Usually are not required.

Treatment Removal of the pericoronal flap eliminates any further episodes of pericoronitis. Use of local antiseptics and analgesics. Good oral hygiene is highly recommended. Systemic antibiotics if complications prevent immediate tooth extraction. Removal of wisdom teeth is the typical treatment after acute symptoms have subsided.

Streptococcal Gingival Infection

Definition A debatable infectious oral disease.

Etiology The infection is usually caused by *b-hemolytic Streptococcus.*

Gingival Involvement Relatively rare. Non-dental biofilm-induced lesion.

Other Sites of Involvement Tongue, tonsils.

Clinical Features

- The infection is usually acute, localized, and rarely involves all of the gingival tissue. Clinically, the inflamed gingiva appears erythematous and edematous, and may demonstrate superficial, round, or linear erosions covered with a white-yellowish smear (Fig. 20.2). The interdental papillae usually remain intact.

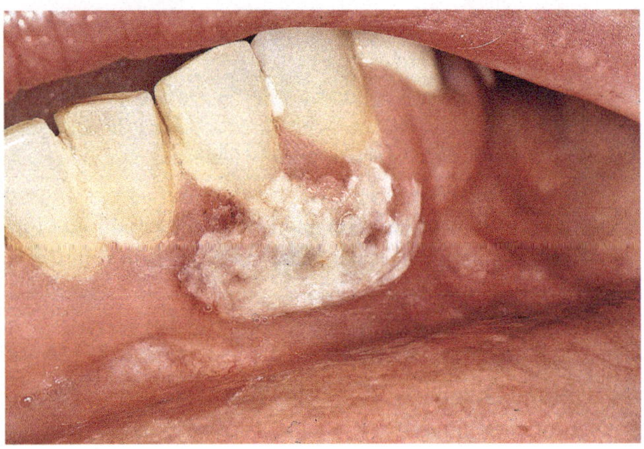

Fig. 20.2 Streptococcal gingival lesion

- Similar lesions may involve other mucosal sites.
- Mild fever and submandibular lymphadenopathy are also present. Sometimes, an upper respiratory infection precedes gingival infection.
- The clinical diagnosis should be confirmed by laboratory tests.

Differential Diagnosis

- Herpetic gingivostomatitis
- Necrotizing gingivitis
- Staphylococcal infection

Laboratory Tests Gram stain and culture for isolation of streptococci.

Treatment Oral antibiotics (penicillin, erythromycin, or clarithromycin).

References

1. Murayama Y, Kurihara H, Nagai A, et al. Acute necrotizing ulcerative gingivitis: risk factors involving host defense mechanisms. Periodontol. 1994;6:116–24.
2. Myoken Y, Sugata T, Kyo T, et al. Pseudomonas-induced necrotizing gingivostomatitis. Oral Surg Oral Med Oral Pathol Oral Radiol Endod. 1999;88:644–5.
3. Novak MJ. Necrotizing ulcerative periodontitis Ann Periodontol. 1999;4:74–8.
4. Wyss C, Dewhirst FE, Gmur R, et al. *Treponema parvum* sp. nov., a small, glucoronic or galacturonic acid-dependent oral spirochaete from lesions of human periodontitis and acute necrotizing ulcerative gingivitis. Int J Syst Evol Microbiol. 2001;51:955–62.
5. Dessirier F, Arnault JP, Denamps J, et al. Actinomycose révélée par Une ulcération du palais et de la gencive [Actinomycosis revealed by ulceration of the palate and gingiva]. Ann Dermatol Venereol. 2018;145(3):173–7. https://doi.org/10.1016/j.annder.2017.11.002. Epub 2017 Nov 28
6. Nuwwareh S. Managing a patient with pericoronitis. J Can Dent Assoc. 2013;79:d169.
7. Ribeiro MHB, Ribeiro PC, Retamal-Valdes B, et al. Microbial profile of symptomatic pericoronitis lesions: a cross-sectional study. J Appl Oral Sci. 2019;28:e20190266. https://doi.org/10.1590/1678-7757-2019-0266.
8. Katsarou T, Kapsalas A, Souliou C, et al. Pericoronitis: a clinical and epidemiological study in Greek military recruits. J Clin Exp Dent. 2019;11(2):e133–7. https://doi.org/10.4317/jced.55383.
9. Katz J, Guelmann M, Rudolph M, Ruskin J. Acute streptococcal infection of the gingiva, lower lip, and pharynx–a case report. J Periodontol. 2002;73(11):1392–5. https://doi.org/10.1902/jop.2002.73.11.1392.
10. Ciçek Y, Ozgöz M, Canakçi V, Orbak R. Streptococcal gingivitis: a report of case with a description of a unique gingival prosthesis. J Contemp Dent Pract. 2004;5(3):150–7.

Viral Gingival Infections

21

Contents

Primary Herpetic Gingivitis

Definition Primary acute, viral infection of the oral mucosa.

Etiology Herpes simplex virus type 1 (*HSV-1*) usually transmitted from saliva. Rarely, oral infection with *HSV-type 2* is transmitted through orogenital contact.

Gingival Involvement Common. Non-dental biofilm-related lesions with no attachment loss.

Other Involvement Tongue, buccal mucosa, palate, lips are often affected. Eyes, pharynx, esophagus, lungs, and brain (meningitis and encephalitis) are rarely involved.

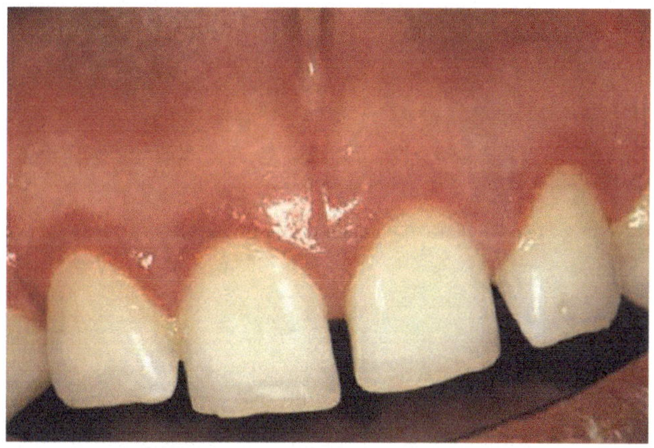

Fig. 21.1 Primary herpetic gingivitis

Clinical Features

- Primary herpetic gingivostomatitis is the most common acute viral infection of the oral mucosa. Mainly affects children and adolescents, and rarely adults.
- Clinically, it presents with erythema and gingival swelling. Coalescing vesicles form, which rapidly rupture, leaving painful small, round, and shallow ulcers, covered by a yellowish-gray pseudomembrane (Figs. 21.1, 21.2, 21.3 and 21.4).
- Multiple oral ulcerations, high fever, and regional bilateral lymphadenopathy are the hallmarks of the disease accompanied by general malaise, headache, and loss of appetite.
- The lesions persist for 1–2 weeks and heal without scarring.
- Diagnosis is based on history and clinical features.

Differential Diagnosis

- Necrotizing gingivitis
- Desquamative gingivitis
- Erythema multiforme
- Pemphigus

G. Laskaris et al., *Periodontal Manifestations of Local and Systemic Diseases*, https://doi.org/10.1007/978-3-031-10828-0_21

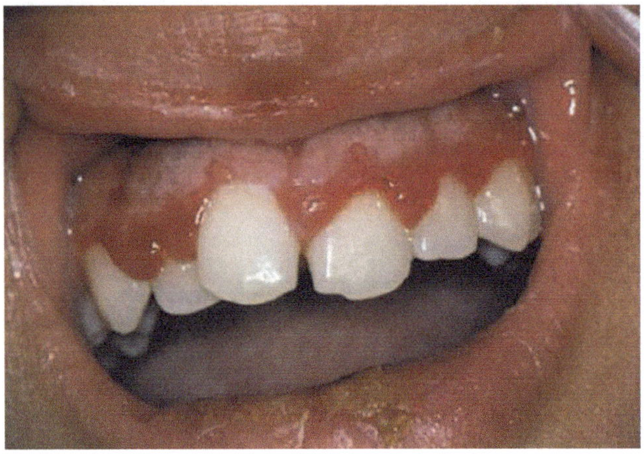

Fig. 21.2 Primary herpetic gingivitis and stomatitis

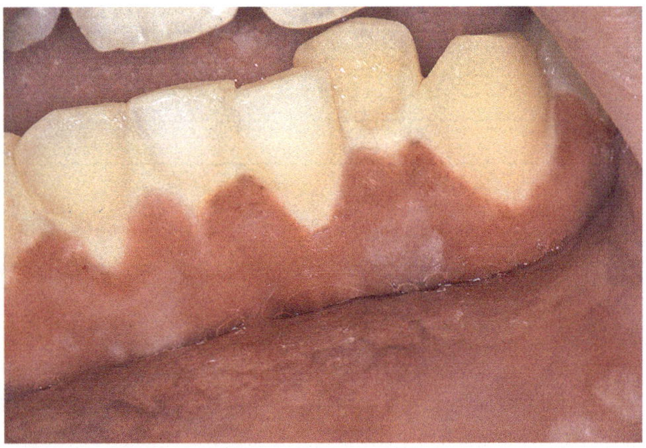

Fig. 21.3 Primary herpetic gingivitis and stomatitis

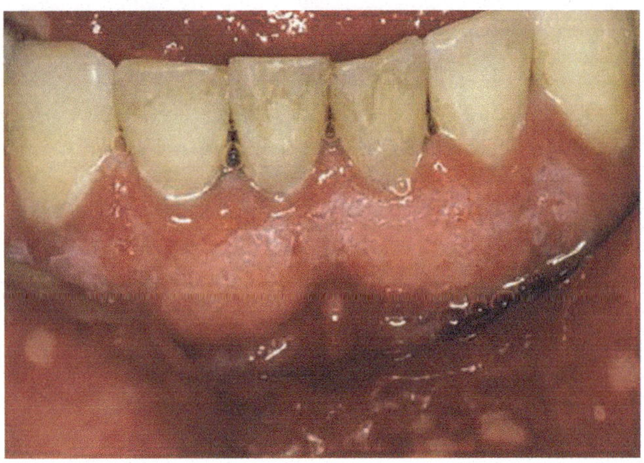

Fig. 21.4 Primary herpetic gingivitis and stomatitis

- Herpetiform aphthous ulcers
- Herpangina
- Hand, foot, and mouth disease
- Drug-induced stomatitis

Laboratory Tests Histopathologic and cytologic examination. Detection of HSV antigen by polymerase chain reaction (PCR) and viral culture may be helpful.

Treatment Symptomatic. Systemic antiviral agents (acyclovir, valacyclovir, famciclovir) should be used as early as possible.

Secondary Herpetic Gingivitis

Definition Recurrent infection with *herpes simplex virus (HSV).*

Etiology Reactivation of HSV-1 following primary herpetic infection. Predisposing factors include emotional or physical stress, febrile illness, cold, sun light, minor trauma, tooth extraction, and local anesthesia.

Gingival Involvement Common. Non-dental biofilm-related lesions.

Other Sites of Involvement Oral mucosa, usually palate, and lips.

Clinical Features
- Multiple localized clustered vesicles and painful round scattered ulcers with yellow slough and erythematous halo on the attached gingival (Figs. 21.5, 21.6 and 21.7).
- Lesions on other oral mucosal sites present similarly as a localized cluster of vesicles, which then rapture leaving small painful ulcers.
- Prodromal symptoms include burning, itching, and erythema, while fever and lymphadenopathy are characteristically absent or mild.
- Diagnosis is based on history and clinical features.

Differential Diagnosis
- Primary herpetic gingivostomatitis
- Early herpes zoster
- Aphthous ulcers

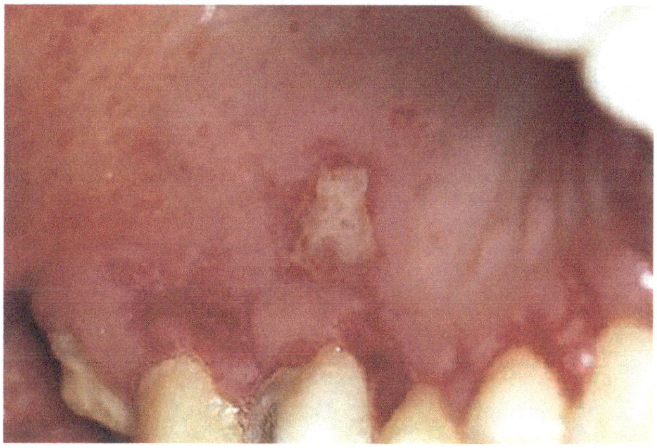

Fig. 21.5 Reccurent herpes simplex gingivitis

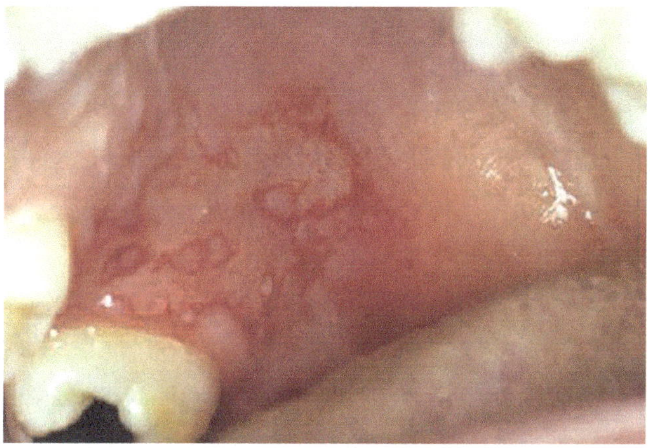

Fig. 21.6 Reccurent herpes simplex gingivitis

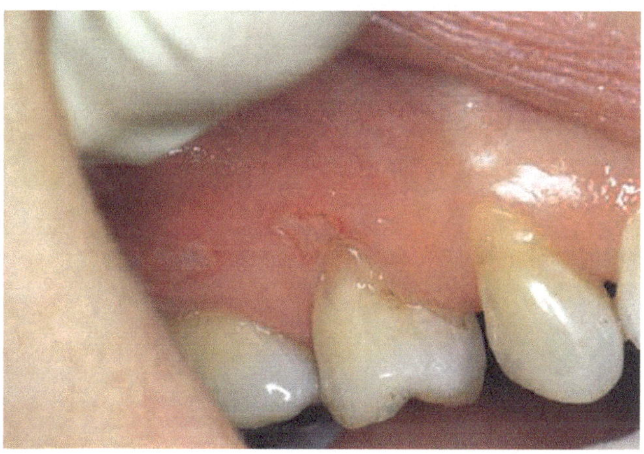

Fig. 21.7 Reccurent herpes simplex gingivitis

- Streptococcal stomatitis
- Traumatic erosions
- Primary and secondary syphilis
- Hand, foot, and mouth disease
- Herpangina

Laboratory Tests Usually not required.

Treatment Soft diet, adequate fluid intake, and local antiseptics. Systemic acyclovir, valacyclovir, and famcyclovir are used particularly in immunocompromised patients.

Human Papilloma Virus Infections

Condyloma Acuminatum

Definition Condyloma acuminatum is a common, sexually transmitted benign lesion.

Etiology *Human papilloma virus (HPV),* mainly the low-risk types 6 and 11, is transmitted through orogenital or oro-anal intercourse.

Gingival Involvement Rare. Non-dental biofilm-related lesion.

Other Sites of Involvement Rare involvement of labial mucosa, buccal mucosa, palate, and tongue. Condylomata accuminata most often appear in the anogenital region.

Clinical Features
- Clinically, gingival lesions may appear as single or multiple, sessile, painless, well-circumscribed, white or normal colored "*cauliflower-like*" projections (Figs. 21.8 and 21.9).
- Similar lesions may be present on other oral mucosal sites.
- The diagnosis is made on history, clinical features, and laboratory tests.

Differential Diagnosis
- Papilloma

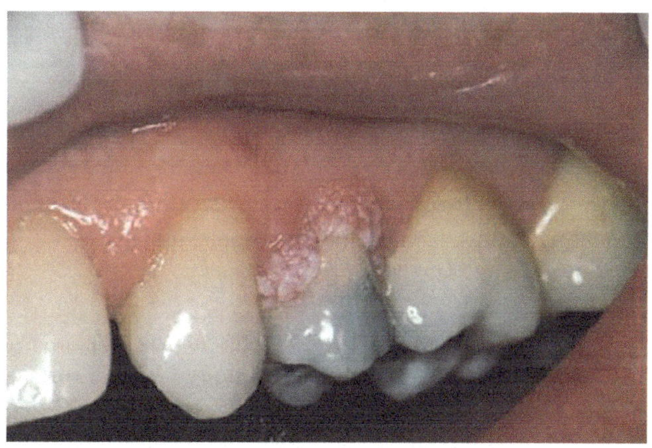

Fig. 21.8 Human papilloma virus, condyloma acuminatum on the gingiva

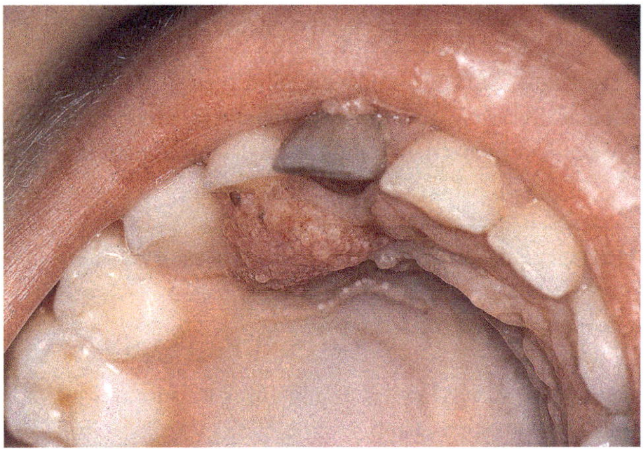

Fig. 21.9 Human papilloma virus, condyloma acuminatum on the gingiva

- Verruca vulgaris
- Verruciform xanthoma
- Verrucous hyperplasia
- Verrucous leukoplakia
- Early verrucous carcinoma
- Sialadenoma papilliferum
- Focal epithelial hyperplasia
- Focal dermal hypoplasia syndrome

Laboratory Tests Histopathologic examination, in situ hybridization, and polymerase chain reaction (PCR) tests.

Treatment Conservative surgical excision and electrosurgery.

Verruca Vulgaris

Definition Verruca vulgaris (common warts) is a common benign skin lesion.

Etiology Infection with human papilloma virus (HPV), mainly types 1, 2, and 4.

Gingival Involvement Rare. Non-dental biofilm-related lesion.

Other Sites of Involvement Lesions develop on the skin, and rarely on lips, labial commissures, and tongue.

Clinical Features
- Clinically, the gingival lesion presents as a painless, small, exophytic growth with a "*cauliflower-like*" surface and whitish or pink-white color (Figs. 21.10, 21.11 and 21.12). The lesions usually appear as single or multiple, sessile or pedunculated.
- Lesions on the other oral mucosal sites and skin present in a similar clinical pattern.

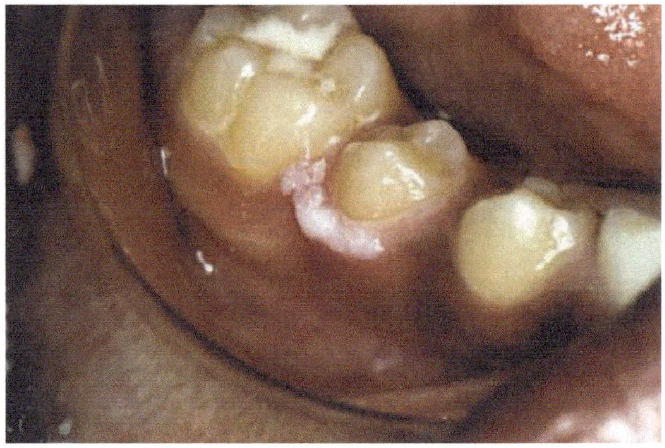

Fig. 21.10 Human papilloma virus, verruca vulgaris on the gingiva

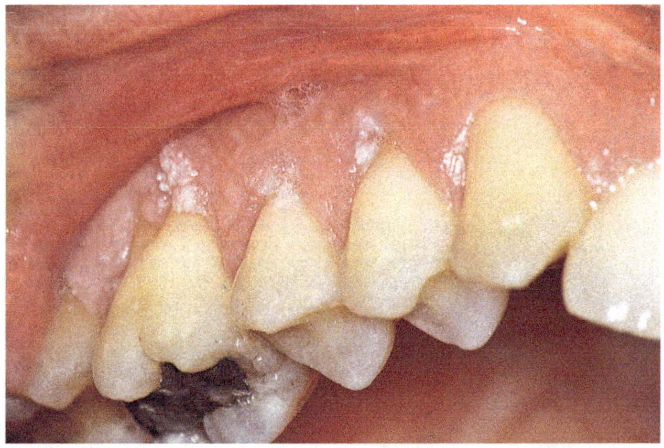

Fig. 21.11 Human papilloma virus, multiple verrucas vulgaris on the gingiva

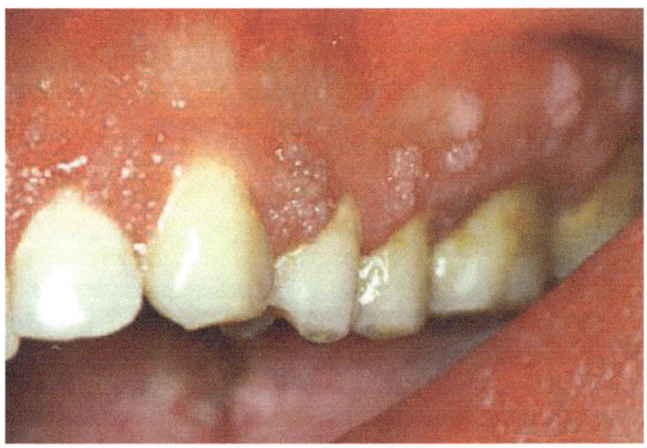

Fig. 21.12 Human papilloma virus, multiple verrucas vulgaris on the gingiva

- The clinical diagnosis should be confirmed by laboratory tests.

Differential Diagnosis
- Papilloma
- Condyloma accuminatum

- Verruciform xanthoma
- Focal epithelial hyperplasia
- Mucosal horn

Laboratory Tests Histopathologic examination, PCR test.

Treatment Conservative surgical excision, electrosurgery.

Papilloma

Definition It is a benign epithelial tumor of the oral mucosa.

Etiology Infection with HPV, types 6 and 11 are usually detected within the lesion.

Gingival Involvement Uncommon. Non-dental biofilm-related lesion.

Other Sites of Involvement Oral mucosa, lip, skin.

Clinical Features
- The most common benign soft tissue neoplasm.
- Clinically, the gingival papilloma presents as asymptomatic, exophytic, well-circumscribed, pendunculated, or sessile tumor with multiple, small *finger-like projections* resembling a *cauliflower whose* color may range from pale pink or white to normal mucosa (Figs. 21.13, 21.14 and 21.15).
- Lesions on the other oral mucosal sites and skin present with similar clinical features.
- Diagnosis is based on history, clinical features, and laboratory tests.

Differential Diagnosis
- Verruca vulgaris
- Condyloma accuminatum
- Sialadenoma papilliferum

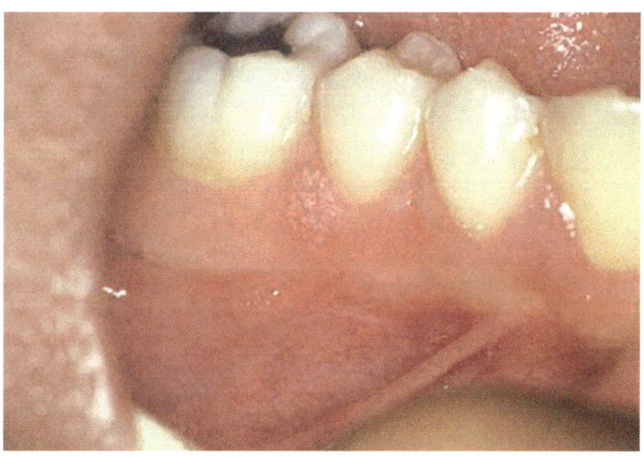

Fig. 21.13 Human papilloma virus, papilloma on the gingiva

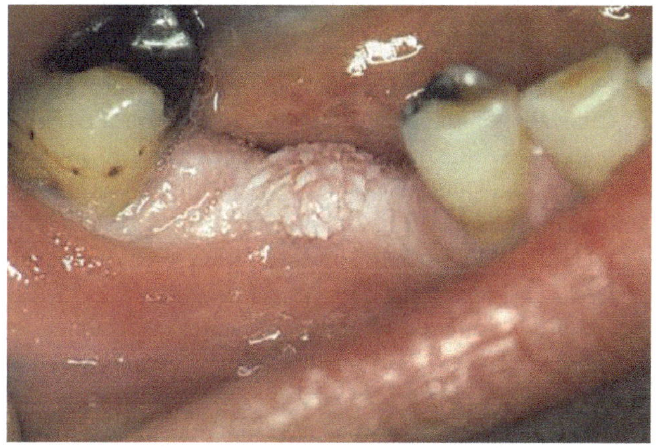

Fig. 21.14 Human papilloma virus, papilloma on the alveolar mucosa

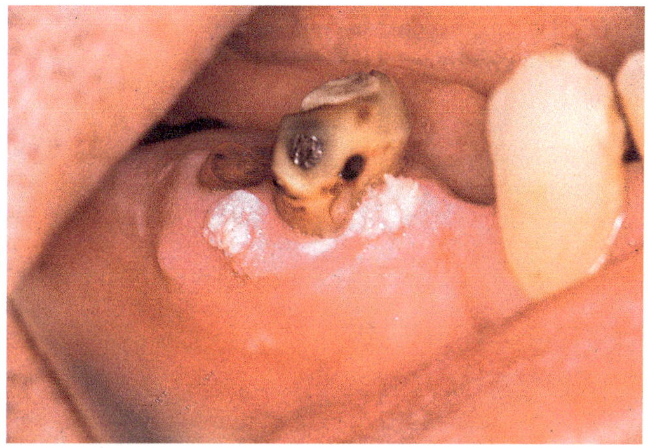

Fig. 21.15 Human papilloma virus, papillomas on the gingiva

- Verruciform xanthoma
- Focal epithelial hyperplasia
- Focal dermal hypoplasia syndrome

Laboratory Tests Histopathologic examination, PCR test.

Treatment Conservative surgical excision, laser surgery, electrosurgery.

Focal Epithelial Hyperplasia

Definition Focal epithelial hyperplasia or Heck's disease is a benign hyperplastic disorder of the oral mucosa.

Etiology *Human papilloma virus (HPV) types 13 and 32.*

Gingival Involvement Rare. Non-dental biofilm-related lesion.

Other Sites of Involvement Lesions primarily involve buccal, labial mucosa, and tongue.

Clinical Features

- The disease is usually observed in several ethnic groups (e.g., Eskimos, American Indians, South Africans, etc.).
- Clinically, on the gingiva the disease is characterized by multiple, sessile, painless, and slightly elevated nodules with a whitish or pale pink color and smooth or slightly granular surface (Figs. 21.16 and 21.17).
- Lesions on the other oral mucosal sites present with similar clinical features.
- Diagnosis is based on clinical features and laboratory tests.

Differential Diagnosis

- Multiple condylomas accuminatum
- Multiple verruca vulgaris
- Multiple papillomas
- Focal dermal hypoplasia syndrome
- Cowden syndrome

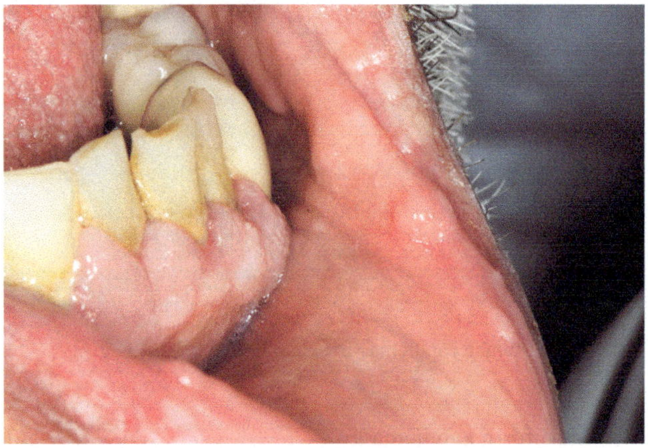

Fig. 21.16 Focal epithelial hyperplasia, papillary nodules on the gingiva and oral mucosa

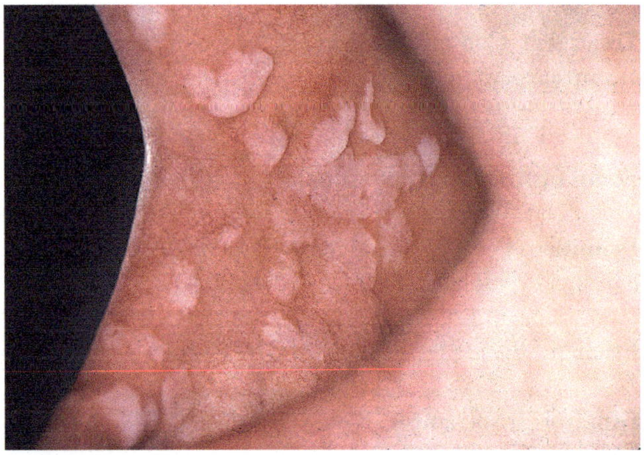

Fig. 21.17 Focal epithelial hyperplasia, papillary nodules on the buccal mucosa

Laboratory Tests Histopathologic examination, in situ hybridization, and PCR detection of HPV.

Treatment Occasionally, the lesions may spontaneously vanish. When lesions cause esthetic problems, conservative management with surgical excision, electrosurgery, or CO_2 laser may be recommended.

Cytomegalovirus Gingival Infection

Definition Oral infection with cytomegalovirus (CMV) is rare and usually occurs in immunosuppressed individuals.

Etiology *CMV* is the cause of the infection. Predisposing conditions are HIV infection, immunosuppressed patients, and transplanted recipients.

Gingival Involvement Rare. Non-dental biofilm-related lesion.

Sites of Involvement Oral mucosa, salivary glands, skin.

Clinical Features

- Clinically, the gingival lesion appears as atypical, usually, painful inflammatory ulcer 0.5–1 cm in diameter that persists for a long time (Figs. 21.18 and 21.19).
- Painful enlargement of the major and minor salivary glands leading to dry mouth.
- Fever, sore throat, cough, pharyngitis, malaise, myalgia, joint pain, abdominal pain, diarrhea, lymphadenopathy, hepatosplenomegaly, meningeal irritation, and less frequently maculopapular and pruritic cutaneous eruptions may occur.

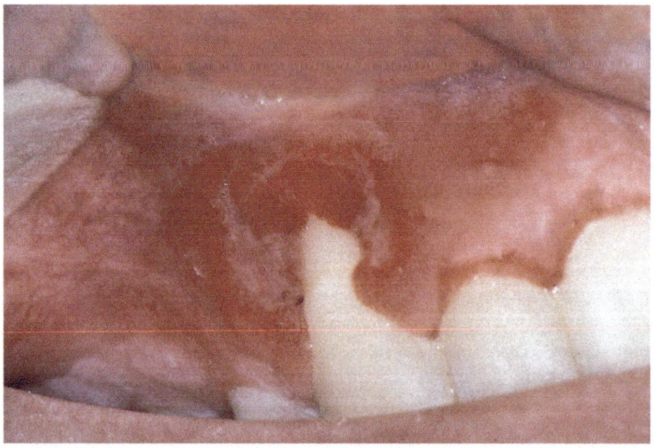

Fig. 21.18 Cytomegalovirus (CMV) infection on the gingiva

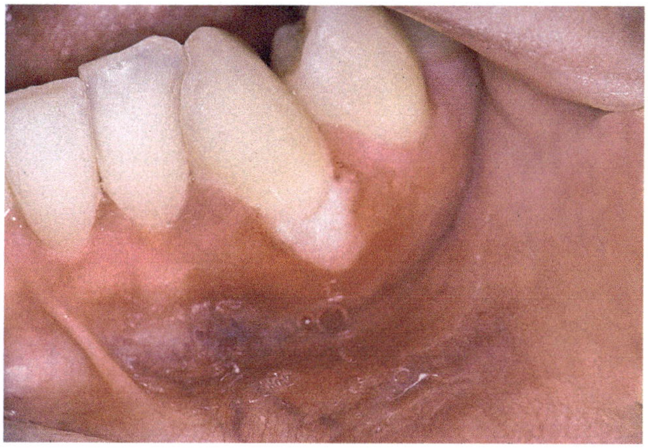

Fig. 21.19 Cytomegalovirus (CMV) infection with gingival ulceration

- Rarely, complications may develop such as eye disorders, pneumonia, myocarditis, gastrointestinal and hematologic disorders, and central nervous system involvement.
- The clinical diagnosis should be confirmed by laboratory tests.

Differential Diagnosis
- Infectious mononucleosis
- Herpes simplex
- Traumatic ulcer
- Chancre
- Aphthous ulcer
- Drug-induced ulceration

Laboratory Tests Monoclonal antibodies against CMV antigen, PCR and ELISA, and histopathologic examination.

Treatment Intravenous ganciclovir and oral valacyclovir.

References

1. Mohan RP, Verma S, Singh U, Agarwal N. Acute primary herpetic gingivostomatitis. BMJ Case Rep. 2013;2013:bcr2013200074. https://doi.org/10.1136/bcr-2013-200074.
2. Baghad B, Benhsaien I, El Fatoiki FZ, et al. Candidose cutanéo-muqueuse chronique avec mutation gain-de-fonction du gène STAT1 associée à des infections herpétiques et à mycobactérie [chronic mucocutaneous candidiasis with STAT1 gain-of-function mutation associated with herpes virus and mycobacterial infections]. Ann Dermatol Venereol. 2020;147(1):41–5. https://doi.org/10.1016/j.annder.2019.09.597. Epub 2019 Oct 31
3. Baez CF, Savassi-Ribas F, Rocha WM, et al. Association of epstein-barr virus (ebv) but not human papillomavirus (hpv) with gingivitis and/or periodontitis in transplanted individuals. Rev Inst Med Trop Sao Paulo. 2016;58:58. https://doi.org/10.1590/S1678-9946201658058.
4. Blevins JY. Primary herpetic gingivostomatitis in young children. Pediatr Nurs. 2003;29:199–202.
5. Epstein JB, Scully C. Herpes simplex virus in immunocompromised patients: growing evidence of drug resistance. Oral Surg Oral Med Oral Pathol. 1991;72:47–50.
6. Epstein JB, Scully C. Cytomegalovirus: a virus of increasing relevance to oral medicine and pathology. J Oral Pathol Med. 1993;22:348–53.
7. Cuberos V, Perez J, Lopez CJ, Castro F, et al. Molecular and serological evidence of the epidemiological association of HPV13 with focal epithelial hyperplasia: a case-control study. J Clin Virol. 2006;37:21–6.
8. dos Santos-Pinto L, Giro EM, Pansani CA, Ferrari J, et al. An uncommon focal epithelial hyperplasia manifestation. J Dent Child (Chic). 2009;76:233–6.
9. Dreyer WP, van der Waal I. Oral medicine case book 15. Intraoral verruca vulgaris SADJ. 2009;64:80–1.
10. Falaki F, Amir Chaghmaghi M, Pakfetrat A, Delavarian Z, et al. Detection of human papilloma virus DNA in seven cases of focal epithelial hyperplasia in Iran. J Oral Pathol Med. 2009;38:773–6.
11. Porter SR, Scully C, Mutlu S. Viral infections affecting periodontal health. Periodon Clin Invest. 1995;15:17–24.

Fungal Gingival Infections

22

Contents

Acute Pseudomembranous Candidiasis

Definition Candidiasis is the most frequent oral fungal infection.

Etiology Fungal infection caused by the yeast Candida. *Candida albicans* is the most prevalent cause of candidiasis. *C. tropicalis, C.glabrata, C. parapsilosis,* and *C. krusei* are implicated less often. Factors that can increase the liability to candidiasis include xerostomia, smoking, local and systemic corticosteroids, broad-spectrum antimicrobials, diabetes mellitus, cytotoxic chemotherapy, irradiation of the head and neck area, malnutrition, appliances, HIV infection, leukemias, lymphomas, cancer, immunosuppressive, and cytotoxic drugs.

Classification Candidiasis is classified into: a. *Primary*, where the condition is exclusively confined to the mouth and perioral tissues, and b. *Secondary* that includes the oral manifestations of systemic mucocutaneous fungal infections.

Gingival Involvement Common. Non-dental biofilm-related lesions.

Other Sites of Involvement Oral mucosa, other mucosae, skin, nails.

Clinical Features

- Clinically, lesions of the gingiva present as white or creamy spots or plaques that can be wiped off leaving an erythematous base (Figs. 22.1 and 22.2).

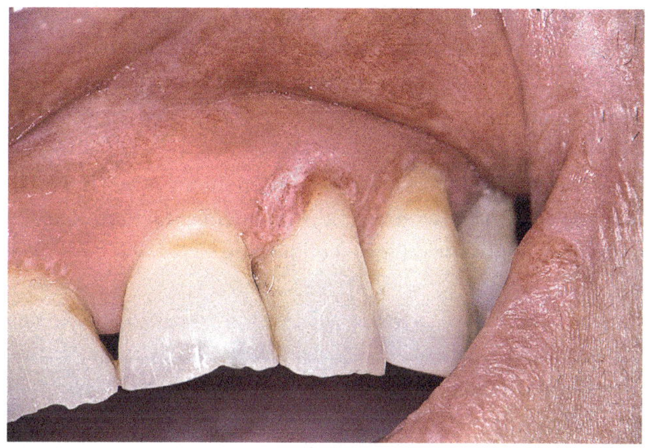

Fig. 22.1 Pseudomembranous candidiasis on the gingiva

- Xerostomia, a burning sensation, unpleasant taste, and difficulty in swallowing are the most common symptoms.
- Similar lesions may appear on other oral mucosal sites.
- Sometimes oral involvement is secondary to a more serious systemic infection.
- The diagnosis is usually based on clinical features and laboratory tests.

Differential Diagnosis

- Koplik spots
- Fordyce spots
- Materia alba
- Cinnamon contact gingivitis
- Chemical burn

G. Laskaris et al., *Periodontal Manifestations of Local and Systemic Diseases*, https://doi.org/10.1007/978-3-031-10828-0_22

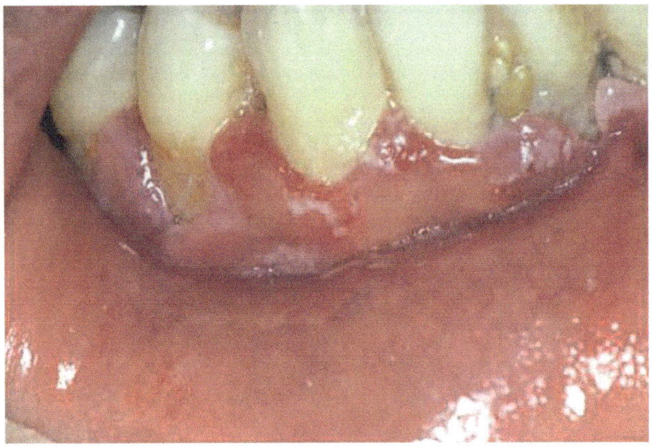

Fig. 22.2 Pseudomembranous candidiasis on the gingiva

- Thermal burn
- Lichen planus
- Leukoplakia
- Lupus erythematosus
- Syphilitic mucous patches

Laboratory Tests The clinical diagnosis is supplemented with results of Gram-stained smear (hyphae) and microbiological culture.

Treatment Systemic triazoles. Meticulous oral hygiene. Topical treatment with nystatin or miconazole can also be used, especially for infants and children.

Erythematous Candidiasis

Definition A relatively rare oral infection caused by *Candida Albicans species*.

Etiology *Candida albicans* and rarely other *Candida* species. Predisposing factors are the same as in the pseudomembranous type. In most cases, it is associated with prolonged use of broad-spectrum antibiotics.

Classification A*cute* or *chronic* (usually seen in HIV patients).

Gingival Involvement Rare. Non-dental biofilm-related lesions.

Other Sites of Involvement Dorsum of the tongue and palate (more common in HIV patients).

Clinical Features

- Clinically, gingival lesions present as diffuse erythematous patches with mild inflammation (Figs. 22.3 and 22.4).
- Similar lesions on other oral mucosal sites can be more severe, localized, or generalized and show a predilection for the palate and the dorsal surface of the tongue.
- Patients may complain of burning sensation, pain, and dry mouth.
- The clinical diagnosis should be confirmed by laboratory tests.

Differential Diagnosis

- Dental biofilm-induced gingivitis
- Plasma cell gingivitis
- Granulomatous gingivitis
- Desquamative gingivitis
- Cinnamon contact gingivitis
- Drug reaction
- Erythroplakia

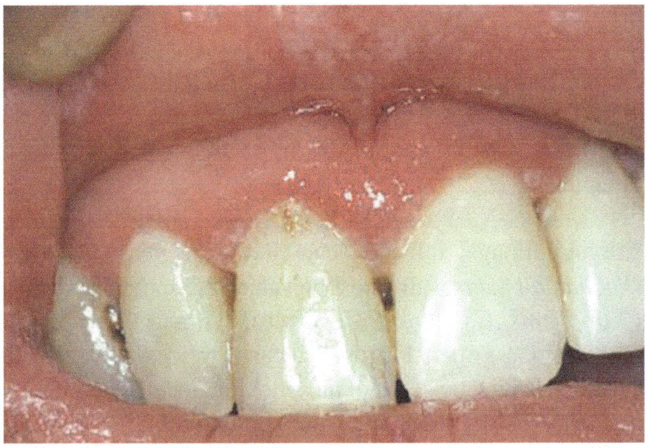

Fig. 22.3 Erythematous candidiasis on the gingiva

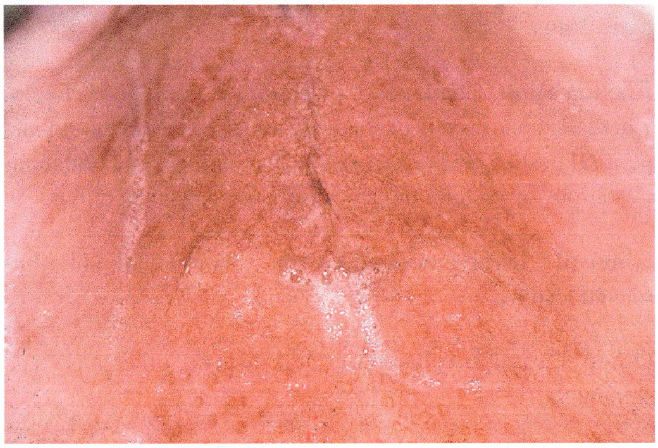

Fig. 22.4 Erythematous candidiasis on the palate

Laboratory Tests Smears, histopathologic examinations, and culture may be helpful.

Treatment Improvement of oral hygiene. Use of topical antifungals such as nystatin oral suspension *or* miconazole gel. Systemic fluconazole or itraconazole are the drugs of choice.

References

1. Hellstein JW, Marek CL. Candidiasis: red and white manifestations in the oral cavity. Head Neck Pathol. 2019;13(1):25–32. https://doi.org/10.1007/s12105-019-01004-6. Epub 2019 Jan 29
2. Mundula T, Ricci F, Barbetta B, et al. Effect of probiotics on oral candidiasis: a systematic review and meta-analysis. Nutrients. 2019;11(10):2449. https://doi.org/10.3390/nu11102449.
3. Baumgardner DJ. Oral fungal microbiota: to thrush and beyond. J Patient Cent Res Rev. 2019;6(4):252–61. https://doi.org/10.17294/2330-0698.1705.
4. Deepa D, Kumar KV, Joshi CS, et al. Fungal infection of gingiva in a patient with hyperimmunoglobulin-E (Job's) syndrome. J Indian Soc Periodontol. 2012;16(2):256–60. https://doi.org/10.4103/0972-124X.99272.
5. Motta-Silva AC, Aleva NA, Chavasco JK, Armond MC, et al. Erythematous oral candidiasis in patients with controlled type II diabetes mellitus and complete dentures. Mycopathologia. 2010;169:215–23.

Aphthous Ulcers

23

Contents

Definition Common recurrent mouth ulcers with onset usually in childhood and adolescence or later.

Etiology Unclear. Autoinflammatory disease. The most probable mechanism is cellular-type immune response.

Classification There are three distinct clinical forms of aphthae: a. *Minor* (common)—small ulcers (<4 mm) on mobile mucosa, healing within 6–8 days, no scarring; b. *Major* (rare)—large ulcers (may be >1 cm), any site including dorsum of tongue and palate, healing within 1–2 months, with scarring; and c. *Herpetiform ulcers* (rare)—multiple, minute ulcers that coalesce to form ragged ulcers, healing within 2–3 weeks.

Gingival Involvement Uncommon. Non-dental biofilm-induced lesion.

Other Sites of Involvement The mobile oral mucosa (tongue, buccal mucosa, soft palate, lip) is common.

Clinical Features

- Aphthous ulcers affect about 15–20% of the population, mostly non-smokers. The onset is usually in childhood or adolescence or later.
- Clinically, aphthous ulcers on the gingiva develop rarely, and they appear as recurrent, round, or ovoid ulcers with a yellowish bottom and red areola and are similar to the lesions located on other mucosal sites (Figs. 23.1, 23.2, 23.3, 23.4, 23.5 and 23.6). They usually last 6–8 days and heal without scarring.
- Diagnosis is based on clinical criteria.

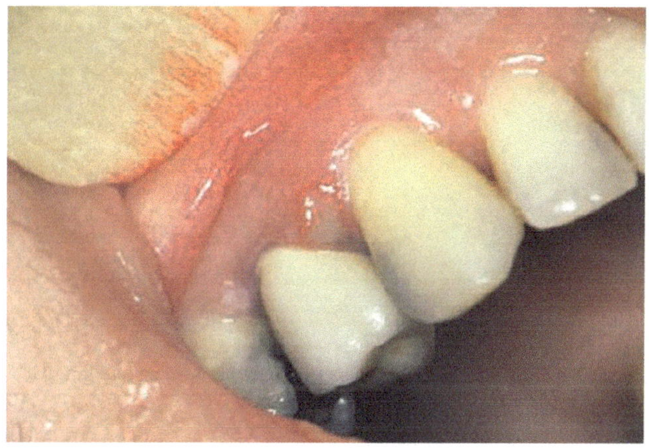

Fig. 23.1 Minor aphthous ulcer on the gingiva

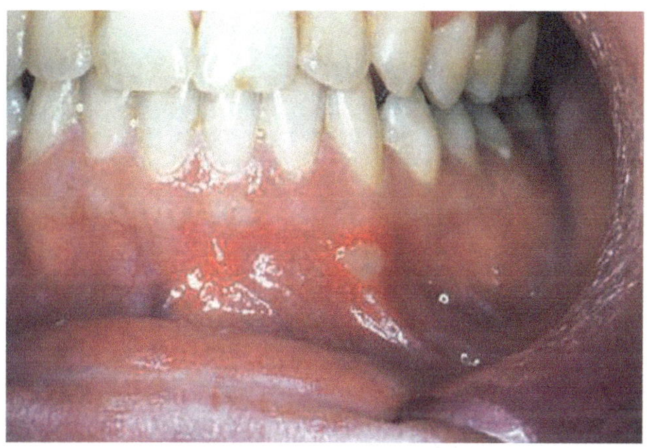

Fig. 23.2 Minor aphthous ulcer on alveolar mucosa

G. Laskaris et al., *Periodontal Manifestations of Local and Systemic Diseases*, https://doi.org/10.1007/978-3-031-10828-0_23

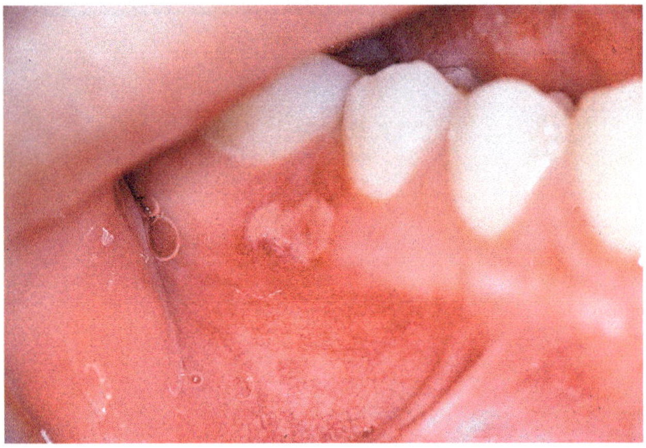

Fig. 23.3 Minor aphthous ulcer on alveolar mucosa and gingiva

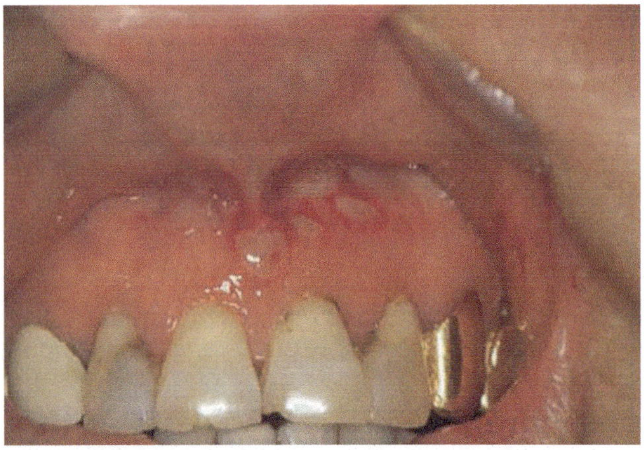

Fig. 23.4 Multiple aphthous ulcers on alveolar mucosa and gingiva

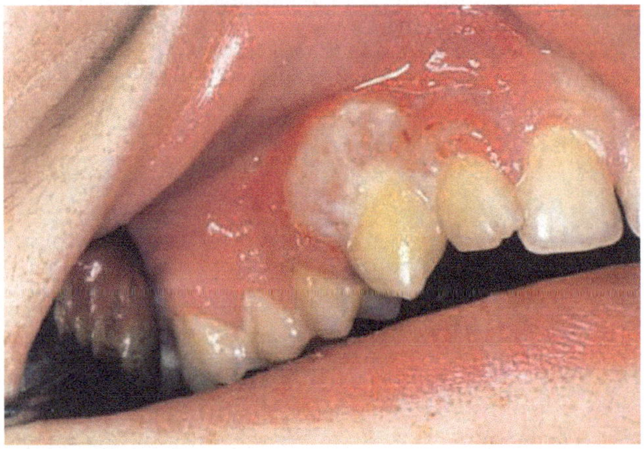

Fig. 23.5 Major aphthous ulcer on alveolar mucosa and gingiva

Differential Diagnosis
- Traumatic ulcers
- PFAPA syndrome

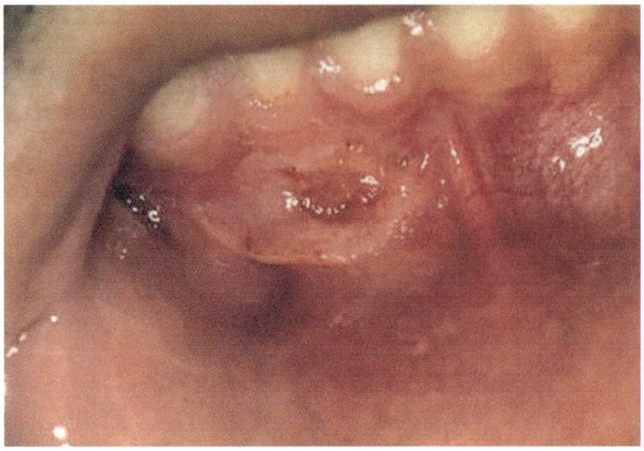

Fig. 23.6 Major aphthous ulcer on alveolar mucosa

- Adamantiades-Behçet disease
- Syphilis (primary ulcer and mucous patches)
- Hematological diseases
- Gastrointestinal disease
- Herpetic stomatitis
- Herpangina
- Erythema multiforme
- Hand, foot, and mouth disease
- Drug reactions

Laboratory Tests There is no specific diagnostic test.

Treatment Treatment of any underlying predisposing factors. Topical corticosteroids (0.1% triamcinolone acetonide in orabase). In severe cases, short-term, low dose, systemic corticosteroids (e.g., prednizolone tabl.10–20 mg/d for 5–10 days).

References

1. Saikaly SK, Saikaly TS, Saikaly LE. Recurrent aphthous ulceration: a review of potential causes and novel treatments. J Dermatolog Treat. 2018;29(6):542–52. https://doi.org/10.1080/09546634.2017.1422079. Epub 2018 Jan 10
2. Mintz GA, Smidansky ED. Aphthous stomatitis with involvement of attached gingiva. Oral Surg Oral Med Oral Pathol. 1985;60(1):122–4. https://doi.org/10.1016/0030-4220(85)90227-0.
3. Ramirez-Amador VA, Esquivel-Pedraza L, Ponce-de-Leon S, et al. Thalidomide as therapy for human immunodeficiency virus-related oral ulcers: a double-blind placebo-controlled clinical trial. Clin Infect Dis. 1999;28:892–4.
4. Laskaris G. Advances in the classification and treatment of recurrent aphthous ulcers. Balk J Stomatol. 1999;3:83–4.
5. Laskaris G. Aphthous stomatitis. In: Katsabas A, Lotti T, editors. European handbook of dermatological treatments. Springer; 2021.

Dental Biofilm as a Risk Factor for Systemic Diseases

24

Contents

Severe periodontitis is the sixth most prevalent disease in the world and the prevalence of gingivitis, manifesting as bleeding upon probing, can exceed 90% on a worldwide basis. The pervasiveness of these two most common periodontal diseases heightens their potential significance for any extra-oral/systemic impact they might have and underscores their possible public health implications.

To date, periodontal disease has been linked to several dozen different diseases and conditions, with the volume and strength of the evidence varying by disease. Severe periodontitis is also significantly associated with all-cause and cardiovascular mortality, independent of other factors. Among the numerous conditions that have been associated with periodontitis, the following will be reviewed here: cardiovascular diseases, pulmonary diseases, diabetes mellitus, and pregnancy outcomes.

Before providing an overview of these periodontal-systemic disease associations, it is important to make the critical distinction between association and causation. The fact that two conditions are strongly associated, based on reliable epidemiological evidence, does not necessarily imply that one is causative of the other. Such associations may simply be the manifestation of common risk factors (e.g., smoking is a risk factor for both periodontitis and cardiovascular diseases). Evidence that one condition is causative for another requires proof that could be obtained from longitudinal investigations and intervention studies, which can be difficult to pursue or properly execute.

When evidence has been reported that periodontitis can be causative for a systemic condition, the proposed plausible biological mechanisms for the association between periodontal disease and systemic disease typically fall under two major categories: effects of the dysbiotic biofilm present in periodontitis and effects of the exacerbated local inflammation and stimulated immune response on distant tissues and organs.

With respect to the periodontitis-associated biofilm, evidence indicates that poorer oral hygiene, i.e., greater plaque accumulation, and increased gingival inflammation significantly increase the prevalence of bacteremia after toothbrushing; this represents just one possible mechanism for the spread of periodontal pathogens to other tissues and organs. Periodontal pathogens have been identified in remote sites, in the course of various disease processes, providing clinical evidence of the potential dissemination and establishment of dental plaque bacteria in distant non-oral tissues.

With respect to the inflammatory and immune processes locally exacerbated in periodontal disease, it is relevant to contemplate the potential magnitude of these changes present in the periodontium. In this context, when one considers the surface area of the dentogingival attachment apparatus in a dentition with periodontitis, the inflamed area has been estimated to be 20 cm^2 on average, with the maximum estimated to be 44 cm^2. This aspect of the disease provides a distinctive perspective regarding the extent of localized inflammation present in a periodontitis patient and how it

G. Laskaris et al., *Periodontal Manifestations of Local and Systemic Diseases*, https://doi.org/10.1007/978-3-031-10828-0_24

can become a significant source of inflammatory mediators and cells that leak into the circulation and another relevant pathway for the penetration and spread of periodontal pathogens or their virulence factors. Clinical evidence, supported by animal studies, indicates that periodontal inflammation exacerbates the systemic immune response and periodontal treatment can reverse these changes. In this manner, periodontitis likely contributes to the inflammatory processes involved in the various chronic diseases that have been associated with periodontitis.

Periodontitis and Cardiovascular Diseases

Periodontitis has been strongly associated with cardiovascular diseases, including endothelial dysfunction, hypertension, coronary artery disease, acute myocardial infarction, and stroke. Evidence indicates that the magnitude of periodontal inflammation, as determined by clinical parameters such as bleeding on probing, correlates with systemic levels of biomarkers, e.g., C-reactive protein (CRP), considered relevant for cardiovascular disease. Furthermore, intervention studies have shown that treatment of periodontitis reduces the levels of such systemic biomarkers, improves endothelial function, reduces systolic and diastolic blood pressure, and can have a positive influence on progression of cardiovascular disease. These findings suggest that periodontitis patients should be informed of their higher risk for cardiovascular diseases and that they should receive proper periodontal treatment along with management of any other cardiovascular disease risk factors, such as smoking and obesity.

Periodontitis and Pulmonary Diseases

Periodontitis has been associated with pulmonary diseases such as pneumonia, asthma, and chronic obstructive pulmonary disease. Pulmonary pathogens residing in the mouth and periodontitis-associated oral bacteria may spread from the periodontium to the lungs, causing infections. Periodontal therapy can decrease the incidence and severity of associated respiratory infections. The mechanisms explaining the reported association between asthma and periodontal diseases (both gingivitis and periodontitis) are less understood, although both bacterial and immunologic processes have been postulated. Obstructive and restrictive pulmonary functions have been significantly associated with the severity of periodontitis. Periodontitis has also been significantly associated with the incidence of lung cancer, after controlling for confounding factors such as smoking.

Periodontitis and Diabetes Mellitus

The association between diabetes and periodontitis is one of the best-documented associations between oral and systemic diseases. An important aspect of the strong relationship between periodontitis and diabetes is its bidirectional nature: periodontitis has an impact on diabetes and vice versa. In fact, diabetes is one of the recognized systemic risk factors for periodontitis, the other being smoking. Non-diabetic periodontitis patients have higher glycated hemoglobin (HbA1C) levels and are more likely to develop prediabetes and diabetes than those without periodontitis. In addition, diabetics with periodontitis have poorer glycemic control and more diabetic complications than diabetics without periodontitis. Poorly controlled diabetic patients have more severe and extensive periodontal destruction, respond less well to periodontal therapy, and are more likely to experience progressive attachment loss during follow-up. In contrast, patients with well-controlled diabetes respond as well as non-diabetic patients to periodontal treatment. These findings indicate that the ideal management of diabetics with periodontitis requires proper measures to control both diseases.

Periodontitis and Pregnancy Outcomes

The association between periodontitis and pregnancy encompasses both maternal and newborn outcomes. Evidence indicates that pregnant women with periodontitis are more likely to develop preeclampsia and to deliver a preterm and/or low-birth-weight baby. However, the evidence of the association between periodontitis and adverse pregnancy outcomes is not as strong as the evidence for the other associations discussed here. Intervention studies have not provided consistent or strong evidence for improved pregnancy outcomes when pregnant women are treated, typically during the second trimester, for periodontitis. In contrast, the available evidence consistently failed to show that periodontal treatment during pregnancy results in any maternal or obstetric negative outcomes, underscoring the general safety of periodontal nonsurgical therapy during the second trimester of pregnancy.

References

1. Albandar JM, Susin C, Hughes FJ. Manifestations of systemic diseases and conditions that affect the periodontal attachment apparatus: case definitions and diagnostic considerations. J Periodontol. 2018;89(Suppl 1):S183–203. https://doi.org/10.1002/JPER.16-0480.

2. Bokhari SA, Khan AA, Butt AK, et al. Non-surgical periodontal therapy reduces coronary heart disease risk markers: a randomized controlled trial. J Clin Periodontol. 2012;39:1065–74.
3. Bokhari SA, Khan AA, Butt AK, et al. Periodontitis in coronary heart disease patients: strong association between bleeding on probing and systemic biomarkers. J Clin Periodontol. 2014;41:1048–54.
4. Cho HJ, Shin MS, Song Y, et al. Severe periodontal disease increases acute myocardial infarction and stroke: a 10-year retrospective follow-up study [published online ahead of print, 2021 Jan 21]. J Dent Res. 2021;100(7):706–13. https://doi.org/10.1177/0022034520986097.
5. Daalderop LA, Wieland BV, Tomsin K, et al. Periodontal disease and pregnancy outcomes: overview of systematic reviews. JDR Clin Trans Res. 2018;3:10–27.
6. Fine N, Chadwick JW, Sun C, et al. Periodontal inflammation primes the systemic innate immune response. J Dent Res. 2021;100:318–25.
7. Gaudilliere DK, Culos A, Djebali K, et al. Systemic immunologic consequences of chronic periodontitis. J Dent Res. 2019;98:985–93.
8. Gomes-Filho IS, da Cruz SS, Castro Trindade S, et al. Periodontitis and respiratory diseases: a systematic review with meta-analysis. Oral Dis. 2020;26:439–46.
9. Hujoel PP, White BA, García RI, Listgarten MA. The dentogingival epithelial surface area revisited. J Periodontal Res. 2001;36:48–55.
10. Kassebaum NJ, Bernabé E, Dahiya M, et al. Global burden of severe periodontitis in 1990-2010: a systematic review and meta-regression. J Dent Res. 2014;93:1045–53.
11. Linden GJ, Lyons A, Scannapieco FA. Periodontal systemic associations: review of the evidence. J Clin Periodontol. 2013;40(Suppl 14):S8–19.
12. Michalowicz BS, Hodges JS, Lussky RC, et al. Maternal periodontitis treatment and child neurodevelopment at 24 to 28 months of age. Pediatrics. 2011;127:e1212–20.
13. Michaud DS, Lu J, Peacock-Villada AY, et al. Periodontal disease assessed using clinical dental measurements and cancer risk in the ARIC study. J Natl Cancer Inst. 2018;110:843–54.
14. Monsarrat P, Blaizot A, Kémoun P, et al. Clinical research activity in periodontal medicine: a systematic mapping of trial registers. J Clin Periodontol. 2016;43(5):390–400.
15. Muñoz Aguilera E, Suvan J, Orlandi M. Association between periodontitis and blood pressure highlighted in systemically healthy individuals: results from a nested case-control study. Hypertension. 2021;77:1765–74.
16. Paraskevas S, Huizinga JD, Loos BG. A systematic review and meta-analyses on C-reactive protein in relation to periodontitis. J Clin Periodontol. 2008;35:277–90.
17. Petersen PE, Ogawa H. Strengthening the prevention of periodontal disease: the WHO approach. J Periodontol. 2005;76:2187–93.
18. Sanz M, Ceriello A, Buysschaert M, et al. Scientific evidence on the links between periodontal diseases and diabetes: consensus report and guidelines of the joint workshop on periodontal diseases and diabetes by the international diabetes federation and the European Federation of Periodontology. Diabetes Res Clin Pract. 2018;137:231–41.
19. Sanz M, Del Castillo AM, Jepsen S, et al. Periodontitis and cardiovascular diseases. Consensus report. Glob Heart. 2020;15(1):1. Published 2020 Feb 3. https://doi.org/10.5334/gh.400.
20. Sharma S, Sridhar S, McIntosh A, et al. Periodontal therapy and treatment of hypertension-alternative to the pharmacological approach. A systematic review and meta-analysis. Pharmacol Res. 2021;166:105511. https://doi.org/10.1016/j.phrs.2021.105511.
21. Teeuw WJ, Slot DE, Susanto H, et al. Treatment of periodontitis improves the atherosclerotic profile: a systematic review and meta-analysis. J Clin Periodontol. 2014;41:70–9.
22. Tomás I, Diz P, Tobías A, et al. Periodontal health status and bacteraemia from daily oral activities: systematic review/meta-analysis. J Clin Periodontol. 2012;39:213–28.
23. Tonetti MS, Jepsen S, Jin L, Otomo-Corgel J. Impact of the global burden of periodontal diseases on health, nutrition and well-being of mankind: a call for global action. J Clin Periodontol. 2017;44:456–62.
24. Gomes-Fihlo IS, Passos JS, Seixas da Cruz S. Respiratory disease and the role of oral bacteria. J Oral Micro. 2010;2:5811.
25. Lalla E, Papapanou PN. Diabetes mellitus and periodontitis: a tale of two common interrelated diseases. Nat Rev Endocrinol. 2011;7:738–48.
26. Lockhart PB, Bolger AF, Papapanou PN, et al. Periodontal disease and atherosclerotic vascular disease: does the evidence support an independent association? A scientific statement from the American Heart Association. Circulation. 2012;125:2520–44.
27. Seymour GJ, Ford PJ, Cullinan MP, et al. Relationship between periodontal infections and systemic disease. Clin Microbiol Infect. 2007;13(Suppl 4):3–10. https://doi.org/10.1111/j.1469-0691.2007.01798.x.
28. Liccardo D, Cannavo A, Spagnuolo G, et al. Periodontal disease: a risk factor for diabetes and cardiovascular disease. Int J Mol Sci. 2019;20(6):1414. Published 2019 Mar 20. https://doi.org/10.3390/ijms20061414.
29. Uwambaye P, et al. Impact of maternal periodontitis on preterm birth and low birth weight in babies: results of a scoping review. Rw J of Med Health Sci. 2020;3(3):372–86.

Gingivitis and Periodontitis as a Source of Oral Malodor

25

Contents

Definition The presence of noticeably unpleasant, socially embarrassing, breath odor is known as halitosis, fetor oris, oral malodor, or putrid breath. Additionally, a person having halitosis may suffer from emotional and psychological distress.

Etiology Oral malodor may be attributed to both *systemic* and *local conditions* (Table 25.1). The unpleasant odor is caused by volatile sulfur compounds (VSCs), e.g., methyl mercaptan and hydrogen sulfide, usually produced by anaerobic bacteria during the proteolytic breakdown of sulfur-containing amino acids (e.g., methionine and cysteine) originating from saliva and exfoliated epithelial cells. Several *Gram-negative bacteria* (e.g., *Tannerella forsythia, Porphyromonas gingivalis, Actinomycetemcomitans Aggregatibacter, and Prevotella intermedia* have been associated with oral malodor. The imbalance of oral microbiome is an important predictor of bad breath.

The prevalence of halitosis is 20–50% among adults or adolescents.

Nearly 85% of cases originate from local conditions characterized by plaque accumulation and inflammation, such as tongue coating, gingivitis and periodontitis, poor oral hygiene, infections, ulcerations, food debris, dry mouth, inadequate restorations, oral cancer, and other chronic painful conditions. Habits, such as smoking and alcohol consumption, can contribute to malodor.

Only 4% of halitosis is related to systemic disorders such as upper and lower respiratory tract infections, nasal, paranasal and/or laryngeal disorders, hepatic, pancreatic, and nephritic insufficiencies, and some medications.

The remaining 11% is attributed to idiopathic causes, as well as pseudo-oral malodor or halitophobia. In idiopathic cases, there are no known risk factors involved, but it is believed that disturbed oral microbial load and increased proportion of gram-negative anaerobic bacteria account for this category of halitosis. In pseudo malodor, there is no obvious malodor perceived by others, but the patient believes he/she has oral malodor, despite reassurance.

Clinical Features

- There are no clinical features. Patient may or may not be aware of the symptom.
- The diagnosis is usually by clinical examination, where the oral health care provider smells the patient's breath (organoleptic examination). Instrumentation that specifically detects VSCs can also be used.

Differential Diagnosis The differential diagnosis pertains to the causative/underlying conditions, whether oral or extra-oral.

Treatment The management of oral malodor when the cause is local and associated with periodontal diseases is a

G. Laskaris et al., *Periodontal Manifestations of Local and Systemic Diseases*, https://doi.org/10.1007/978-3-031-10828-0_25

Table 25.1 Classification of oral malodor according to etiology

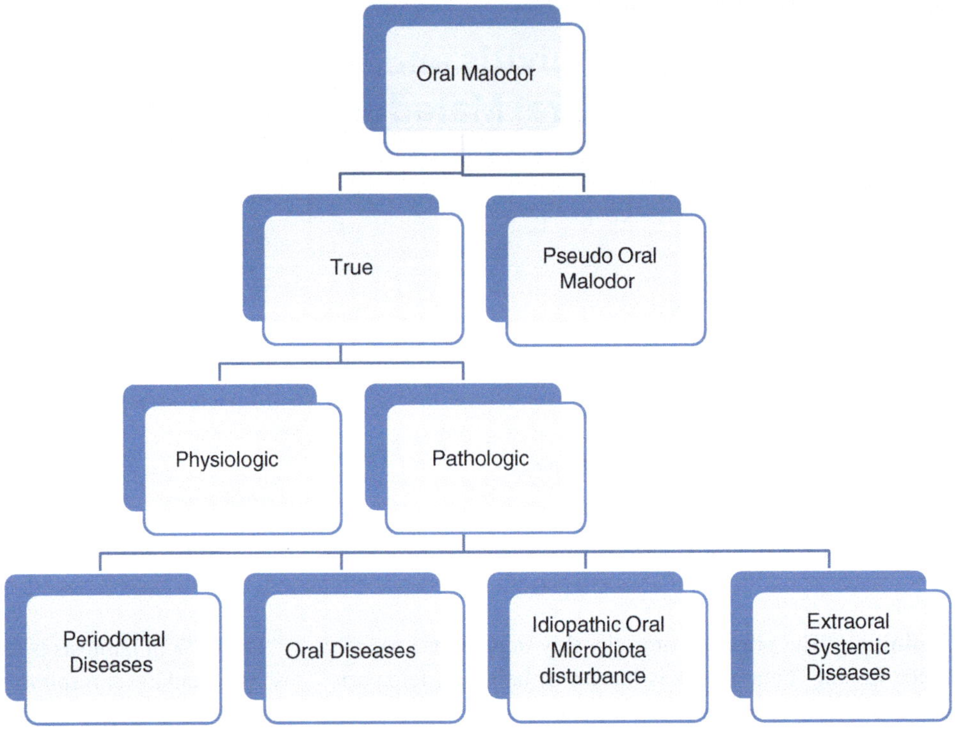

combination of good oral hygiene (effective plaque control, tongue cleaning), scaling and root planing, and use of antimicrobial oxygenating mouthwashes for 1–2 months. Treatment of underlying oral (e.g., periodontitis, defective restorations) or non-oral conditions will provide resolution. Studies on adjunctive use of fluoride-containing toothpastes and probiotics have shown encouraging results.

In severe cases, systemic antibiotics (metronidazole 500 mg, three times daily, for 5–7 days) followed by oxygenating antimicrobial mouthrinses, may be considered.

References

1. Foo LH, Balan P, Pang LM, et al. Role of the oral microbiome, metabolic pathways, and novel diagnostic tools in intra-oral halitosis: a comprehensive update. Crit Rev Microbiol. 2021;3:1–17. https://doi.org/10.1080/1040841X.2021.1888867. Epub ahead of print
2. Wu J, Cannon RD, Ji P, Farella M, Mei L. Halitosis: prevalence, risk factors, sources, measurement and treatment–a review of the literature. Aust Dent J. 2020;65:4–11. https://doi.org/10.1111/adj.12725. Epub 2019 Nov 15
3. Mogilnicka I, Bogucki P, Ufnal M. Microbiota and malodor—etiology and management 1. Int J of Mol Sci. 2020;21(8):2886.

Part IV

Systemic Diseases Affecting Periodontal Tissues

Genetic Diseases

26

Contents

G. Laskaris et al., *Periodontal Manifestations of Local and Systemic Diseases*, https://doi.org/10.1007/978-3-031-10828-0_26

Chédiak-Higashi Syndrome

Definition Chédiak-Higashi syndrome is a rare autosomal recessive disorder, that causes primary immunodeficiency.

Etiology Genetic. It is caused by mutation of the lysosomal trafficking regulatory gene (LYST1q42.3).

Periodontal Involvement Common. Severe gingival inflammation associated with early-onset and rapidly progressive periodontitis and immunologic disorders.

Other Sites of Involvement Oral mucosa, skin, hair, eyes, respiratory tract, liver, spleen, lymph nodes, and other internal organs.

Clinical Features

- Clinically, the syndrome usually presents in infancy. Severe gingivitis and early-onset rapidly progressive periodontitis (Figs. 26.1, 26.2 and 26.3). Early loss of the primary and permanent teeth. Dental caries may also occur. Oral mucosal ulcerations, bleeding, and petechiae.
- Early and common findings include mild and diffuse pigmentary dilution of the skin, hair, and eyes (Fig. 26.4). In sun-exposed skin, areas of bronze or slate-grey hyperpig-

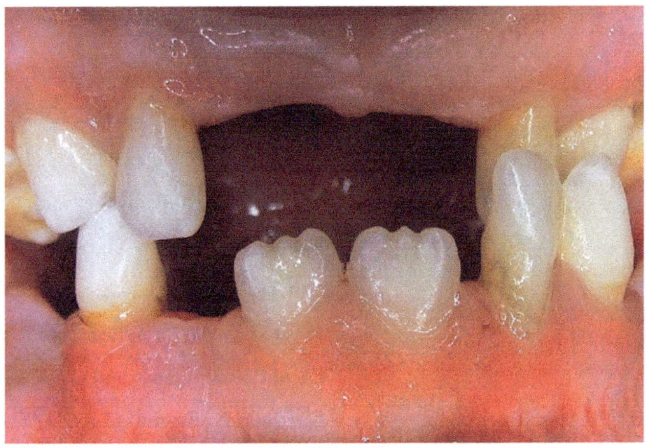

Fig. 26.2 Chédiak-Higashi syndrome, gingival recession and loss of upper centrals due to periodontitis

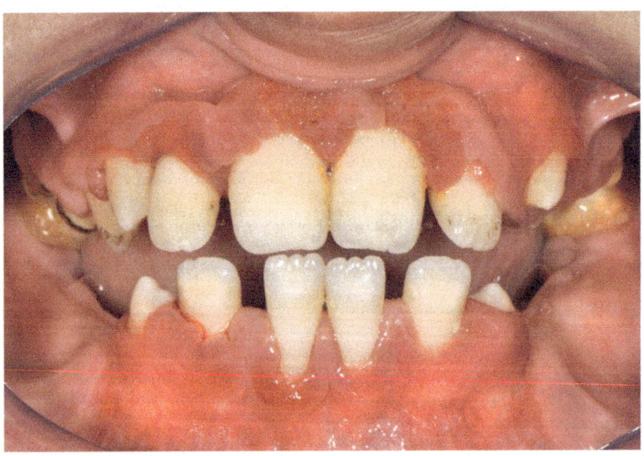

Fig. 26.1 Chédiak-Higashi syndrome, severe gingival inflammation and teeth mobility

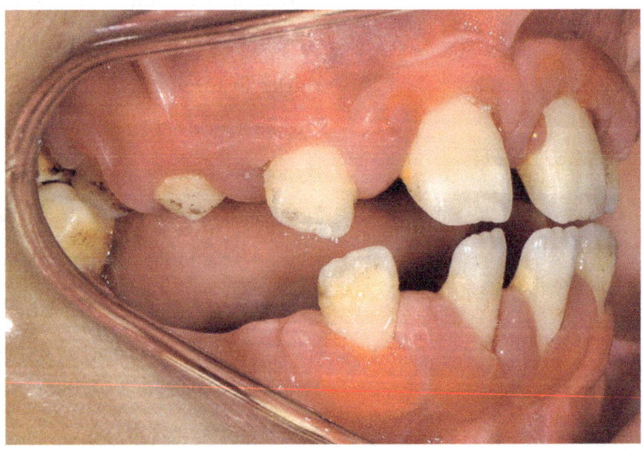

Fig. 26.3 Chédiak-Higashi syndrome, gingival enlargement, inflammation and teeth staining

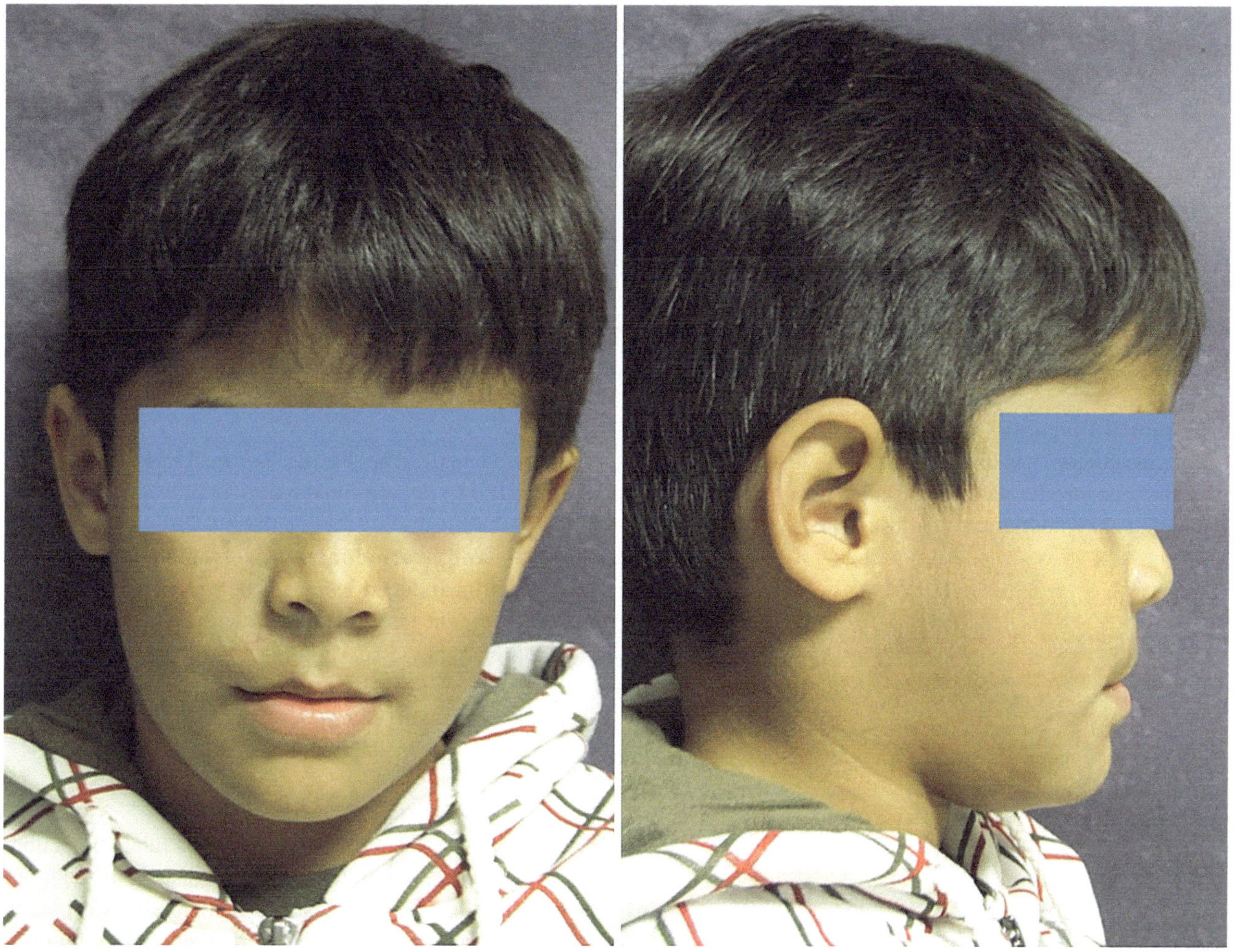

Fig. 26.4 Chédiak-Higashi syndrome, skin hypochromia

mentation usually mixed with guttate hypopigmented macules may occur. Silver hair is a typical feature.

- Decreased ocular pigment results in photophobia, nystagmus, and strabismus without visual problems. Other common findings are epistaxis, petechiae, and ecchymoses.
- Bacterial infections by *Staphylococcus aureus* and *Streptococcus pyogenes* are common on skin and lungs.
- Most of the children affected reach a stage known as the *"accelerated phase"* or *"lymphoma-like syndrome"* which can be life-threatening.

Differential Diagnosis

- Other primary immunodeficiencies
- Griscelli syndrome
- Hermansky-Pudlak syndrome
- Neutropenia
- Leukemia

Laboratory Tests Histopathologic and Immunologic examination. Examination of peripheral blood smears. Genetic testing.

Treatment Should be left to Pediatric specialists. Hematopoietic stem cell transplantation is the treatment of choice followed by corticosteroids, cyclosporine, and others, in order to prevent the onset of the *"accelerated phase."* Prophylactic antibiotics. Good oral hygiene for effective biofilm control.

Chondroectodermal Dysplasia

Definition Chondroectodermal dysplasia or Ellis-van Creveld syndrome is a rare disorder of the osteochondrodysplasia group of defects.

Etiology Genetic. It is inherited as an autosomal recessive trait.

Gingival Involvement Common. Mucogingival deformities (aberrant frenum) and non-dental biofilm-induced gingivitis.

Other Sites of Involvement Teeth, skeleton, eyes, heart, central nervous system, hair, and nails.

Clinical Features

- Fusion of the middle portion of the lower or upper lip to the gingiva, leading to the disappearance of the mucolabial fold and multiple frenula is the most characteristic oral manifestation (Figs. 26.5 and 26.6).
- Oligodontia and small teeth with conical crowns may occur.
- Chondrodysplasia of the long bones, bilateral polydactyly, shortened extremities, thin and sparse hair, dystrophic nails, heart defects, and genital abnormalities are common.
- Diagnosis is mainly based on clinical criteria.

Differential Diagnosis

- Orofaciodigital syndrome type 1
- Other chondrodysplasia syndromes
- Hereditary epidermolysis bullosa, type3

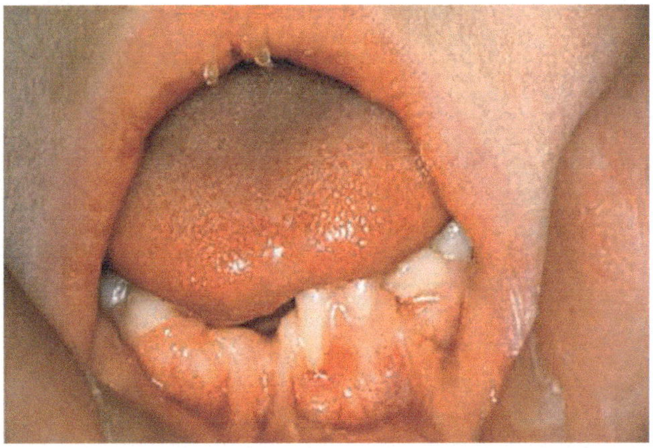

Fig. 26.5 Chondroectodermal dysplasia, multiple frenula and loss of mandibular fold

Laboratory Tests Radiographic examination, genetic testing.

Treatment Supportive.

Chronic Granulomatous Disease

Definition Chronic granulomatous disease is a rare genetic life-threatening group of primary immunodeficiencies associated with the inability of neutrophils and monocytes to effectively kill bacteria and fungi by generating oxidative metabolites.

Etiology Genetic. The disorder is inherited by an X-linked recessive (80%) or autosomal recessive (20%) trait.

Gingival and Periodontal Involvement Rare. Non-dental biofilm-induced lesions. The severity of periodontal involvement is correlated with the severity of immunodeficiency.

Other Sites of Involvement Oral mucosa, skin, lungs, liver, spleen, bones, brain, and lymph nodes.

Clinical Features

- Recurrent life-threatening bacterial and fungal infections are the most common features of the disease.
- The periodontal manifestations include gingival inflammation to generalized severe periodontitis depending on the severity of the immune deficiency (Fig. 26.7). Nonspecific gingival and oral ulcerations are common (Fig. 26.8). Additionally, fungal and bacterial infections of the oral cavity, salivary gland swelling, granulomatous cheilitis, and perioral dermatitis may occur.

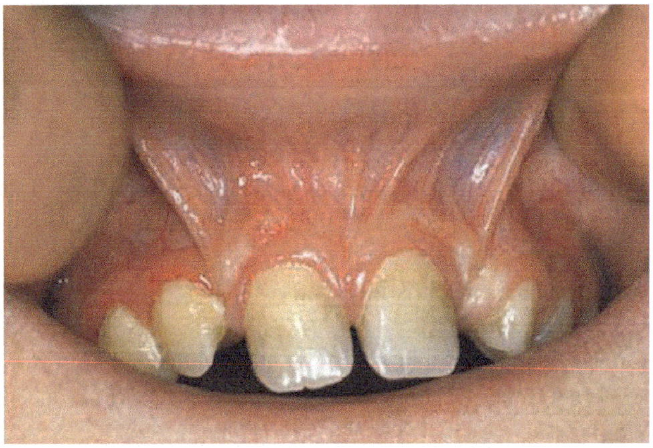

Fig. 26.6 Chondroectodermal dysplasia, multiple gingivolabial frenula

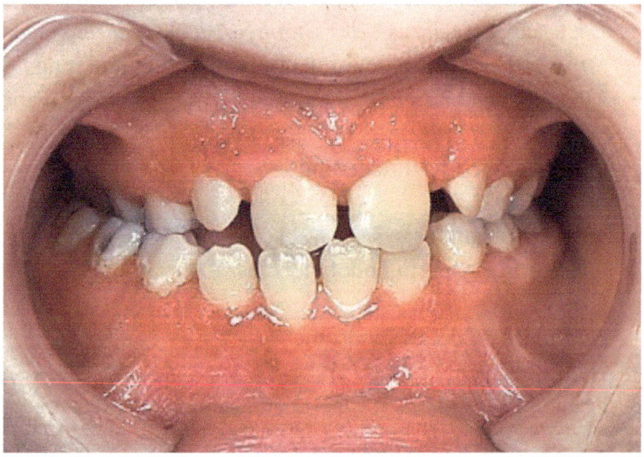

Fig. 26.7 Chronic granulomatous disease, gingival inflammation and early periodontitis

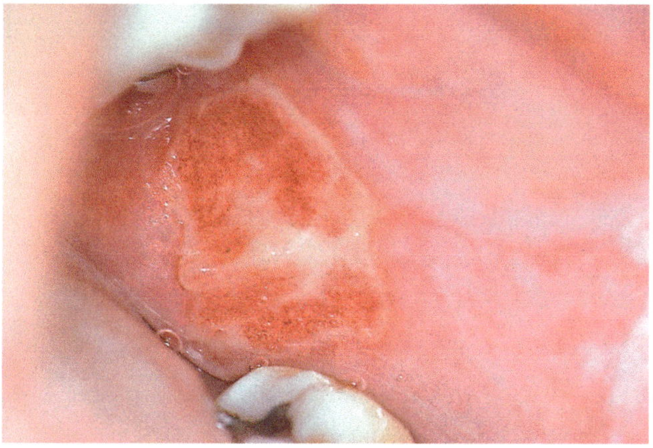

Fig. 26.8 Chronic granulomatous disease, ulceration on the buccal mucosa

- Cutaneous lesions include seborrheic dermatitis, lupus erythematosus-like lesions, scalp folliculitis, ulcerations, and granulomas.
- Infections, granulomas, and abscesses in several internal organs are common.
- Diagnosis is based on history and clinical features. However, it should be confirmed by laboratory tests.

Differential Diagnosis
- Other primary immunodeficiencies
- Congenital neutropenia
- Cyclic neutropenia
- Chédiak-Higashi syndrome
- Wiskott-Aldrich syndrome

Laboratory Tests Genetic testing. Nitroblue tetrazolium slide test, Cytochrome c reductase assay, Neutrophil function tests, histopathologic examination.

Treatment Patient should be referred to specialists who will work to prevent bacterial and fungal infections. Treatment may include antibiotic and antifungal drugs. Good oral hygiene for effective biofilm control is highly recommended.

Cowden Disease

Definition Cowden disease or Cowden syndrome or multiple hamartoma syndrome is an uncommon disorder characterized by a wide spectrum of mucocutaneous lesions usually associated with breast, thyroid, and other organ disorders.

Etiology Genetic. It is inherited as an autosomal dominant trait.

Gingival Involvement Relatively common. Non-dental biofilm-induced gingival lesions.

Other Sites of Involvement Oral mucosa (lips, tongue, buccal mucosa) and skin (neck, nasolabial folds, dorsum of hand, and forearm), breast, and thyroid gland are commonly involved. Other organs (e.g., genitourinary system, gastrointestinal tract, skeletal, eye) may also be involved.

Clinical Features
- Lesions occur on both free and attached gingiva as well as on the edentulous alveolar mucosa. They appear as multiple, small, smooth, pale or whitish, painless papules or nodules that may be isolated or coalesce in a cobblestone pattern (Figs. 26.9 and 26.10).
- Oral mucosal lesions are similar to those found on gingiva.
- Skin lesions appear as multiple papillomatous papules and small nodules that are hair follicle hamartomas (*trichilemmomas*). Dermal fibromas are also common.
- Several breast and thyroid gland abnormalities, including benign and malignant tumors, are common.
- Clinical diagnosis should be confirmed by laboratory tests.

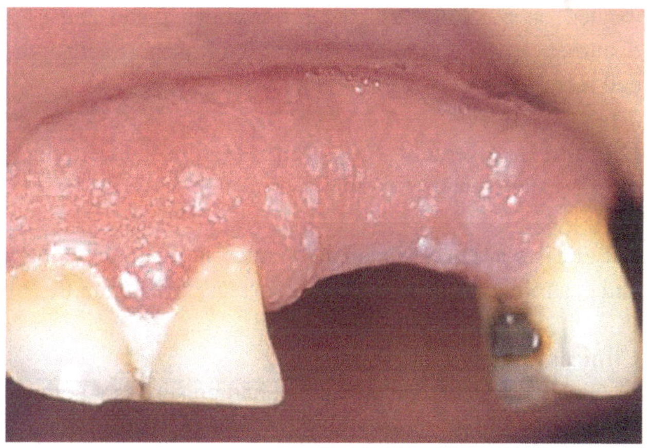

Fig. 26.9 Cowden disease, multiple, small nodules on the gingiva

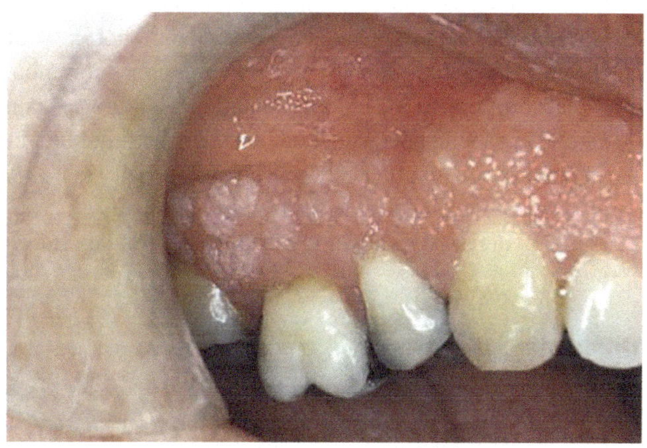

Fig. 26.10 Cowden disease, multiple, small nodules coalescing in a cobblestone pattern on the gingiva and alveolar mucosa

Differential Diagnosis
- Focal epithelial hyperplasia
- Familial acanthosis nigricans
- Tuberous sclerosis
- Multiple endocrine neoplasia syndromes
- Darier disease
- Lipoid proteinosis

Laboratory Tests Histopathologic examination of cutaneous biopsies is the preferable option. Genetic testing.

Treatment There is no treatment.

Cystic Fibrosis

Definition Cystic fibrosis is a relatively common, multisystemic, life-threatening disorder characterized by a dysfunction of the exocrine glands.

Etiology Genetic. It is inherited as an autosomal recessive trait. The pathological gene known as the *CFTR* gene is located on the long arm of chromosome 7 and causes a disturbance in chloride and sodium ion transport across the cell membrane.

Gingival Involvement Rare. Dental biofilm-induced gingivitis associated with xerostomia.

Other Sites of Involvement Oral mucosa (lips), pulmonary and gastrointestinal tracts, liver, pancreas, sweat glands.

Clinical Features
- Gingival lesions are uncommon and present as a nonspecific, diffuse erythema on both free and attached gingiva (Fig. 26.11). They may be due to oral dryness and increased dental biofilm accumulation.
- Oral manifestations include lip enlargement, erythema of the oral mucosa, and occasionally mild xerostomia.
- Chronic coughing, pulmonary infections, shortness of breath, bronchitis, and hemoptysis are common. Malabsorption, bulky, greasy stools, and failure to gain weight even with adequate food intake are common. Liver and pancreatic insufficiency, sweating with salty taste are also common. The disease starts early in infancy.
- Clinical diagnosis should be confirmed by laboratory tests.

Differential Diagnosis
- Dental biofilm-induced gingivitis
- Lipoid proteinosis
- Cheilitis glandularis
- Cheilitis granulomatosa

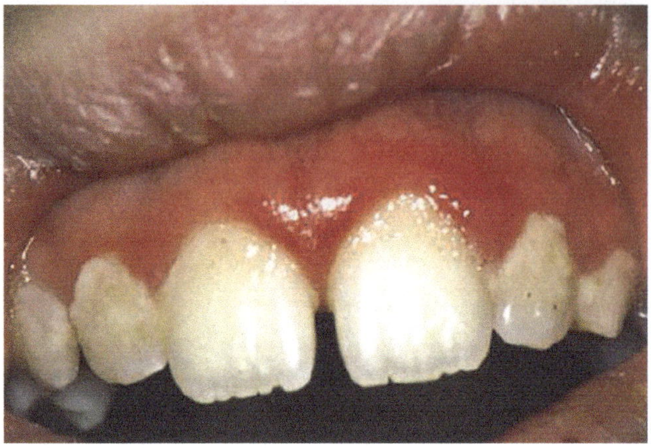

Fig. 26.11 Cystic fibrosis, gingivitis

Laboratory Tests Histopathologic examination of the lip. Elevated chloride, sodium, and potassium levels in sweat. Absence of pancreatic enzymes in the intestinal fluid. Airflow obstruction on spirometry and pulmonary CT scanning. Genetic testing.

Treatment Effectivedental biofilm control for the gingival lesions. Palliative high-calorie diet is indicated for the systemic manifestations. Patient should be referred to specialists who may use antibiotics, inhaled bronchodilators, and lung transplantation.

Darier Disease

Definition Darier disease or dyskeratosis follicularis is a relatively rare mucocutaneous disorder.

Etiology Genetic. It is inherited as an autosomal dominant trait.

Gingival Involvement Relatively common. Non-dental biofilm-induced gingival lesions.

Other Sites of Involvement Oral mucosa (20–40%). Other mucosae (genitalia, rectum, pharynx), skin (always), and nails.

Clinical Features
- Gingival lesions appear as small, multiple, whitish, and confluent papules. They may become hypertrophic typically shown a reticular pattern or developing a cobblestone appearance (Fig. 26.12).
- Similar lesions appear on other oral mucosal sites (e.g., palate, tongue, and buccal mucosa). Oral lesions usually follow cutaneous lesions.

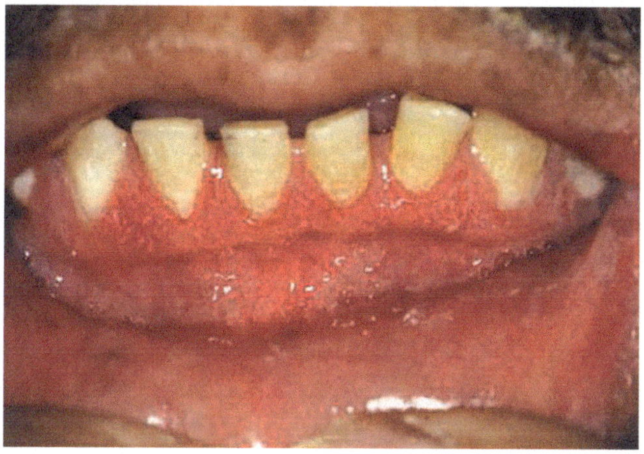

Fig. 26.12 Darier disease, multiple, small whitish papules on the gingiva

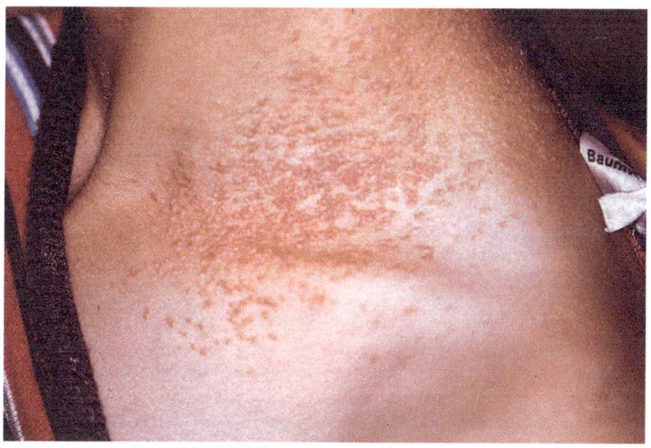

Fig. 26.13 Darier disease, multiple red papules on the skin

- Skin lesions appear as multiple, brownish-red, painless papules that usually coalesce into plaques (Fig. 26.13). Forehead, neck, ears, scalp, chest, and back are most often affected. Nails exhibit subungual keratosis and longitudinal ridges and lines.
- Clinical diagnosis should be confirmed by laboratory tests.

Differential Diagnosis
- Familial acanthosis nigricans
- Cowden disease
- Wegener granulomatosis
- Lichen planus

Laboratory Tests Histopathologic examination of oral and skin lesions. Genetic testing.

Treatment Good oral hygiene. Use of systemic aromatic retinoids for skin and other lesions.

Down Syndrome

Definition Down syndrome, or trisomy 21, is a common disorder with variable clinical manifestations with an incidence in the general population of 1 in 600–800 live births.

Etiology Chromosomal disorder of chromosome 21. Most patients with Down syndrome exhibit full trisomy 21. Few cases are mosaic and fewer are the result of translocation. Intrinsic immune system defects contribute to disturbed immune function and respiratory infection.

Gingival Involvement Common. Dental biofilm-induced gingival lesions and frequent periodontitis are associated with a high risk for periodontal supporting tissue loss, probably induced by immune system intrinsic abnormalities.

Other Sites of Involvement Oral cavity, common. Dysmorphic changes in craniofacies, thorax, abdomen, pelvis, hands, and feet.

Clinical Features
- Clinically, gingival tissues are red, swollen, and bleed easily. (Fig. 26.14). Gingival hyperplasia may occur due to chronic mouth breathing, poor oral hygiene, and other local irritating factors. Gingivitis frequently progresses to generalized early periodontitis, which commences in the deciduous dentition and continues into the permanent dentition. Bone loss, mobility, and migration of the teeth are common. All these factors predispose to the premature loss of teeth. Macroglossia, fissured and geographic tongue, high-arched palate, cleft palate, delayed tooth eruption, and hypoplastic teeth are the most frequent oral lesions.

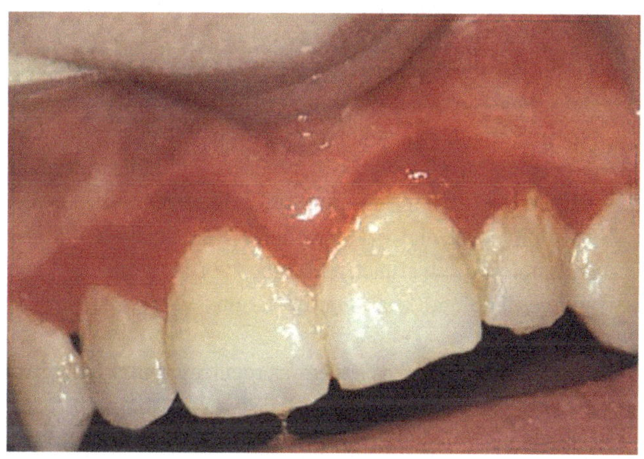

Fig. 26.14 Down syndrome, severe gingivitis

- Follicular hyperkeratosis, facial flushing, alopecia areata, and dry skin are common.
- Polydactyly, syndactyly, clinodactyly, hyperextensibility of joints, other skeletal abnormalities, congenital heart anomalies, hormonal disturbances, learning disability, abnormal slanting of the eye, short ears, and flat face are common findings.
- Diagnosis is usually based on clinical criteria.

Differential Diagnosis
- Cyclic neutropenia
- Agranulocytosis
- Leukemias
- Glycogen storage disease type Ib

Laboratory Tests Chromosomal analysis.

Treatment Good oral hygiene for effective dental biofilm control prevent or reduce the progression of ginigival lesions.

Dyskeratosis Congenita

Definition Dyskeratosis congenita is a rare genodermatosis characterized by mucocutaneous and bone marrow disorders.

Etiology Genetic. It is usually transmitted via an x-linked recessive pattern of inheritance (90%) and rarely via an autosomal dominant and autosomal recessive trait. The x-linked recessive form is caused by a mutation in the DKC1 gene, which encodes the dyskerin protein that interacts with the telomerase enzyme.

Gingival Involvement Rare, non-dental biofilm-induced lesions.

Other Sites of Involvement Oral and other mucosae, skin, nails, bone marrow, peripheral cells, liver, and lungs.

Clinical Features
- The clinical mainstay of the disorder is reticulated skin hyperpigmentation, which is occasionally associated with epidermal atrophy and telangiectasias (poikiloderma), wrinkled skin, skin and mucosal bullous formation, nail dystrophy, eye and ear disorders, bone marrow failure, immunologic dysfunction, other organ and system involvement and oral manifestations (Figs. 26.15 and 26.16).
- Clinically, oral lesions appear as recurrent bullae that rapture leaving a raw ulcerated surface on the tongue, buccal mucosa, and palate. Atrophy of the oral mucosa and development of leukoplakia may occur. Malignant transformation of oral leukoplakia may develop, especially on the dorsum of the tongue.

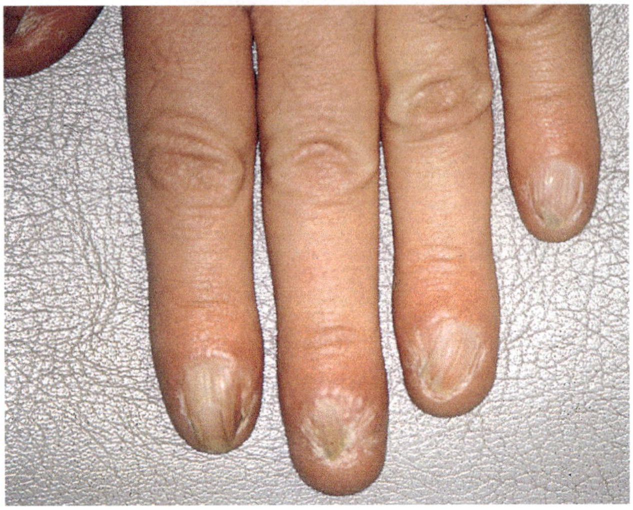

Fig. 26.15 Dyskeratosis congenita, nail dystrophy

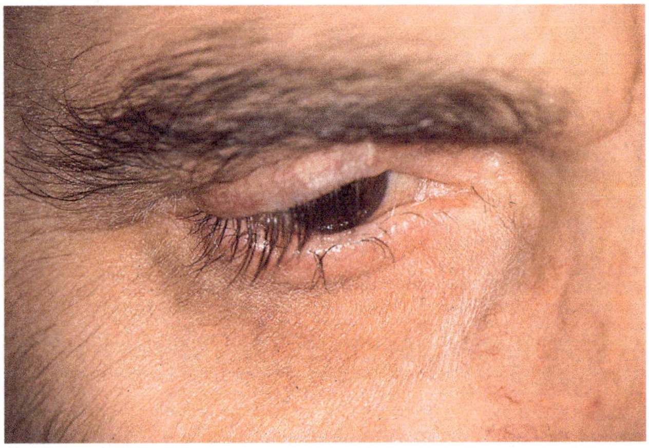

Fig. 26.16 Dyskeratosis congenita, blepharitis

- Gingival lesions are rare and characterized by leukoplakia (Fig. 26.17) and early-onset severe periodontal disease. Dental anomalies (e.g., decreased dental crown to root ratio, taurodontism, hypodontia, large interdental spaces) may be observed.
- Patients have an increased risk of developing mucosal squamous cell carcinoma, acute myelogenous leukemia, and Hodgkin's disease.
- Clinical diagnosis should be supported by laboratory tests.

Differential Diagnosis
- Pachyonychia congenita
- Epidermolysis bullosa
- Coltz syndrome
- Fanconi anemia
- Chronic Graft-Versus-Host Disease
- Lichen planus, hypertrophic type
- Oral leukoplakia

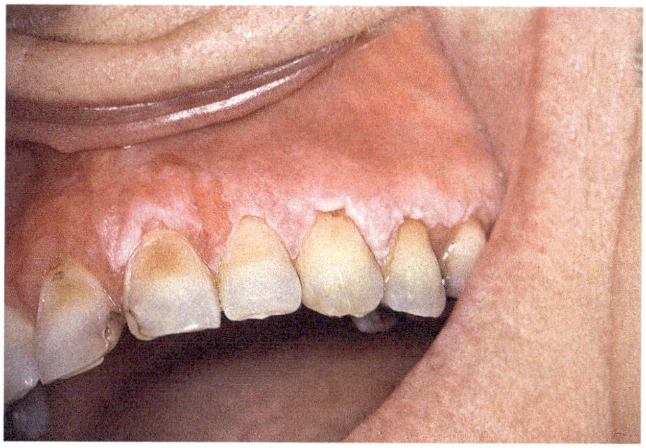

Fig. 26.17 Dyskeratosis congenita, gingival leukoplakia

Laboratory Tests Histopathologic examination, flow fluorescence in situ hybridization (flow-FISH), genetic testing.

Treatment The management of the disorder should be left to a multidisciplinary team of specialists. The management of oral lesions is symptomatic. Surgical excision of leukoplakia and periodic follow-up is recommended.

Ehlers-Danlos Syndrome

Definition Ehlers-Danlos syndrome includes a group of connective tissue disorders, that are characterized by defects in collagen synthesis.

Etiology Genetic. It is mainly inherited as an autosomal dominant trait. Mutations in genes encoding fibrillar collagens or enzymes are involved in the biosynthesis of these proteins.

Classification On the basis of clinical features and the mode of inheritance, ten types of disorders are recognized.

Gingival Involvement Generalized, severe, early-onset periodontitis and gingival recession, relatively common. Mainly types IV and VIII have an increased susceptibility to periodontitis. Possibly multigene disorder influenced by dental biofilm levels.

Other Sites of Involvement Oral mucosa, teeth, skin, joints, heart.

Clinical Features

- Periodontal lesions usually appear in the form of generalized, severe periodontitis with clinical attachment loss and bone destruction, leading to premature loss of the primary and permanent teeth (Fig. 26.18). Gingival recession and bleeding are also common.
- Oral manifestations include thin and fragile mucosa, prolonged bleeding on minor trauma, and decreased wound healing. About 50% of patients can touch their nose with the tip of the tongue compared with 10% of normal people (Fig. 26.19). Temporomandibular joint hypermobility, multiple pulp stones, enamel, dentin, and cementum defects may occur.
- Skin manifestations include thin and fragile skin, hypermobility, and hematomas. Scarring formation, especially over the knees, elbows, and chin.
- Joint hypermobility, cardiovascular and ocular abnormalities may occur, (especially mitral valve prolapsed).
- Diagnosis is mainly based on clinical criteria.

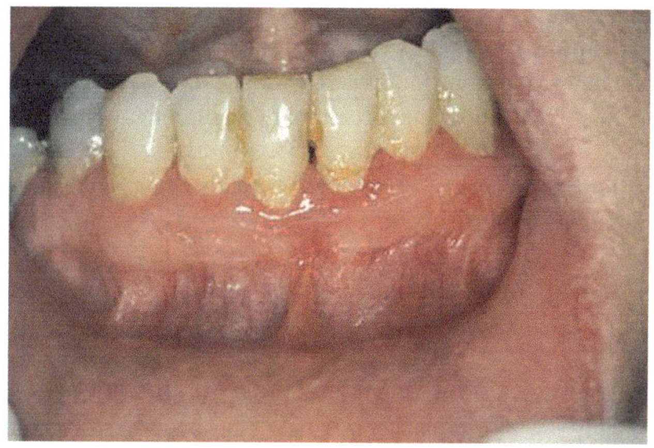

Fig. 26.18 Ehlers-Danlos syndrome, generalized periodontitis

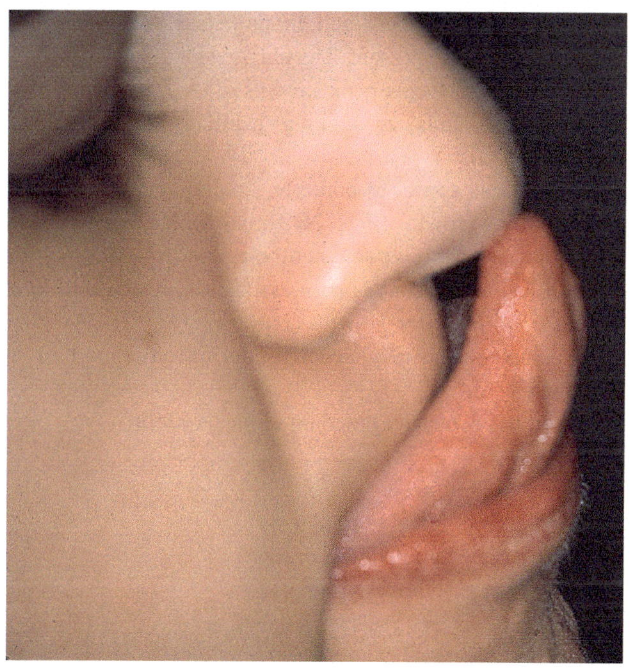

Fig. 26.19 Ehlers-Danlos syndrome, increased tongue mobility

Differential Diagnosis

- Severe periodontitis associated with other genetic disorders
- Marfan syndrome
- Cutis laxa

Laboratory Tests Radiographic examination, dental scan. Genetic testing for mutations in collagen type V (COL5A1 and COL5A2).

Treatment Dental biofilm control. Symptomatic management of other manifestations.

Familial Acanthosis Nigricans

Definition Familial or juvenile acanthosis nigricans is an uncommon benign mucocutaneous disorder, characterized by papillary lesions and occasional skin discoloration.

Etiology Genetic. It is inherited by an irregular autosomal dominant trait.

Gingival Involvement Relatively common. Non-dental biofilm-induced lesions.

Other Sites of Involvement Oral mucosa in 10–25% of cases, mainly on tongue, palate, and lips. Skin is always involved (axillae, groins, neck, umbilicus, genitalia, perianal region).

Clinical Features

- Gingival enlargement and in particular the interdental papillae may be present. The enlargement is occasionally so severe that it covers the crowns of teeth. Enlarged gingiva often ends up looking papillary in appearance (Fig. 26.20).
- Oral lesions appear as multiple, small, painless, and papillomatous growths (Figs. 26.21 and 26.22). Gingival and oral lesions exhibit normal color.
- Skin lesions present as painless, dark, velvety, multiple, and small papillary growths (*skin tags*) (Fig. 26.23).
- The disorder usually develops during childhood or at puberty.
- Diagnosis is usually based on clinical criteria.

Differential Diagnosis

- Hereditary gingival fibromatosis
- Drug-induced gingival hyperplasia
- Malignant acanthosis nigricans

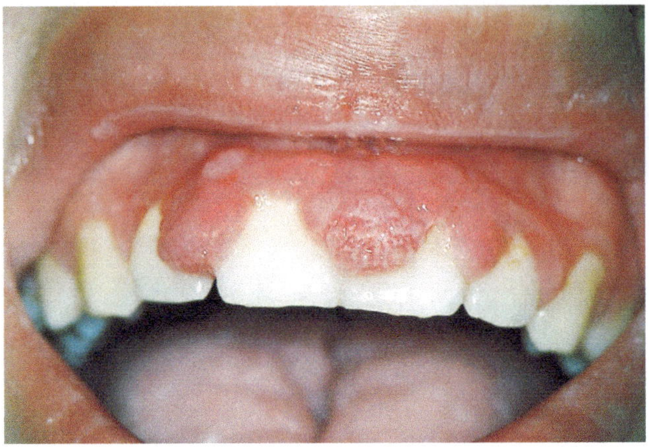

Fig. 26.20 Familiar acanthosis nigricans, papillary enlargement of interdental papillae of the gingiva

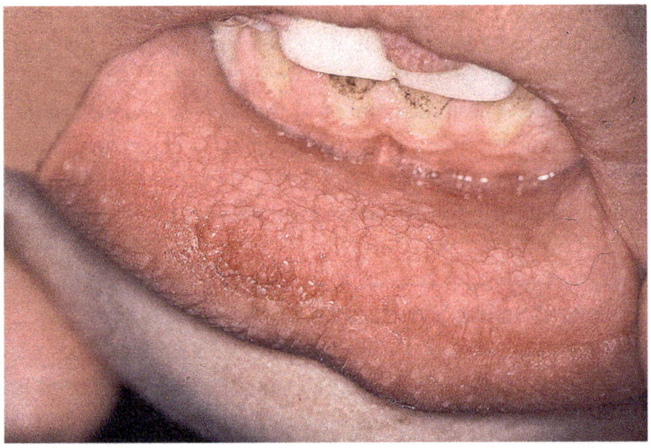

Fig. 26.21 Familiar acanthosis nigricans, multiple lesions on the lower lip

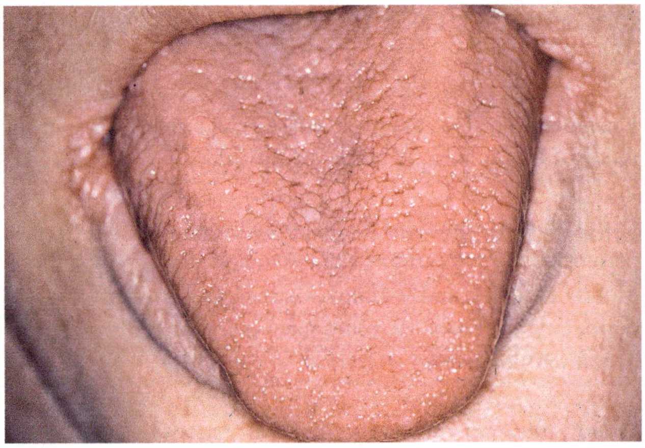

Fig. 26.22 Familiar acanthosis nigricans, small papillomatous growth on the tongue

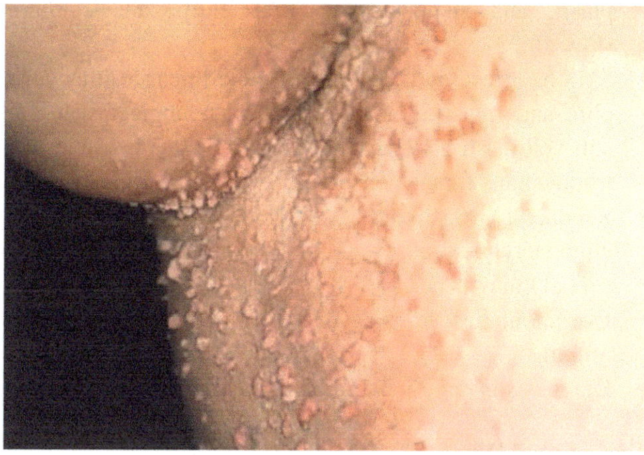

Fig. 26.23 Familiar acanthosis nigricans, multiple, papillary growths on the skinon the skin (skin tags)

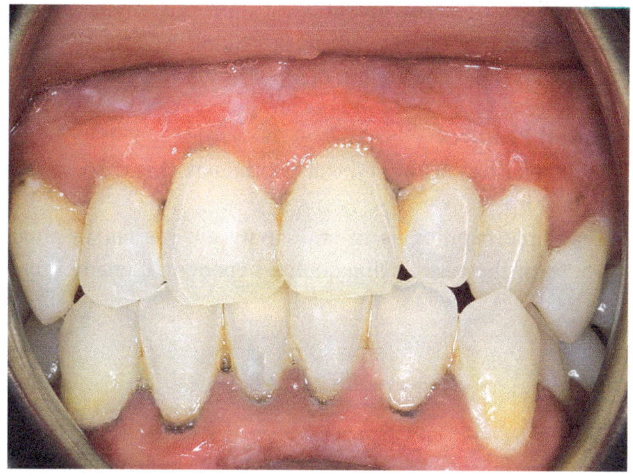

Fig. 26.24 Fanconi anemia, gingivitis and periodontitis

- Endocrine-related acanthosis nigricans
- Cowden disease
- Darier disease

Laboratory Tests Histopathologic examination of oral and skin lesions are supportive. Genetic testing.

Treatment Gingivectomy and good oral hygiene for the gingival lesions. Surgical reconstruction of skin lesion in cases of severe esthetic problems.

Fanconi Anemia

Definition Fanconi anemia is a rare genetic disorder characterized by pancytopenia and several congenital abnormalities.

Etiology Genetic. It can be inherited in an autosomal recessive manner, and rarely an x-linked manner.

Gingival Involvement Rare. Dental biofilm-induced gingival lesions modified by defective hemopoiesis.

Other Sites of Involvement Skin, bones, bone marrow, endocrine glands, heart, kidney.

Clinical Features

- The clinical hallmarks are generalized diffuse hyperpigmentation, pancytopenia (anemia, leucopenia, thrombocytopenia), skeletal malformations, heart and kidney abnormalities, increased risk for malignancies (acute myelogenous leukemia, Hodgkin disease, skin and oral squamous cell carcinoma, breast and pancreatic carcinomas), and chromosomal fragility.
- Periodontal and oral manifestations are characterized by gingivitis and severe periodontitis, gingival and mucosal bleeding, ulcerations, microdontia, tooth mobility, and halitosis (Fig. 26.24).
- Patients are at high risk for squamous cell carcinoma, most frequently on the tongue and gingiva. The clinical onset of the disease appears during the first decade of life and rarely later.
- Diagnosis should be confirmed by laboratory tests, although there is no definitive diagnostic test.

Differential Diagnosis

- Dyskeratosis congenita
- Chronic Graft-Versus-Host Disease
- Naegeli-Franceschetti-Jadassohn syndrome
- Xerodermapigmentosum

Laboratory Tests Chromosome breakage tests, mutation analyses, bone marrow chromosome tests, histopathologic examination, micro-CT (micro-computed tomography) scans of tibia bone.

Treatment Good oral hygiene for periodontal lesions. The management must be left to a multidisciplinary team of specialists.

Focal Dermal Hypoplasia Syndrome

Definition Focal dermal hypoplasia syndrome or Goltz-Gorlin syndrome is an uncommon disorder characterized by multiple abnormalities.

Etiology Genetic. It is inherited as an X-linked dominant trait. However, most of the reported cases are sporadic.

Gingival Involvement Rare. Non-dental biofilm-related lesions.

Other Sites of Involvement Oral mucosa (tongue, palate, buccal mucosa, lips) and teeth. Skin, hair, and nails. Musculoskeletal and central nervous systems, eyes.

Clinical Features

- Gingival lesions are typical papillomas (Figs. 26.25 and 26.26).
- Multiple papillomas in oral cavity are present in about 50% of the cases. Oligodontia, hypodontia, enamel dysplasia and malocclusion, oral clefts are common (Fig. 26.27).
- Skin manifestations include atrophic linear lesions, atrophic and hyperpigmented plaques, telangiectasias, and soft yellowish nodules (Fig. 26.28). Sparse hair and dystrophic nails may be observed.
- Syndactyly, brachydactyly, oligodactyly or polydactyly, clinodactyly extremity, asymmetry, scoliosis, and microcephaly may occur.
- Eye anomalies, learning disability are the less common findings.
- Diagnosis is mainly based on clinical criteria.

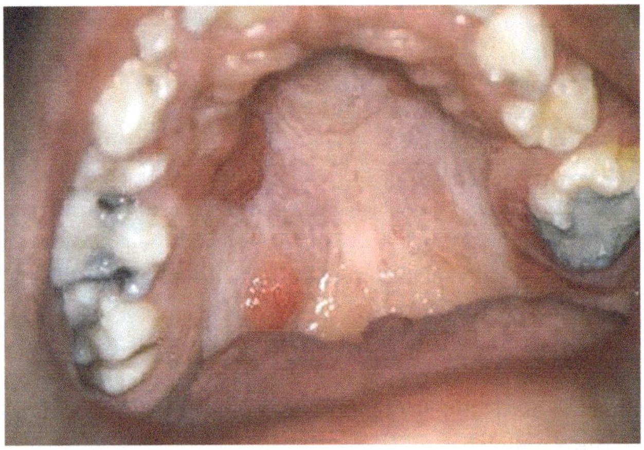

Fig. 26.25 Focal dermal hypoplasia syndrome, multiple papillomas on the gingiva and the palate

Differential Diagnosis

- Multiple oral papillomas
- Multiple oral condylomas acuminata
- Focal epithelial hyperplasia
- Incontinentia pigmenti

Laboratory Tests Radiographic examination. Histopathologic examination of skin and oral lesions. Genetic testing.

Treatment Surgical excision of oral papillomas. Supportive for the skin and other lesions.

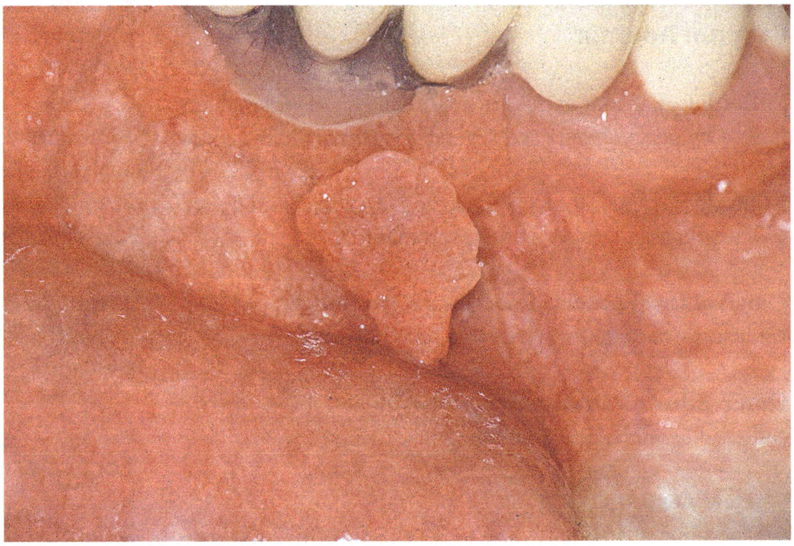

Fig. 26.26 Focal dermal hypoplasia syndrome, papilloma on the alveolar mucosa

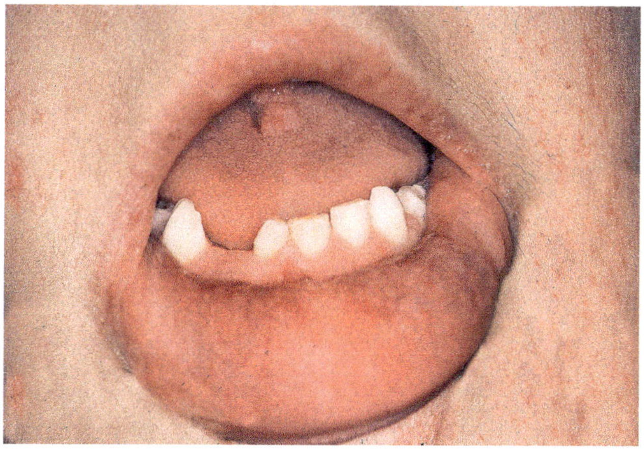

Fig. 26.27 Focal dermal hypoplasia syndrome, teeth deformity

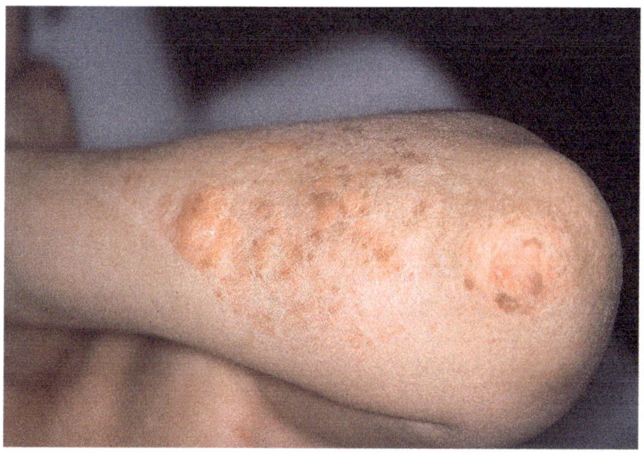

Fig. 26.28 Focal dermal hypoplasia syndrome, skin pink-yellowish papules and nodules

Focal Palmoplantar and Oral Mucosa Hyperkeratosis Syndrome

Definition Focal palmoplantar and oral mucosa hyperkeratosis syndrome or hyperkeratosis palmoplantaris and attached gingival hyperkeratosis is an unusual genetic disorder characterized by oral mucosal and dermal hyperkeratosis.

Etiology Genetic. It is inherited as an autosomal dominant trait.

Gingival Involvement Always present, mainly attached gingiva, without involvement of periodontal apparatus. Non-dental biofilm-induced lesions.

Other Sites of Involvement Oral mucosa (sites subjected to mechanical pressure or friction such as hard palate, retromolar pad mucosa, alveolar mucosa, lateral border of the tongue). Skin (mainly on the weight-bearing and pressure-related areas such as soles and palms) and nails.

Clinical Features

- Marked white hyperkeratosis of the attached gingiva, presenting clinically as leukoplakia, is a consistent finding (Fig. 26.29). There is no inflammation or attachment loss.
- White hyperkeratotic lesions in other mucosal sites are less frequently observed.
- Hyperkeratotic lesions on the weight-bearing and pressure-related areas of the palms and soles are always present (Figs. 26.30 and 26.31). Nail dystrophy and hyperhidrosis may also occur.
- Hyperkeratosis develops early in childhood and the severity increases with age.
- Diagnosis is mainly based on clinical criteria.

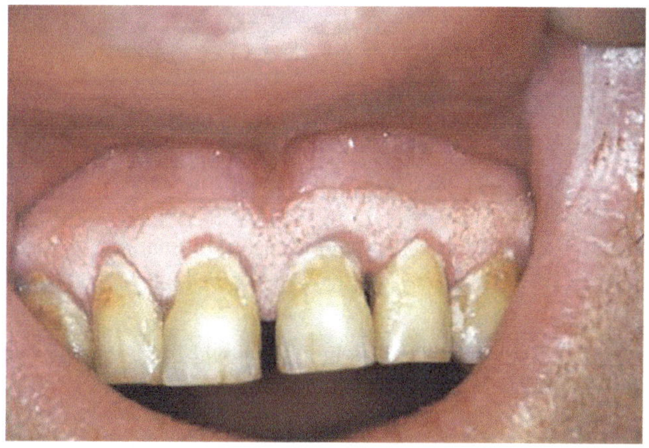

Fig. 26.29 Focal palmoplantar and oral mucosa hyperkeratosis syndrome, generalized white hyperkeratosis of the gingiva

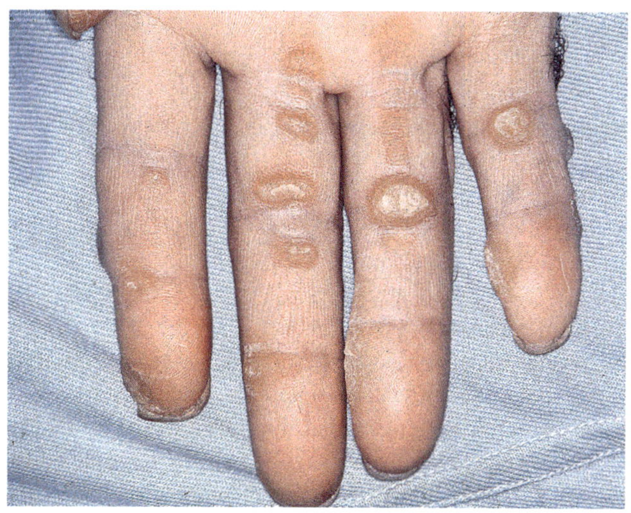

Fig. 26.30 Focal palmoplantar and oral mucosa hyperkeratosis syndrome, hyperkeratosis on the palms

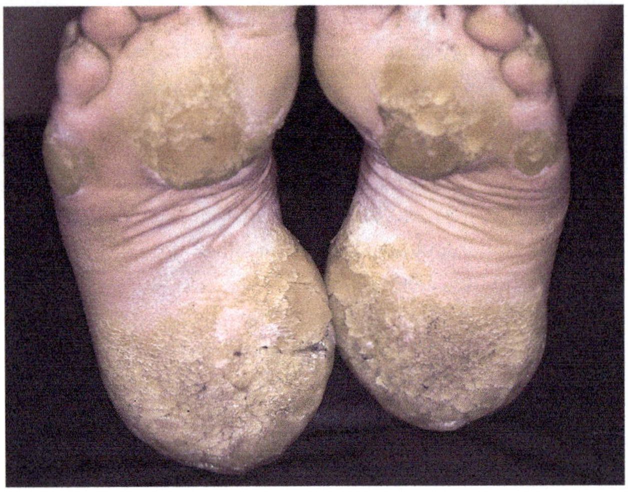

Fig. 26.31 Focal palmoplantar and oral mucosa hyperkeratosis, hyperkeratosis on the soles

Differential Diagnosis
- Leukoplakia
- White sponge nevus
- Pachyonychia congenita
- Dyskeratosis congenita

Laboratory Tests Histopathologic examination, genetic testing.

Treatment Local and systemic aromatic retinoids with partial success.

Gardner Syndrome

Definition Gardner syndrome is a rare disorder in the group of familial colorectal polyposis syndromes.
Etiology Genetic. It is inherited as an autosomal dominant trait.

Alveolar Bone Involvement Relatively common. The gingival tissue is normal.

Other Sites of Involvement Bones (skull, calvaria), skin, gastrointestinal tract.

Clinical Features
- The alveolar bone lesions are characterized by multiple osteomas that present as painless, hard masses covered by normal attached gingival and alveolar mucosa (Fig. 26.32). Central osteomas in other sites of the jaws, multiple odontomas, multiple impacted supernumerary teeth, and rarely benign oral soft tissue tumors may occur (Fig. 26.33). It is important for Dentists to diagnose the oral lesions of the syndrome as early as possible and to refer the patient to a gastroenterologist.
- Multiple osteomas of the skull, paranasal sinuses, and calvaria may also develop.
- Gastrointestinal manifestations are common and appear as multiple polyps of the colon and rectum that are characterized by a high rate of malignant transformation into adenocarcinoma.
- Skin lesions are epidermoid cysts, multiple fibromas, and hyperpigmentation (Fig. 26.34).
- Clinical diagnosis should be confirmed by laboratory tests.

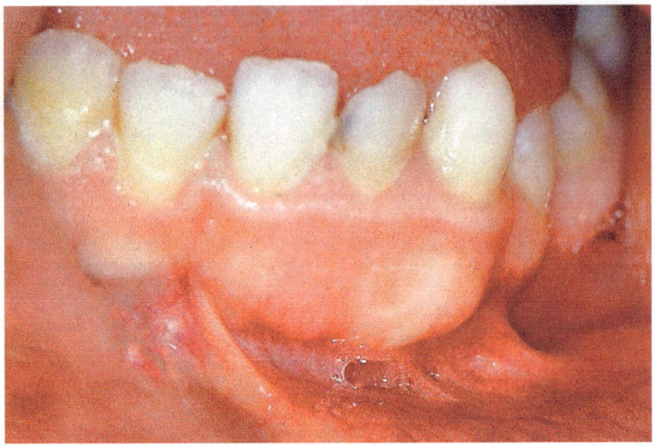

Fig. 26.32 Gardner syndrome, multiple osteomas on the mandible

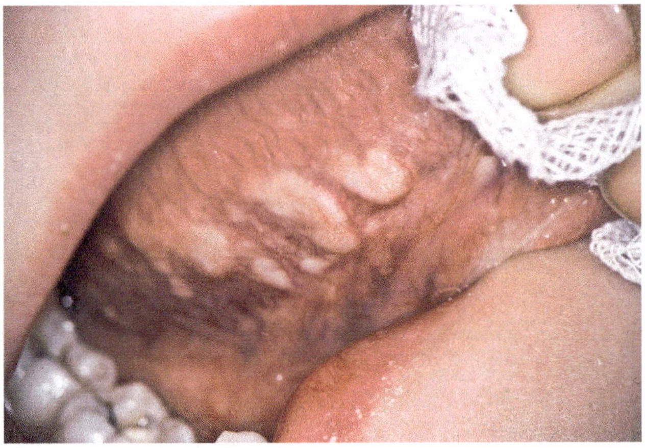

Fig. 26.33 Gardner syndrome, fibromyxoma on the tongue

Differential Diagnosis
- Isolated osteomas and exostoses
- Odontogenic tumors
- Peutz-Jeghers syndrome
- Cowden disease

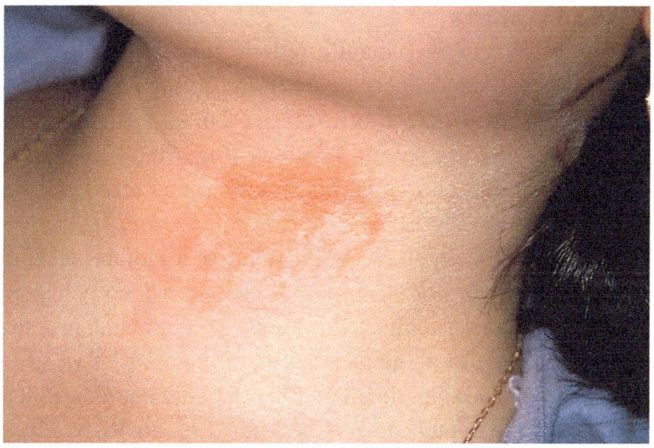

Fig. 26.34 Gardner syndrome, skin pigmentation on the neck

Laboratory Tests Radiographic examination of the jaws, skull, and intestinal tract. Biopsy and histopathologic examination of tumors and polyps.

Treatment Osteomas do not require excision unless they cause symptoms or cosmetic problems. The intestinal polyps must be under observation by the specialist.

Glycogen Storage Disease Type 1b

Definition Glycogen storage disease type 1bis a rare metabolic disorder with severe prognosis.

Etiology Genetic. It is inherited as an autosomal recessive trait. Deficiency in SLC37A4 (11q23.3) gene. This is a defect of the microsomal glucose-6-phosphate translocase. The disorder is associated with neutropenia and neutrophil dysfunction.

Periodontal Involvement Relatively common. Severe periodontitis associated with genetic, metabolic, and endocrine disorders.

Other Sites of Involvement Oral mucosa, liver, kidneys, skeleton, and many other organs.

Clinical Features

- Early-onset chronic gingivitis soon leads to severe periodontitis with alveolar bone loss and teeth migration (Figs. 26.35 and 26.36). The oral mucosa lesions present as discrete, deep, irregular, recurrent ulcers that are usually covered by a whitish pseudomembrane. Vaulted palate and recurrent oral infection may occur.
- Characteristic face (*doll's face*), liver and kidney enlargement, hypoglycemia, hyperlipidemia, growth retardation, and recurrent bacterial infection are common (Fig. 26.37).
- Clinical diagnosis should be confirmed by laboratory tests.

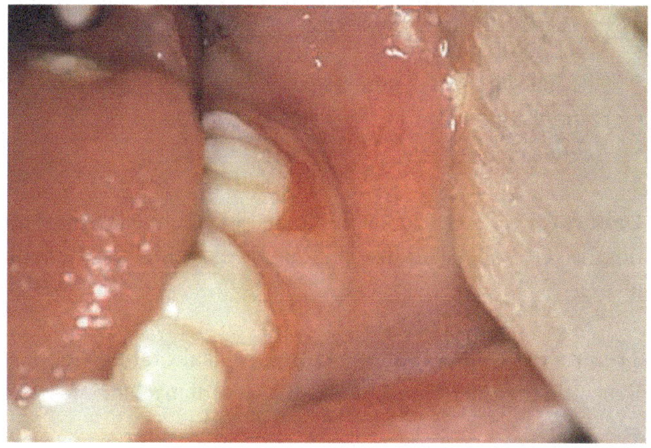

Fig. 26.35 Glycogen storage disease type 1b localized early onset gingivitis

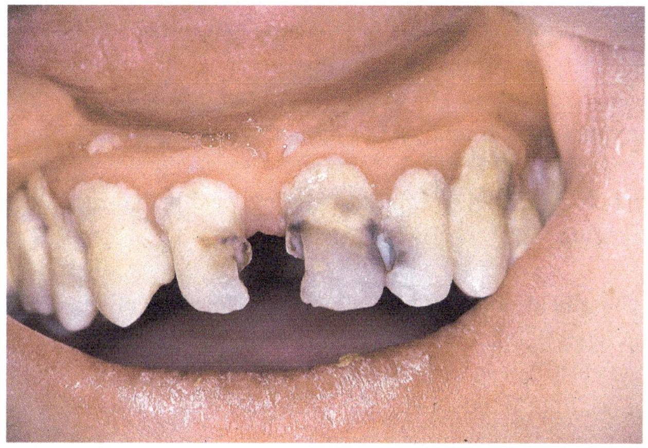

Fig. 26.36 Glycogen storage disease type 1b periodontitis and teeth decay

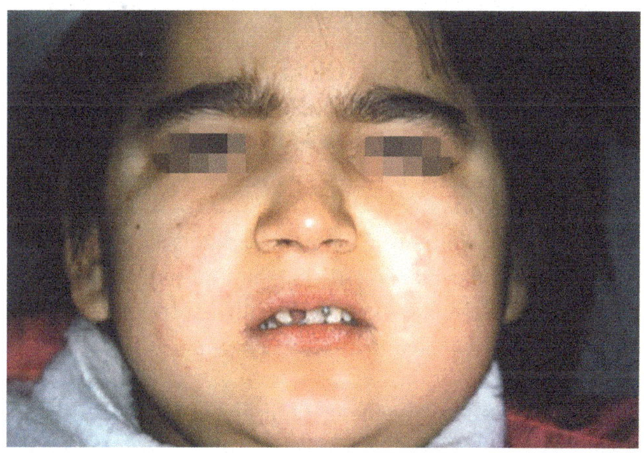

Fig. 26.37 Glycogen storage disease type 1b characteristic "doll's face"

Differential Diagnosis

- Neutropenia
- Neutrophil dysfunction.
- Congenital neutropenia

- Cyclic neutropenia
- Myeloid dysfunctions
- Chédiak-Higashi syndrome
- Hypophosphatasia
- Acatalasia

Laboratory Tests Hematologic and biochemical examination. Liver biopsy and histopathologic examination. Genetic testing.

Treatment Dental biofilm control, topical oral antiseptics. Systemic treatment must be left to the pediatrician.

Hereditary Epidermolysis Bullosa

Definition Hereditary epidermolysis bullosa (HEB) is a rare chronic, recurrent, mechanobullous group of genetic mucocutaneous disorders, that share three characteristics: a. *genetic transmission, b. mechanical fragility of the skin,* and c. *mucosal and skin bullous formation.*

Etiology Genetic. The exact etiology and pathogenesis are obscure.

Classification Four major types and numerous clinical phenotypes of epidermolysis bullosa have been described. They are classified according to a. *the ultrastructural level of bulla formation;* b. *the mode of inheritance;* c. *the antigenic target;* and d. *the clinical phenotype.*

- *Type I*, epidermolysis bullosa *simplex.* Inherited in an autosomal dominant and x-linked recessive trait.
- *Type II*, epidermolysis bullosa *junctional*. Inherited in an autosomal recessive trait.
- *Type III*, epidermolysis bullosa *dystrophic*. Inherited in an autosomal dominant or recessive trait.
- *Type IV*, *Kindler syndrome*. Inherited in an autosomal recessive trait.

Gingival Involvement Common, particularly types II, III, and mainly type IV. Non-dental biofilm-induced gingival lesions, occasionally associated with severe periodontitis with alveolar bone and tooth loss.

Other Sites of Involvement Oral mucosa (tongue, buccal mucosa, palate, lips). Other mucosae (eyes, larynx, esophagus, genitals, gastrointestinal). Skin, always (hands, feet, fingers, toes, knee, elbows, scalp, nails), mainly in areas of mechanical friction.

Clinical Features

- Typically, gingival manifestations usually follow skin lesions and may appear in the form of *desquamative gingivitis* or as localized or extensive bullae formation that ruptures leaving painful erosions (Fig. 26.38). Gingival recession and periodontal destruction may also occur in severe cases (Fig. 26.39).
- The oral mucosa shows bullae that soon rapture, leaving painful erosions or ulcerations which occasionally lead to scarring. Microstomia, symphyses and epithelial atrophy, elimination of tongue movement, elimination of vestibular and buccal sulci, lobulated hyperplastic nodules, pitted enamel and dental caries may occur (Fig. 26.40).
- Occasionally, leukoplakia and squamous cell carcinoma may develop on the atrophic lesions; mainly in the dystrophic type and Kindler syndrome (Fig. 26.41).

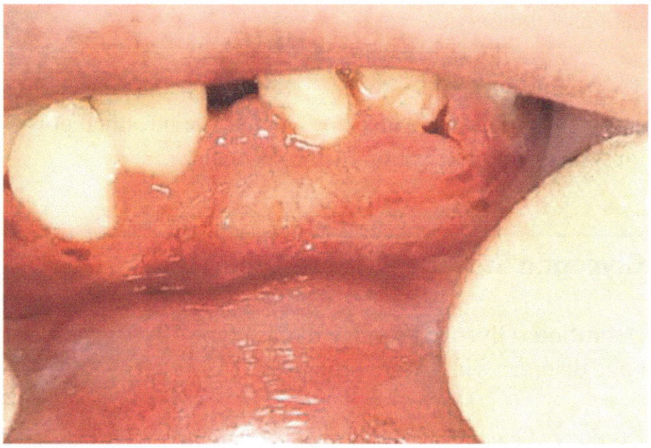

Fig. 26.38 Hereditary epidermolysis bullosa type II gingival erosions and enlargement

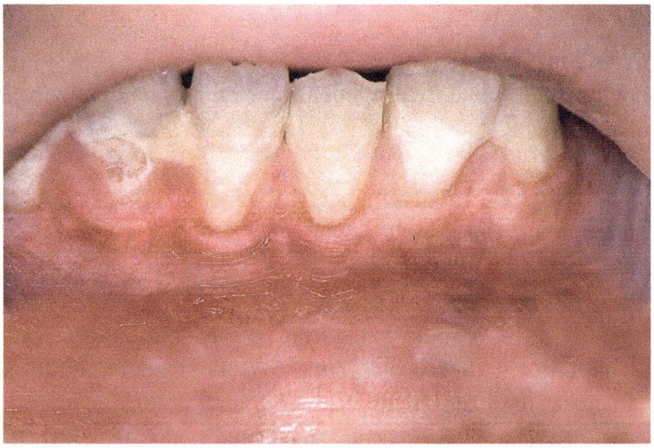

Fig. 26.39 Epidermolysis bullosa, dystrophic type, gingival recession and periodontitis

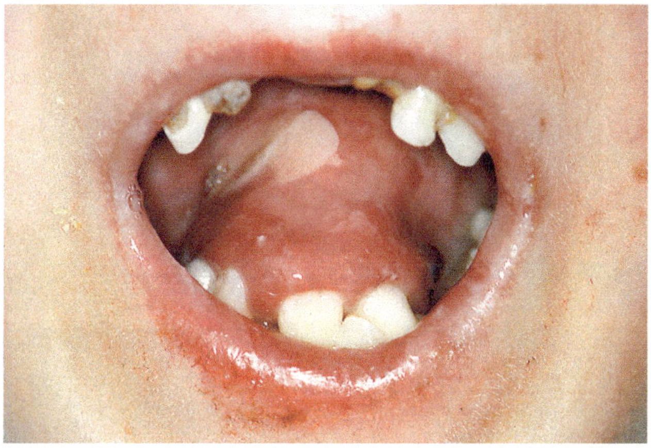

Fig. 26.40 Epidermolysis bullosa, dystrophic type, scaring on the tongue, lips and mouth stenosis

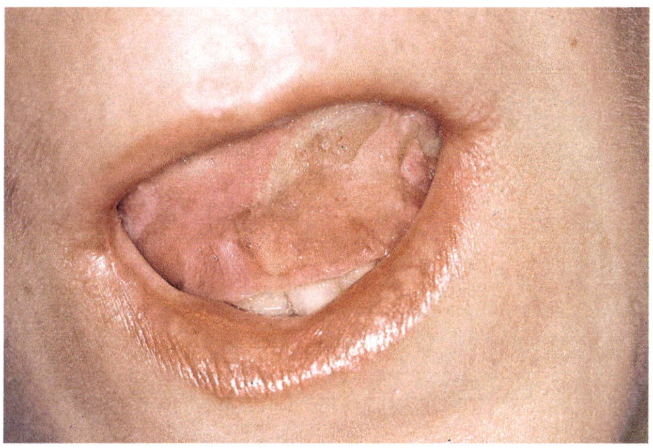

Fig. 26.41 Epidermolysis bullosa, dystrophic type, squamous cell carcinoma on the tongue

- Clinically, cutaneous manifestations are characterized by bullae formation, ulcerations, scarring, deformities, milia, nail dystrophy, and several others (Figs. 26.42 and 26.43). All occur mainly in areas of mechanical friction and pressure.
- The clinical manifestations of the disorder present early in life (infants and children) and the severity of skin and mucosal lesions depend on the type of the disease.
- Diagnosis is based on clinical and laboratory criteria.

Differential Diagnosis

- Mucous membrane pemphigoid
- Bullous pemphigoid
- Pemphigus vulgaris
- Linear IgA disease
- Epidermolysis bullosa acquisita
- Bullous dermatoses of childhood

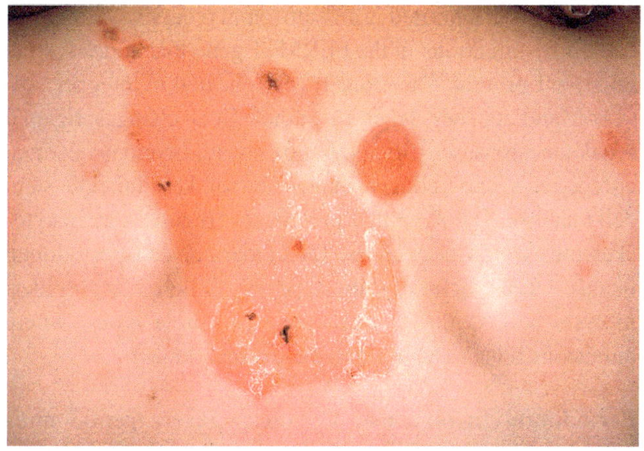

Fig. 26.42 Epidermolysis bullosa, dystrophic type, skin erythema, atrophy and ulcerations

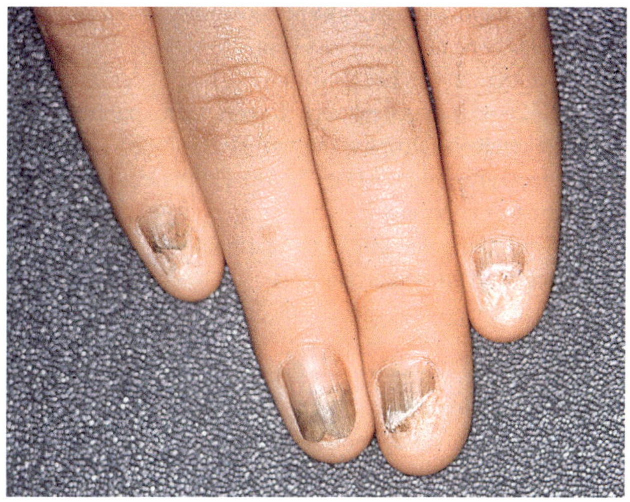

Fig. 26.43 Epidermolysis bullosa, dystrophic type, nail dystrophy

Laboratory Tests Histopathologic examination, immunofluorescent antigen mapping. Electron microscopic examination. Immunohistochemical examination. Molecular and genetic testing for mutations in the COL7A1 gene.

Treatment Supportive. There is no effective treatment for any of the types of the disease. Avoid pressure on the gingiva and oral mucosa. Good oral hygiene. Topical corticosteroid application. Use of systemic corticosteroids in severe cases.

Kindler Syndrome

Definition It is the type IV of hereditary epidermolysis bullosa, with some specific characteristics, which have been described by T. Kindler (1954) and later by P. Weary (1974).

Etiology It is inherited in an autosomal recessive trait and is caused by mutations in the FERMT1 gene that codes for the Kindlin-1 protein. This protein is implicated in integrin activation and its lack leads to pathological changes beyond focal adhesions, with disruption of several hemidesmosomal components and reduced expression of keratinocyte stem cell markers. The Kindlin-1 protein also regulates actin cytoskeleton, which is essential for epidermal and periodontal health. Ultrastructurally, the type IV of hereditary epidermolysis bullosa differs from the other three types, where cutaneous blisters form (mixed cleavage planes).

Periodontal Involvement Common. Severe periodontitis with alveolar bone loss that progresses rapidly, independently of dental biofilm-induced lesions.

Clinical Features

- Severe, rapidly progressive periodontitis, associated with alveolar bone and tooth loss (Fig. 26.44).
- Poikiloderma, photosensitivity and conjunctivitis (Fig. 26.45), mechanically fragile skin, palmoplantar hyperkeratosis, atrophy, and wrinkling of the skin (hands and feet) are common (Fig. 26.46). Colitis, ectropion, and phimosis may occur.
- Ep (oral, skin, bladder) may occasionally develop in association with Kindler syndrome.
- Clinical diagnosis should be confirmed by laboratory tests.

Differential Diagnosis

- Other types of epidermolysis bullosa
- Rothmund-Thomson syndrome
- Cockayne syndrome

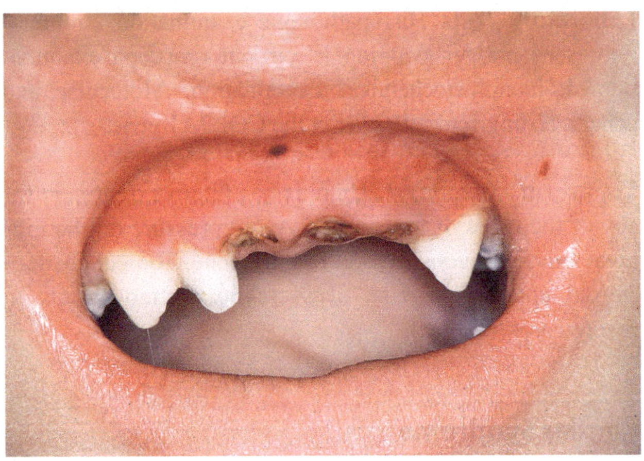

Fig. 26.44 Kindler syndrome, severe periodontitis and tooth loss

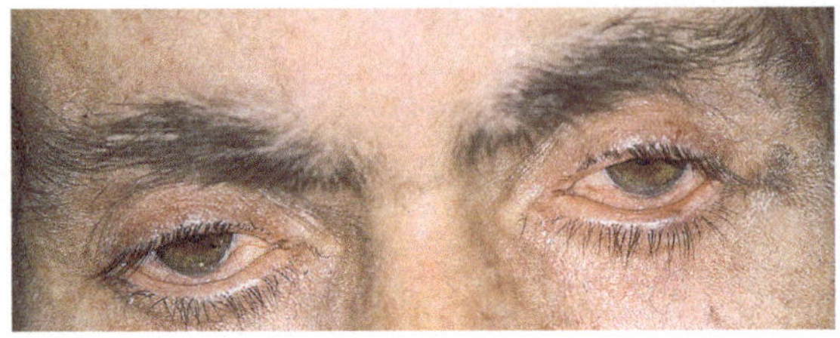

Fig. 26.45 Kindler syndrome, conjunctivitis

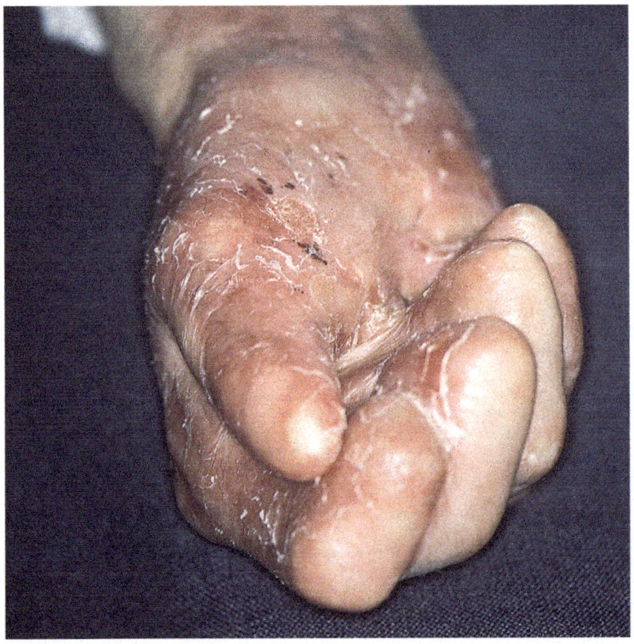

Fig. 26.46 Kindler syndrome, palmoplantar hyperkeratosis with scarring and dystrophy

Laboratory Tests Histopathologic and Immunohistochemical examination, genetic testing for mutations in the FERMT1 gene.

Treatment It is symptomatic. Regular periodontal examination is recommended. Recently, promising treatments include: pluripotent stem cells, revertant mosaicism, bone marrow stem cells, injection of allogeneic fibroblasts, and gene therapy. All of them must be left to specialists.

Hereditary Gingival Fibromatosis

Definition Hereditary gingival fibromatosis is a rare genetic disorder that may exist as an isolated disease entity or as part of a syndrome.

Etiology Genetic. As a single disease entity, it may be sporadic or may be transmitted as an autosomal dominant or rarely autosomal recessive trait.

Gingival Involvement Exclusively present. Non-dental biofilm-induced gingival lesions.

Other Sites of Involvement No other involvement in isolated cases. May vary according to the syndrome it is associated with.

Clinical Features

- The characteristic clinical feature is severe generalized gingival overgrowth covering the teeth (Figs. 26.47 and 26.48). The gingiva is smooth, usually normal in color, and of firm consistency.
- Appear during childhood and occasionally delay eruption of teeth.
- Clinical diagnosis should be confirmed by laboratory tests.

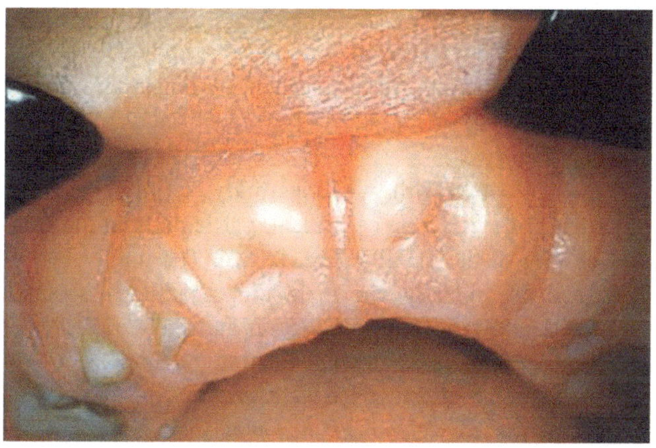

Fig. 26.47 Hereditary gingival fibromatosis, generalized gingival enlargement covering the teeth

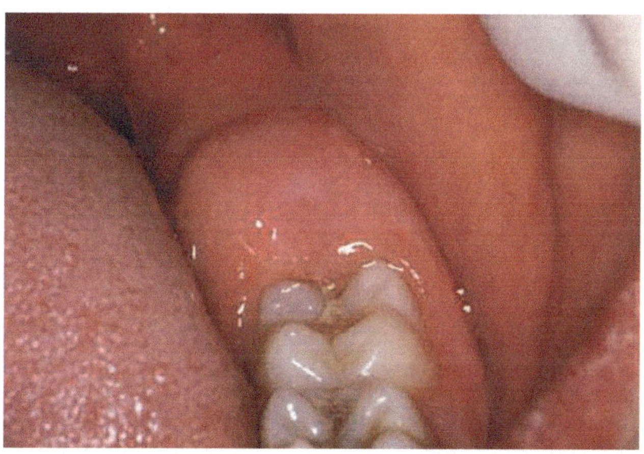

Fig. 26.48 Hereditary gingival fibromatosis, localized early gingival enlargement

Differential Diagnosis

- Several syndromes associated with gingival fibromatosis (e.g., Zimmermann-Laband, Cross, Ramon, Rutherford)
- Drug-induced gingival overgrowth
- Familial acanthosis nigricans
- Orofacial granulomatosis
- Crohn disease
- Amyloidosis
- Leukemia
- Wegenergranulomatosis

Laboratory Tests Histopathologic examination. Genetic testing.

Treatment Gingivectomy. Good oral hygiene for dental biofilm control.

Hereditary Hemorrhagic Telangiectasia

Definition Hereditary hemorrhagic telangiectasia, or Osler-Rendu-Weber disease, is a relatively rare disorder characterized by permanent small dilations of vessels.

Etiology Genetic. It is inherited as an autosomal dominant trait.

Gingival Involvement Rare, Non-dental biofilm-induced lesions.

Other Sites of Involvement Oral mucosa (tongue, lips, buccal mucosa, palate). Other mucosae (nasal, esophagus, genital), skin, internal organ (liver, spleen, gastrointestinal tract, lungs).

Clinical Features

- The gingival lesions appear as small (usually 1–3 mm in size), localized or multiple, bright red macules or nodules, which characteristically disappear when pressure is applied (Figs. 26.49 and 26.50). Frequent gingival bleeding, usually during or after tooth brushing.
- Oral manifestations are characterized by multiple telangiectasias with rare bleeding (Fig. 26.51). Persistent or frequent nose bleeding is usually the first and most common clinical sign of the disease.
- Multiple telangiectasias on the skin and gastrointestinal tract are common.
- Liver and spleen vascular abnormalities may be less frequent.
- The disease usually manifests during the second or third decade of life.
- Diagnosis is mainly based on clinical criteria.

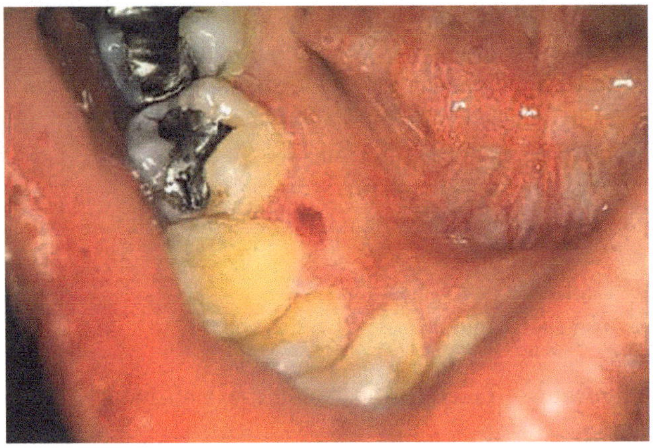

Fig. 26.49 Hereditary hemorrhagic telangiectasia, solitary red lesion on the gingiva

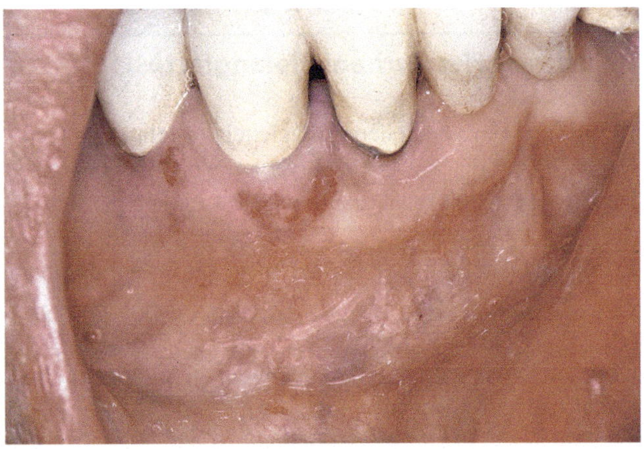

Fig. 26.50 Hereditary hemorrhagic teleangiectasia, small, multiple gingival lesions

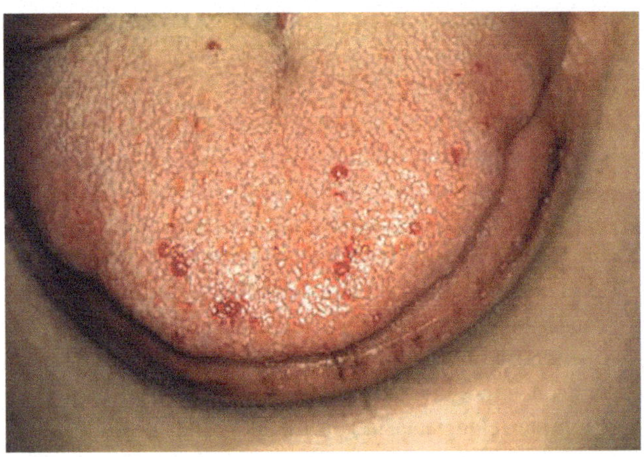

Fig. 26.51 Hereditary hemorrhagic telangiectasia, multiple red lesions on the tongue

Differential Diagnosis

- CREST syndrome
- Fabry disease
- Maffucci syndrome

Laboratory Tests Histopathologic examination.

Treatment Usually no treatment is required for oral lesions. If lesions often bleed, surgical excision or laser therapy is recommended.

Hurler Syndrome

Definition Hurler syndrome is a rare disorder—the most common and severe—in the group of mucopolysaccharide metabolic disorders.

Etiology Genetic. It is inherited as an autosomal recessive trait. The basic defect is the deficiency of the enzyme alpha-L-iduronidase which results in an accumulation of heparan and dermatan sulfates within the tissues and their excessive excretion in the urine.

Gingival Involvement Common. Dental and non-dental biofilm-induced lesions.

Other Sites of Involvement Oral mucosa and teeth, skeletal, cornea, internal organs (liver, spleen, heart, lungs, and others).

Clinical Features

- Gingival overgrowth, which partially or fully covers the crowns of teeth, may be present, particularly in the anterior area of the maxilla (Fig. 26.52). The gingival overgrowth is probably due to mouth breathing associated with dental biofilm accumulation and the deposition of heparan and dermatan sulfates within the gingiva.
- Other oral manifestations include macrocheilia, macroglossia, open mouth with protruding tongue, numerous impacted teeth, large interdental spaces, and teeth dislocation.
- Growth retardation, craniofacial malformations, characteristic facies, scoliosis, stiff joints, and chondrodystrophy are common.

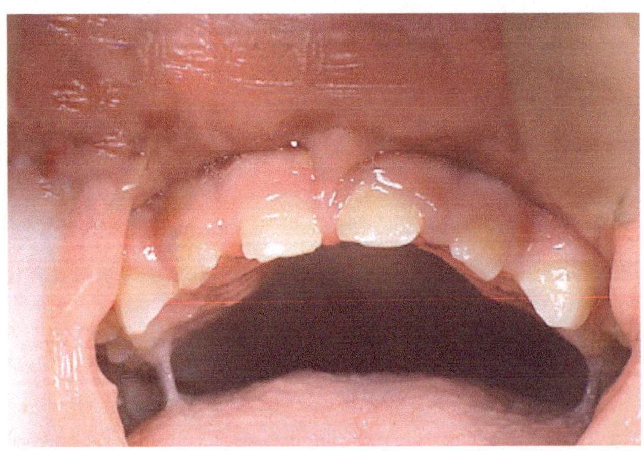

Fig. 26.52 Hurler syndrome, mild gingival enlargement

- Corneal clouding that frequently leads to blindness, learning disability, cardiac failure, hypertension, and lung infection may also occur.
- The disease presents during infancy and often leads to death usually before the patient reaches 10 years of age.
- Diagnosis is based on clinical and laboratory criteria.

Differential Diagnosis
- Hereditary gingival fibromatosis
- Mouth-breathing gingivitis
- Other forms of mucopolysaccharidoses
- Alpha-mannosidosis

Laboratory Tests Histochemical evaluation of alpha-L-iduronidase. Detection of heparan and dermatan sulfates in the urine. Radiographic examination, genetic testing.

Treatment Good oral hygiene and gingivectomy. Management of dental problems. Supportive for the other manifestations.

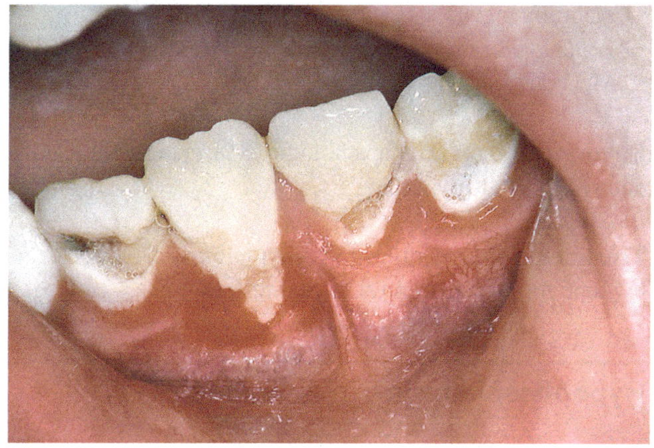

Fig. 26.53 Hypomelanosis of Ito, gingival inflammation, enamel hypoplasia and teeth decay

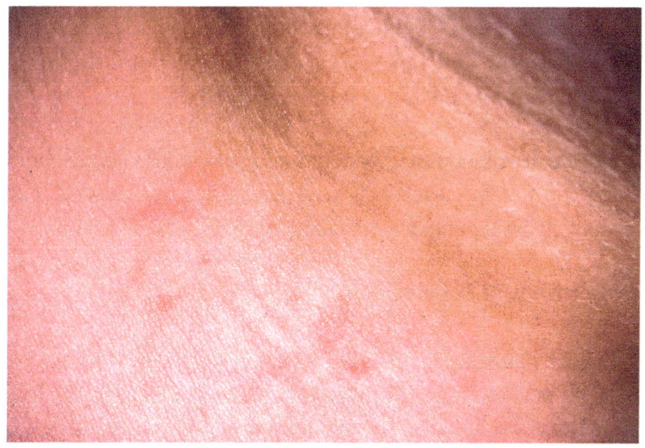

Fig. 26.54 Hypomelanosis of Ito, cutaneous hypopigmented area

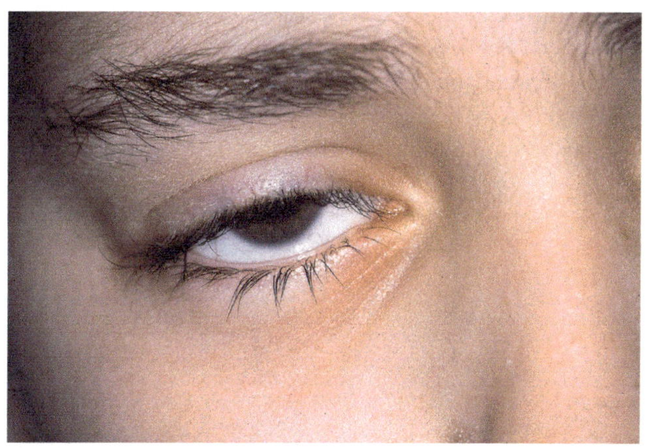

Fig. 26.55 Hypomelanosis of Ito, conjuctivitis

Hypomelanosis of Ito

Definition Hypomelanosis of Ito is a descriptive term for hypopigmentation distributed along *Blaschko's lines.*

Etiology It may be the result of chromosomal *mosaicism* without a clear genetic causative fingerprint.

Gingival Involvement Rare. Usually dental biofilm-induced gingivitis.

Other Sites of Involvement Dentition, skin, musculoskeletal, ocular, cardiac, CNS.

Clinical Features
- The disease usually appears after birth or during infancy and early childhood.
- Gingival lesions present as nonspecific inflammatory gingivitis, usually dental biofilm-induced (Fig. 26.53).
- Other oral disorders are dental anomalies, e.g., enamel and dentin hypoplasia, conical and pitted anterior deciduous teeth, multiple cusps teeth, brown-yellow crowns.
- The main clinical features are cutaneous lesions, such as hypopigmented whorls or lines or plaques that follow *Blaschko's lines* (Fig. 26.54). The lesions can be bilateral or unilateral and are common on the trunk and extremities. Hypertrichosis, alopecia, lentigines, nail, and hair abnormalities may occur.
- Extracutaneous abnormalities such as ocular, cardiac, musculoskeletal, and CNS may develop (Fig. 26.55).
- The clinical diagnosis should be confirmed by laboratory tests.

Differential Diagnosis
- Other genetic forms of hypomelanosis
- Vitiligo
- Leukoderma

- Achromicnevus
- Goltz syndrome
- McCune-Albright syndrome

Laboratory Tests Histopathologic examination of the cutaneous lesions. Karyotyping.

Treatment The treatment is symptomatic. Good oral hygiene for biofilm control, dental restorations.

Hypophosphatasia

Definition Hypophosphatasia is a rare inherited enzyme deficiency disorder, characterized by decreased serum and tissue alkaline phosphate production and activity.

Etiology Genetic. It is usually inherited as an autosomal recessive trait and rarely as an autosomal dominant trait. Mutations in the alkaline phosphatase (ALPL) gene.

Gingival Involvement Very common, particularly in the childhood form of the disease. Severe periodontitis associated with genetic disorder, unrelated to dental biofilm-induced lesions.

Other Sites of Involvement Skeleton, skull, eyes.

Clinical Features
- The periodontal manifestations include early severe loss of alveolar bone and premature loss of deciduous and permanent teeth in the absence of an inflammatory response (Fig. 26.56). Patients experience early exfoliation of primary teeth, especially anterior teeth, which may be the only clinical sign of the disease.
- Skeletal abnormalities, growth retardation, craniosynostosis, intracranial hypertension may occur.
- Diagnosis is made by history and clinical features and may be supplemented by laboratory tests.

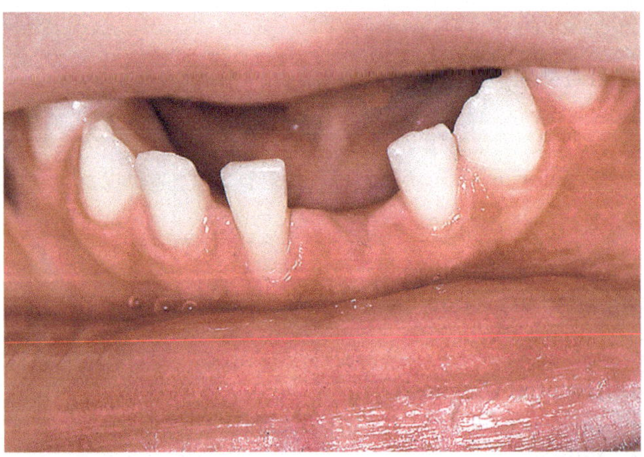

Fig. 26.56 Hypophosphatasia, tooth loss in a 10-year-old child

Differential Diagnosis
- Localized severe periodontitis
- Acatalasia
- Papillon-Lefèvre syndrome
- Chédiak-Higashi syndrome
- Glycogen storage disease Ib

Laboratory Tests Panoramic dental radiography and radiographic examination of the skeleton and skull. Measurement of serum alkaline phosphatase as well as of phosphoethanolamine levels in blood and urine. Genetic testing for mutations in the ALPL gene.

Treatment Good oral hygiene. Vitamin D, phosphorus, and parathormone have been used with poor results.

Juvenile Hyaline Fibromatosis and Infantile Systemic Hyalinosis

Definition Juvenile hyaline fibromatosis and infantile systemic hyalinosis are rare severe autosomal recessive inherited disorders characterized by hyaline accumulation, mainly in skin, oral mucosa, and other organs.

Etiology Genetic. Mutations in the gene (ANTXR2), that encodes capillary morphogenesis protein-2 (CMG2) are responsible for the development of these two disorders. However, there is a different expression to severity and involvement of internal organs.

Gingival Involvement Common. Gingival overgrowth unrelated to dental biofilm for both varieties.

Other Sites of Involvement Oral mucosa, skin, joints, bones, viscera.

Clinical Features
- There are numerous similarities and clinical overlap between juvenile hyaline fibromatosis and infantile systemic hyalinosis which suggest that both disorders are a spectrum of the same disease entity with varying phenotypic expression.
- Clinically, severe generalized gingival overgrowth is one of the most common and classic manifestation in both varieties of the disorder (Figs. 26.57 and 26.58). Palatal mucosa overgrowth, limited mouth opening, eating and speech difficulties, and temporomandibular joint dysfunction are also common.
- The skin lesions are common and are characterized by firm pearly papules and nodules on hands, fingers, toes, knees, face (usually perioral and perinasal region), trunk, and ears and diffuse skin thickening (Figs. 26.59 and 26.60).

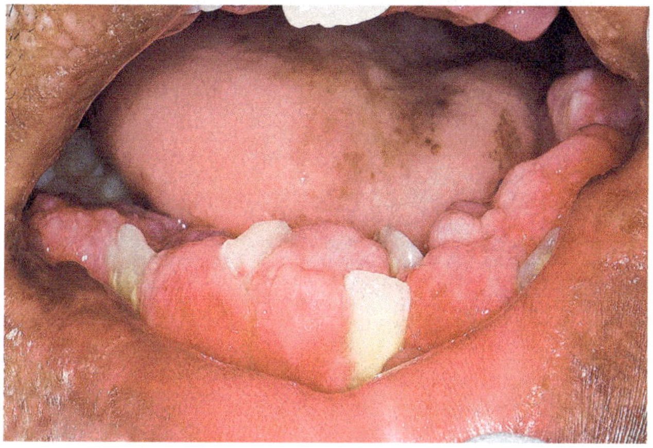

Fig. 26.57 Juvenile hyaline fibromatosis, generalized gingival enlargement

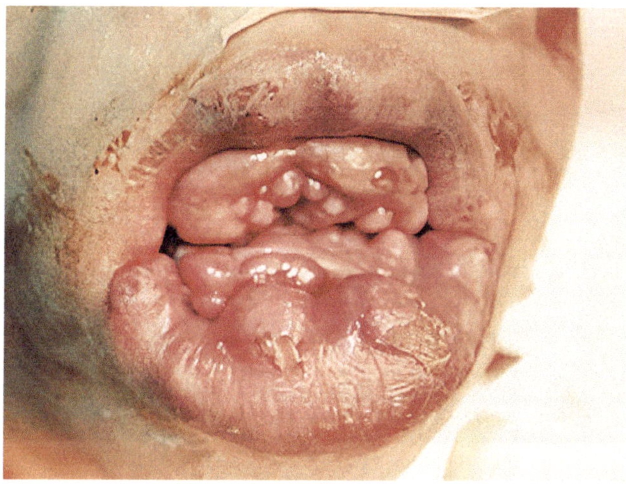

Fig. 26.58 Infantile systemic hyalinosis, severe gingival enlargement and lip nodules

- Infantile systemic hyalinosis is the severe variant involving multiple internal organs, usually associated with recurrent infections, starting in infancy and commonly conduct to death during early childhood. Juvenile hyaline fibromatosis starts during childhood and has a better prognosis.
- Diagnosis is mainly based on the history and clinical features but should be confirmed by laboratory tests.

Differential Diagnosis
- Hereditary gingival fibromatosis.
- Zimmermann-Laband syndrome.
- Drug-induced gingival overgrowth.
- Winchester syndrome.
- Nodulosis–arthropathy–osteolysis syndrome.

Laboratory Tests Histopathologic examination, genetic testing.

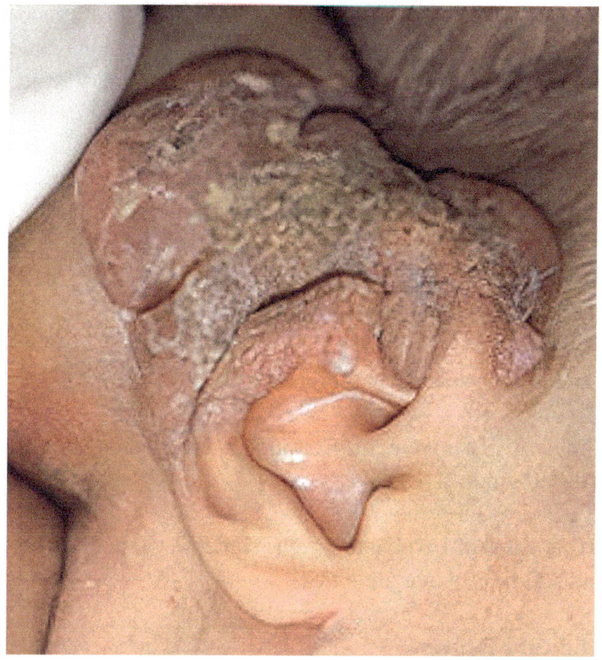

Fig. 26.59 Juvenile hyaline fibromatosis, enormous nodules on the ear and the skin

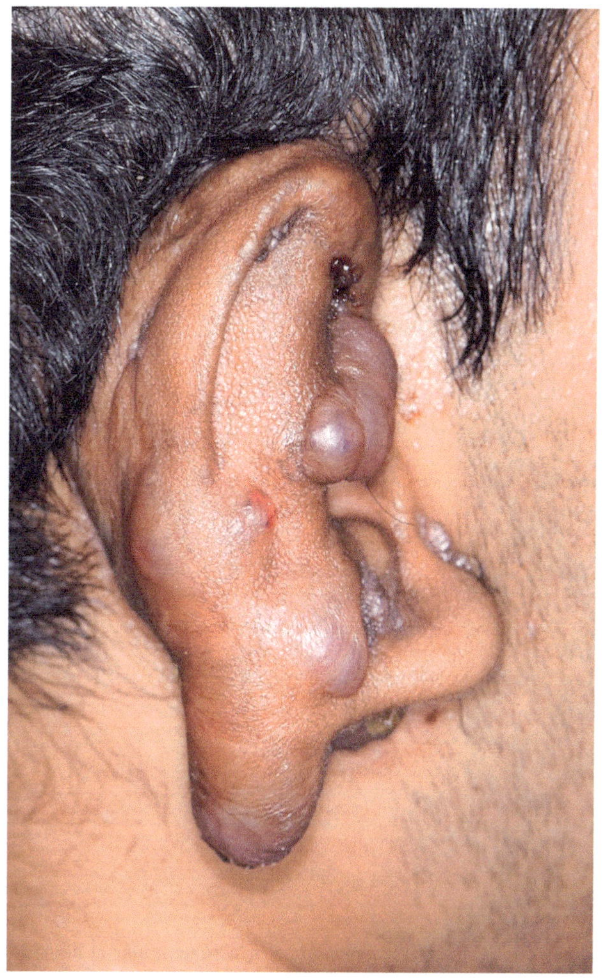

Fig. 26.60 Juvenile hyaline fibromatosis, multiple nodules on the ear

Treatment Surgical excision of gingival and oral mucosal overgrowth and high level of oral hygiene. The management of the other manifestations need a multidisciplinary team of specialists to improve the patient's quality of life.

Klippel-Trénaunay-Weber Syndrome

Definition Klippel-Trénaunay-Weber syndrome is an uncommon dysplastic vascular disorder.

Etiology Dysplastic malformation.

Gingival Involvement Common. Non-dental biofilm-induced gingival lesions.

Other Sites of Involvement Oral mucosa, skin, eyes, bone, and soft tissues of extremities.

Clinical Features

- Gingival lesions appear as capillary or cavernous hemangiomas, occasionally leading to gingival overgrowth that may cover the crown of the teeth (Fig. 26.61). Premature tooth eruption and alveolar bone overgrowth may occur. Oral lesions are mainly hemangiomas, especially on the hard and soft palate.
- Multiple facial hemangiomas, ocular disorders (scleral pigmentation, glaucoma, cataract, iris heterochromia), vascular masses that involve soft tissue and bone leading to asymmetrical enlargement of the extremities, hemangiomas in internal organs are common (Figs. 26.62 and 26.63).
- Diagnosis is mainly based on clinical criteria.

Differential Diagnosis

- Isolated hemangiomas
- Sturge-Weber angiomatosis
- Maffucci syndrome

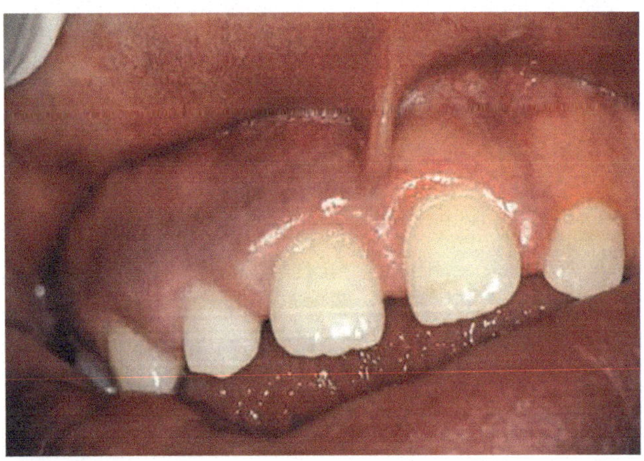

Fig. 26.61 Klippel-Trénaunay-Weber syndrome, gingival hemangiomas leading to gingival overgrowth

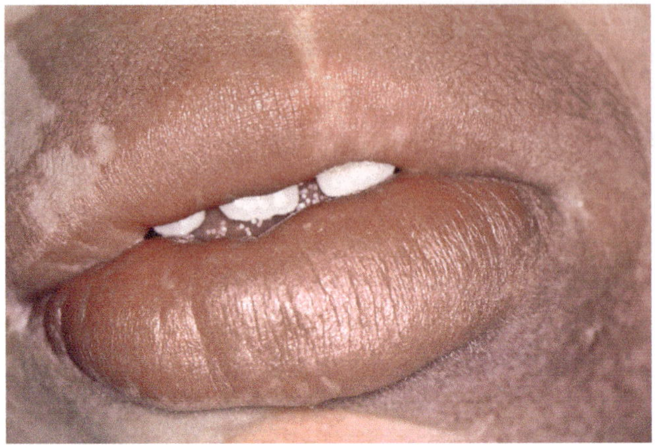

Fig. 26.62 Klippel-Trénaunay-Weber syndrome, hemangiomas of the lips and face

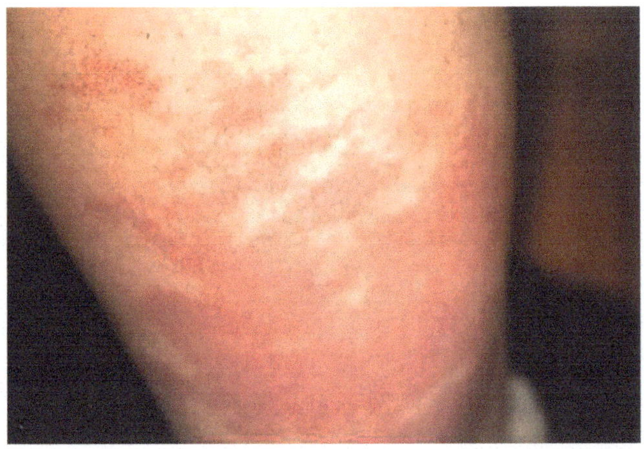

Fig. 26.63 Klippel-Trénaunay-Weber syndrome, skin hemangiomas of the leg

Laboratory Tests Histopathologic examination, CT scan.

Treatment Palliative. Laser may improve skin lesions.

Leukocyte Adhesion Deficiency Syndromes

Definition Leukocyte adhesion deficiency (LAD) syndromes consist of three autosomal disorders that affect the ability of leukocytes to adhere to blood vessel walls, preventing migration to tissue infection resulting in recurrent infections.

Etiology Genetic. LAD-1 is caused by mutations in the ITGB2 gene that encodes CD18. LAD-2 is caused by mutations in the FUCT1 gene that encodes a GDP-fucose transporter and LAD-3 is caused by loss of function, leading to mutations in the FERMT3 gene that encodes kindling-3.

Gingival Involvement Common. Dental biofilm-induced lesions associated with selective immune dysfunction that helps dental biofilms to flourish, causing severe periodontitis.

Other Sites of Involvement Severe recurrent bacterial and fungal infections mainly of the skin, mucosae, lungs, and other organs.

Clinical Features

- Severe recurrent infections of the skin, pneumonia, and otitis media, usually associated with bleeding.
- Severe gingival inflammation and early-onset rapidly progressive severe periodontitis leading to the loss of primary and permanent teeth are the most common manifestations of LAD (Figs. 26.64 and 26.65).
- The clinical hallmark of the disease is the absence of pus formation of the lesions (non-purulent infections).

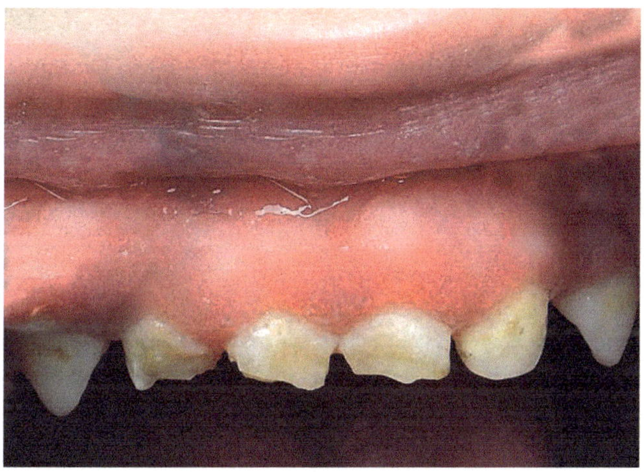

Fig. 26.64 Leukocyte adhesion deficiency (LAD) syndrome, severe gingival inflammation and enamel hypoplasia

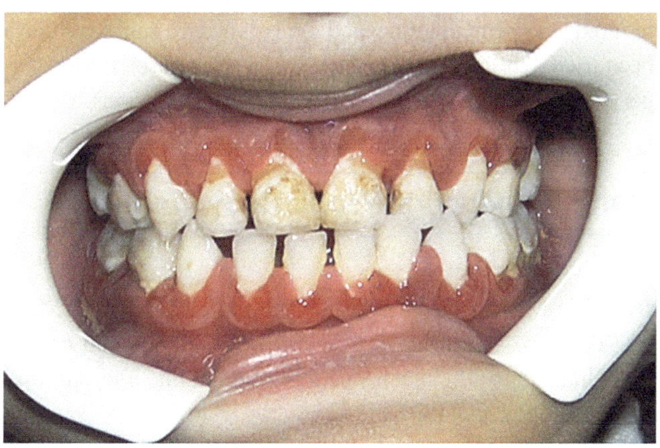

Fig. 26.65 Leukocyte adhesion deficiency (LAD) syndrome, generalized gingival inflammation and periodontitis

- Minor skin trauma may lead to formation of large necrotic ulcerations, clinically similar to *pyoderma gangrenosum*. Delayed wound healing and separation of the umbilical stump, developmental bone disorders, and mental retardation are common findings. The prognosis is poor.
- The clinical diagnosis should be confirmed by laboratory tests.

Differential Diagnosis

- Other forms of acute early-onset severe periodontitis
- Chédiak-Higashi syndrome
- Severe combined immunodeficiency
- Severe congenital neutropenia
- Other primary immunodeficiency disorders

Laboratory Tests Genetic testing, flow cytometry analysis.

Treatment Antibiotics. Stem cell transplant in severe cases. High level of periodontal and oral hygiene is suggested. Systemic treatment must be handled by a team of specialists.

Lipoid Proteinosis

Definition Lipoid proteinosis or hyalinosis cutis et mucosae or Urbach-Wiethe disease is a rare genetic metabolic disorder affecting the skin and mucosae.

Etiology Genetic. An autosomal recessive metabolic disorder due to mutations in the extracellular matrix protein 1 (ECM1) gene. It is characterized by hyaline-like material deposition around blood vessels and in the connective tissue of the skin and mucous membranes.

Gingival Involvement Rare. Non-dental biofilm-induced gingival lesions.

Other Sites of Involvement Oral mucosa, larynx, skin, brain.

Clinical Features

- Clinically, the first clinical sign of the disease is hoarseness and the inability of the baby to cry, due to infiltration of a glycoprotein and lipids containing amorphous material of the laryngeal mucosa.
- Cutaneous lesions usually develop during the second year of life and are characterized by blisters and hemorrhagic crusts mainly on the face and extremities. Papules, nodules, and plaques of yellow discoloration are common, particularly on the face, eyelids, neck, axillae, hands and elbows, knees, scalp, and scrotum (Figs. 26.66 and 26.67).

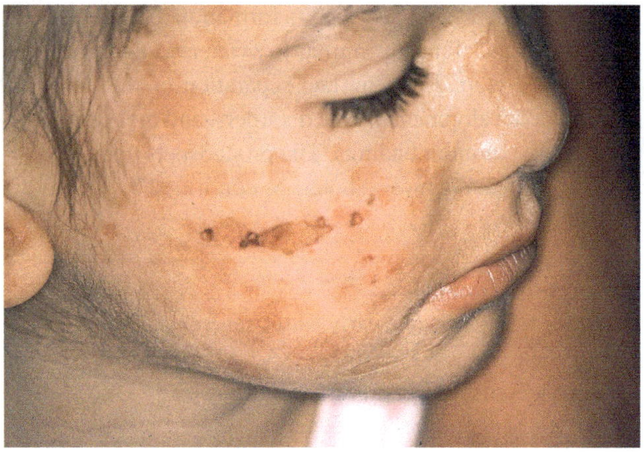

Fig. 26.66 Lipoid proteinosis, skin papules, nodules and plaques

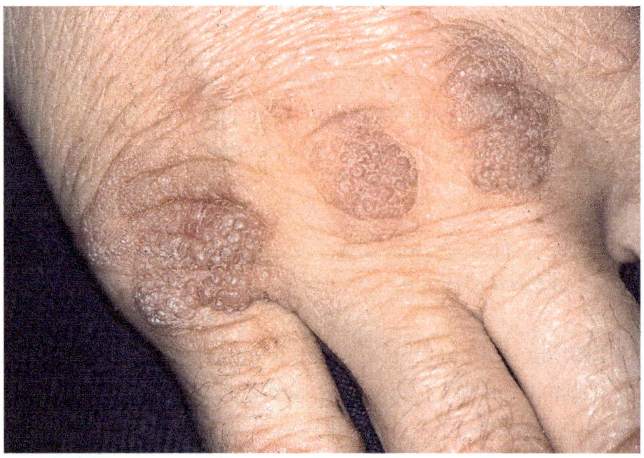

Fig. 26.67 Lipoid proteinosis, nodules on the hands

Later, verrucous lesions and scars are formed that are the typical skin changes.

- The oral mucosa lesions are characterized by vesicles, erosions, tongue and lips induration, short and thick lingual frenum resulting in reduced mobility of the tongue (Fig. 26.68). Occlusion of the salivary ducts, hypodontia, dental hypoplasia, or aplasia may occur.
- Gingival involvement appears as enlargement mainly of the interdental papillae and the free gingiva (Fig. 26.69).
- Finally, neurologic disorders (seizures, abnormal behavior) are common.
- Diagnosis is based predominantly on the history and clinical features and less on laboratory tests.

Differential Diagnosis

- Systemic sclerosis
- Erythropoietic protoporphyria
- Primary systemic amyloidosis
- Juvenile hyaline fibromatosis
- Infantile systemic hyalinosis
- Papular mucinosis

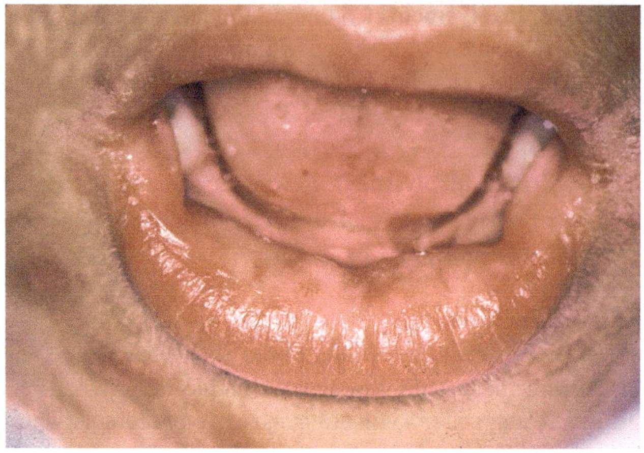

Fig. 26.68 Lipoid proteinosis, erosions on the lips and tongue

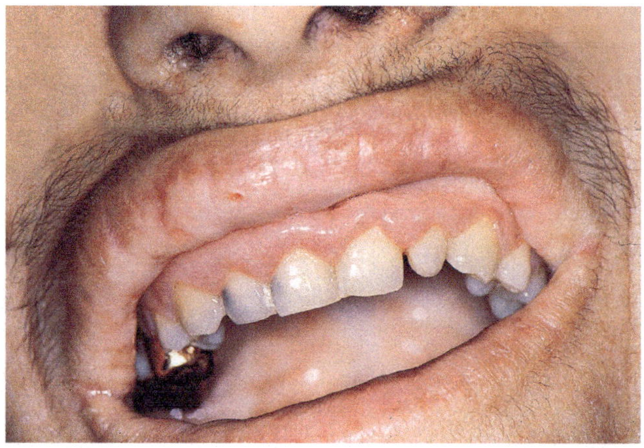

Fig. 26.69 Lipoid proteinosis, gingival enlargement and lip induration

Laboratory Tests Genetic testing, histopathologic examination.

Treatment Good periodontal and oral hygiene. Systemic treatment is symptomatic as there is no effective therapy. Systemic retinoids, D-penicillamine and oral dimethyl sulfoxine have been used, but they must be handled by specialists. Plastic surgery and dermabrasion have been used for skin lesions.

Multiple Endocrine Neoplasia Syndrome, Type 2B

Definition Multiple endocrine neoplasia, type 2B (MEN 2B) is a rare syndrome in the endocrine glands and causes medullary thyroid cancer, pheochromocytoma, and parathyroid gland cancer.

Etiology Genetic. It is transmitted by an autosomal dominant trait with high penetrance, but variable expressivity and it is caused by missense mutation in the RET proto-oncogene, which is located on chromosome sub-band 10q11.2 and encodes a tyrosine kinase receptor expressed in tissues and tumors derived from neural crest.

Gingival Involvement Rare. Non-dental biofilm-related lesions.

Other Sites of Involvement Oral mucosa (buccal, tongue, and lips), other mucosae, thyroid and adrenal glands, and bone.

Clinical Features

- Multiple neuromas involve gingiva and other areas of the oral cavity. They present the most distinct, characteristic, and constant clinical feature.
- Clinically, multiple neuromas appear as small, soft, asymptomatic papules or nodules, which are present in almost all patients and are usually the first sign of the disease and may develop during infancy (Fig. 26.70).
- Similar lesions are observed on the eyelid ridge, conjunctivae, cornea, laryngeal, and nasal mucosa.
- The most characteristic finding is the development of medullary thyroid carcinoma (>90%) and pheochromocytoma in the adrenal glands (50%), usually during the second or third decade of life.
- Clinical diagnosis should be confirmed by laboratory tests.

Differential Diagnosis

- Other types of this syndrome
- Neurofibromatosis
- Werner syndrome

Laboratory Tests Histopathologic examination, elevated levels of serum and urinary calcitonin (thyroid carcinoma), increased level of urinary vanillylmandelic acid (pheochromocytoma), genetic analysis.

Treatment Conservative surgical excision of oral neuromas only if they cause functional or esthetic problems. For the management of MEN 2B patients should be referred to a specialized clinic.

Neurofibromatosis, Type 1

Definition Neurofibromatosis type 1 or von Recklinghausen disease is the most common of the eight subtypes of neurofibromatosis and accounts for 80–90% of cases.

Etiology Genetic. It is inherited in an autosomal dominant trait.

Gingival Involvement Rare. Non-dental biofilm-induced lesions and no periodontal apparatus involvement.

Other Sites of Inv olvement Relatively common in oral mucosa (buccal mucosa, tongue, palate), but relatively rare in jaws. Skin is always involved. Various internal organs (stomach, heart, intestine, renal, bladder, etc.) are affected.

Clinical Features

- Gingival lesions are neurofibromas, which clinically present as slowly developing, painless, firm, and well circumscribed tumors that are usually covered by normal or whitish mucosa (Fig. 26.71). The size varies from several millimeters to centimeters.
- Similar lesions develop more often on the tongue, buccal mucosa, palate, and alveolar mucosa. Malocclusion, displaced teeth, and very rare jaw bone lesions may occur.
- Skin lesions are the major clinical feature and are always present. They usually appear as multiple cutaneous neurofibromas and *café au lait* macules and patches (Fig. 26.72).

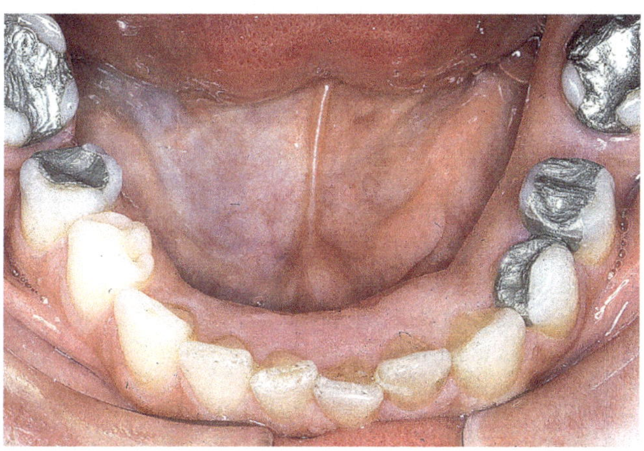

Fig. 26.70 Multiple endocrine neoplasia syndrome, type 2B (MEN), multiple small nodules on the lingual gingiva

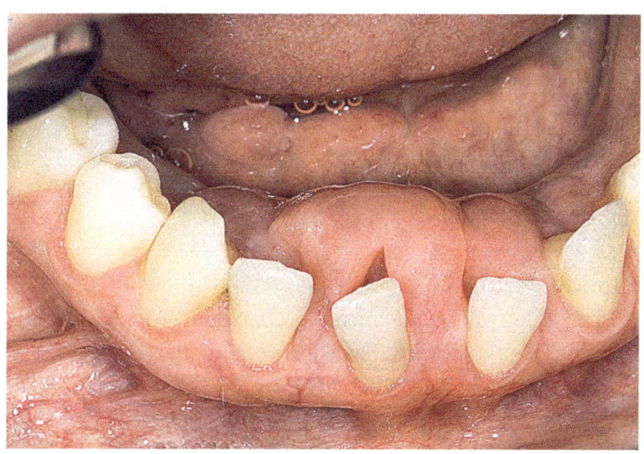

Fig. 26.71 Neurofibromatosis type I, multiple tumors (neurofibromas) on the lingual gingiva

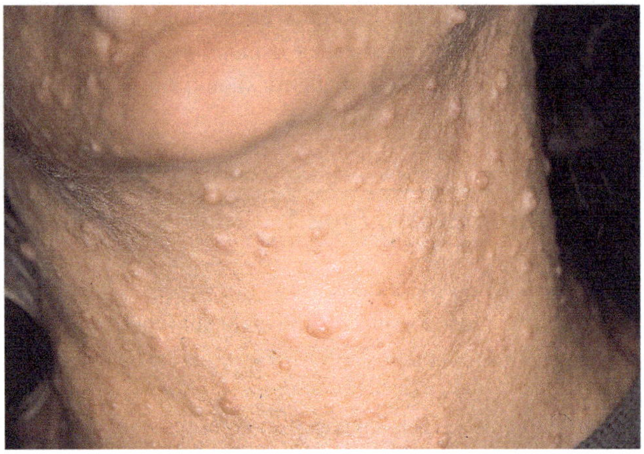

Fig. 26.72 Neurofibromatosis type I, multiple neurofibromas of the skin

Differential Diagnosis

- Other types of neurofibromatosis
- Multiple endocrine neoplasia syndrome types 1 and 2B
- Tuberous sclerosis
- Cowden disease
- McCune-Albright syndrome

Laboratory Tests Histopathologic examination. Computed tomography (CT) scan monitoring. Genetic testing.

Treatment Conservative surgical excision of oral neurofibromas.

Orofaciodigital Syndrome Type I

Definition Orofaciodigital syndrome type I is an uncommon disorder in the group of orofaciodigital syndrome.

Etiology Genetic It is inherited as an X-linked dominant trait. It predominantly affects females and is lethal in males.

Gingival Involvement Common. Mucogingival deformities. Aberrant and non-dental biofilm-related gingivitis.

Other Sites of Involvement Oral mucosa, teeth, facies, digits, skin.

Clinical Features

- The gingival involvement is characterized by multiple hyperplastic fibrous bands traversing the gingivolabial and gingivobuccal fold, hypertrophy and shortening of the frenulum of the lips and tongue (Fig. 26.73). These may result in hyperplastic gingivitis and gingival recession (Fig. 26.74).

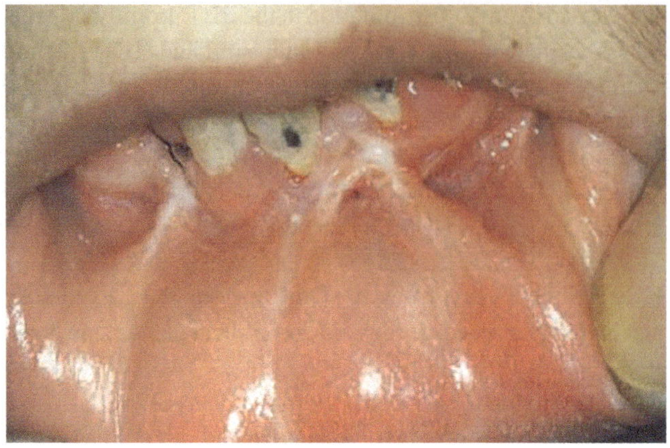

Fig. 26.73 Orofaciodigital syndrome type I, multiple gingivolabial frenula

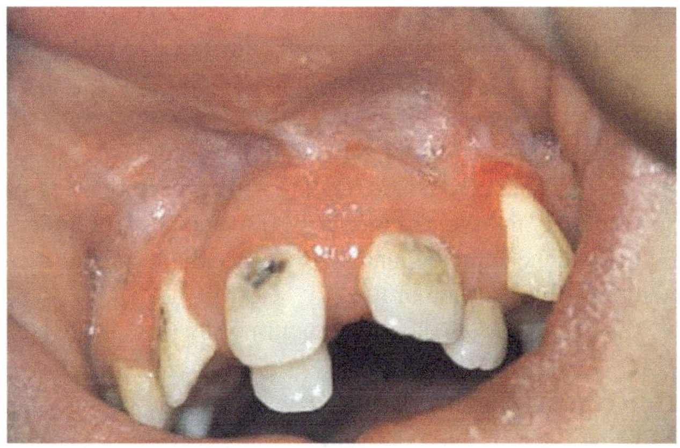

Fig. 26.74 Orofaciodigital syndrome type I, gingivitis and gingival enlargement

- Oral lesions include multilobed or bifid tongue with multiple hamartomas, lips and palate clefts, supernumerary teeth, tooth malposition and missing teeth, and hypoplastic mandible.
- Frontal bossing, ocular hypertelorism, short upper lip, broad nasal root, asymmetry of the nostrils, polydactyly, brachydactyly, clinodactyly, and syndactyly are common (Figs. 26.75 and 26.76).
- Skin manifestations include xeroderma, milia, alopecia, and sparse hair. Learning disability and polycystic kidneys may occasionally occur.
- Diagnosis is mainly based on clinical criteria.

Differential Diagnosis

- Orofaciodigital syndrome type II
- Chondroectodermal dysplasia
- Oculodento digital syndrome

Laboratory Tests Radiographic examination, skin biopsy, and histopathologic examination.

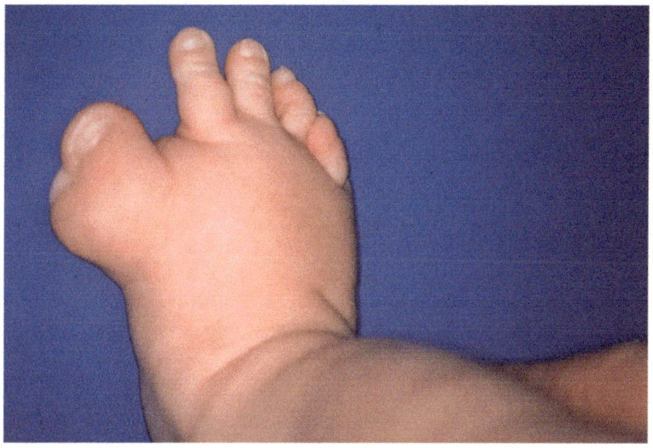

Fig. 26.75 Orofaciodigital syndrome type I, syndactyly

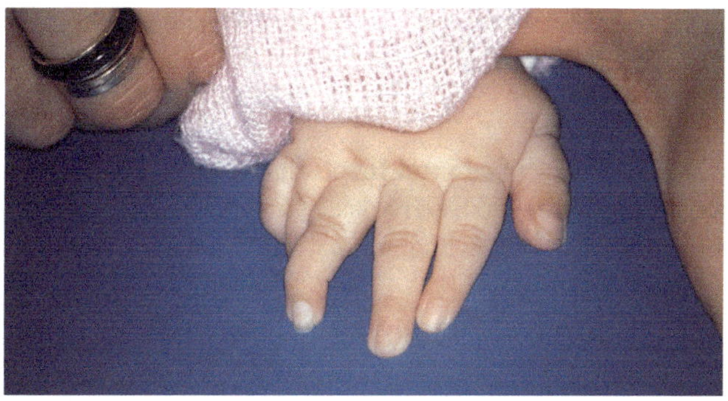

Fig. 26.76 Orofaciodigital syndrome type I, polydactyly and clinodactyly

Treatment Surgical reconstruction of oral frenulum and gingivolabial and gingivobuccal folds. Symptomatic for the rest of the lesions.

Papillon-Lefèvre Syndrome

Definition Papillon-Lefèvre syndrome (PLS) is a rare genetic disorder characterized by periodontal and skin manifestations.

Etiology Genetic. It is inherited as an autosomal recessive trait. The genetic mutation is within cathepsin C (CTSC), an enzyme that coordinates activation of proteases necessary for immune cell function. Periodontal lesions are due to multiple leukocyte dysfunctions. Subgingival plaque samples from periodontal pockets of PLS cases contain primarily *Actinobacillus actinomycetemcomitans*.

Gingival Involvement Always present. Periodontitis associated with genetic and immunologic disorders, unrelated to dental biofilm-induced lesions.

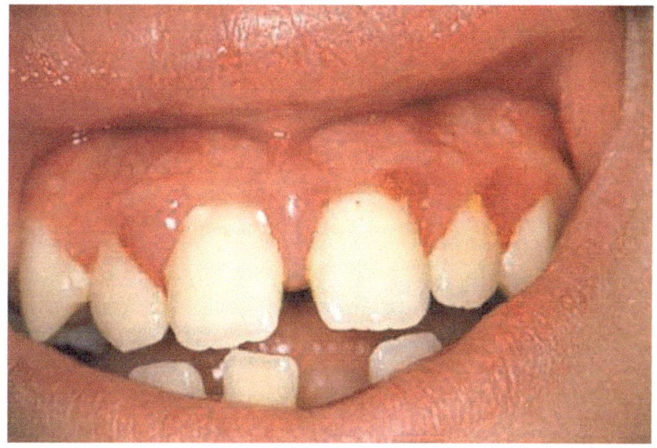

Fig. 26.77 Papillon-Lefèvre syndrome, severe periodontitis in a 13 year old boy

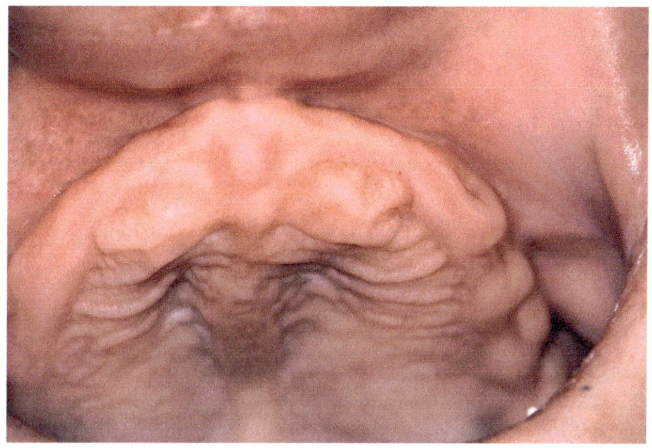

Fig. 26.78 Papillon-Lefèvre syndrome, premature tooth loss

Other Sites of Involvement Skin, always present (palms, soles, elbows, knees, dorsum of the fingers and toes), liver, kidney, and brain.

Clinical Features

- Clinically, the gingiva appears red, swollen, and bleeds easily. Early onset of severe generalized periodontitis with deep periodontal pockets and bone loss is the characteristic clinical feature (Fig. 26.77). Mobility, migration, and premature loss of deciduous and permanent teeth in the order of their eruption is the rule (Fig. 26.78).
- Skin lesions are characterized by hyperkeratosis of palms and soles.
- (Figs. 26.79 and 26.80). Hyperkeratosis and diffuse red and scaly patches may occur in other skin areas.
- Diagnosis is mainly based on clinical criteria.

Differential Diagnosis

- Generalized severe periodontitis
- Haim-Munk syndrome

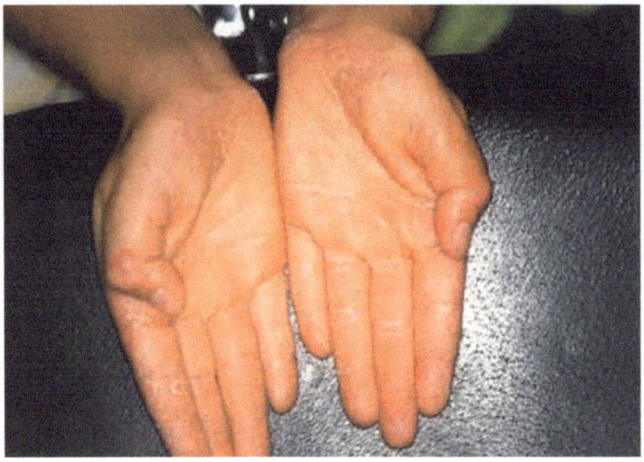

Fig. 26.79 Papillon-Lefèvre syndrome, hyperkeratosis of the palms

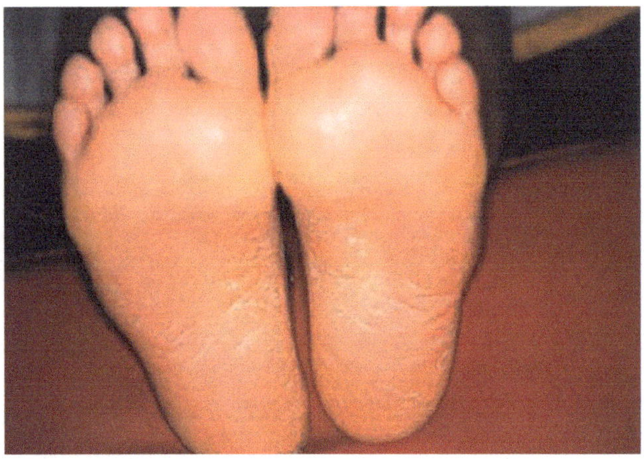

Fig. 26.80 Papillon-Lefèvre syndrome, hyperkeratosis of the soles

- Hypophosphatasia
- Acatalasia
- Chédiak-Higashi syndrome
- Langerhans cell histiocytosis
- Glycogen storage disease Ib
- Congenital neutropenia
- Cyclic neutropenia

Laboratory Tests Panoramic radiography. Skin biopsy and histopathologic examination. Genetic testing for mutations in the lysosomal protease cathepsin C (CTSC) gene on chromosome 11q14.

Treatment Good oral hygiene for dental biofilm control. Aromatic retinoids for skin lesions.

Haim-Munk Syndrome

Definition Haim-Munk syndrome is a rare genetic disorder of keratinization related to Papillon-Lefèvre syndrome.

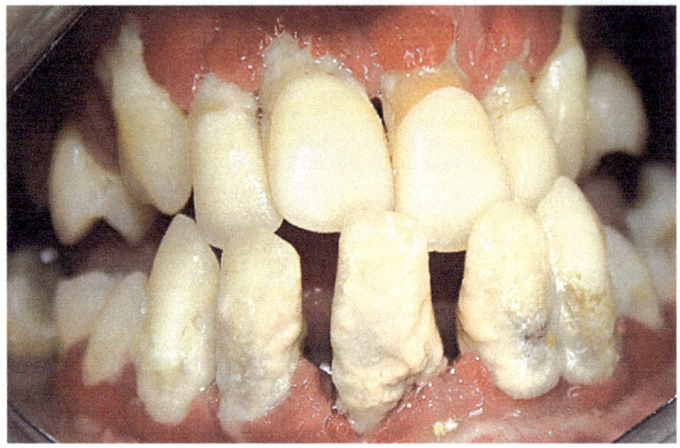

Fig. 26.81 Haim-Munk syndrome, severe periodontitis

Etiology Genetic. It is transmitted by an autosomal recessive trait. Mutation in the lysosomal protease cathepsin C (CTSC) gene mapped to chromosome11q14.1-q14.3.

Gingival and Periodontal Involvement Common. Severe, dental biofilm-related, early-onset gingivitis and severe periodontitis associated with immunologic disorders.

Other Sites of Involvement Skin, nails, skeletal manifestations.

Clinical Features

- The periodontal manifestations in Haim-Munk syndrome are common and are characterized by early gingival inflammation soon after eruption of teeth and severe periodontitis associated with attachment loss and early loss of teeth in both deciduous and permanent dentition (Fig. 26.81).
- Other classic clinical features include palmoplantar hyperkeratosis (Fig. 26.82), arachnodactyly, onychogryphosis, and acro-osteolysis.
- Diagnosis is based on the history and clinical features as well as on laboratory tests.

Differential Diagnosis

- Papillon-Lefèvre syndrome
- Hypohidrotic ectodermal dysplasia
- Hypophosphatasia
- Accatalacia
- Severe early-onset periodontitis
- Chédiak-Higashi syndrome

Laboratory Tests Genetic testing. Radiographic examination.

Treatment Good oral hygiene for dental biofilm control, root scaling, and planning for periodontitis. The lesions in other organs should be treated by specialists.

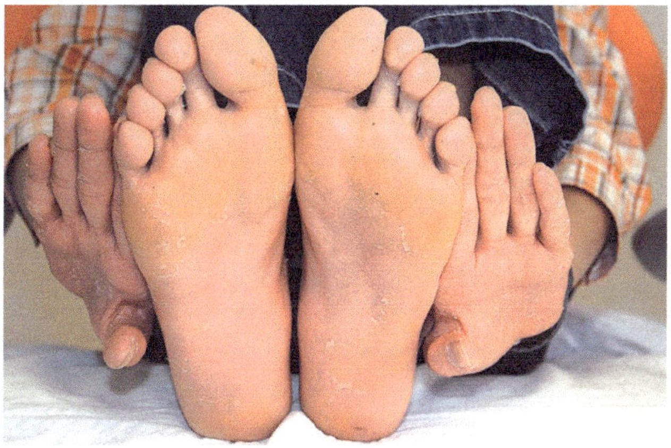

Fig. 26.82 Haim-Munk syndrome, palmoplantar hyperkeratosis

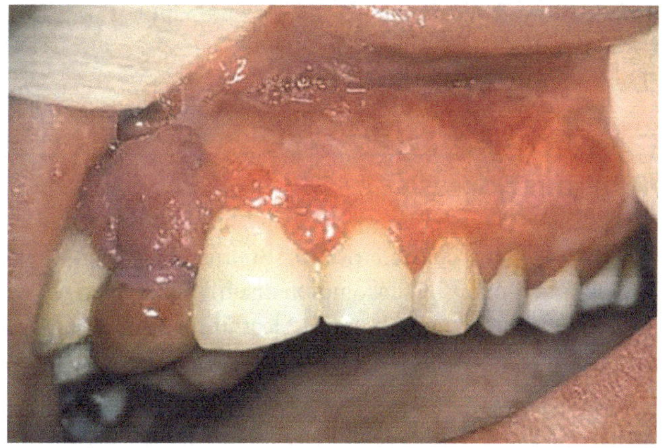

Fig. 26.83 Sturge-Weber angiomatosis, unilateral gingival hemangiomas of the maxilla

Sturge-Weber Angiomatosis

Definition Sturge-Weber angiomatosis or encephalotrigeminal angiomatosis is a rare sporadic congenital hamartomatous vascular disorder typically involving areas innervated by the trigeminal nerve.

Etiology Obscure; developmental abnormality.

Gingival Involvement Relatively common. Non-dental biofilm-induced gingival lesions.

Other Sites of Involvement Oral mucosa, skin, eyes, central nervous system.

Clinical Features

- Hemangiomas tend to be unilateral, and usually are capillary. Lesions arise from attached gingiva or alveolar mucosa and they may occasionally lead to gingival hyperplasia and premature or delayed eruption (Figs. 26.83 and 26.84). Lesions have a bright red or purple color and are usually flat. Dentists must be careful during tooth extraction and periodontal surgery to avoid bleeding complications. Unilateral oral hemangiomas on the buccal mucosa, tongue, and lips may occur.
- Unilateral facial hemangioma is the most common lesion. It is clinically evident at birth and is limited to the area supplied by the trigeminal nerve (Fig. 26.85).
- Hemangiomas of the leptomeninges, brain calcification, epilepsy, and ocular disorders may also be present.
- Diagnosis is usually based on clinical criteria.

Differential Diagnosis

- Solitary hemangioma
- Klippel-Trénaunay-Weber syndrome

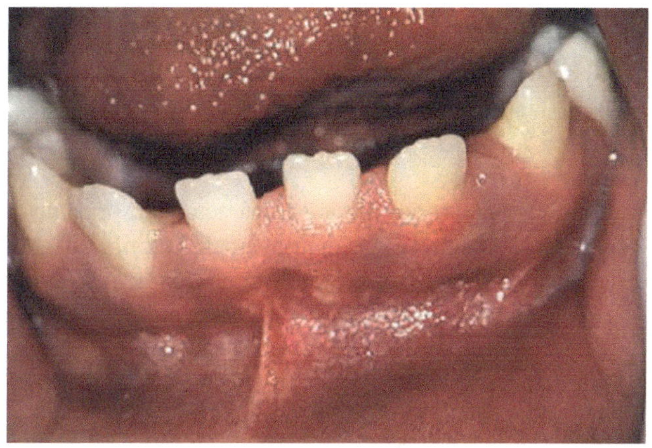

Fig. 26.84 Sturge-Weber angiomatosis, unilateral gingival hemangiomas of the mandible

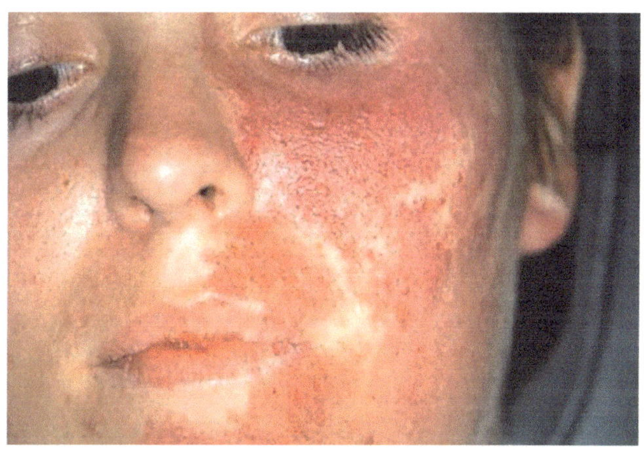

Fig. 26.85 Sturge-Weber angiomatosis, unilateral facial hemangiomas

Laboratory Tests Histopathologic examination, CT scan.

Treatment Laser therapy is recommended.

Tuberous Sclerosis

Definition Tuberous sclerosis or Bourneville-Pringle syndrome or epiloia, is an uncommon disorder characterized by mucocutaneous angiofibromas, learning disability, and seizures.

Etiology Genetic. It is inherited as an autosomal dominant trait with variable expressivity.

Gingival Involvement Relatively common (10–15%). Non-dental biofilm-induced gingival lesions.

Other Sites of Involvement Oral mucosa, rare. Skin, always. Central nervous system and others (retinal, heart, kidneys, lungs).

Clinical Features

- Gingival lesions are the most characteristic oral manifestations and present as multiple, painless, fibrous nodules with smooth surface and normal or whitish color (Figs. 26.86 and 26.87). The anterior gingiva is more frequently affected. Oral mucosal lesions, although less often, are similar to those seen on gingiva. Cleft palate and lip, vaulted palate, macroglossia, and enamel pits may occur.
- Skin disorders are common and present as multiple, small, red to brown nodules (*angiofibromas*), mainly in the nasolabial folds and elsewhere in the face (Fig. 26.88). Periungual fibromas can also be seen.

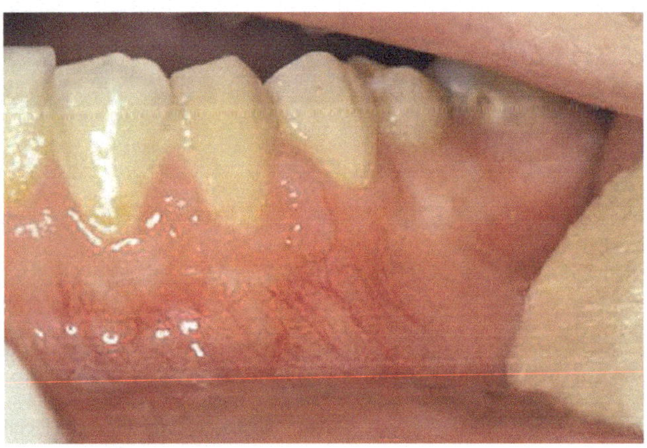

Fig. 26.86 Tuberous sclerosis, solitary nodule on the gingiva

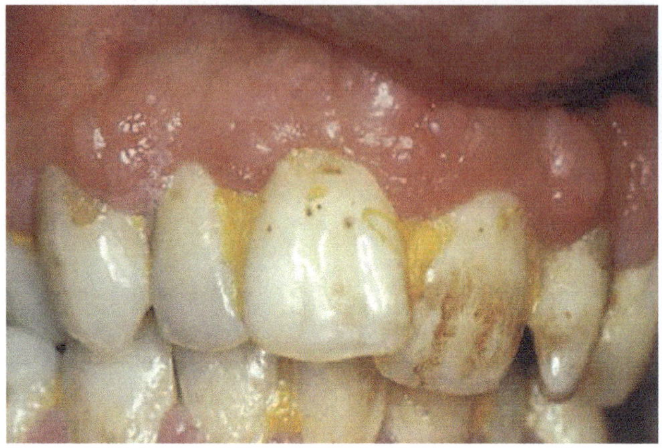

Fig. 26.87 Tuberous sclerosis, multiple nodules on the gingiva

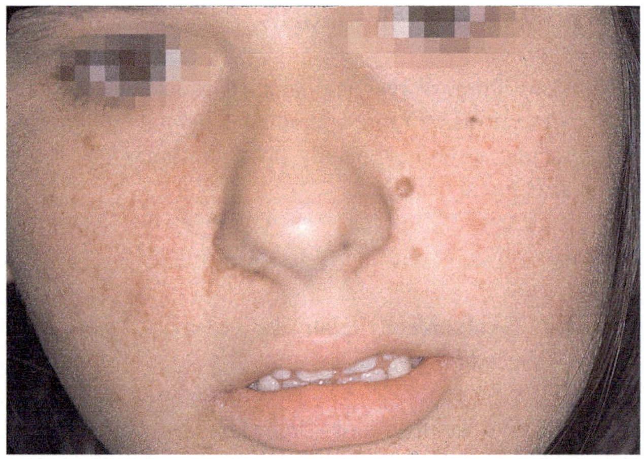

Fig. 26.88 Tuberous sclerosis, brown skin nodules on the face (angiofibromas)

- Learning disability, seizures, and neural hamartomas are common.
- Cardiac rhabdomyoma, multiple retinal hamartomata, lung, and renal abnormalities may also occur.
- Diagnosis is based on clinical and laboratory criteria.

Differential Diagnosis

- Cowden disease
- Neurofibromatosis
- Lipoid proteinosis
- Acanthosis nigricans, familial
- Focal dermal hypoplasia syndrome

Laboratory Tests Histopathologic examination of cutaneous and oral lesions. Brain CT scan, electroencephalography, genetic testing.

Treatment Symptomatic. Surgical excision of gingival lesions only for esthetic purposes.

White Sponge Nevus

Definition White sponge nevus, or Cannon disease, is a relatively uncommon genetic disorder that primarily affects the oral mucosa.

Etiology Genetic. It is inherited as an autosomal dominant trait.

Gingival Involvement Rare. Non-dental biofilm-induced lesions.

Other Sites of Involvement Oral mucosa (buccal, tongue, floor of the mouth, lips) is always affected. Other mucosae (vaginal, rectal, esophageal, nasal), rarely.

Clinical Features

- Gingival lesions present as painless, white or grey-white thickenings with multiple furrows, or diffuse plaques with a spongy texture (Fig. 26.89).
- Similar lesions appear, more often, in other sites of the oral mucosa (Fig. 26.90).
- Oral lesions become fully fledged by the second decade of life and remain relatively stable thereafter.
- Diagnosis is based on clinical and laboratory criteria.

Differential Diagnosis

- Leukoplakia
- Focal palmoplantar and oral mucosa hyperkeratosis syndrome
- Pachyonychia congenita
- Dyskeratosis congenita

Laboratory Tests Histopathologic examination. Cytology is also useful.

Treatment No treatment is available. Surgical excision of gingival lesions only for esthetic purposes.

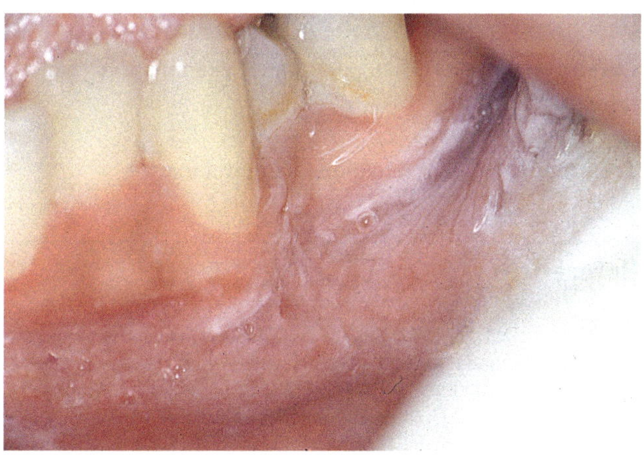

Fig. 26.89 White sponge nevus, white lesions on the alveolar mucosa and gingiva

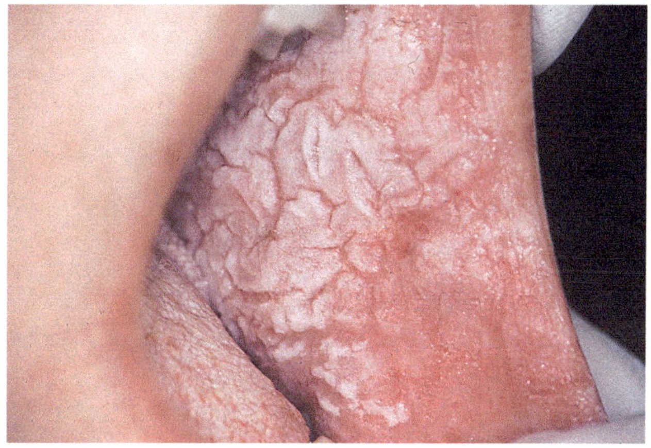

Fig. 26.90 White sponge nevus, white lesions on the buccal mucosa

Wiskott-Aldrich Syndrome

Definition Wiskott-Aldrich syndrome is a rare inherited disease characterized by immune dysregulation and congenital thrombocytopenia and small platelets.

Etiology Genetic. It is inherited in an X-linked recessive trait, arising from mutation in WASp gene.

Gingival Involvement Rare. Non-dental biofilm-related lesions, modified by primary immunodeficiency.

Other Sites of Involvement Blood, skin, kidney, lymphoreticular malignancy, autoimmune diseases.

Clinical Features

- The main disorders of Wiskott-Aldrich syndrome are congenital thrombocytopenia (70.000 platelets/mm^3) and small platelets (mean platelet volume < 5.0 fL). The clinical features associated with the syndrome include skin eczema, recurrent bacterial and viral infections, IgA nephropathy, high incidence of autoimmune diseases, lymphoreticular malignancies, and hemolytic anemia.
- The periodontal manifestations are not specific and include gingival inflammation, ulcerations, and increased tendency for bleeding (Fig. 26.91). Oral mucosal petechiae are common.
- The clinical diagnosis should be confirmed by laboratory tests.

Differential Diagnosis

- Other thrombocytopenic diseases
- Von Willebrand disease
- Antithrombotic drug therapy
- Myelodysplastic syndrome

Laboratory Tests Genetic testing. Blood and bone marrow molecular tests.

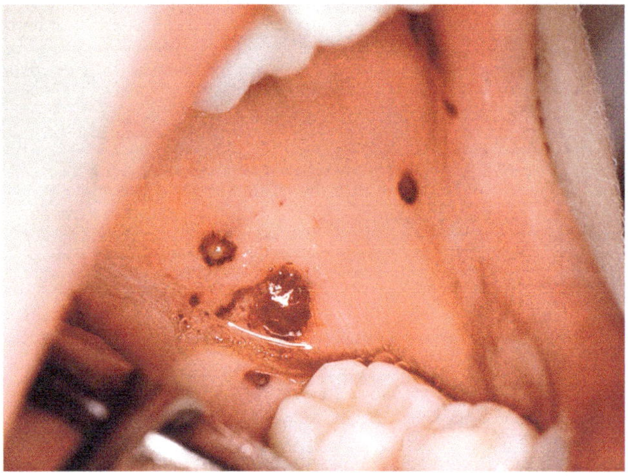

Fig. 26.91 Wiskott-Aldrich syndrome, gingival and buccal hemorrhagic lesions

Treatment Good oral hygiene. The systemic treatment should be left to specialists.

Zimmermann-Laband Syndrome

Definition Zimmermann-Laband syndrome is a rare disorder characterized by a broad spectrum of lesions.

Etiology Genetic. It is inherited as an autosomal dominant trait.

Gingival Involvement Always present. Non-dental biofilm-induced gingival lesions with no attachment loss.

Other Sites of Involvement Oral mucosa, skin, facies, skeletal, liver, spleen.

Clinical Features

- Gingival fibromatosis is the predominant intraoral feature. It is manifested at birth or within the first 2 months of life. The excess gingival tissue covers the crowns of the teeth partially or completely (Fig. 26.92). The enlarged gingiva is usually lobulated and slightly firm on palpation.
- Macroglossia and enlargement of the lips are less common.
- Large nose and pinnae, hypoplastic or absent thumb nails, rudimentary or missing terminal phalanges, pes cavus, joint hypermobility and hirsutism are common (Fig. 26.93).
- Hepatomegaly, splenomegaly, and learning disability may be noted.
- Diagnosis is mainly based on clinical criteria.

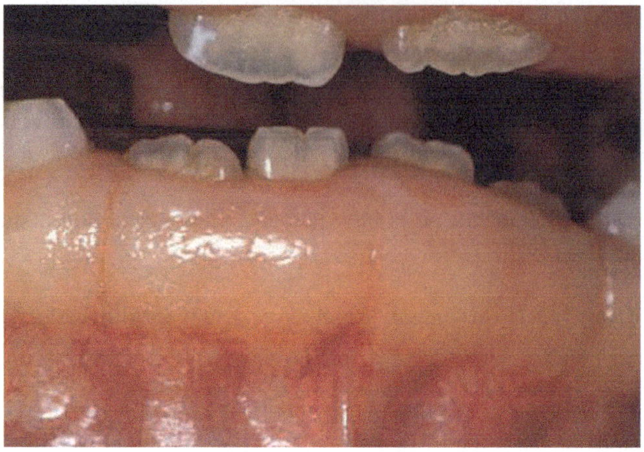

Fig. 26.92 Zimmermann-Laband syndrome, gingival enlargement, covering the crowns of the teeth

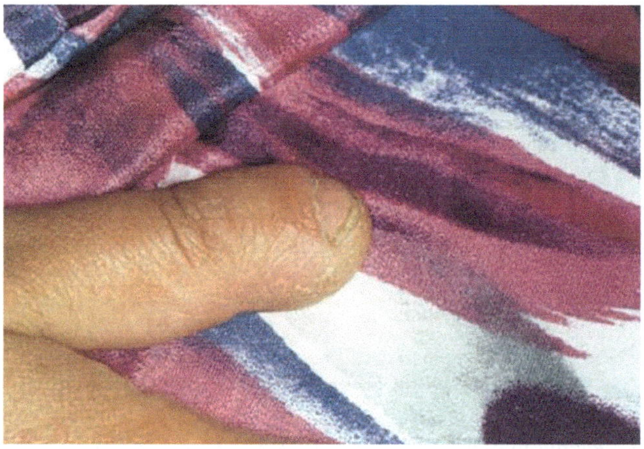

Fig. 26.93 Zimmermann-Laband syndrome, hypoplastic thumb nails

Differential Diagnosis

- Hereditary gingival fibromatosis
- Drug-influenced gingival enlargement
- Several syndromes associated with gingival fibromatosis (Rutherford, Murray-Puretic-Drescher, Cross and Ramon)
- Alpha-mannosidosis

Laboratory Tests Histopathologic examination, genetic testing.

Treatment Good oral hygiene. Gingivectomy.

References

1. Albandar JM, Susin C, Hughes FJ. Manifestations of systemic diseases and conditions that affect the periodontal attachment apparatus: case definitions and diagnostic considerations. J Periodontol. 2018;89:S183–203. https://doi.org/10.1002/JPER.16-0480.
2. Hanisch M, Hoffmann T, Bohner L, Hanisch L, Benz K, Kleinheinz J, Jackowski J. Rare diseases with periodontal manifestations. Int J

Environ Res Public Health. 2019;16(5):867. https://doi.org/10.3390/ijerph16050867. PMID: 30857312; PMCID: PMC6427617
3. Shankargouda P, Roopa SR, Barnali M. Chromosomal and multifactorial genetic disorders with oral manifestations. J Int Oral Health. 2014;6(5):118–25.
4. Nualart-Grollmus ZC, Morales-Chávez MC, Silvestre-Donat FJ. Periodontal disease associated to systemic genetic disorders. Med Oral Patol Oral Cir Bucal. 2007;12:E211–5.
5. Kanjanapongkul S. Chediak-Higashi syndrome: report of a case with uncommon presentation and review literature. J Med Assoc Thail. 2006;89:541–4.
6. Rezende KM, Canela AH, Ortega AO, et al. Chediak-Higashi syndrome and premature exfoliation of primary teeth. Braz Dent J. 2013;24(6):667–70. https://doi.org/10.1590/0103-6440201302258. PMID: 24474367
7. Ward DM, Shiflett SL, Kaplan J. Chediak-Higashi syndrome: a clinical and molecular view of a rare lysosomal storage disorder. Curr Mol Med. 2002;2(5):469–77. https://doi.org/10.2174/1566524023362339. PMID: 12125812
8. Aminabadi NA, Ebrahimi A, Oskouei SG. Chondroectodermal dysplasia (Ellis-van Creveld syndrome): a case report. J Oral Sci. 2010;52:333–6.
9. Dar-Odeh NS, Hayajneh WA, Abu-Hammad OA, et al. Orofacial findings in chronic granulomatous disease: report of twelve patients and review of the literature. BMC Res Notes. 2010;3:37.
10. Buduneli N, Baylas H, Aksu G, Kütükçüler N. Prepubertal periodontitis associated with chronic granulomatous disease. J Clin Periodontol. 2001;28(6):589–93. https://doi.org/10.1034/j.1600-051x.2001.028006589.x. PMID: 11350528
11. Donadieu J, Fenneteau O, Beaupain B, et al. Congenital neutropenia: diagnosis, molecular bases and patient management. Orphanet J Rare Dis. 2011;19(6):26. https://doi.org/10.1186/1750-1172-6-26. PMID: 21595885; PMCID: PMC3127744
12. Scheper MA, Nikitakis NG, Sarlani E, et al. Cowden syndrome: report of a case with immunohistochemical analysis and review of the literature. Oral Surg Oral Med Oral Pathol Oral Radiol Endod. 2006;101:625–31.
13. Chen Y, Fang L, Yang X. Cyclic neutropenia presenting as recurrent oral ulcers and periodontitis. J Clin Pediatr Dent. 2013;37(3):307–8. https://doi.org/10.17796/jcpd.37.3.n8k0111177074828. PMID: 23855177
14. Naehrig S, Chao CM, Naehrlich L. Cystic fibrosis. Dtsch Arztebl Int. 2017;114(33–34):564–74.
15. Elborn JS. Cystic fibrosis. Lancet. 2016;388(10059):2519–31.
16. Frezzini C, Cedro M, Leao JC, Porter S. Darier disease affecting the gingival and oral mucosal surfaces. Oral Surg Oral Med Oral Pathol Oral Radiol Endod. 2006;102:e29–33.
17. Rafii MS, Kleschevnikov AM, Sawa M, Mobley WC. Down syndrome. Handb Clin Neurol. 2019;167:321–36.
18. Rosso M, Fremion E, Santoro SL, et al. Down syndrome disintegrative disorder: a clinical regression syndrome of increasing importance. Pediatrics. 2020;145(6):e20192939.
19. Ashwinirani SR, Suragimath G. Oral and perioral manifestations in Down's syndrome patients. BLDE Univ J Health Sci. 2020;5:77–82.
20. Karunakaran A, Ravindran R, Arshad M, et al. Dyskeratosis congenita: a report of two cases. Case Rep Dent. 2013;2013:845125. https://doi.org/10.1155/2013/845125. Epub 2013 Aug 6. PMID: 23984114; PMCID: PMC3748431
21. Mitakides J, Brad D, Tinkle T. Oral and mandibular manifestations in the Ehlers–Danlos syndromes. Am J Med Genet. 2017.;Part C (Seminars in Medical Genetics);175C:220–5.
22. Kapferer-Seebacher I, Lundberg P, Malfait F, Zschocke J. Periodontal manifestations of Ehlers-Danlos syndromes: a systematic review. J Clin Periodontol. 2017;44(11):1088–100. https://doi.org/10.1111/jcpe.12807. Epub 2017 Sep 25. PMID: 28836281
23. Rahman N, Dunstan M, Teare MD, et al. Ehlers-Danlos syndrome with severe early-onset periodontal disease (EDS-VIII) is a distinct, heterogeneous disorder with one predisposition gene at chromosome 12p13. Am J Hum Genet. 2003;73(1):198–204. https://doi.org/10.1086/376416. Epub 2003 May 29. PMID: 12776252; PMCID: PMC1180581
24. de Araujo MR, et al. Fanconi's anemia: clinical and radiographic oral manifestations. Oral Dis. 2007;13(3):291–5. https://doi.org/10.1111/j.1601-0825.2006.01282.x. PMID: 17448211
25. Goswami M, Bhushan U, Goswami M. Dental perspective of rare disease of Fanconi anemia: case report with review. Clin Med Insights Case Rep. 2016;17(9):25–30. https://doi.org/10.4137/CCRep.S37931. PMID: 27013901; PMCID: PMC4798261
26. Touil D, Bouhouch R, Chebil RB, et al. Gingival bleeding in a child with Fanconi anemia: a case report and literature review. Case Rep Dent. 2020;9(2020):3161053. https://doi.org/10.1155/2020/3161053. PMID: 32231808; PMCID: PMC7085353
27. Laskaris G, Vareltzidis A, Avgerinou G. Focal palmoplantar and oral mucosa hyperkeratosis syndrome: a report concerning five members of a family. Oral Surg Oral Med Oral Pathol. 1980;50:250–3.
28. Bethke G, Kolde G, Bethke G, Reichart PA. Fokales palmoplantares und orales Mukosa-Hyperkeratose-Syndrom [focal palmoplantar and oral mucosa hyperkeratosis syndrome]. Mund Kiefer Gesichtschir. 2001;5(3):202–5. https://doi.org/10.1007/s100060100306. PMID: 11432338
29. Lyra ALCO, Razo LM, Estrella RR, Pantaleão L. Juvenile hyaline fibromatosis: an unusual clinical presentation. Dermatol Online J. 2019;25(7):13030/qt75082292. PMID: 31450278
30. Knežević P, Tarle M, Fratrić LI, et al. Gingival hypertrophy in a child with hyaline fibromatosis syndrome. Acta Stomatol Croat. 2020;54(1):69–74. https://doi.org/10.15644/asc54/1/8. PMID: 32523159; PMCID: PMC7233120
31. Bilkay U, Erdem O, Ozek C, Helvaci E, et al. Benign osteoma with Gardner syndrome: review of the literature and report of a case. J Craniofac Surg. 2004;15:506–9.
32. Bali DS, Chen YT, Austin S, Goldstein JL. Glycogen storage disease type I. [updated 2016 Aug 25]. In: Adam MP, Ardinger HH, Pagon RA, Wallace SE, Bean LJH, Stephens K, Amemiya A, editors. GeneReviews® [Internet]. Seattle (WA): University of Washington; 1993–2020. PMID: 20301489.
33. Salapata Y, Laskaris G, Drogari E, et al. Oral manifestations in glycogen storage disease type 1b. J Oral Pathol Med. 1995;24(3):136–9. https://doi.org/10.1111/j.1600-0714.1995.tb01154.x. PMID: 7776266
34. Mariath LM, Santin JT, Schuler-Faccini L, Kiszewski AE. Inherited epidermolysis bullosa: update on the clinical and genetic aspects. An Bras Dermatol. 2020;95(5):551–69.
35. Wiebe CB, Larjava HS. Do mutations in the basement membrane zone affect the human periodontium? Review with special reference to epidermolysis bullosa. J West Soc Periodontol Periodontal Abstr. 1998;46(1):5–18. PMID: 9709672
36. Coletta RD, Graner E. Hereditary gingival fibromatosis: a systematic review. J Periodontol. 2006;77(5):753–64.
37. Gawron K, Łazarz-Bartyzel K, Potempa J, Chomyszyn-Gajewska M. Gingival fibromatosis: clinical, molecular and therapeutic issues. Orphanet J Rare Dis. 2016;27(11):9. https://doi.org/10.1186/s13023-016-0395-1. PMID: 26818898; PMCID: PMC4729029
38. Sakuru R, Bollu PC. Hurler Syndrome. Treasure Island (FL): Stat Pearls Publishing; 2020.
39. Pascual-Castroviejo I, Roche C, Martinez-Bermejo A, Arcas J, et al. Hypomelanosis of Ito. A study of 76 infantile cases. Brain and Development. 1998;20:36–43.
40. Bartholomew DW, Jabs EW, Levin LS, Ribovich R. Single maxillary central incisor and coloboma in hypomelanosis of Ito. Clin Genet. 1987;31:370–3.
41. Reibel A, Maniere MC, Clauss F, Droz D, et al. Orodental phenotype and genotype findings in all subtypes of hypophosphatasia. Orphanet J Rare Dis. 2009;4:6.

42. Lai-Cheong JE, McGrath JA. Kindler syndrome. Dermatol Clin. 2010 Jan;28(1):119–24.
43. Wiebe CB, Petricca G, Häkkinen L, et al. Kindler syndrome and periodontal disease: review of the literature and a 12-year follow-up case. J Periodontol. 2008;79(5):961–6. https://doi.org/10.1902/jop.2008.070167. PMID: 18454678; PMCID: PMC2697853
44. Penagos H, Jaen M, Sancho MT, et al. Kindler syndrome in native Americans from Panama: report of 26 cases. Arch Dermatol. 2004;140(8):939–44. https://doi.org/10.1001/archderm.140.8.939. PMID: 15313809
45. Sciubba JJ, Brown AM. Oral-facial manifestations of Klippel-Trenaunay-weber syndrome. Report of two cases. Oral Surg Oral Med Oral Pathol. 1977;43:227–32.
46. Toomarian L, Hashemi N. Periodontal manifestation of leukocyte adhesion deficiency type I. Arch Iran Med. 2010;13(4):355–9.
47. Moutsopoulos NM, Konkel J, Sarmadi M, et al. Defective neutrophil recruitment in leukocyte adhesion deficiency type I disease causes local IL-17-driven inflammatory bone loss. Sci Transl Med. 2014;6(229):229ra40. https://doi.org/10.1126/scitranslmed.3007696. PMID: 24670684; PMCID: PMC4090608
48. Majidi M, Haghpanah V, Hedayati M, et al. A family presenting with multiple endocrine neoplasia type 2B: a case report. J Med Case Rep. 2011;20(5):587. https://doi.org/10.1186/1752-1947-5-587. PMID: 22185228; PMCID: PMC3287411
49. MacIntosh RB, Shivapuja PK, Krzemien MB, Lee M. Multiple endocrine neoplasia type 2B: maxillofacial significance in 5 cases. J Oral Maxillofac Surg. 2014;72(12):2498.e1–17. https://doi.org/10.1016/j.joms.2014.08.032. Epub 2014 Sep 10. PMID: 25454714
50. Bongiorno MR, Pistone G, Arico M. Manifestations of the tongue in neurofibromatosis type 1. Oral Dis. 2006;12:125–9.
51. Cunha KS, Barboza EP, Dias EP, Oliveira FM. Neurofibromatosis type I with periodontal manifestation. A case report and literature review. Br Dent J. 2004;196:457–60.
52. Driva T, Franklin D, Crawford PJ. Variations in expression of Oral-facial-digital syndrome (type i): report of two cases. Int J Paediatr Dent. 2004;14:61–8.
53. da Silva Santos PS, Fernandes KS, Magalhães MH. Osler-weber-Rendu syndrome--dental implications. J Can Dent Assoc. 2009;75(7):527–30. PMID: 19744364
54. Hart TC, Hart PS, Michalec MD, et al. Haim-Munk syndrome and Papillon-Lefèvre syndrome are allelic mutations in cathepsin C. J Med Genet. 2000;37(2):88–94. https://doi.org/10.1136/jmg.37.2.88. Erratum in: J Med Genet 2001 Jan;38(1):79. Zlorogorski, A [corrected to Zlotogorski, A]. PMID: 10662807; PMCID: PMC1734521
55. Pallos D, Acevedo AC, Mestrinho HD, Cordeiro I, et al. Novel cathepsin c mutation in a Brazilian family with Papillon-Lefévre syndrome: case report and mutation update. J Dent Child (Chic). 2010;77:36–41.
56. Vassilopoulou A, Laskaris G. Papillon-Lefévre syndrome: report of two brothers. ASDC J Dent Child. 1989;56:388–91.
57. Etoz OA, Ulu M, Kesim B. Treatment of patient with Papillon-Lefévre syndrome with short dental implants: a case report. Implant Dent. 2010;19:394–9.
58. Yang Z, He TY, Zhao XD, Yang J. Clinical and genetic analysis of 11 cases with periodic fever, aphthous stomatitis, pharyngitis and adenitis syndrome. Zhonghua Er Ke Za Zhi. 2018;56(7):524–8. Chinese. https://doi.org/10.3760/cma.j.issn.0578-1310.2018.07.010.
59. Pahwa P, Lamba AK, Faraz F, Tandon S. Haim-Munk syndrome. J Indian Soc Periodontol. 2016;14(3):201–3.
60. Bhansali RS, Yeltiwar RK, Agrawal AA. Periodontal management of gingival enlargement associated with Sturge-weber syndrome. J Periodontol. 2008;79:549–55.
61. Martelli H, Lima LS, Bonan PR, Coletta RD. Oral manifestations leading to the diagnosis of familial tuberous sclerosis. Indian J Dent Res. 2010;21:138–40.
62. Lopez JP. White sponge nevus: presentation of a new family. Pediatr Dermatol. 2008;25:116–7.
63. Shirian S, Shahabinejad H, Saeedzadeh A, et al. Zimmermann-Laband syndrome: clinical and cytogenetic study in two related patients. J Clin Exp Dent. 2019;11(5):e452–6.
64. Castaman G, Linari S. Human von Willebrand factor/factor VIII concentrates in the management of pediatric patients with von Willebrand disease/hemophilia a. Ther Clin Risk Manag. 2016;30(12):1029–37. https://doi.org/10.2147/TCRM.S87543.
65. Kubaski F, de Oliveira PF, Michelin-Tirelli K, et al. Mucopolysaccharidosis type I. Diagnostics (Basel). 2020;10(3):161.

Bacterial Infections

27

Contents

Tuberculosis

Definition Tuberculosis is a chronic granulomatous infectious disease.

Etiology *Mycobacterium tuberculosis.*

Gingival Involvement Rare. Non dental biofilm-induced gingival lesions.

Other Sites of Involvement Oral mucosa (tongue, palate, uvula, buccal, lips), rare. Lungs, almost always. Gastrointestinal tract.

Clinical Features

- Gingival lesions may present as chronic, irregular, usually painless ulcers with vegetating red surface or covered by grey-yellowish exudates (Figs. 27.1 and 27.2). Vegetating diffuse gingival enlargement may also occur.
- Oral lesions manifest as irregular, vegetating ulcers with thin borders (Fig. 27.3). The surrounding tissue is slightly indurated with inflammation. Regional lymphadenopathy accompanies oral lesions.
- Tuberculous osteomyelitis of the jaws may rarely occur.

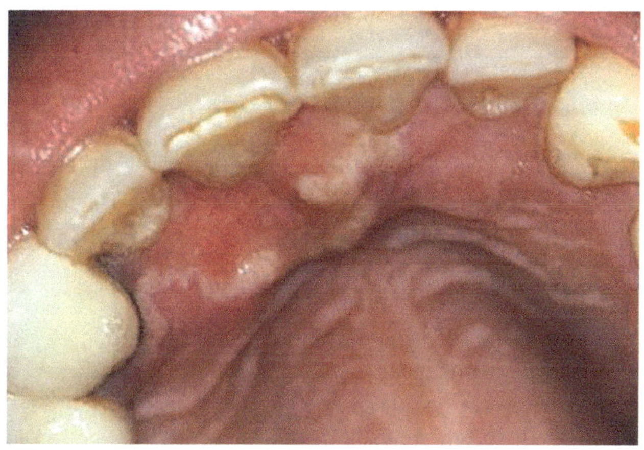

Fig. 27.1 Tuberculosis, small ulcer on the upper gingiva

- Gingival and oral manifestations usually represent secondary infection from the initial pulmonary infection and the oral prevalence ranges from 0.5 to 1.5%. Rarely, oral tuberculosis may be the only manifestation of otherwise silent tuberculosis.
- Low-grade fever, anorexia, malaise, cough, night sweats are early and common symptoms. Chest pain and hemoptysis are also common.
- The clinical diagnosis should be confirmed by laboratory tests.

G. Laskaris et al., *Periodontal Manifestations of Local and Systemic Diseases*, https://doi.org/10.1007/978-3-031-10828-0_27

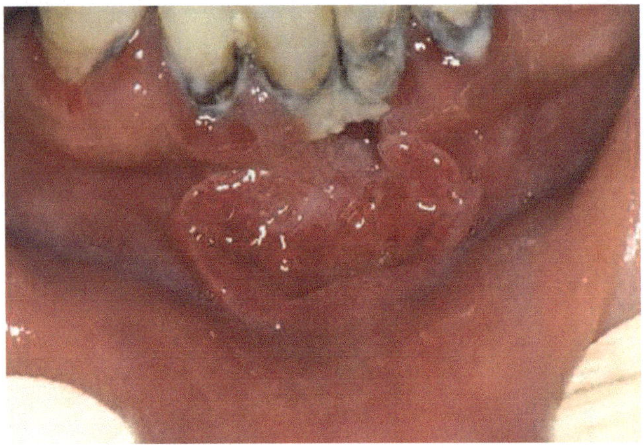

Fig. 27.2 Tuberculosis, vegetative irregular ulceration on the gingiva

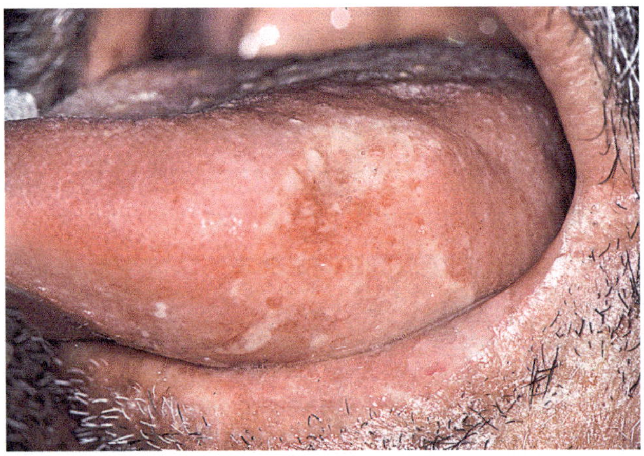

Fig. 27.3 Tuberculosis, ulceration on the lateral border of the tongue

Differential Diagnosis

- Traumatic ulcer.
- Squamous cell carcinoma.
- Primary and secondary syphilis.
- Major aphthous ulcer.
- Non-Hodgkin lymphoma.
- Wegener granulomatosis.
- Pyostomatitis vegetans.

Laboratory Tests Histopathologic examination of oral lesions. Chest radiographs. Mycobacterial examination or culture of infected sputum and tissues. Mantoux tuberculin skin test.

Treatment Anti-tuberculosis regimens containing multiple drugs used by specialists.

Syphilis

Definition Syphilis is a sexually transmitted disease involving several organs and systems.

Etiology *Treponema pallidum.*

Classification Congenital and acquired. Acquired syphilis develops in three stages: *Primary, Secondary, and Tertiary.*

Gingival Involvement Rare. Non-dental biofilm-induced gingival lesions.

Other Sites of Involvement Oral mucosa, common. Approximately 5–10% of the primary and over 40% of secondary syphilis appear in the oral cavity. Genitalia, very common. Skin, common (secondary and tertiary stages).

Clinical Features

- *Primary syphilis* is characterized by the development of *chancre* at the site of inoculation of *treponema pallidum.* Chancre begins as an inflammatory papule that ulcerates to form a painless round ulcer with a raised border and indurated base. Chancre on the gingiva is extremely rare (Figs. 27.4 and 27.5). The lips, tongue, soft palate, and tonsils are the most common oral sites affected. Regional lymph node enlargement is a constant finding. Direct oro-genital contact is necessary for the development of an oral chancre.
- *Secondary syphilis* begins 6–8 weeks after the appearance of the chancre. Oral lesions are common in this stage and are mainly characterized by the appearance of *mucous patches*, which are painless, slightly raised, oval or round erosions or superficial ulcers covered by a greyish-white membrane. Gingival involvement is relatively rare (Fig. 27.6).
- The tongue, buccal mucosa, palate, tonsils, and lips are most frequently affected (Fig. 27.7).
- The classic signs and symptoms of secondary syphilis are headache, malaise, fever, generalized painless lymph node enlargement, and maculopapular skin eruption.

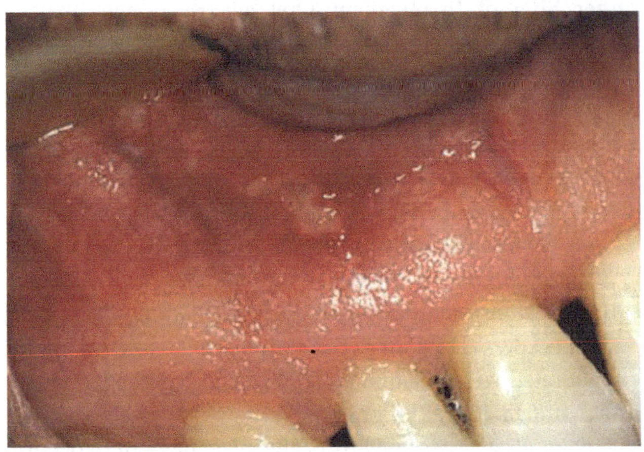

Fig. 27.4 Primary syphilis, small chancre on the border of attached gingiva and alveolar mucosa

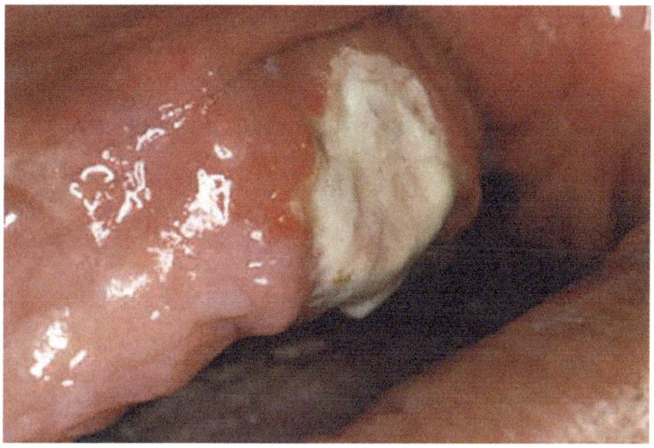

Fig. 27.5 Primary syphilis, large chancre on the edentulous alveolar mucosa

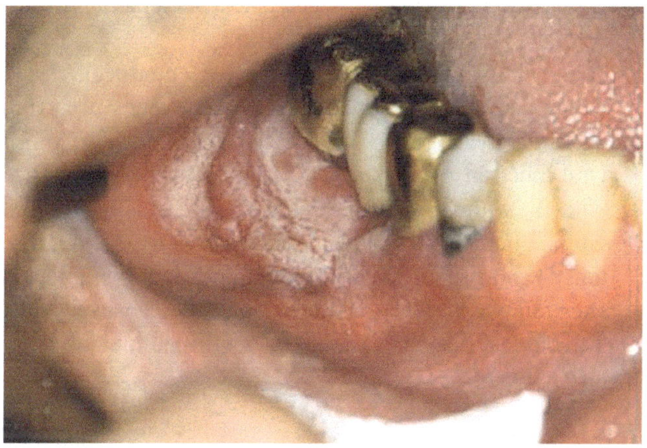

Fig. 27.6 Secondary syphilis, mucous patches on the gingiva

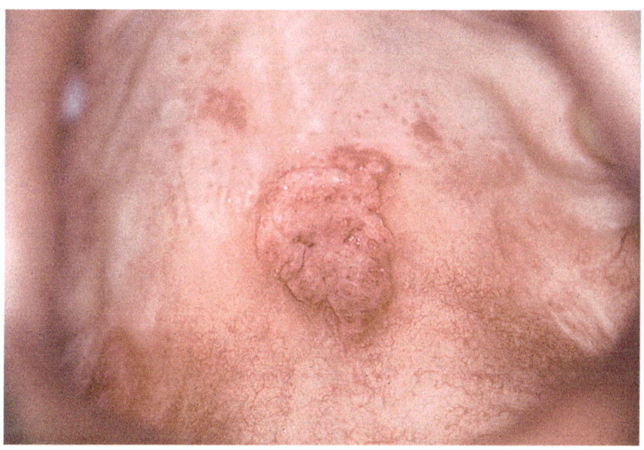

Fig. 27.7 Secondary syphilis, mucous patches on the palate

- *Tertiary syphilis (late syphilis)* develops in about 30% of untreated patients and is characterized by multisystem involvement and broad spectrum of manifestations. The *gumma* is the most characteristic oral lesion of this stage, and the hard palate is the most common site of involvement followed by tongue and lips. Gingiva is not involved.
- The clinical diagnosis of syphilis should be confirmed by laboratory tests.

Differential Diagnosis
- Herpetic oral lesions.
- Traumatic oral lesions.
- Aphthous ulcer.
- Candidiasis.
- Erythema multiforme.
- Infectious mononucleosis.
- Non-Hodgkin lymphoma.
- Squamous cell carcinoma and other malignant tumors.
- Others.

Laboratory Tests Serologic tests (VDRL, RPR, FTA-ABS, TPI, TPHA), dark field microscopy.

Treatment Penicillin G is the treatment of choice for all stages of syphilis, but it must be left to the specialist physicians.

Actinomycosis

Definition Actinomycosis is a chronic granulomatous infectious disease.

Etiology Mainly *Actinomyces israelii* and rarely other species.

Classification Actinomycosis is divided into three clinical types:
(a) *cervicofacial*, (b) *pulmonary*, and (c) *abdominal*.

Gingival Involvement Rare. Non-dental biofilm-induced gingival lesions.

Other Sites of Involvement Jaws, oral mucosa, cervical lymph nodes, gastrointestinal tract, lungs, and other organs.

Clinical Features
- Oral manifestations are part of the cervicofacial actinomycosis.
- Gingival lesions are rare and may present as localized atypical gingivitis or more commonly as painless alveolar bone swelling covered by slightly erythematous gingiva, usually with draining sinuses (Fig. 27.8).
- Involvement of the jaws is common but soft tissues (tongue, palate, buccal) may be less frequently involved. A slow-growing and painless hard swelling is the classic feature of the disease. It is usually followed by multiple

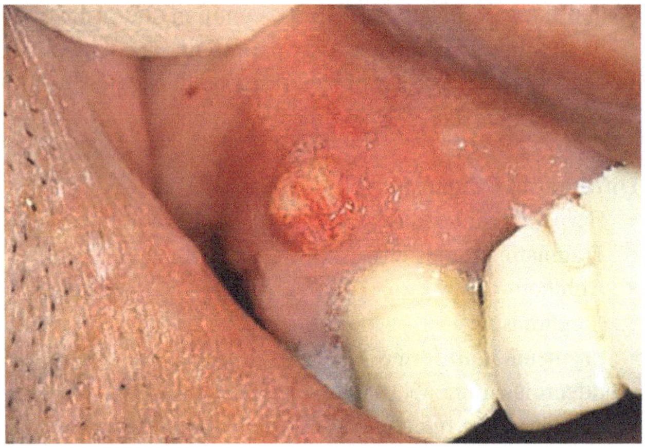

Fig. 27.8 Actinomycosis, draining sinus on the gingiva

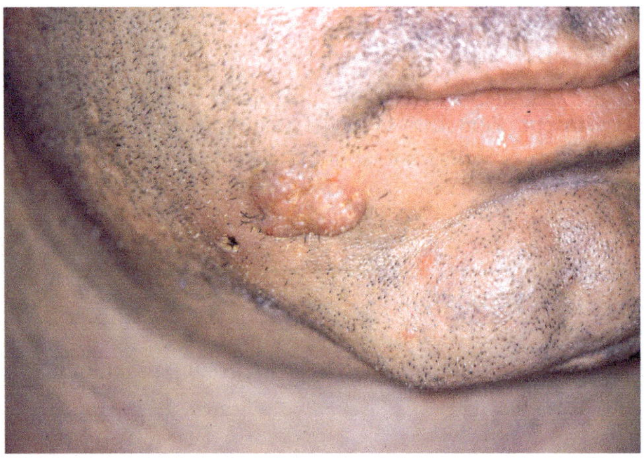

Fig. 27.9 Actinomycosis, draining sinus on the skin of the face

abscesses that drain to the surface by sinus tracts (Fig. 27.9). Sinus tracts carry exudates to the outside, which often contains the characteristic *"sulfur granules"* filled with microorganisms.
- The clinical diagnosis should be confirmed by laboratory tests.

Differential Diagnosis
- Periodontal and dental abscess.
- Tuberculosis.
- Systemic mycoses.

Laboratory Tests Direct bacteriologic examination and culture, histopathologic examination.

Treatment Penicillin is the drug of choice. Erythromycin or tetracyclines may be used as alternative drugs. Surgery is suggested for localized oral lesions in combination with penicillin.

Gonococcal Infection

Definition Gonococcal infection is a sexually transmitted disease that primarily involves mucous membranes of genitals, anus, and rectum.

Etiology *Neisseria gonorrhoeae.*

Gingival Involvement Rare. Non-dental biofilm-induced gingival lesions.

Other Sites of Involvement Oral mucosa, relatively rare. Urethra, anus, and cervix, common.

Clinical Features
- Gingival and oral mucosal lesions are more common among homosexuals and heterosexuals practicing oral sex.
- Gingival involvement may present as nonspecific erythema and slight edema with painful erosions occurring occasionally (Fig. 27.10).
- Oral mucosal manifestations present as a fiery erythema with or without superficial ulceration, usually covered with a greyish or yellowish exudates (Fig. 27.11). The tonsils and the soft palate are the most common affected sites followed by the tongue and buccal mucosa.
- The clinical diagnosis should be confirmed by laboratory tests.

Differential Diagnosis
- Desquamative gingivitis.
- Herpetic gingivitis.
- Granulomatous gingivitis.
- Streptococcal gingivitis.

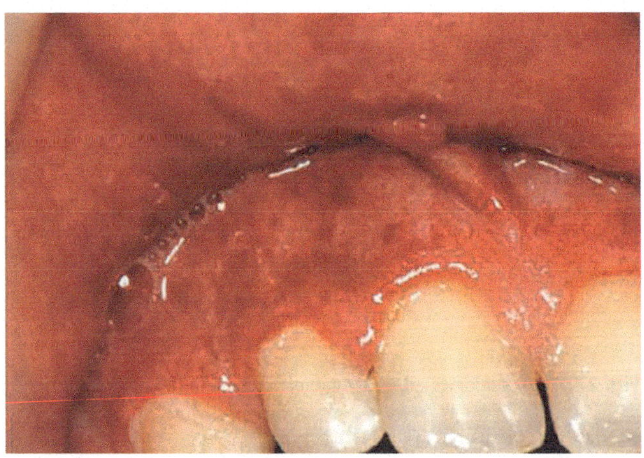

Fig. 27.10 Gonococcal gingivitis, localized erythema and edema

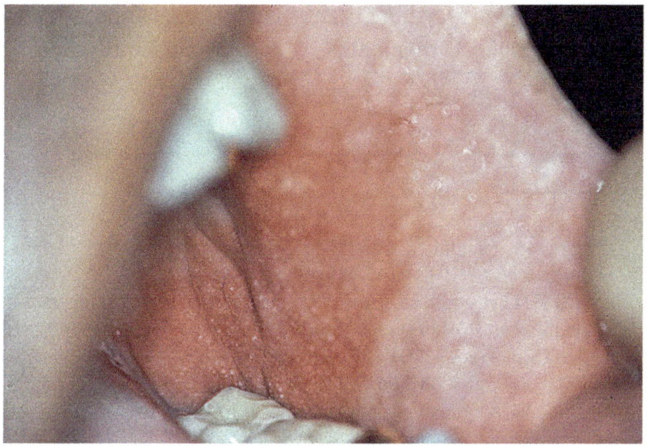

Fig. 27.11 Gonococcal stomatitis, erythema on the buccal mucosa

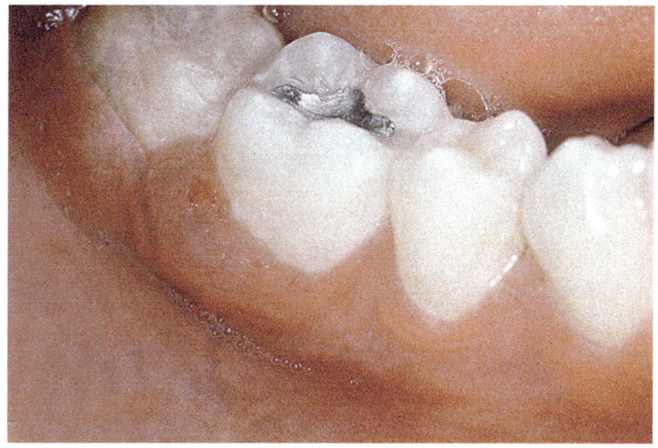

Fig. 27.12 Bacillary angiomatosis, red swelling on the gingiva of an AIDS patient

- Erythematous candidiasis.
- Cinnamon contact gingivitis.

Laboratory Tests Culture and microscopic identification of the microorganism. Fluorescent antibody test, molecular biological testing.

Treatment Systemically administered penicillin or third-generation cephalosporins are the drugs of choice.

Bacillary Angiomatosis

Definition Bacillary angiomatosis is a rare, opportunistic bacterial infection which occurs mainly in patients with AIDS and other immunosuppressed patients.

Etiology The gram-negative bacteria *Bartonella quintana* and *Bartonella henselae* are the cause. A vascular proliferation is provoked by an angiostimulating factor(s).

Gingival Involvement Very rare. Non-dental biofilm-induced gingival lesions.

Other Sites of Involvement The most frequent site of involvement is the skin followed by bones and liver. Extracutaneous lesions, including oral mucosa, are less common and may develop with or without skin lesions.

Clinical Features
- Gingival lesions may appear as a painless,elevated, atypical, and red swelling that cannot be diagnosed clinically (Fig. 27.12).
- Skin lesions appear as asymptomatic, single or multiple, deep red papules or macules or plaques with a smooth surface, which may be ulcerated. The clinical diagnosis should be confirmed by laboratory tests.

Differential Diagnosis
- Kaposi sarcoma.
- Pyogenic granuloma.
- Leiomyoma.
- Hemangioma.
- Angiosarcoma.
- Amyloidosis.

Laboratory Test Histopathologic examination.

Treatment The drugs of choice include erythromycin, clarithromycin, and doxycycline. Treatment must be left to the specialist physicians.

Donovanosis

Definition Donovanosis is a rare,chronic, relapsing, granulomatous anogenital bacterial infection.

Etiology The bacterium *Klebsiella granulomatis* (formerly known as *Calymmatobacterium granulomatis)* is the cause. It is sexually transmitted.

Gingival Involvement Relatively rare. Non-dental biofilm-induced gingival lesions.

Other Sites of Involvement Mainly on the skin and mucous membranes. The oral mucosa is rarely affected. Extragenital lesions on the skin, larynx, pharynx, nose, genitalia, and perineal region.

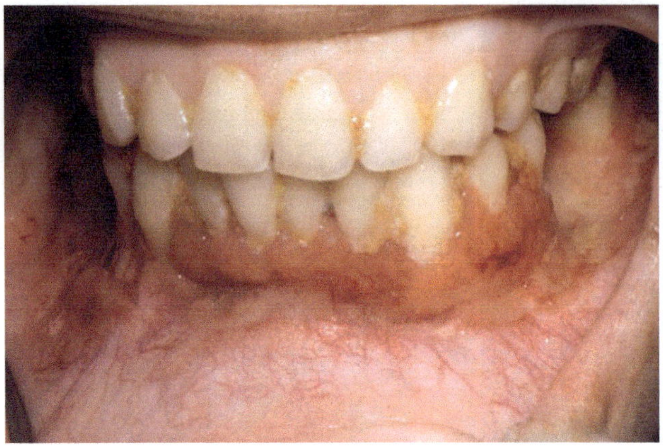

Fig. 27.13 Donovanosis, red granular ulcerations with spongy bleeding areas

Clinical Features

- The incubation period ranges from 1 to 10 weeks or more.
- Clinically, gingival lesions appear as painful or painless, localized or generalized, chronic red granulomatous ulcerations or papillary granulomatous swellings (Fig. 27.13). Similar ulcerations may develop on the buccal mucosa, palate, and tongue.
- Clinically, lesions affect the anogenital skin, the inguinal area and mucous membranes.They present as a small, painless papules or nodules leading progressively to sharply demarcated ulcers with a beefy-red granulomatous surface and increased bleeding tendency.
- Donovanosis is usually restricted to India, South Africa, New Guinea, Papua, and Australia.
- The clinical diagnosis should be confirmed by laboratory tests.

Differential Diagnosis

- Syphilis.
- Chancroid.
- Systemic mycosis.
- Wegener granulomatosis.
- Tuberculosis.
- Orofacial granulomatosis.
- Crohn disease.
- Pyostomatitis vegetans.

Laboratory Tests Histopathologic examination, tissue smear microscopy.

Treatment Doxycycline, azithromycin, and ciprofloxacin are recommended treatments, which should be handled by specialists.

References

1. Kapoor S, Gandhi S, Gandhi N, Singh I. Oral manifestations of tuberculosis. CHRISMED J Health Res. 2014;1:11–4.
2. Sezer B, Zeytinoglu M, Tuncay U, Unal T. Oral mucosal ulceration: a manifestation of previously undiagnosed pulmonary tuberculosis. J Am Dent Assoc. 2004;135:336–40.
3. Bansal R, Jain A, Mittal S. Orofacial tuberculosis: clinical manifestations, diagnosis and management. J Family Med Prim Care. 2015;4(3):335–41. https://doi.org/10.4103/2249-4863.161312. PMID: 26288770; PMCID: PMC4535091
4. Smolka W, Burger H, Lizuka T, Smolka K. Primary tuberculosis of the oral cavity in an elderly non immunosuppressed patient: case report and review of the literature. Arch Otolaryngol Head Neck Surg. 2008;134:1107–9.
5. Bruce AJ, Rogers RS. Oral manifestations of sexually transmitted diseases. Clin Dermatol. 2004;22(6):520–7. https://doi.org/10.1016/j.clindermatol.2004.07.005. PMID: 15596324
6. Ramos-E-Silva M. Facial and oral aspects of some venereal and tropical diseases. Acta Dermatovenerol Croat. 2004;12(3):173–80. PMID: 15369643
7. Matias MDP, Oliveira de Jesus A, Gonçalves Resende R, et al. Diagnosing acquired syphilis through oral lesions: the 12 year experience of an oral medicine center. Braz J Otorhinolaryngol. 2020;86(3):358–63.
8. Compilato D, Amato S, Campisi G. Resurgence of syphilis: a diagnosis based on unusual oral mucosa lesions. Oral Surg Oral Med Oral Pathol Oral Radiol Endod. 2009;108:e45–9.
9. Queirós C, Borges da Costa J. Oral transmission of sexually transmissable infections: a narrative review. Acta Medica Port. 2019;32(12):776–81.
10. Balmelli C, Gunthard HF. Gonococcal tonsillar infection–a case report and literature review. Infection. 2003;31:362–5.
11. Hook EW, Bernstein K. Kissing, saliva exchange, and transmission of Neisseria gonorrhoeae. Lancet Infect Dis. 2019;19(10):e367–9.
12. Doddridge M, Muirhead R. Donovanosis of the oral cavity. Aust Dent J. 1994;39(4):203–5. https://doi.org/10.1111/j.1834-7819.1994.tb04776.x. PMID: 7945045
13. Ramírez Ramírez CR, Saavedra S, Ramírez Ronda CH. Bacillary angiomatosis: microbiology, histopathology, clinical presentation, diagnosis and management. Bol Asoc Med PR. 1996;88:46–51.
14. Veeranna S, Raghu TY. Oral donovanosis. Int J STD AIDS. 2002;13:855–6.
15. Ahmed N, Pillay A, Lawler M, Bobat R, Archary M. Donovanosis causing lymphadenitis, mastoiditis, and meningitis in a child. Lancet. 2015;385(9987):2644. https://doi.org/10.1016/S0140-6736(15)60992-8. PMID: 26122163
16. Laskaris G. Color atlas of oral diseases, 4th, Thieme 2017.

28 Viral Infections

Contents

Measles

Definition Measles is a highly communicable infectious disease of childhood.

Etiology RNA *paramyxovirus* belonging to the *Morbillivirus* genus.

Gingival Involvement Rare. Non-dental biofilm-related lesions.

Other Sites of Involvement Oral mucosa, relatively rare. Skin, always.

Clinical Features

- Gingival lesions may present as small round ulcers on the attached gingiva or the alveolar mucosa, and occasionally as gingival erythema (Figs. 28.1 and 28.2.). The gingival lesions are not diagnostic.
- Oral lesions present as *"Koplik's spots"* on the buccal mucosa, redness, petechiae, and small round ulcers.

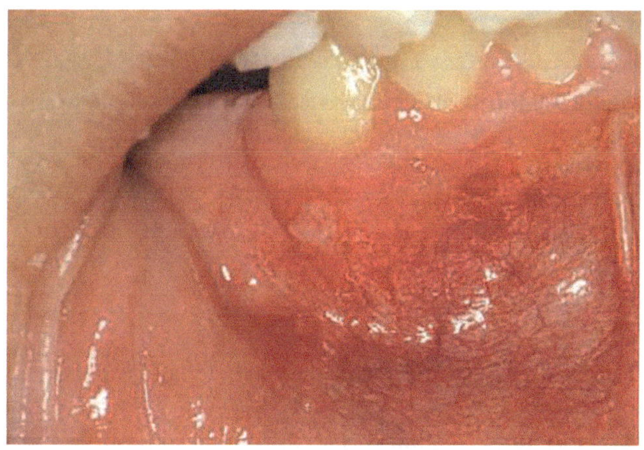

Fig. 28.1 Measles, small, round ulcer on the attached gingiva

- Skin manifestations present as maculopapular dull red eruptions (Fig. 28.3).
- Constitutional symptoms, such as fever, chills, cough, photophobia, conjunctivitis, and myalgias, begin 3–4 days prior to skin eruption.
- Diagnosis is mainly based on clinical criteria.

G. Laskaris et al., *Periodontal Manifestations of Local and Systemic Diseases*, https://doi.org/10.1007/978-3-031-10828-0_28

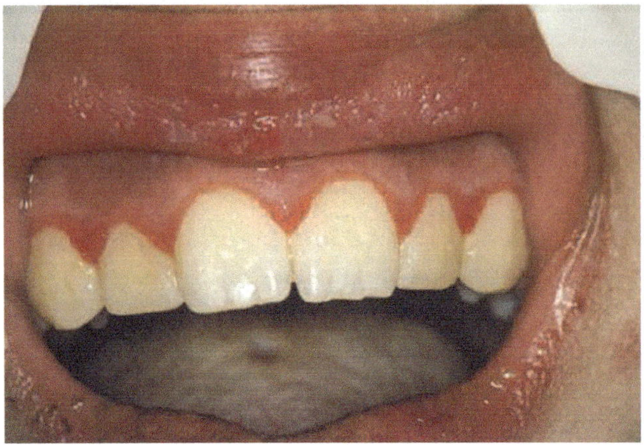

Fig. 28.2 Measles, gingival erythema

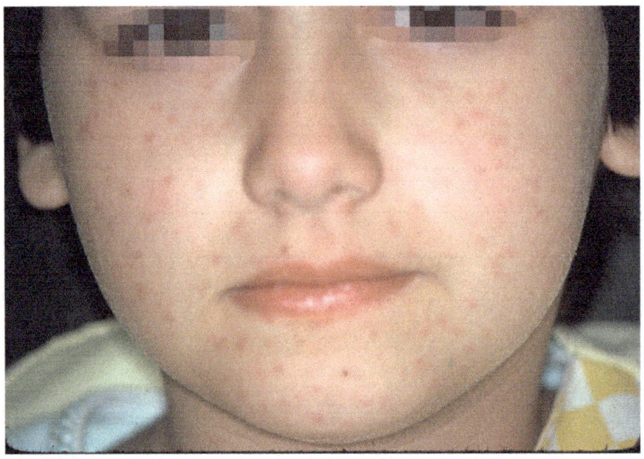

Fig. 28.3 Measels, maculopapular red skin rush and conjunctivitis

Differential Diagnosis

- Varicella.
- Herpetic gingivostomatitis.
- Herpetiform ulcers.
- Infectious mononucleosis.

Laboratory Tests Serologic tests only for atypical cases.

Treatment No treatment is needed for the gingival and oral lesions. The general management of patients must be left to pediatricians.

Chickenpox

Definition Chickenpox or varicella is a highly contagious, self-limited, and primary infection that occurs chiefly among children.

Etiology *Varicella-zoster virus* or HHV-3.

Gingival Involvement Rare. Non-dental biofilm-related lesions.

Other Sites of Involvement Oral mucosa (palate, buccal, lip), relatively rare. Skin (face, head, and neck), always.

Clinical Features

- Gingival lesions present usually as diffuse erythema and isolated small vesicles that rupture quickly leaving round shallow ulcerations on an erythematous area (Fig. 28.4).
- Oral mucosal lesions also present as small vesicles, which rupture quickly leaving small ulcerations.
- Skin manifestations include a pruritic red maculopapular rash, vesicles, and pustules that rupture, crust, and later exfoliate (Fig. 28.5).
- The prodromal symptoms are malaise, fever, anorexia, and irritability.
- Diagnosis is mainly based on clinical criteria.

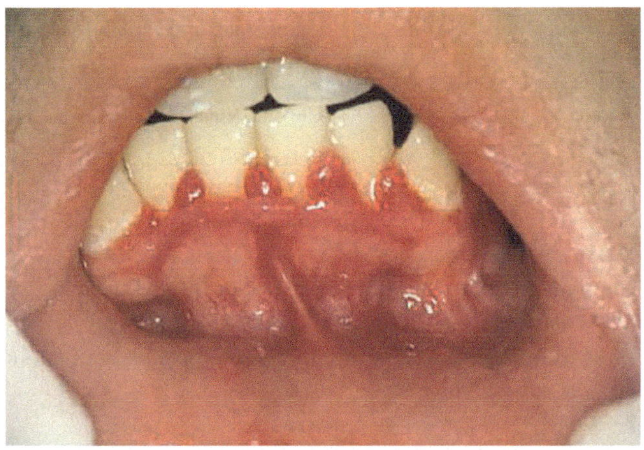

Fig. 28.4 Chickenpox, diffuse gingival erythema

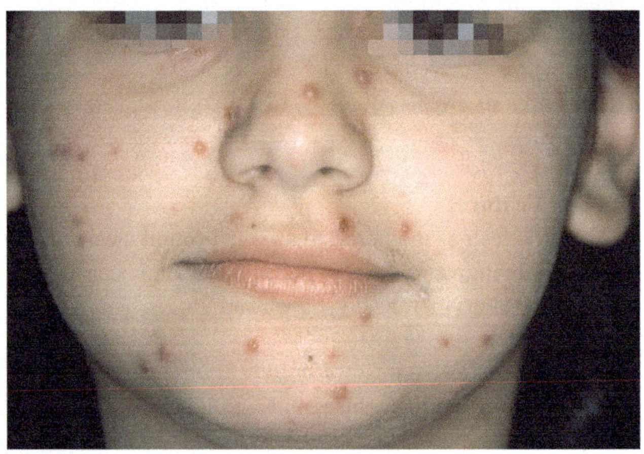

Fig. 28.5 Chickenpox, skin maculopapular lesions

Differential Diagnosis

- Herpes simplex oral infection.
- Minor aphthous ulcers.
- Measles.
- Herpangina.
- Hand, foot, and mouth disease.

Laboratory Tests Cytologic smear examination. Polymerase chain reaction (PCR) for detection of *varicella-zoster virus*.

Treatment No treatment is needed for oral lesions. Supportive treatment should be left to pediatricians.

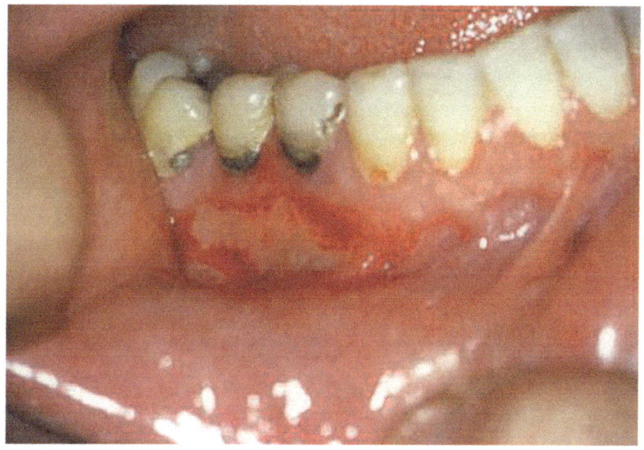

Fig. 28.6 Herpes zoster, ulceration of the attached gingiva of mandible

Herpes Zoster

Definition Herpes zoster is an acute viral disease caused by reactivation of a latent *varicella-zoster virus* that is transported via sensory nerve axons to mucosa and/or skin.

Etiology Reactivation of *varicella-zoster virus*, especially in immunocompromised patients.

Gingival Involvement Relatively common, non-dental biofilm-related lesions. Gingival and oral mucosal lesions may occur when second or third division of the trigeminal nerve is involved.

Other Sites of Involvement Oral mucosa (palate, buccal, tongue, lip), skin.

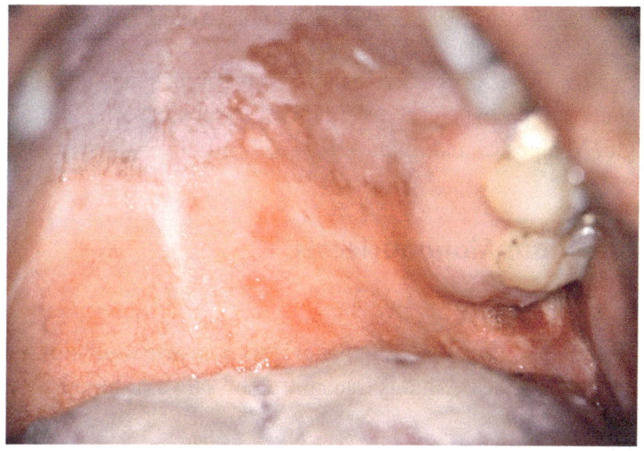

Fig. 28.7 Herpes zoster, unilateral ulceration of the palate and gingiva

Clinical Features

- Gingival lesions present as unilateral clusters of vesicles, which rupture within 2–3 days, leaving painful ulceration with irregular borders (Figs. 28.6 and 28.7). Necrosis of the periodontium and alveolar bone may be seen. The ulcers usually heal after 2–3 weeks without scarring.
- Similar unilateral lesions may appear on other oral sites, depending on which division of the trigeminal nerve is involved. An itching sensation and pain, which may simulate pulpitis, may precede oral lesions.
- Skin manifestations (trigeminal involvement) appear on the face and are characterized by unilateral clusters of maculopapules on an erythematous base, which will soon form vesicles and will evolve into pustules within 2–3 days. The pustules usually form crust within 5–8 days and persist for 10–20 days (Fig. 28.8). New lesions continue to appear for several days.
- Tenderness and pain are always present. Constitutional symptoms, such as fever, malaise, and headache, are common. Postherpetic trigeminal neuralgia is the most common complication.
- Diagnosis is mainly based on clinical criteria.

Differential Diagnosis

- Oral herpes simplex infection.
- Necrotizing gingivitis and periodontitis.
- Erythema multiforme.
- Leukemia.
- Agranulocytosis.

Laboratory Tests Viral culture, cytology smear, serological tests, and viral DNA studies may be necessary only in atypical cases.

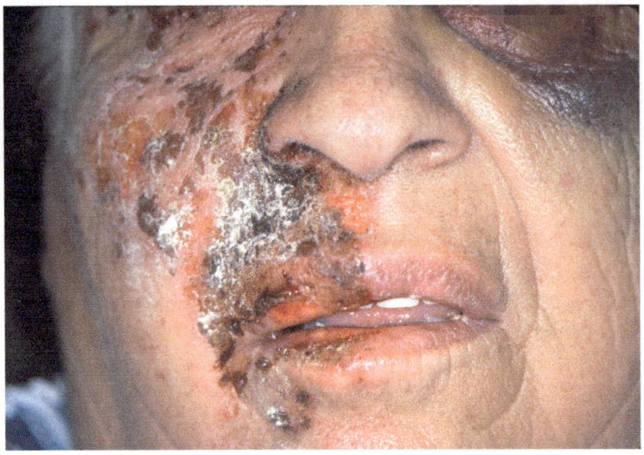

Fig. 28.8 Herpes zoster, severe typical unilateral lesions of the skin and lips

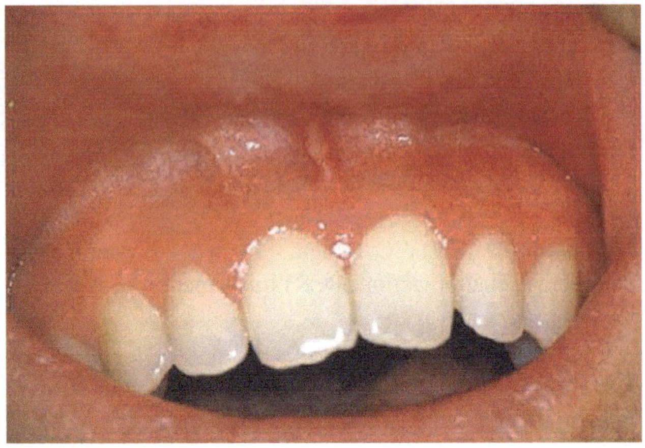

Fig. 28.9 Infectious mononucleosis, diffuse erythema on the gingiva and lip

Treatment Antiviral drugs (brivudine, valaciclovir, famciclovir, acyclovir).

Low-dose corticosteroids for about 2 weeks may alleviate acute symptoms and reduce the risk for postherpetic neuralgia. Analgesics and sedatives.

Infectious Mononucleosis

Definition Infectious mononucleosis is an acute self-limited infectious disease that is transmitted by saliva or blood.

Etiology *Epstein-Barr* or HHV-4 virus.

Gingival Involvement Rare. Non-dental biofilm-related lesions.

Other Sites of Involvement Oral mucosa (soft palate, uvula, buccal), relatively common. Skin, lymph nodes.

Clinical Features

- Gingival lesions may present as localized or diffuse erythema, and less frequently as small ulcerations, particularly at the interdental papillae, mimicking necrotizing gingivitis (Figs. 28.9 and 28.10).
- Oral manifestations include palatal petechiae, facial edema, tonsillar exudates, pericoronitis, and occasionally ulcerations.
- A generalized maculopapular rash causes flat and raised lesions on the skin.
- Generalized lymphadenopathy, profound malaise, sore throat, fever, anorexia, and headache are common signs and symptoms.
- Clinical diagnosis should be confirmed by laboratory tests.

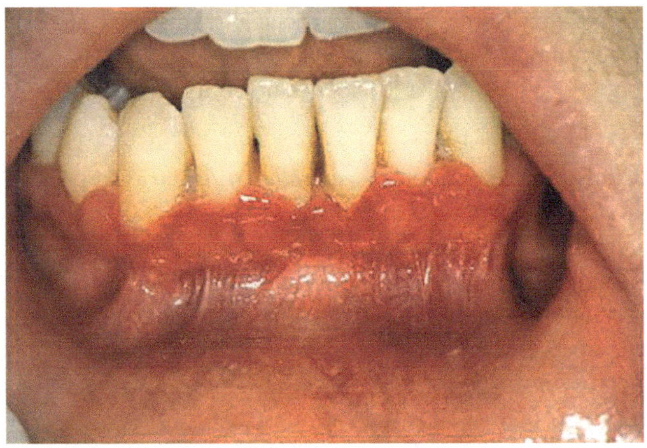

Fig. 28.10 Infectious mononucleosis, localized erythema on the gingiva and necrotizing gingivitis

Differential Diagnosis

- Herpetic gingivostomatitis.
- Streptococcal gingivitis.
- Necrotizing gingivitis.
- Leukemia.
- Aplastic anemia.

Laboratory Tests Monospot test, increased plasma EBV DNA levels in serum.

Treatment Supportive. Antiviral drugs in combination with low doses of corticosteroids may be used.

Hand, Foot, and Mouth Disease

Definition Hand, foot, and mouth disease is an acute viral infection that usually affects children and young adults.

Etiology *Coxsackie virus A16* and occasionally other types (A5, A9, A10,) are responsible.

Gingival Involvement Rare. Non-dental biofilm-related lesions.

Other Sites of Involvement Oral mucosa (buccal, labial, tongue, soft palate, uvula), common. Skin (hands, feet, back, buttocks), common.

Clinical Features

- Gingival lesions are characterized by small vesicles that soon rupture, leaving slightly painful, shallow ulcers surrounded by a red halo (Figs. 28.11 and 28.12).
- Similar lesions appear in the oral cavity. Oral lesions are usually multiple (3–20), 2–6 mm in diameter.
- Skin lesions present as multiple small vesicles (Figs. 28.13 and 28.14).
- Low-grade fever, malaise, and headache precede oral and skin lesions. The disease lasts 5–8 days.
- Diagnosis is mainly based on clinical criteria.

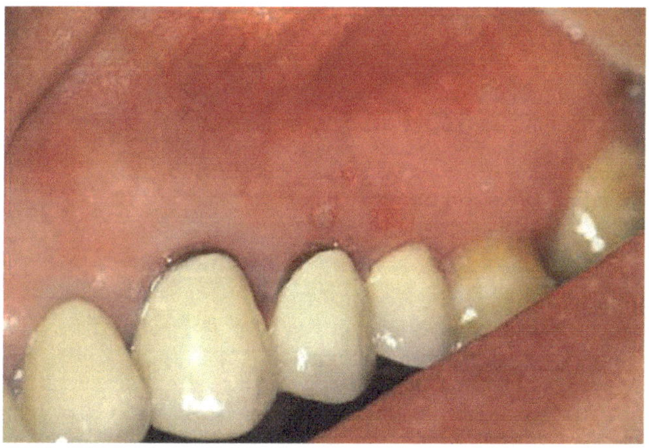

Fig. 28.11 Hand-foot-and-mouth disease, small erosions on the gingiva

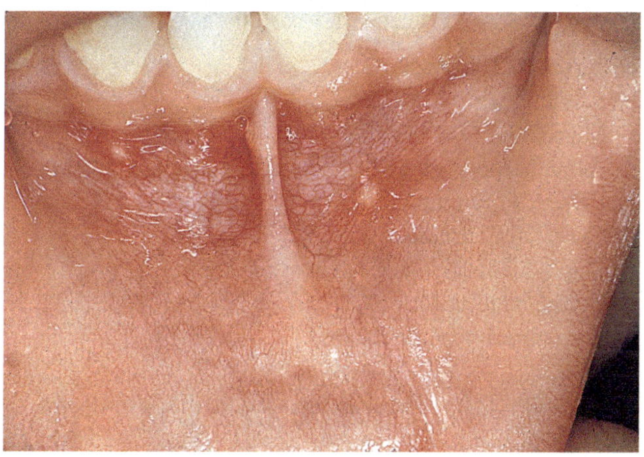

Fig. 28.12 Hand-foot-and-mouth disease, small erosions on the gingiva and alveolar mucosa

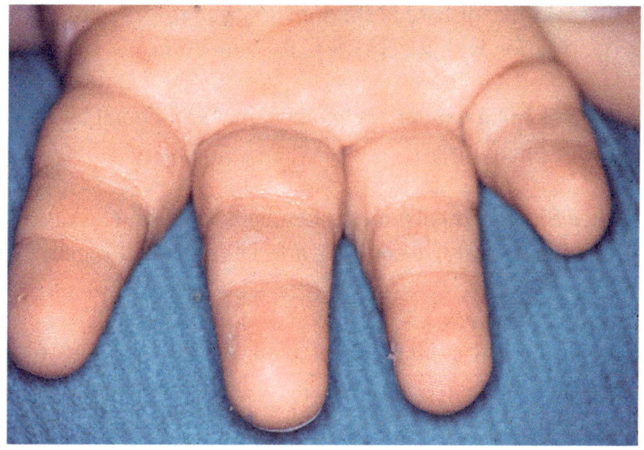

Fig. 28.13 Hand-foot-and-mouth disease, multiple skin vesicles on the fingers

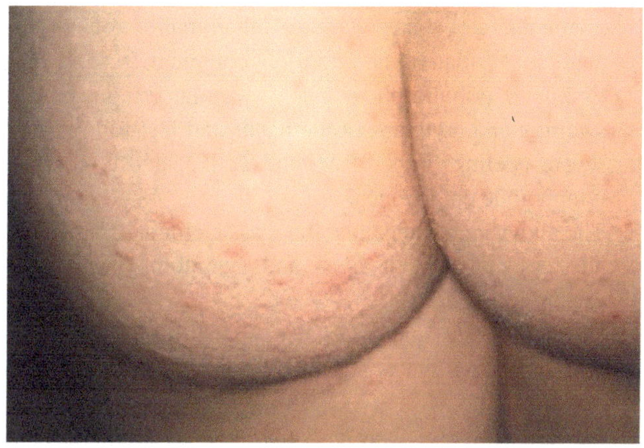

Fig. 28.14 Hand-foot-and-mouth disease, multiple small vesicles on the buttocks

Differential Diagnosis

- Minor aphthous ulcers.
- Herpetic stomatitis.
- Herpangina.
- Erythema multiforme.

Laboratory Tests Viral cultures and serologic investigation needed only in doubtful cases.

Treatment Symptomatic.

Kawasaki Disease

Definition Kawasaki disease (KD) is an acute, self-limited, febrile multisystemic vasculitis that primarily affects infants and children. It was described by Tomisaku Kawasaki in 1960.

Etiology It remains unknown. However, an infectious agent with tropism to vascular tissue, likely a virus, could be linked to KD in genetically predisposed individuals. An outbreak of

Kawasaki-like disease in children has been recorded recently in association with the SARS-CoV-2 infection.

Gingival Involvement Relatively rare. Non-dental biofilm-induced gingivitis.

Other Sites of Involvement Oral and ocular mucosa, skin, lymph nodes, cardiac coronary arteries, and other organs.

Clinical Features

- The clinical course of the disease is divided into four stages: *a. acute, b. subacute, c. convalescent, and d. chronic.*
- The disease is characterized by sudden high fever (39–40 °C) lasting at least 5 days and five important clinical signs: a. erythema, edema, and fissuring of the lips (Fig. 28.15) and oral mucosa, associated with gingival erythema, strawberry tongue, inflammation of lingual papillae; b. bilateral non-purulent conjunctivitis and choroiditis; c. polymorphous, maculopapular skin lesions; d. swelling and erythema of the hands and feet followed by severe peeling (Figs. 28.16 and 28.17); and e. cervical lymph node enlargement.
- The above signs constitute the classic clinical frame usually associated with signs and symptoms from other organs and systems.
- Gingival lesions appear usually as localized, and nonspecific erythema that is not associated with dental biofilm (Fig. 28.18).
- Kawasaki disease represents the most common cause of acquired cardiovascular disorders in children due to the development of coronary artery aneurysms and thrombosis.
- Diagnosis is mainly based on history and clinical features.

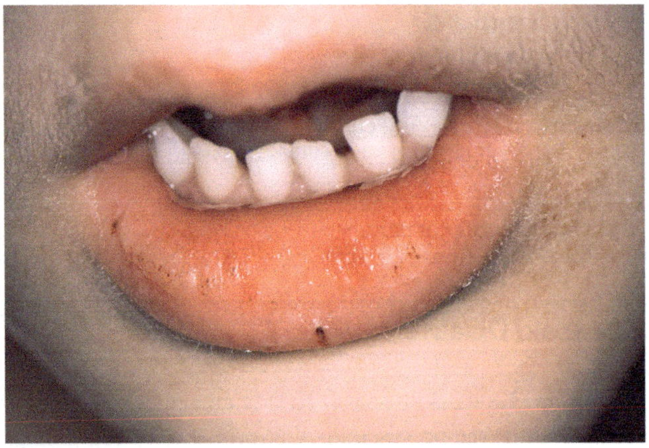

Fig. 28.15 Kawasaki disease, erythema and fissuring of the lower lip

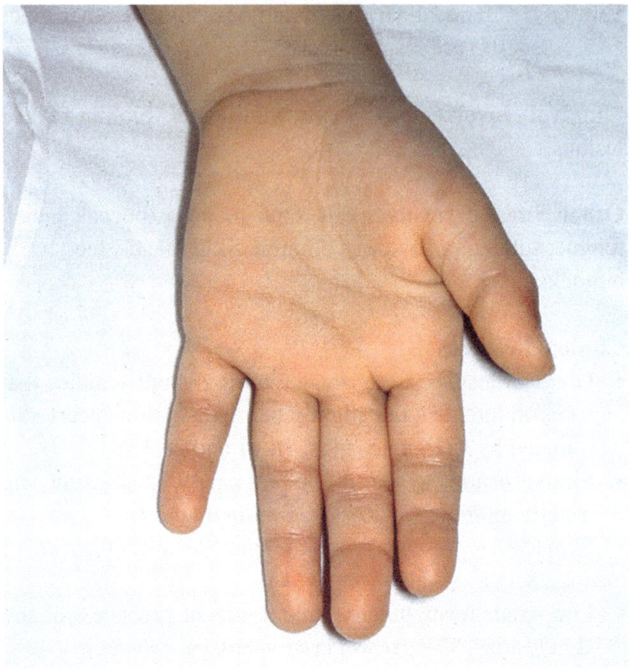

Fig. 28.16 Kawasaki disease, erythema and peeling of the palm and fingers

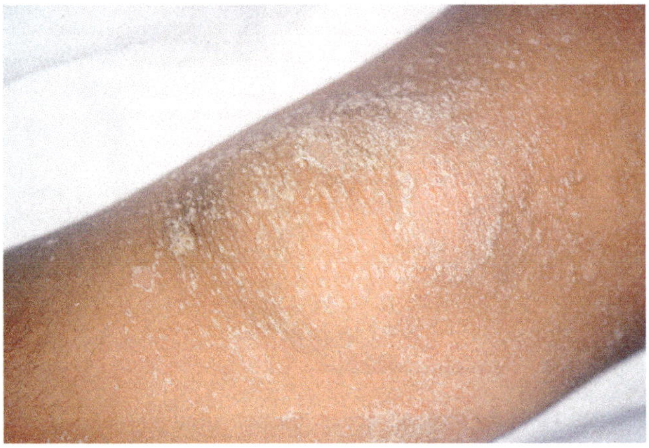

Fig. 28.17 Kawasaki disease, peeling of the skin on the knee

Differential Diagnosis

- Scarlet fever.
- Measles.
- Acute herpetic gingivostomatitis.
- PFAPA syndrome.
- COVID-19 disease.
- Staphylococcal scalded skin syndrome.
- Erythema multiforme.
- Stevens-Johnson syndrome.

Laboratory Tests There are no specific diagnostic tests.

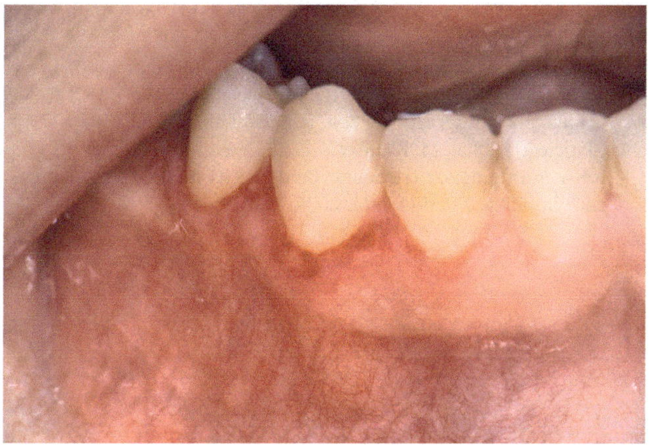

Fig. 28.18 Kawasaki disease, gingivitis

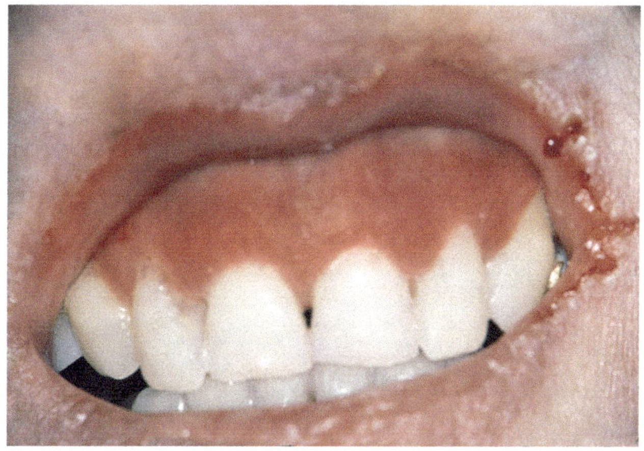

Fig. 28.19 Chronic viral hepatitis, diffuse gingival erythema

Treatment Intravenous administration of high dose of gamma globulin is the treatment of choice. Adding steroids and high doses of aspirin to standard therapy may improve initial treatment success. Therapy should be left to the specialist pediatricians.

Chronic Viral Hepatitis

Definition Chronic viral hepatitis is a chronic necroinflammatory disorder of the liver with characteristic histopathologic and serologic findings, lasting more than 6 months. Chronic active hepatitis is a type of chronic viral hepatitis that gradually progresses to cirrhosis.

Etiology The causes are mainly hepatitis B virus (HBV), hepatitis C virus (HCV), and hepatitis D virus (HDV) infections as well as autoimmune and other liver disorders.

Gingival Involvement Rare. Non-dental biofilm-induced gingival lesions.

Other Sites of Involvement Liver, skin, bones, central nervous system.

Clinical Features

- The main clinical features include jaundice, pruritus, diarrhea, skin manifestation, xanthomas, hemorrhages, encephalopathy, osteomalacia, and others.
- Oral manifestations include thin and erythematous mucosa with telangiectasias that mostly affect the lips.
- Rarely, the gingiva appears deep erythematous and edematous, hemorrhagic and sensitive, and is not detached by friction (Fig. 28.19).
- The clinical diagnosis should be confirmed by laboratory tests.

Differential Diagnosis

- Plasma cell gingivitis.
- Desquamative gingivitis.
- Granulomatous gingivitis.
- Soft tissue plasmacytoma.

Laboratory Tests Specific serologic and immunologic tests, liver biopsy, and histopathologic examination.

Treatment Good oral hygiene. The systemic treatment must be left to the specialists.

References

1. Holmstrup P, Plemons J, Meyle J. Non-plaque-induced gingival diseases. J Clin Periodontol. 2018;45(Suppl 20):528–43. https://doi.org/10.1111/jcpe.12938.
2. Katz J, Guelmann M, Stavropolous F, Heft M. Gingival and other oral manifestations in measles virus infection. J Clin Periodontol. 2003;30:665–8.
3. Famularo G. Koplik's spots and measles. Am J Med. 2018;131(6):e249–50. https://doi.org/10.1016/j.amjmed.2018.01.030. Epub 2018 Feb 21. PMID: 29476743
4. Chopra A, Sivaraman K, Thomas BS. Herpes zoster of gingiva in an older woman: a rare case report. Gerodontology. 2017;34(2):280–3. https://doi.org/10.1111/ger.12246. Epub 2016 Jul 19. PMID: 27435832
5. Kolokotronis A, Louloudiadis K, Fotiou G, Matiakis A. Oral manifestations of infections of infections due to varicella zoster virus in otherwise healthy children. J Clin Pediatr Dent. 2001;25(2):107–12. https://doi.org/10.17796/jcpd.25.2.p255673211764073. PMID: 11314207
6. Courant P, Sobkov T. Oral manifestations of infectious mononucleosis. J Periodontol. 1969;40(5):279–83.
7. Kimmis BD, Downing C, Tyring S. Hand-foot-and-mouth disease caused by coxsackievirus A6 on the rise. Cutis. 2018;102(5):353–6. PMID: 30566537
8. Laskaris G. Oral manifestations of infectious diseases. Dent Clin N Am. 1996;40(2):395–423. PMID: 8641529
9. Scully C, Epstein J, Porter S, Cox M. Viruses and chronic disorders involving the human oral mucosa. Oral Surg Oral Med

Oral Pathol. 1991;72(5):537–44. https://doi.org/10.1016/0030-4220(91)90490-4. PMID: 1745511
10. Chen KT, Chang HL, Wang ST, Cheng YT, et al. Epidemiologic features of hand-foot-mouth disease and herpangina caused by enterovirus 71 in Taiwan, 1998-2005. Pediatrics. 2007;120:244–52.
11. Hosoya M, Kawasaki Y, Sato M, et al. Genetic diversity of coxsackievirus a16 associated with hand, foot, and mouth disease epidemics in Japan from 1983 to 2003. J Clin Microbiol. 2007;45:112–20.
12. Rowley AH. Kawasaki disease: novel insights into etiology and genetic susceptibility. Ann Rev Med. 2011;62:69–77.
13. Verdoni L, Mazza A, Gervasoni A, et al. An outbreak of severe Kawasaki-like disease at the Italian epicentre of the SARS-CoV-2 epidemic: an observational cohort study. Lancet. 2020;395:1771–8.
14. Maticic M, Poljak M, Kramar B, et al. Detection of hepatitis C virus RNA from gingival crevicular fluid and its relation to virus presence in saliva. J Periodontol. 2001;72(1):11–6.

HIV Infection and AIDS

29

Contents

The spectrum of oral clinical signs and symptoms in HIV-infected patients is wide and its study is of great importance. Information concerning the nature, clinical and laboratory significance, and treatment of oral lesions in HIV-infected patients has accumulated over the past four decades. Oral lesions in HIV-positive patients are often the first clinical symptoms of the disease and have been used as indicators for its progression and as entry criteria into clinical trials. Emphasis should be placed on the fact that oral lesions in HIV infection are indicative of and not truly specific to the disease as several of those lesions can also be found in non-HIV-infected patients. They should always be regarded as markers of HIV disease in correlation with the medical history and other clinical and laboratory studies, especially in cases of unknown HIV status. Oral lesions are mainly a result of cellular immunodeficiency due to HIV infection and are etiologically divided into five major groups. These include:

(a) Infections (bacterial, viral, fungal); (b) Neoplasms; (c) Drug reactions; (d) Neurological manifestations; and (e) Lesions of unknown cause.

Lesions may represent early or late manifestations of HIV disease, they may be common or rare, and the oral physician should be familiar with all of them. Oral lesions are classified according to their relationship to HIV infection into three groups: (a) *Group I:* lesions that are strongly associated with HIV infection; (b) *Group II*: lesions less commonly associated with HIV infection; and (c) *Group III*: lesions rarely observed in HIV infection.

A dramatic reduction of oral lesions, including periodontal manifestations, has been observed over the past 20 years in HIV-infected patients due to successful therapeutic regimens with new anti-HIV drugs that reduced viral replication and increase immune cells. It is of great importance for the periodontist to be familiar with periodontal manifestations of HIV infection, as the periodontium is a crucial anatomical region in dental practice.

The most common gingival lesions follow.

Bacterial Infections

Necrotizing Gingivitis (see also p. 33)

Necrotizing gingivitis is a common early manifestation in HIV-infected patients with a prevalence rate of 4–16%. A high possibility for HIV infection exists, particularly if high-risk behavior is associated with necrotizing gingivitis.

G. Laskaris et al., *Periodontal Manifestations of Local and Systemic Diseases*, https://doi.org/10.1007/978-3-031-10828-0_29

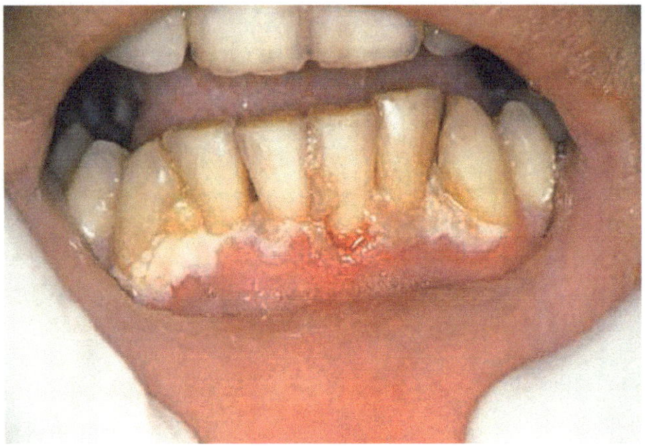

Fig. 29.1 HIV infection, necrotizing gingivitis

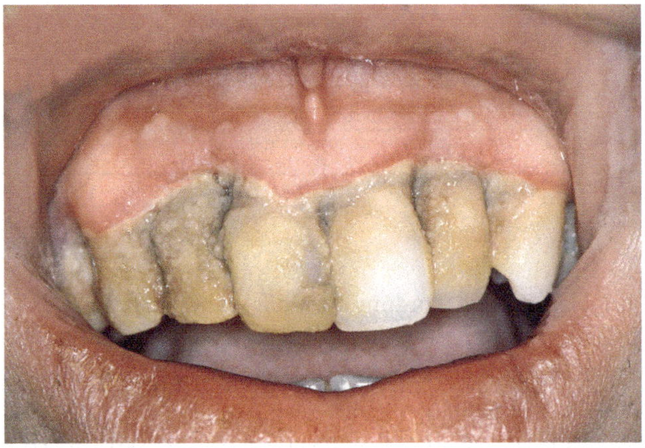

Fig. 29.2 HIV infection, necrotizing periodontitis

Clinical Features

- Clinically, the onset of the disease is either acute or subacute and it presents with fiery red and swollen gingiva and characteristic destruction of one or more interdental papillae. In the acute stage, ulceration, necrosis, and sloughing of both the margin of the gingiva and the tip of the interdental papillae are common findings (Figs. 29.1 and 29.2). Pain, bleeding, and halitosis are also common symptoms. The anterior gingiva is most frequently affected. Necrotizing gingivitis should be limited to lesions only involving gingival tissue with no loss of periodontal attachment. Necrotizing gingivitis may rarely progress to necrotizing periodontitis and stomatitis in HIV-infected patients.

Treatment In the acute phase, treatment of necrotizing gingivitis should include metronidazole for 6–8 days and topical use of oxygen-releasing mouthwashes. Conventional periodontal treatment (biofilm control measures, root planning and scaling) should follow.

Necrotizing Periodontitis (see also p. 34)

Necrotizing periodontitis is the most severe form of periodontitis associated with HIV infection that develops in patients with marked immunosuppression. The prevalence is 5% or less. This low prevalence may be related to the improved quality of patient care and medical treatment.

Clinical Features

- Necrotizing periodontitis is characterized by gingival ulceration, necrosis, rapid loss of clinical attachment and alveolar bone, and loosening or shifting of the teeth in the affected area (Figs. 29.3 and 29.4). Spontaneous bleeding, deep-seated pain, halitosis, erythema, and edema are prominent features (Fig. 29.5). The lesions may be localized or less often generalized. They are usually not associated with deep pocket formation, because extensive gingival necrosis often coincides with the loss of crestal alveolar bone.

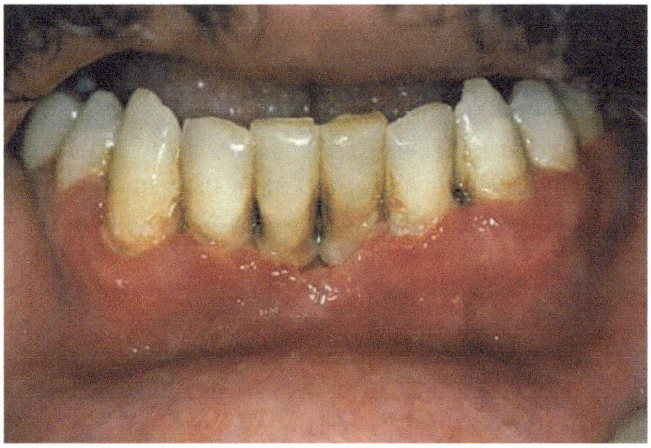

Fig. 29.3 HIV infection, necrotizing periodontits

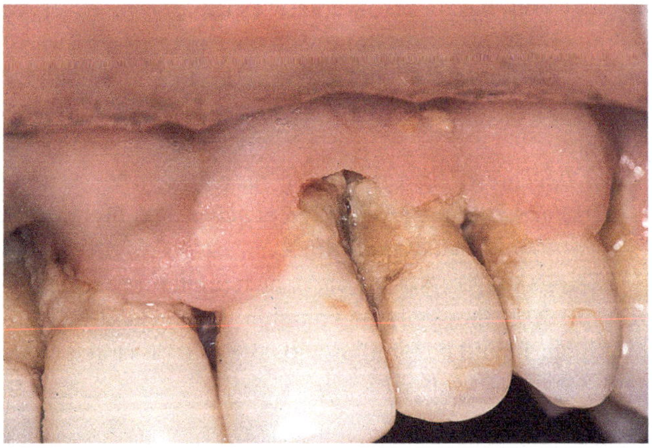

Fig. 29.4 HIV infection, severe necrotizing periodontitis

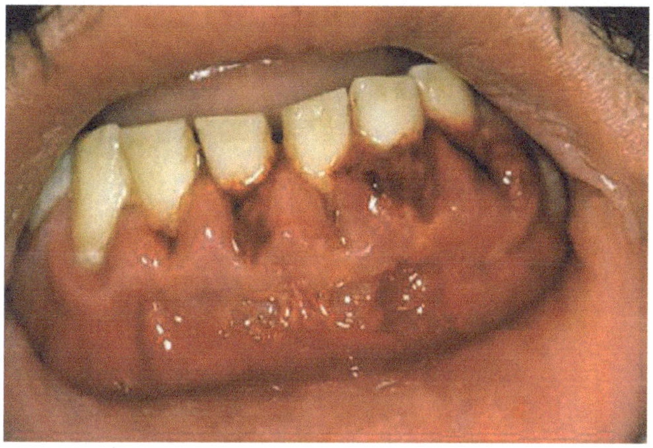

Fig. 29.5 HIV infection, severe periodontitis with severe edema, multiple abscesses and bleeding

Treatment The treatment of necrotizing periodontitis includes systemic administration of metronidazole or tetracycline in association with topical antibacterial mouthwashes. Conventional periodontal treatment maintenance and prevention should follow.

Bacillary Angiomatosis (see also p. 157)

Bacillary angiomatosis is a recently described bacterial infection due to *Bartonella henselae* and *Bartonella quintana.* It is characterized by vascular proliferation and occurs more frequently in HIV-infected patients, and rarely in other immunosuppressed individuals or patients with malignancies. Skin, visceral, and rarely gingival and other oral lesions may occur. Oral bacillary angiomatosis should be regarded as an important prediction marker for HIV infection.

Other Bacterial Infections (see also p. 153)

- *Oral syphilis* is a relatively common infection occurring in HIV-infected patients. Both primary and secondary syphilis can occur in oral cavity, and rarely on the gingiva. In patients with HIV disease, lesions may have a malignant and protracted course.
- *Oral tuberculosis* should also be regarded in the differential diagnosis of oral lesions in HIV-infected patients, particularly after the recent dramatic increase of tuberculosis in this group of patients. Gingival involvement is rare and present as atypical and irregular ulceration.
- Some *other oral infections* caused by *Mycobacterium avium-intracellulare, Klebsiella pneumoniae, Enterobacter cloacae, Escherichia coli, Actinomyces israelii,* and *Pseudomonas aeruginosa* have also been reported predominantly during the later stages of HIV disease. Lesions caused by all of these microorganisms may develop on the gingiva (Fig. 29.6).

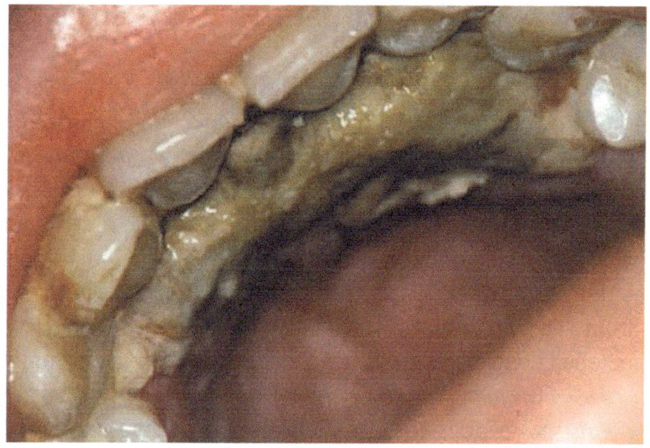

Fig. 29.6 HIV infection, diffuse necrotizing ulceration on the gingiva due to pseudomonas aeruginosa

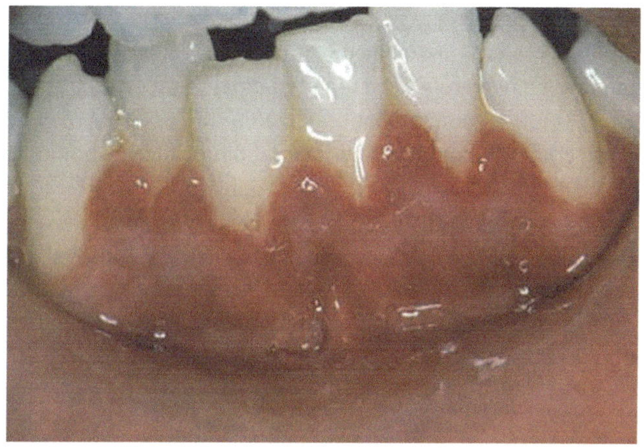

Fig. 29.7 HIV infection, herpetic gingivitis

Viral Infections

The most frequent viral oral lesions in HIV-infected patients are caused by members of the herpes virus group. Less frequent lesions may be caused by various types of human papilloma virus.

Herpes Simplex Virus (see also p. 95)

Primary and recurrent intraoral and perioral herpes simplex is a relatively frequent viral infection with a prevalence of 5–10%. The clinical features of oral herpes virus infection are usually similar to those seen in non-HIV-infected patients. However, in HIV-infected patients with severe immune suppression (CD4 cell counts usually below 100 cells/mm), widespread, severe, and prolonged lesions resemble primary herpetic gingivostomatitis (Fig. 29.7). In addition, recurrences are also common.

Herpes Zoster (see also p. 161)

Herpes zoster is one of the earliest clinical signs of HIV infection, particularly in individuals under 40 years of age with severe lesions, but without a history of immunosuppression. It would be more accurate to classify oral herpes zoster in young persons as a lesion "strongly associated with HIV infection." In addition, HIV-infected individuals with herpes zoster develop acquired immunodeficiency syndrome (AIDS) more frequently than do HIV-negative matched controls, but the prevalence of oral herpes zoster is low (1–2%). Gingival lesions may occur when herpes zoster affects the second and third division of the trigeminal nerve (Fig. 29.8).

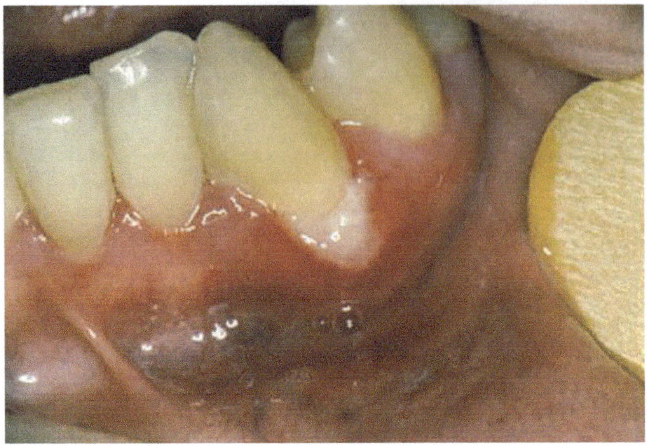

Fig. 29.9 HIV infection, gingival ulcer due to cytomegalovirus (CMV)

Cytomegalovirus (see also p. 100)

Oral ulcerations associated with cytomegalovirus (CMV) infection have rarely been reported in HIV-infected patients. However, it is thought that oral lesions due to CMV may be more common, and thus the final laboratory tests should be based on histological verification and molecular biology testing. These oral lesions are usually early signs of disseminated CMV infection and usually involve the gingival tissue (Figs. 29.9 and 29.10) Oral CMV infection is associated with severe immune suppression. Intravenous (IV) ganciclovir and acyclovir in high doses can be used for treatment.

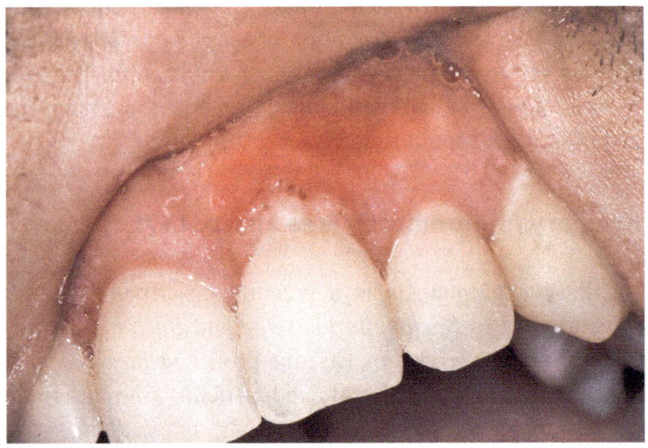

Fig. 29.10 HIV infection, localized erosion and deep erythema on the gingiva due to cytomegalovirus (CMV)

Condyloma Acuminatum (see also p. 97)

Condyloma acuminatum is relatively common in HIV-infected patients and the gingiva is the most commonly affected area (Fig. 29.11).

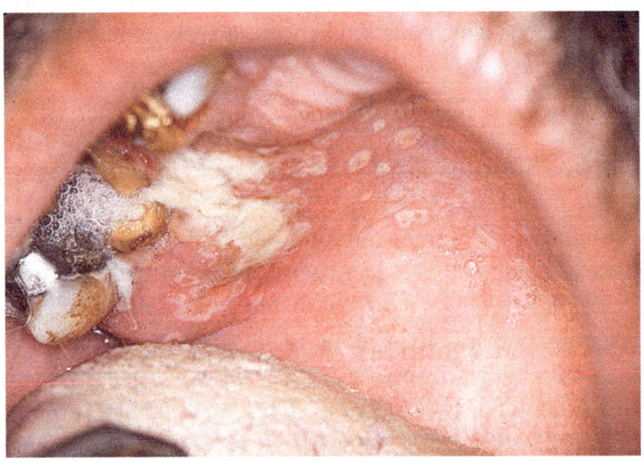

Fig. 29.8 HIV infection, severe herpes zoster on the palate and gingiva

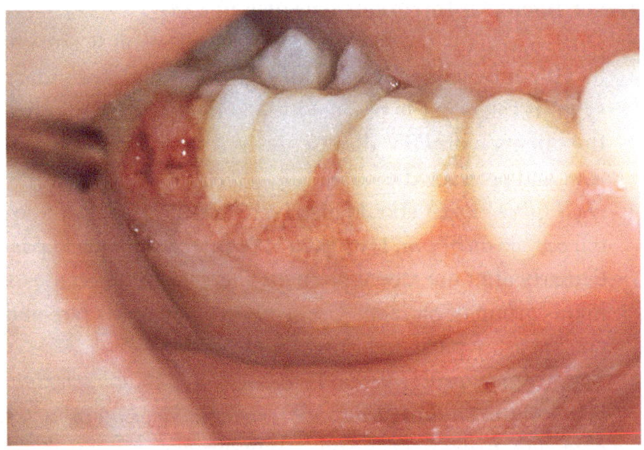

Fig. 29.11 HIV infection, multiple condylomas acuminatum on the gingiva

Mycoses

Linear Gingival Erythema

Linear gingival erythema is a relatively uncommon gingival lesion presumably indicative of an underlying HIV infection. The lesion has received little attention in the literature and its exact prevalence rate in HIV-infected patients is not yet clear. Although the exact etiology remains unclear a close association between oral candidiasis and linear gingival erythema exists.

Clinical Features

- Clinically, linear gingival erythema is characterized by a fiery red band along the margin of the gingiva and a punctate or diffuse erythema of the attached gingiva (Figs. 29.12 and 29.13). There is no ulceration and evidence of pocket formation or attachment loss. Gingival bleeding may occur spontaneously or on probing. However, an important clinical sign of linear gingival erythema is now considered to be the absence of bleeding on probing. The lesion does not respond well to biofilm control measures or scaling and root planing. Good oral hygiene for biofilm control is the treatment being recommended. Persistent lesions may be related to Candida infection and should be managed with antifungals.

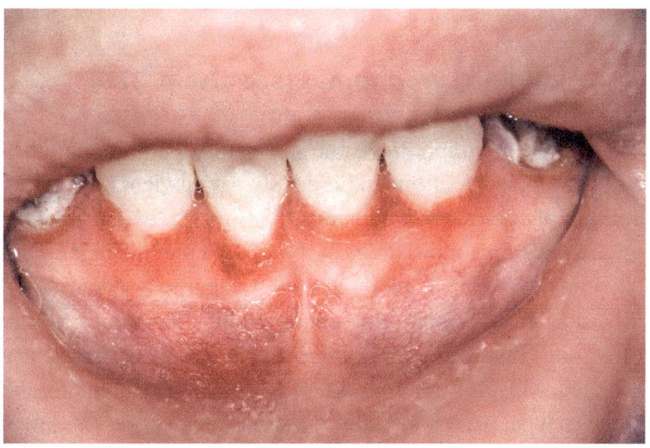

Fig. 29.12 HIV infection, linear gingival erythema

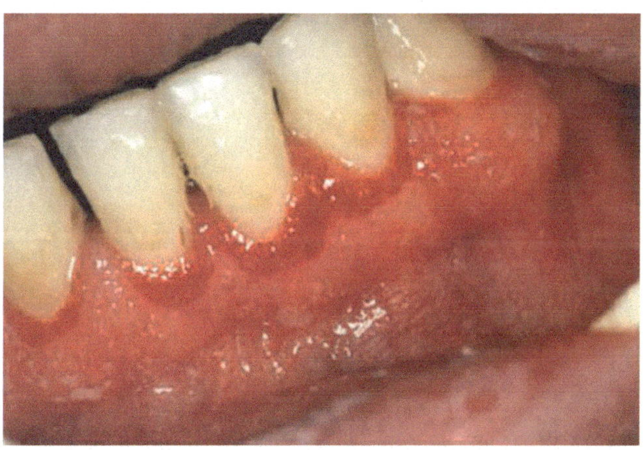

Fig. 29.13 HIV infection, linear gingival erythema

Candidiasis (see also p. 103)

Oral candidiasis is the most common oral manifestation among patients with HIV, predominantly caused by *Candida albicans* and rarely by other *Candida* species. It may be the initial sign of HIV infection in patients who appear otherwise healthy. In addition, oral candidiasis is usually associated with an increased risk for progression to HIV disease. A significant interaction between oral candidiasis and higher rate of CD4 cell count decline has also been detected. In one study of 700 HIV-infected patients, 70% with oral candidiasis had a CD4 cell count below 200 cells/mm^3. The prevalence of the lesions ranges between 11% and 95%, depending on the study design and the patient group. Except for HIV infection, other predisposing, systemic and local factors can also influence the development of oral candidiasis.

In HIV-infected patients, candida infection can occur in two major forms: (a) *pseudomembranous* and (b) *erythematous*. Pseudomembranous candidiasis presents as white or yellowish spots or plaques that can be wiped off, revealing an erythematous surface. Gingival lesions are not common (Figs. 29.14 and 29.15). The soft palate, buccal mucosa, lateral borders of the tongue, and commissures of lips are more frequently affected.

Erythematous candidiasis presents as a red area usually on the palate and the dorsum of the tongue. Less often, gingival involvement may occur (Figs. 29.16 and 29.17). White spots and plaques may be seen, but these are not usually conspicuous.

The treatment of oral candidiasis includes azole (ketoconazole, fluconazole, itraconazole) and polyene drugs (nystatin and amphotericin B). Resistance of oral candidiasis to those drugs in HIV-infected patients is a common finding and recurrences are frequently seen.

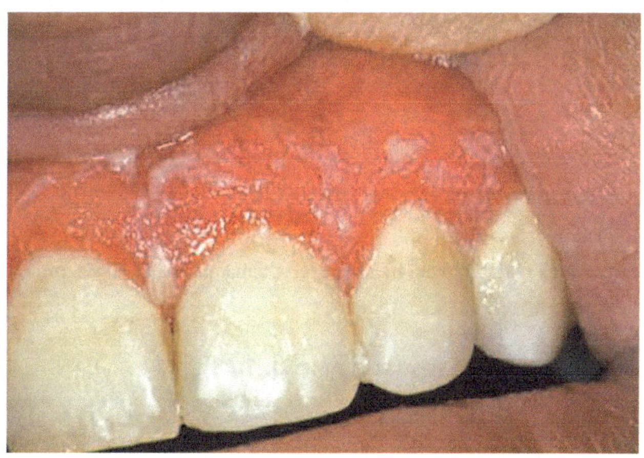

Fig. 29.14 HIV infection, pseudomembranous candidiasis on the gingiva

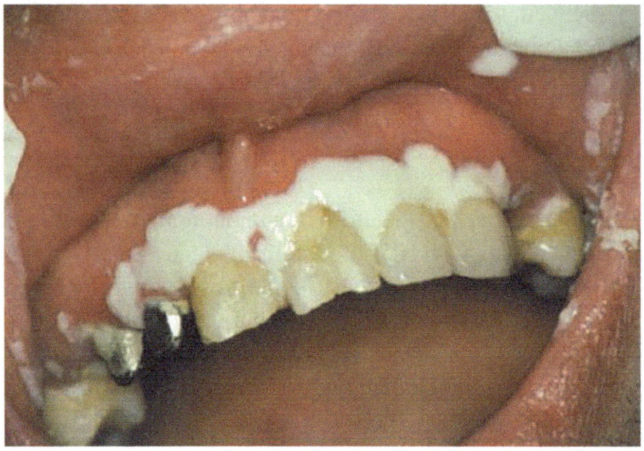

Fig. 29.15 HIV infection, severe pseudomembranous candidiasis on the gingiva

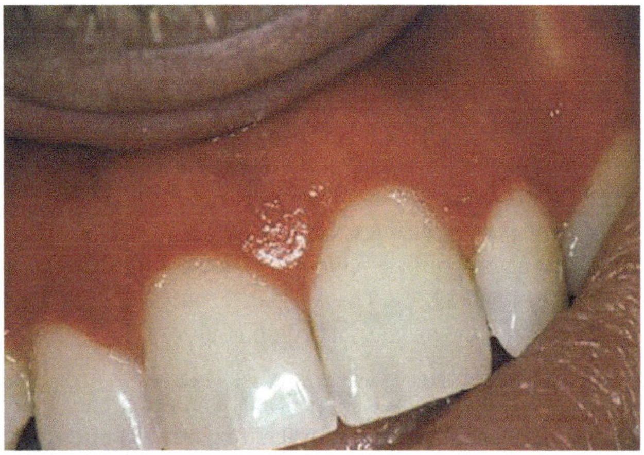

Fig. 29.16 HIV infection, erythematous candidiasis on the gingiva

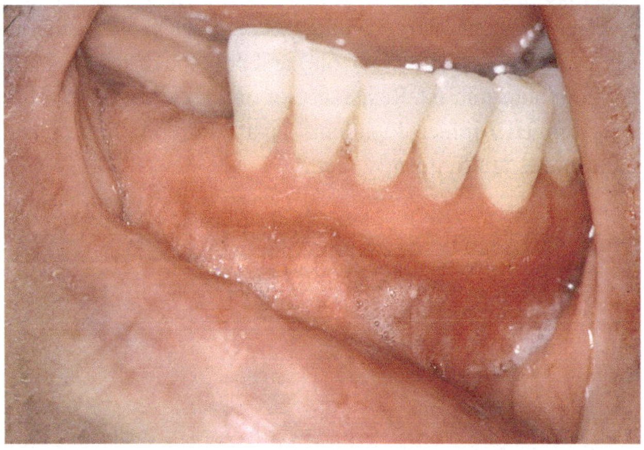

Fig. 29.17 HIV infection, severe erythematous candidiasis on the gingiva

Systemic Mycoses (see also p. 175)

Systemic or deep mycoses have, traditionally, been seen mainly in endemic areas as well as in developing countries. They are now increasing in immunocompromised individuals, including HIV-infected patients.

Gingival and oral lesions caused by systemic mycoses may occasionally be the primary or even the only manifestation, but they are usually associated with systemic signs and symptoms. HIV-infected patients are at particular risk of disseminating systemic mycoses.

Of the systemic mycoses with oral manifestations, *histoplasmosis* and *cryptococcosis* have been most frequently encountered in HIV-infected patients.

Sporadic cases of other systemic mycoses with oral manifestations have also been described in HIV-infected patients.

Neoplasms

Kaposi Sarcoma (see also p. 267)

Kaposi's sarcoma (KS) is the most common HIV-associated neoplasm, occurring after new therapeutic regimens in approximately 3–5% of the patients with AIDS. It is a potentially multicentric neoplasm that may manifest only with regional involvement in the oropharynx or with multiple-site involvement, including viscera. Up to 60% of AIDS patients with Kaposi's sarcoma have oral and gingival lesions (Figs. 29.18 and 29.19).

Non-Hodgkin Lymphomas (see also p. 279)

Non-Hodgkin lymphoma is the second most common malignancy in HIV infection, and it develops in patients with CD4 cell counts below 100 cells/mm^3. Up to 3% of the patients would develop a non-Hodgkin lymphoma and the oral cavity accounts for 3% of all malignant lymphomas occurred in HIV-positive patients. Not uncommonly, the mouth is the only site involved. The posterior gingival is frequently affected. Most lymphomas are of B cell origin, including the Burkitt type. Rarely, Hodgkin disease may present intra-

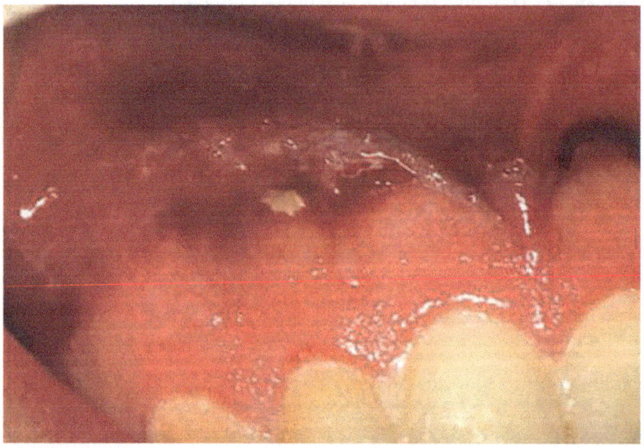

Fig. 29.18 AIDS, early Kaposi sarcoma, red patch on the alveolar mucosa

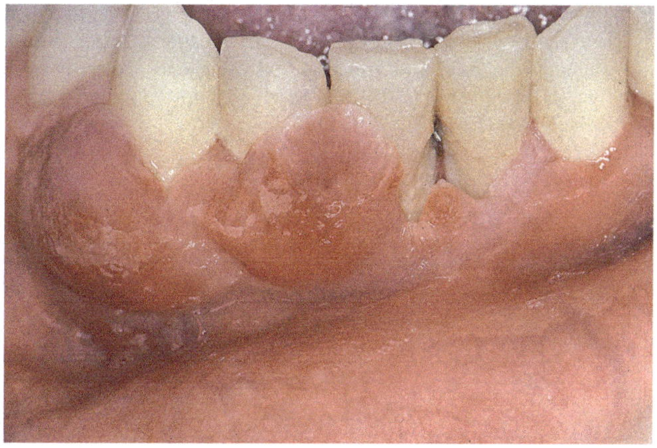

Fig. 29.19 AIDS, multiple Kaposi sarcomas on the gingiva

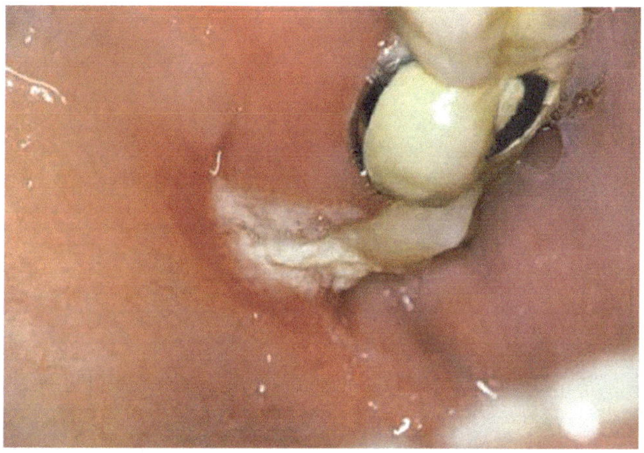

Fig. 29.20 AIDS, non-Hodgkin lymphoma presenting as small ulceration on the upper gingiva

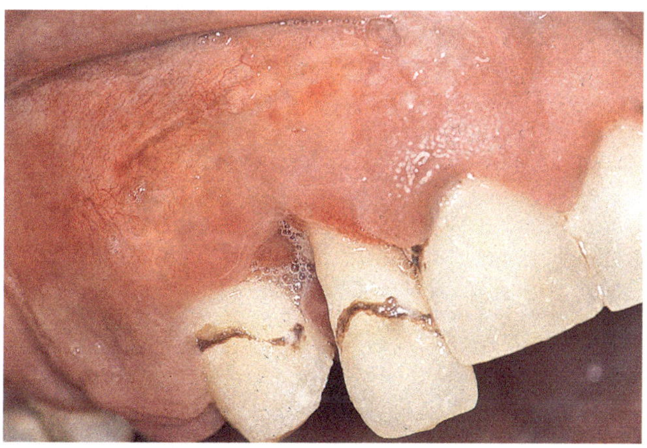

Fig. 29.21 AIDS, Burkitt lymphoma, swelling on the upper gingiva

orally and affect gingiva. Epstein-Barr virus is implicated as a cause for up to 50% of AIDS-associated lymphomas. Clinically, oral lymphoma usually presents as a slowly or more often rapidly growing red or purplish, painless, or painful mass that may be ulcerated (Figs. 29.20 and 29.21). Tooth loosening and paresthesia are often the presenting symptoms. The posterior gingiva and the soft palate are the most commonly affected sites, while jaw involvement may also occur.

References

1. Winkler JR, Robertson PB. Periodontal disease associated with HIV infection. Oral Surg Oral Med Oral Pathol. 1992;73(2):145–50. https://doi.org/10.1016/0030-4220(92)90186-t.
2. Yeung SC. HIV infection and periodontal disease. Ann R Austr Coll Dent Surg. 2000;15:331–4. PMID: 11709967
3. Patil K, Mahima VG, Srikanth HS. Extranodal non-Hodgkin's lymphoma of the gingiva in an HIV seropositive patient. Indian J Sex Transm Dis AIDS. 2010;31(2):112–5. https://doi.org/10.4103/0253-7184.75008.
4. Shah JS, Prajapati MN. Gingival mass in acquired immune deficiency syndrome patient: an unusual manifestation. Indian J Sex Transm Dis AIDS. 2016;37(1):78–80. https://doi.org/10.4103/0253-7184.176219.
5. Fokam J, Geh BKN, Sosso SM, et al. Determinants of periodontitis according to the immunological and virological profiles of HIV-infected patients in Yaoundé. Cameroon BMC Oral Health. 2020;20:359.
6. Laskaris G, Potouridou I, Laskaris M, Stratigos J. Gingival lesions of HIV infection in 178 Greek patients. Oral Surg Oral Med Oral Pathol. 1992b;74:168–71.
7. Laskaris G, Stergiou G, Kittas C, Scully C. Hodgkin's disease involving the gingiva in AIDS. Eur J Cancer Oral Oncol. 1992c;28B:39–41.
8. Laskaris G, Hadjivassiliou M, Stratigos J. Oral signs and symptoms in 160 Greek HIV-infected patients. J Oral Pathol Med. 1992a;21(3):120–3. https://doi.org/10.1111/j.1600-0714.1992.tb00994.x. PMID: 1316436
9. Laskaris G. Oral manifestations of HIV disease. Clin Dermatol. 2000;18(4):447–55. https://doi.org/10.1016/s0738-081x(99)00140-6. PMID: 11024312
10. Scully C, Laskaris G, Pindborg J, Porter SR, Reichart P. Oral manifestations of HIV infection and their management. I. More common lesions. Oral Surg Oral Med Oral Pathol. 1991a;71(2):158–66. https://doi.org/10.1016/0030-4220(91)90459-p. PMID: 2003011
11. Scully C, Laskaris G, Pindborg J, Porter SR, Reichart P. Oral manifestations of HIV infection and their management. II. Less common lesions. Oral Surg Oral Med Oral Pathol. 1991b;71(2):167–71. https://doi.org/10.1016/0030-4220(91)90460-t. PMID: 2003012
12. Economopoulou P, Laskaris G, Kittas C. Oral histoplasmosis as an indicator of HIV infection. Oral Surg Oral Med Oral Pathol Oral Radiol Endod. 1998;86(2):203–6. https://doi.org/10.1016/s1079-2104(98)90126-3. PMID: 9720097
13. Nakou M, Kamma J, Gargalianos P, Laskaris G, et al. Periodontal microflora of HIV infected patients with periodontitis. Anaerobe. 1997;3:97–102.
14. Chebbi F, Poveda JD, Suzuki T, et al. Search for infectious HIV in gingival crevicular fluid and saliva of advanced AIDS patients with severe periodontitis. AIDS. 1997; 11:927–8.
15. Reichart PA. Oral manifestations in HIV infection: fungal and bacterial infections, Kaposi's sarcoma. Med Microbiol Immunol. 2003;192:165–9.
16. Kaur J, Singh P, Levine D. Cytomegalovirus-induced gingival hyperplasia. Clin Infect Dis. 2003;37:44–6.
17. Gonçalves LS, Gonçalves BM, Fontes TV. Periodontal disease in HIV-infected adults in the HAART era: clinical, immunological, and microbiological aspects. Arch Oral Biol. 2013;58(10):1385–

96. https://doi.org/10.1016/j.archoralbio.2013.05.002. Epub 2013 Jun 10. PMID: 23755999

18. Silva-Boghossian CM, Boscardini BAB, Pereira CM, Moreira EJL. Evaluation of oral care protocols practice by dentists in Rio de Janeiro towards HIV/AIDS individuals. BMC Oral Health. 2020;20(1):13. https://doi.org/10.1186/s12903-020-0999-7. PMID: 31937291; PMCID: PMC6961293

19. Sanadhya YK, Sanadhya S, Nagarajappa R, et al. Correlation between oral lesions and opportunistic infections among human immunodeficiency virus–infected individuals in Indian population. Int Marit Health. 2014;65(3):124–30. https://doi.org/10.5603/IMH.2014.0026. PMID: 25471161

Systemic Mycoses

30

Contents

Histoplasmosis

Definition Histoplasmosis is a granulomatous systemic mycosis that is mainly endemic in the Ohio and Mississippi valleys in the USA, Latin America, India, east Asia, and in Australia. However, sporadic cases may occur in other parts of the world, particularly in HIV-positive patients.

Etiology *Histoplasma capsulatum.*

Classification Three main forms are recognized: (a) *Primary acute pulmonary;* (b) *Chronic pulmonary;* and (c) *Disseminated form.*

Oral lesions occur mainly in patients with disseminated disease and less frequently with pulmonary histoplasmosis, especially in patients with AIDS.

Gingival Involvement Relatively common. Non-dental biofilm-associated lesions.

Other Sites of Involvement Oral mucosa, skin, lung, and other organs.

Clinical Features

- Gingival lesions present as a chronic vegetative painful ulcer with a tendency to increase in size and less frequently as nodules (Figs. 30.1, 30.2).

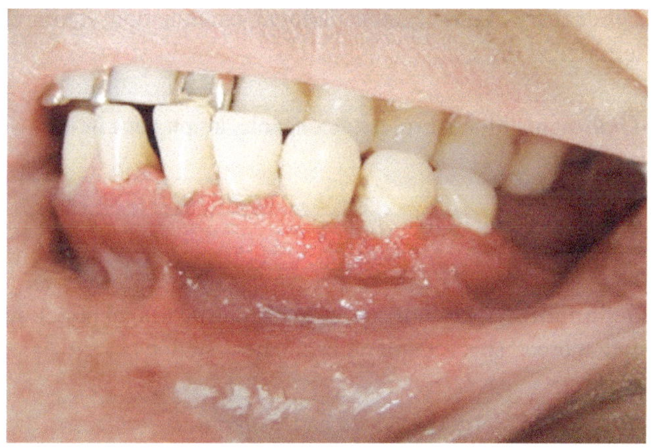

Fig. 30.1 Histoplasmosis, erythematous ulcerated swelling of the gingiva

- Oral lesions present also as painful ulcers or nodules usually on the tongue, palate, and buccal mucosa. Oral lesions of histoplasmosis may be found in a patient without evidence of systemic histoplasmosis.
- Systemic manifestations include cough, fever, weight loss, chest pain, weakness, fatigue and involvements of lymph nodes, spleen, liver, kidneys, gastrointestinal tract, and central nervous system.
- Clinical diagnosis should be confirmed by laboratory tests.

G. Laskaris et al., *Periodontal Manifestations of Local and Systemic Diseases*, https://doi.org/10.1007/978-3-031-10828-0_30

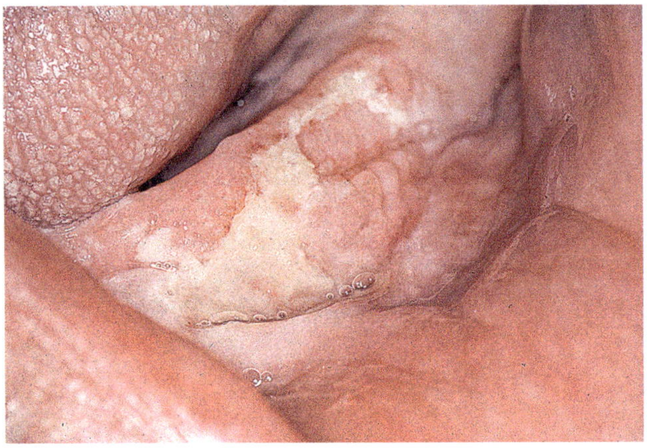

Fig. 30.2 Histoplasmosis, irregular ulceration on the alveolar mucosa and edema

Differential Diagnosis

- Oral tuberculosis.
- Squamous cell carcinoma.
- Other systemic mycoses.
- Eosinophilic ulcer.
- Wegener granulomatosis.
- Non-Hodgkin lymphoma.

Laboratory Tests Histopathologic examination, culture, serological tests.

Treatment Fluconazole, itraconazole, amphotericin B.

Aspergillosis

Definition Aspergillosis is an opportunistic fungal infection with a broad spectrum of clinical manifestations.

Etiology *Aspergillus flavus* and *aspergillus fumigatus* are the causative agents. Predisposing factors are hematologic malignancies, organ transplantations, immunosuppressives, and HIV infection.

Classification Five main forms are recognized: (a) *Allergic bronchopulmonary*; (b) *Aspergilloma* (or fungus balls); (c) *Invasive*; (d) *Chronic necrotizing pulmonary*; and (e) *Cutaneous*.

Gingival Involvement Relatively common. Non-dental biofilm-induced lesions.

Other Sites of Involvement Oral mucosa, nasal mucosa, skin, lungs.

Clinical Features

- Gingival lesions are commonly secondary to systemic infection and present as a violaceous surface, which progressively becomes necrotic covered by a brownish-black pseudomembrane containing fungal hyphae (Fig. 30.3).
- Oral lesions present as irregular ulcerations with a tendency to spread with a characteristic brownish-black surface of necrotic tissues (Fig. 30.4). Rarely, oral lesions are early and they are observed after endodontic therapy or tooth extraction.
- Prodromal symptoms of infection are dry cough, fever, dyspnea, chest pain, and cardiac problems.
- Clinical diagnosis should be confirmed by laboratory tests.

Differential Diagnosis

- Mucormycosis.
- Cryptococcosis.
- Nasal NK/T Non-Hodgkin lymphoma.

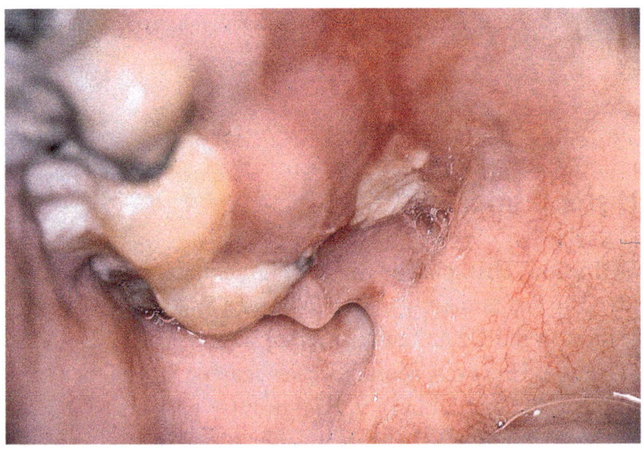

Fig. 30.3 Aspergillosis, ulceration on the palate and localized gingival enlargement of a patient with leukemia

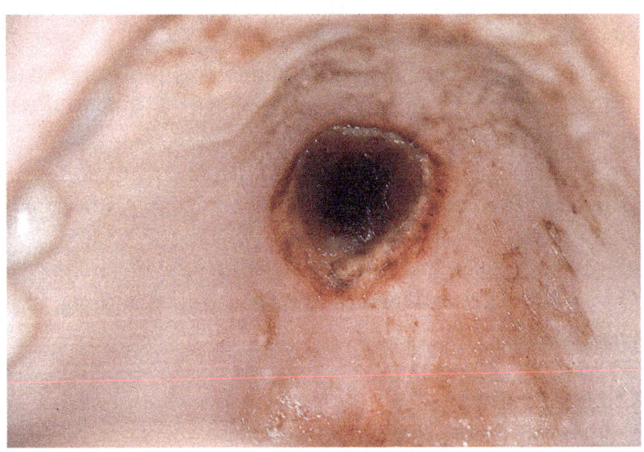

Fig. 30.4 Aspergillosis, necrotic ulceration on the palate of a patient with leukemia

- Leukemia.
- Agranulocytosis.
- Malignant neoplasms.

Laboratory Tests Histopathologic examination, microbiologic culture, computed tomography.

Treatment Drugs of choice are voriconazole and posaconazole or intravenous amphotericin B. Therapy should be left to the infectious diseases specialists.

Mucormycosis

Definition Mucormycosis or zygomycosis or phycomycosis is a relatively rare systemic mycosis that mainly affects immunocompromised patients (patients with leukemia, non-Hodgkin lymphoma, severe poorly controlled diabetes mellitus, AIDS).

Etiology Species that belong to the genera *Mucor*, *Rhizopus*, and *Absidia.*

Classification There are five major clinical forms: (a) *Rhino-orbito-cerebral*; (b) *Pulmonary*; (c) *Gastrointestinal*; (d) *Cutaneous;* and (e) *Disseminated.*

Gingival Involvement Relatively common. Non-dental biofilm-related lesions.

Other Sites of Involvement Oral mucosa, nasal cavity and paranasal sinuses, lung, gastrointestinal tract, cardiovascular and central nervous system.

Clinical Features

- Oral manifestations occur in rhino-orbito-cerebral mucormycosis, which is the most common form of the disease.
- Gingival lesions present as erythematous and edematous areas, which soon progress to black necrotic ulcerations with severe alveolar bone destruction (Fig. 30.5).
- Oral lesions usually appear as palatal, black necrotic ulcers, which quickly spread, creating extensive bone destruction.
- The disease usually commences in the nasal cavity or paranasal sinuses with pain, nasal discharge, and fever. Facial swelling and headache are also common. Without proper treatment, mucormycosis may spread to the orbits and brain, eventually leading to death.
- Clinical diagnosis should be confirmed by laboratory tests.

Differential Diagnosis

- Severe necrotizing ulcerative gingivitis and stomatitis.
- Malignant granuloma.

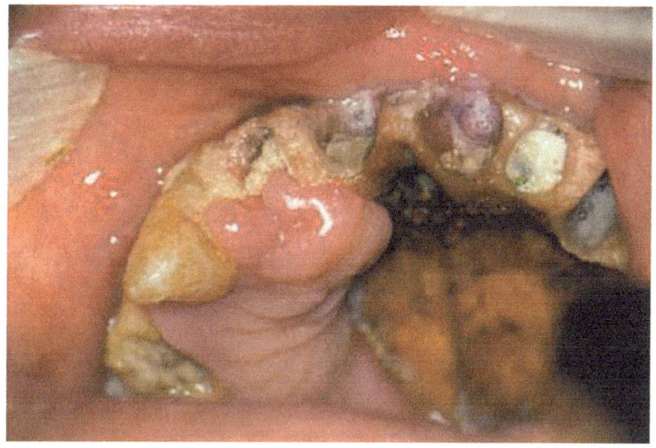

Fig. 30.5 Mucormycosis, necrotic ulcerations and severe alveolar bone and palatal destruction

- Wegener granulomatosis.
- Tuberculosis.
- Non-Hodgkin lymphoma.
- Extranodal NK/T cell lymphoma, nasal type.
- Other systemic mycoses.

Laboratory Tests Histopathologic examination. Smear examination, CT scan.

Treatment Surgical debridement and systemic amphotericin B.

Blastomycosis

Definition Blastomycosis is a rare systemic fungal infection, endemic in certain areas of North America (Mississippi river valley, Ohio river valley, Great Lakes region) but sporadic cases have been reported in South America, India, and Africa.

Etiology *Blastomyces dermatitidis,* a thermally dimorphic fungus.

Gingival Involvement Rare. Non-dental biofilm-induced lesions.

Other Sites of Involvement Lungs (mainly), bone, skin, oral and nasal mucosa (20–25%).

Clinical Features

- Clinically, oral blastomycosis appears as solitary or multiple atypical ulcerations with a slightly verrucous and irregular surface and thin border that mimic squamous cell carcinoma. The palate, tongue, lips, and gingiva are most frequently involved (Fig. 30.6). The gingival ulcerations are also not specific.

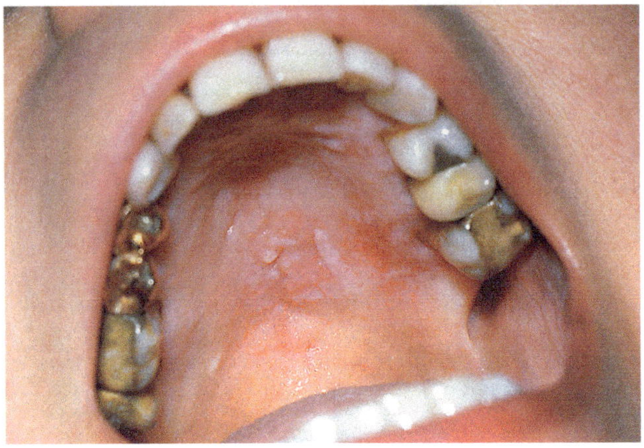

Fig. 30.6 Blastomycosis, ulcerations on the palate and adjacent gingiva

- Skin lesions can be solitary or multiple and present as papulopustules and well-circumscribed, verrucous plaques covered by scale-crust. Central ulceration may occur mimicking *pyoderma gangrenosum*.
- The pulmonary infection may mimic tuberculosis and is associated with fever, weight loss, nocturnal sweats, and cough. In about 50% of patients, the infection is subclinical.
- Clinical diagnosis should be confirmed by laboratory tests.

Differential Diagnosis
- Squamous cell carcinoma.
- Tuberculosis.
- Syphilis.
- Other systemic mycoses.

Laboratory Tests Histopathologic examination, smear and culture examination, PCR assays are also useful.

Treatment The treatment of choice is systemic itraconazole or liposomal amphotericin B. Alternative treatments are fluconazole, ketoconazole, and voriconazole.

Paracoccidioidomycosis

Definition Paracoccidioidomycosis or South American blastomycosis is a chronic granulomatous systemic mycosis, which is endemic in Brazil and less common in Venezuela, Uruguay, Argentina, and Colombia.

Etiology *Paracoccidioides brasiliensis*, a temperature-dependent dimorphic fungus.

Gingival Involvement Relatively common. Non-dental biofilm-related lesions.

Other Sites of Involvement Oral mucosa, lungs, skin, internal organs.

Clinical Features
- Gingival lesions present as painful, chronic, granular vegetative ulcer with severe erythema, which may be localized or generalized (Figs. 30.7, 30.8, and 30.9).
- Oral lesions also present as painful exophytic ulcerations with granular surface, usually occurring on the palate, tongue, and lips.
- In several cases, oral lesions follow tooth extraction.
- The presenting features of chronic pulmonary disease include cough, dyspnea, hemoptysis, fever, and weight loss.
- Clinical diagnosis should be confirmed by laboratory tests.

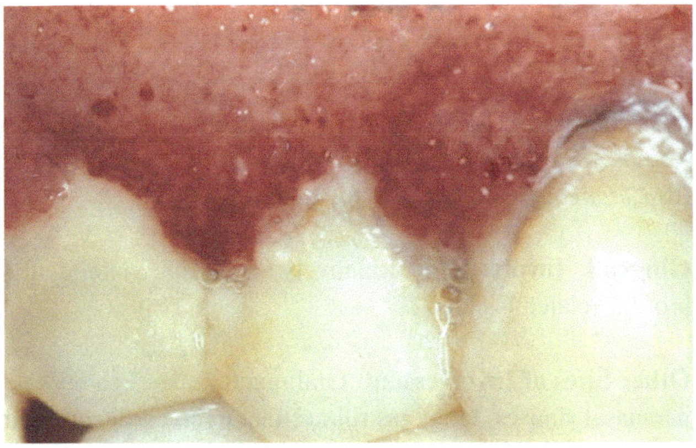

Fig. 30.7 Paracoccidioidomycosis, erythematous granular lesions on the upper gingiva

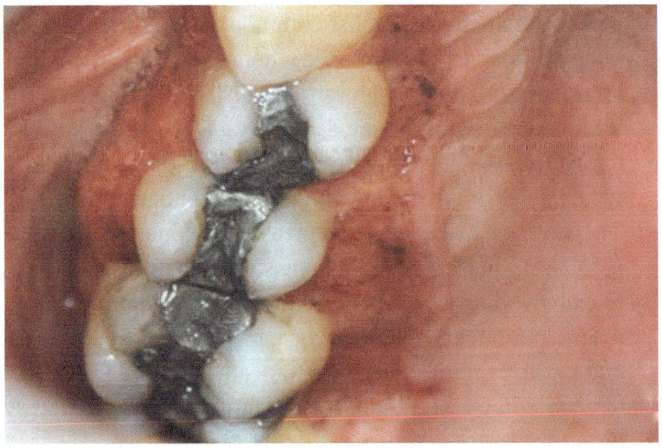

Fig. 30.8 Paracoccidioidomycosis, hemorrhagic erosions on the buccal and palatal gingiva

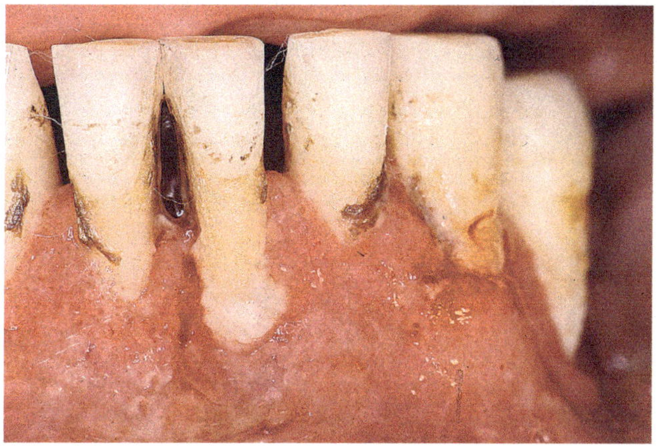

Fig. 30.9 Paracoccidioidomycosis, severe papillary gingival ulceration and erythema

Differential Diagnosis

- Pyostomatitis vegetans.
- Wegener granulomatosis.
- Tuberculosis.
- Sarcoidosis.
- Other systemic mycoses.
- Squamous cell carcinoma.
- Extranodal NK/T cell lymphoma, nasal type.

Laboratory Tests Histopathologic examination. Smear examination or culture, serological tests.

Treatment Fluconazole, itraconazole, amphotericin B.

References

1. Scully C, Almeida OP. Orofacial manifestations of the systemic mycoses. J Oral Pathol Med. 1992:21–7.
2. Akin L, Herford AS, Cicciu M. Oral presentation of disseminated histoplasmosis: a case report and literature review. J Oral Maxillofac Surg. 2011;69:535–41.
3. Broome WC, Hutchinson RA, Mays EE. Histoplasmosis of the gingiva. Report of a case. J Periodontol. 1976;47(2):95–7. https://doi.org/10.1902/jop.1976.47.2.95. PMID: 1062555
4. Cho H, Lee KH, Colquhoun AN, Evans SA. Invasive oral aspergillosis in a patient with acute myeloid leukaemia. Aust Dent J. 2010;55:214–8.
5. Kruse AL, Zwahlen RA, Bredell MG, et al. Primary blastomycosis of oral cavity. J Craniofac Surg. 2010;21(1):121–3. https://doi.org/10.1097/SCS.0b013e3181c4680c. PMID: 20072023
6. Brazao-Silva MT, Andrade MF, Franco T, et al. Paracoccidioidomycosis: a series of 66 patients with oral lesions from an endemic area. Mycoses. 2011;54:189–95.
7. Silva CO, Almeida AS, Pereira AA, et al. Gingival involvement in oral paracoccidioidomycosis. J Periodontol. 2007;78:1229–34.
8. Lee DH, Lim SC. Maxillary fungus ball caused by retained foreign bodies for 25 years. J Craniofac Surg. 2012;23(3):e176–7.
9. Mutalik VS, Bissonnette C, Kalmar JR, McNamara KK. Unique oral presentations of deep fungal infections: a report of four cases. Head Neck Pathol. 2020; https://doi.org/10.1007/s12105-020-01217-0. Epub ahead of print. PMID: 32889592
10. Economopoulou P, Laskaris G, Ferekidis E, Kanelis N. Rhinocerebral mucormycosis with severe oral lesions: a case report. J Oral Maxillofac Surg. 1995;53(2):215–7. https://doi.org/10.1016/0278-2391(95)90407-7. PMID: 7830193
11. Dogan MC, Leblebisatan G, Haytac MC, et al. Oral mucormycosis in children with leukemia: report of 2 cases. Quintessence Int. 2007;38(6):515–20. PMID: 17625636

Protozoa and Infestations

31

Contents

Leishmaniasis

Definition Leishmaniasis is a chronic protozoal infection with a broad spectrum of clinical manifestations and a worldwide distribution, especially in the Mediterranean basin, South America, and parts of Africa and Asia.

Etiology It is caused by different *protozoan parasites* of the genus Leishmania. The parasites are spread by the bite of female *sandflies* of the genus *Phlebotomus* and *Lutzomyia.*

Classification Clinically, leishmaniasis is divided into four major types: (a) *cutaneous* or *oriental sore,* which is usually caused by *Leishmania tropica*and primarily involves the skin (b) *mucocutaneous,* which is caused by *Leismania braziliensis* and involves the skin and mucous membranes (c) *Diffuse cutaneous,* caused by *Leishmania amazonensis* and (d) *Visceral (also known as kala-azar),* which involves internal organs and bone marrow.

Gingival Involvement Rare. More commonly in the mucocutaneous and diffuse cutaneous types. Non-dental biofilm-induced lesions.

Other Sites of Involvement Oral and nasal mucosa, skin, viscera.

Clinical Features

- Clinically, the skin lesions evolve from papules at the site of parasite inoculation to erythematous nodular plaques and to ulcerative lesions surrounded by inflammatory skin.
- Oral lesions are more common on the lips and commissures. Clinically, they are characterized by erythematous elevated nodules, which soon evolve into an atypical ulcer.
- Gingival lesions are uncommon and they clinically present as erythematous nonspecific gingivitis, which soon progresses to ulcerative periodontal tissue destruction (Figs. 31.1 and 31.2).
- Clinical diagnosis should be confirmed by laboratory tests.

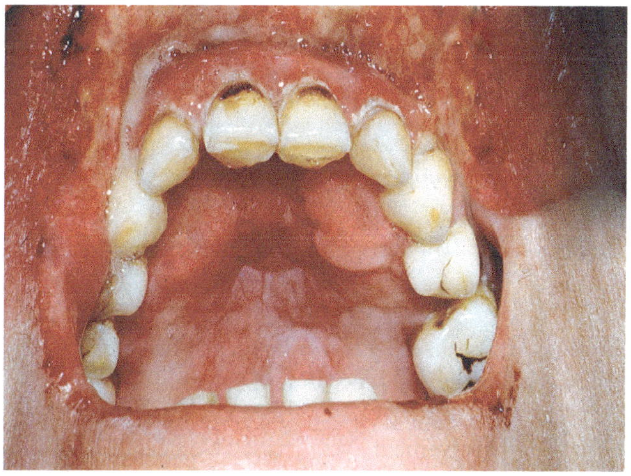

Fig. 31.1 Leishmaniasis, severe ulcerative lesions and nodules on the upper gingiva, the palate and the upper lip

G. Laskaris et al., *Periodontal Manifestations of Local and Systemic Diseases*, https://doi.org/10.1007/978-3-031-10828-0_31

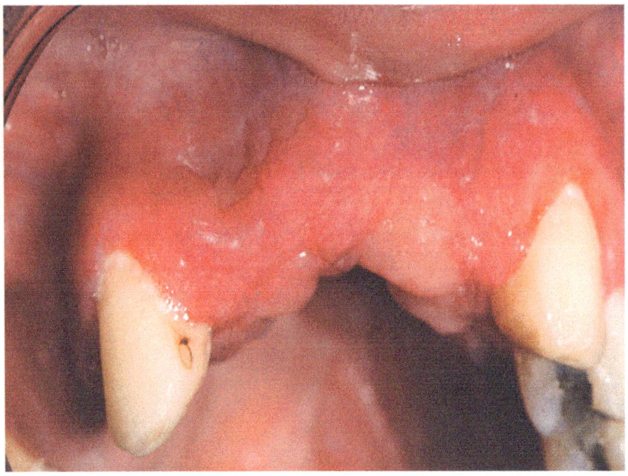

Fig. 31.2 Leishmaniasis on the upper gingiva presenting with erythema and atypical swellings

Differential Diagnosis

- Ulcerative gingivitis.
- Ulcerative periodontitis.
- Systemic mycoses.
- Squamous cell carcinoma.
- Non-Hodgkin lymphoma.
- Other nonspecific ulcerations.
- HIV infection.

Laboratory Tests Histopathologic examination. Isolation and culture of the parasite using specific stains (Giemsa, Wright, Feulgen). Smear examination, leishmanin skin test.

Treatment The first-line treatment for the cutaneous type is the use of parenteral pentavalent antimonials (meglumine or sodium stibogluconate or miltefosine). The second line treatment is the use of fluconazole, liposomal amphotericin B, allopurinol, and pentamidine. The treatment must be left to specialists.

Gingival Myiasis

Definition Oral myiasis is a rare infestation of the oral mucosa.

Etiology It is caused by *larvae (maggots)* of a variety of fly species within the anthropod order Diptera.

Gingival Involvement Very rare. Non-dental biofilm-induced lesions, associated with poor oral hygiene.

Other Sites of Involvement Oral mucosa, nose, ears, anus, vagina (rare), and skin (more common).

Clinical Features

- The disease is more common in tropical and subtropical regions of Africa and South America, and is associated with warm and humid environments as well as with very poor hygiene.
- Intraorally, the eggs of various species *(Cochliomyia hominivorax, Chrysomya bezziana)* of flies can be deposited in a preexisting ulcer, postextraction socket and periodontal disease bedding in people who breathe through their mouths when they sleep outside during the summer.
- The flies are attracted to bad odors from food remnants and debris due to very poor oral hygiene. The eggs hatch within 24 hours and the developing larvae can be seen (Fig. 31.3). The lesions are associated with purulent discharge, edema, bad odor, and lymphadenopathy. Malaise and fever are common.
- Diagnosis is usually based on history and clinical features.

Differential Diagnosis

- Osteomyelitis.
- Necrotizing periodontitis.
- Noma.

Laboratory Tests Usually they are not necessary. The larvae may be seen macroscopically.

Treatment Surgical removal and debridement with irrigation to eliminate the larvae is the first choice. This and other treatments should be left to specialists.

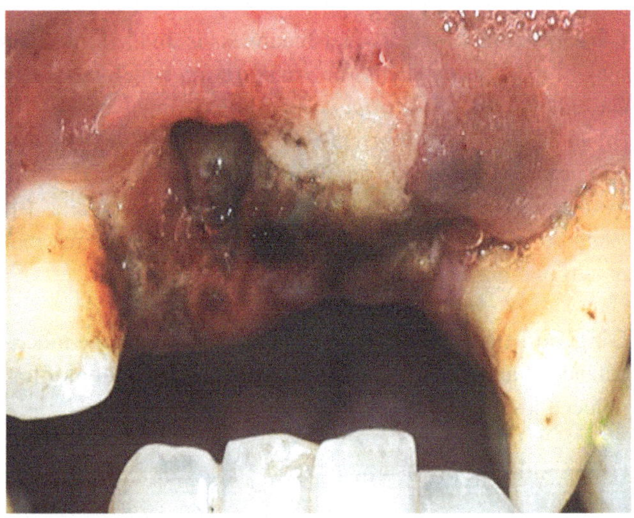

Fig. 31.3 Myiasis on the upper gingiva, multiple larvae within an ulcerated area of the upper gingiva

References

1. Almeida TF, da Silveira EM, Dos Santos CR, et al. Exclusive primary lesion of oral eishmaniasis with immunohistochemical diagnosis. Head Neck Pathol. 2016;10(4):533–7. https://doi.org/10.1007/s12105-016-0732-7. Epub 2016 Jun 3. PMID: 27260217; PMCID: PMC5082056
2. Mignogna MD, Celentano A, Leuci S, et al. Mucosal leishmaniasis with primary oral involvement: a case series and a review of the literature. Oral Dis. 2015;21(1):e70–8. https://doi.org/10.1111/odi.12268. Epub 2014 Jul 12. PMID: 24939442
3. Sharma D, Kumar S, Parashar P, Naphade VV. Oral gingival myiasis: a rare case report and literature review. Contemp Clin. Dent. 2015;6(4):548–51.
4. Özdemır EÇ, et al. A case of gingival myiasis caused by Wohlfahrtia magnifica. Mikrobiyoloji Bulteni. 2014;48(3):512–7.
5. Sankari LS, Ramakrishnan K. Oral myiasis caused by chrysomya bezziana. J Oral Maxillofac Pathol. 2010;14:16–8.
6. Sharma J, Mamatha GP, Acharya R. Primary oral myiasis: a case report. Med Oral Patol Oral Cir Bucal. 2008;13:714–6.
7. Hassona Y, Scully C, Aguida M, de Almeida OP. Flies and the mouth. J Investig Clin Dent. 2014;5(2):98–103. https://doi.org/10.1111/jicd.12076. Epub 2013 Dec 20. PMID: 24574273

Hematologic Diseases Non-Neoplastic

32

Contents

Severe Congenital Neutropenia

Definition Congenital neutropenia or Kostmann syndrome is a rare hematological disorder characterized by quantitative decrease of neutrophils in the peripheral blood due to their improper release from the bone marrow. Patients with congenital neutropenia become more susceptible to bacterial infections.

Etiology Genetic. It is inherited as an autosomal dominant and recessive trait. Mutations in the ELANE gene that codes for neutrophil elastase are involved in the pathogenesis of periodontitis.

Periodontal Involvement Common. Dental biofilm-induced, modified by quantitative leukocyte disorders are responsible for the periodontal lesions.

Other Sites of Involvement Oral mucosa, skin, ear, respiratory tract, urinary system.

Clinical Features

- The main clinical manifestations are recurrent infections and are usually present at birth.
- Periodontal manifestations include fiery red edematous gingivitis, severe periodontal lesions with deep periodontal pockets, and extensive generalized bone loss leading to tooth mobility and loss (Figs. 32.1 and 32.2).
- Recurrent oral ulceration, which may lead to scar formation, is common.
- Recurrent skin infections, otitis media, and pneumonia are constant manifestations.
- The severity of infections depends on quantitative neutrophil decrease. Affected children tend to improve with age and some undergo total remission in late childhood.
- Clinical diagnosis should be confirmed by laboratory tests.

Differential Diagnosis

- Severe periodontitis.
- Cyclic neutropenia.
- Agranulocytosis.

G. Laskaris et al., *Periodontal Manifestations of Local and Systemic Diseases*, https://doi.org/10.1007/978-3-031-10828-0_32

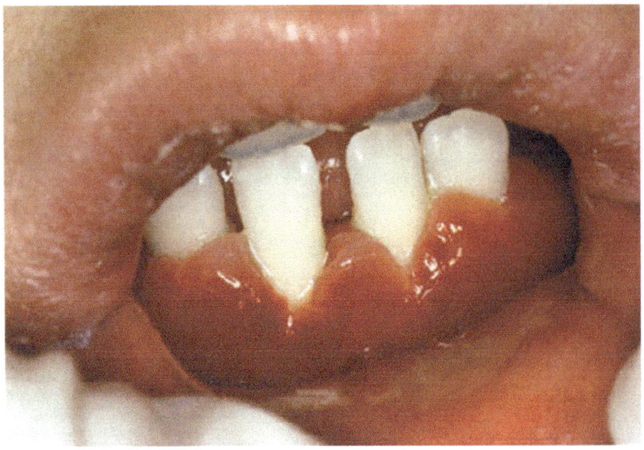

Fig. 32.1 Severe congenital neutropenia, diffuse erythematous gingivitis on the upper gingiva

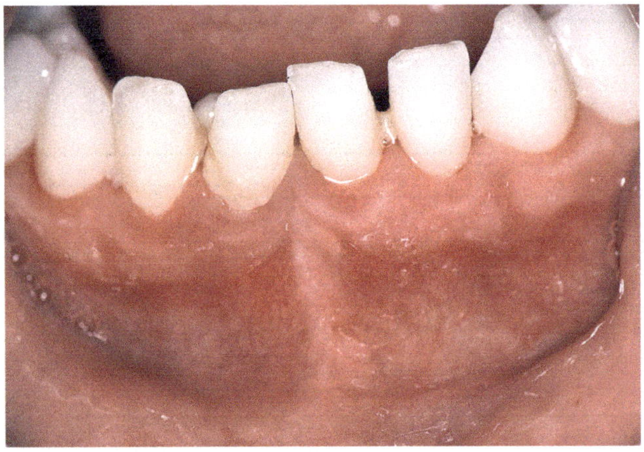

Fig. 32.2 Severe congenital neutropenia, generalized periodontitis at a 6 years -old- child

- Leukemia.
- Chediak-Higashi syndrome.
- Glycogen storage disease type 1b.
- Infantile genetic agranulocytosis.
- Hypophosphatasia.
- Acatalasemia

Laboratory Tests Complete blood count, bone marrow test, radiographic examination. Genetic testing for mutations in the ELANE gene

Treatment Good oral hygiene. Periodontal treatment (scaling, surgery, antimicrobial agents). The systemic treatment should be left to hematologists.

Acquired Neutropenia

Definition Neut000ropenia is a hematological disorder characterized by a decrease in the number of circulating neutrophils below 1800/μL in an adult with increased susceptibility to bacterial and fungal infections.

Etiology It is classified into two forms: (a) *hereditary* and (b) *acquired*. The cause of the acquired form may be drugs, bone marrow malignancies, HIV infection, other viral infections, systemic lupus erythematosus, and other autoimmune diseases. However, many acquired neutropenias have an unknown cause.

Gingival and Periodontal Involvement Common. Non-dental biofilm-induced lesions with increased risk for periodontal apparatus destruction depending on the severity of neutropenia.

Other Sites of Involvement Oral mucosa, skin, ear, respiratory and uropoetic systems, and other organs.

Clinical Features

- The risk of infection is related to the severity of neutropenia.
- Gingival and periodontal lesions consist of abnormal ulcerations covered by yellow-dark pseudomembranes with lack of red halo around them (Fig. 32.3). Occasionally, gingival inflammation and periodontal bone loss are noted with increased risk of tooth loss (Fig. 32.4).

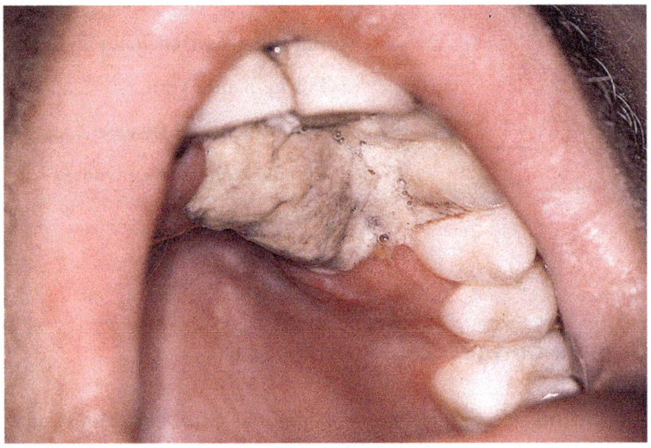

Fig. 32.3 Aquired neutropenia, ulcerations covered by pseudomembranes on the gingiva and palate

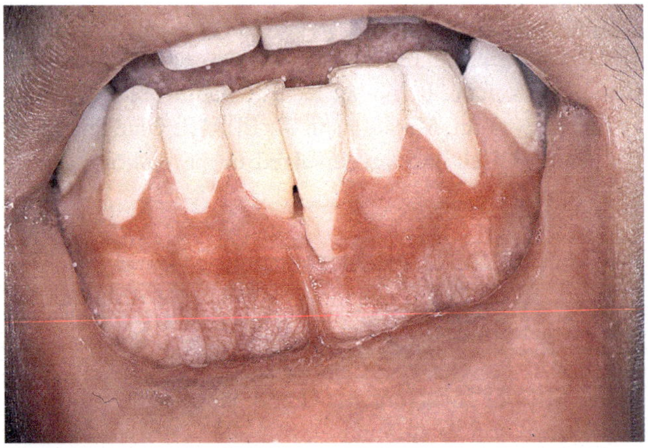

Fig. 32.4 Aquired neutropenia, erythematous gingivitis and periodontal bone loss

- Oral lesions are characterized by multiple abnormal ulcers with characteristic absence of peripheral inflammation. Oral and gingival lesions often present as the first or early manifestation of the disease.
- Systemic symptoms are high fever, malaise, and loss of appetite. Additional signs and symptoms appear in respiratory and urinary systems, inner ear, and skin. Systemic mycoses may also develop.
- Clinical diagnosis should be confirmed by laboratory tests.

Differential Diagnosis
- Congenital neutropenia.
- Cyclic neutropenia.
- Agranulocytosis.
- Aplastic anemia.
- Leukemia.
- Myelodysplastic syndromes.

Laboratory Tests Peripheral blood examination, histopathologic examination, bone marrow examination.

Treatment Appropriate systemic antibiotics and antifungal medication, and granulocyte colony-stimulating factor (G-CSF) are the first line of treatment, which should be left to hematologists. In persistent severe cases, hematopoietic stem cell transplantation is recommended. Good oral hygiene for decrease of bacterial and fungal load in the mouth is necessary.

Cyclic Neutropenia

Definition Cyclic neutropenia is a rare blood disorder characterized by regular episodes—on a cycle of approximately every 3 weeks—of low levels of neutrophils. The duration of neutropenia is usually short and may persist for 5–10 days. Following the episode, the counts of neutrophils gradually return to normal.

Etiology The etiology remains unknown. The disorder is thought to be due to a defect of hematopoietic regulation. An autosomal dominant trait has been recorded in some cases.

Periodontal Involvement Relatively common. Dental biofilm-induced, modified by quantitative leukocyte disorders are responsible for the periodontal lesions.

Other Sites of Involvement Oral mucosa, skin, ear.

Clinical Features
- Periodontal manifestations include diffuse gingival inflammation and ulcerations. Increased risk for periodontal attachment and bone loss (Fig. 32.5).

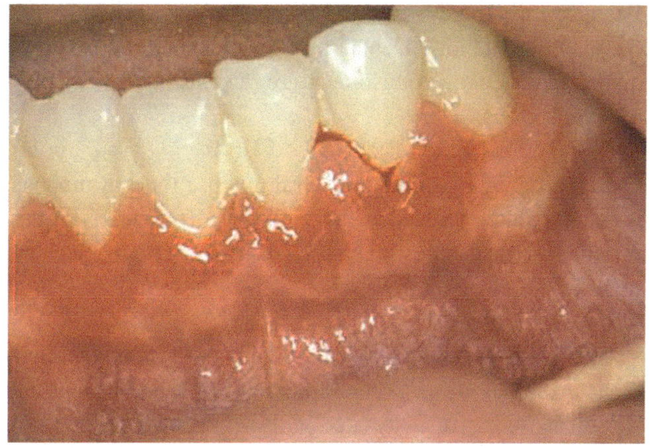

Fig. 32.5 Cyclic neutropenia, diffuse gingival erythema and edema

- Painful, recurrent, oval oral ulcerations covered by a whitish membrane on an erythematous base usually occur.
- Skin infections and otitis media may also occur during an episode of profound neutropenia.
- Low-grade fever, malaise, headache, arthralgia, and cervical adenitis may occur. The disease usually begins after 10 years of age.
- Clinical diagnosis should be confirmed by laboratory tests.

Differential Diagnosis
- Severe periodontitis.
- Congenital neutropenia.
- Agranulocytosis.
- Chediak-Higashi syndrome.
- Glycogen storage disease type 1b.
- Infantile genetic agranulocytosis.
- Leukemia.
- Aphthous ulcers.
- Herpeticstomatitis.

Laboratory Tests Repeated complete blood count, bone marrow examination during periods of neutropenia shows decreased numbers of neutrophil precursors. Genetic testing.

Treatment Good oral hygiene. Periodontal treatment (scaling and root planing, surgery, antimicrobial agents). The systemic treatment must be left to the specialist hematologist.

Agranulocytosis

Definition Agranulocytosis is an acute hematological disorder characterized by severe depletion of neutrophils or all granulocytes in blood.

Etiology It is often due to adverse drug reactions. Idiopathic cases or cases induced by infections may also occur.

Periodontal Involvement Common as generalized periodontal destruction. Dental biofilm-induced, modified by quantitative leukocyte disorders are responsible for the periodontal lesions.

Other Sites of Involvement Oral mucosa (buccal mucosa, tongue, palate, tonsils), other mucosae (pharynx, larynx, esophagus, gastrointestinal tract), respiratory tract.

Clinical Features

- Periodontal lesions are early manifestations and are characterized by ulceration and necrosis of the marginal and attached gingiva associated with hemorrhage (Fig. 32.6). Severe generalized bone loss may also occur (Fig. 32.7).
- Necrotic ulcers covered by grey-white or dark, friable pseudomembranes are common findings in oral mucosa. The ulcers do not have a red halo around them. Halitosis, sialorrhoea, dysphagia, fever, malaise, and headache are common.
- Pulmonary and gastrointestinal infections are common.
- Clinical diagnosis should be confirmed by laboratory tests.

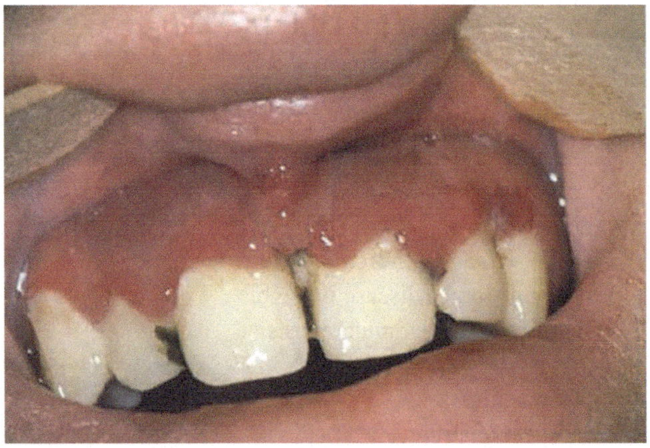

Fig. 32.6 Agranulocytosis, severe erythema and necrotic ulcerations on the gingiva

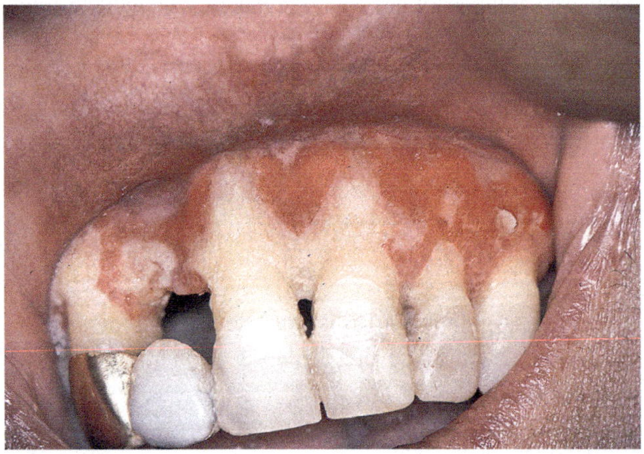

Fig. 32.7 Agranulocytosis, severe periodontitis and osteonecrosis

Differential Diagnosis

- Necrotizing gingivitis and stomatitis.
- Severe periodontitis.
- Congenital neutropenia.
- Cyclic neutropenia.
- Acuteleukemia.
- Other types of neutropenia.
- Infectious mononucleosis.
- Aplastic anemia.

Laboratory Tests Complete blood count and bone marrow aspiration.

Treatment Good oral hygiene. Periodontal treatment should follow systemic treatment. Systemic treatment must be left to hematologists.

Aplastic Anemia

Definition Aplastic anemia is a severe hematological disorder characterized by acellular or markedly hypocellular bone marrow resulting in pancytopenia.

Etiology Drugs, chemicals, radiation, infections are usually associated with the disease. Idiopathic cases may also occur.

Gingival Involvement Common. Dental biofilm-induced, modified by quantitative leukocyte disorders are responsible for the gingival lesions.

Other Sites of Involvement Oral mucosa, other mucosae, skin.

Clinical Feature

- Gingival bleeding is a common early sign. Localized necrotic ulcerations of the marginal gingiva and interdental papillae mimic necrotizing gingivitis (Figs. 32.8 and 32.9).

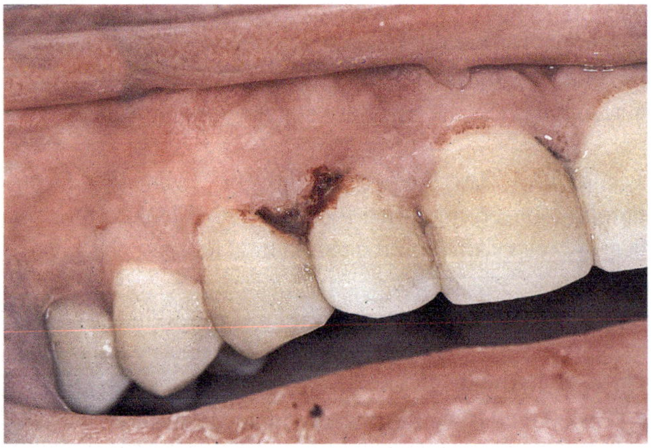

Fig. 32.8 Aplastic anemia, ulceration and gingival hemorrhage

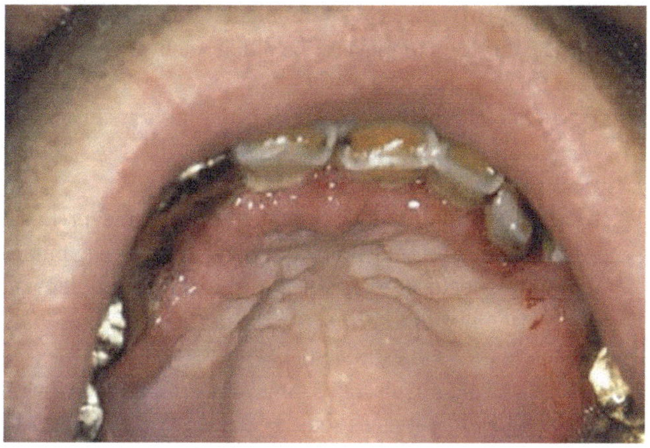

Fig. 32.9 Aplastic anemia, early necrotic ulceration on the gingiva

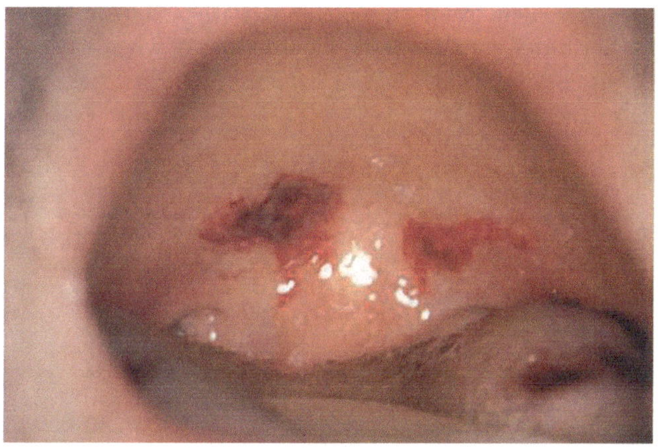

Fig. 32.10 Aplastic anemia, ecchymoses on the palate and tongue

- Oral lesions appear as necrotic ulcers, petechiae, ecchymoses, and pallor of oral mucosa (Fig. 32.10).
- Pallor, petechiae or ecchymoses, and purpuric spots of the skin and other mucous membranes are also early signs.
- The onset of the disease is usually insidious, and the most common symptoms are fever, weakness, fatigue, and mild hemorrhage. The course of the disease depends on the severity of aplasia.
- Clinical diagnosis should be confirmed by laboratory tests.

Differential Diagnosis
- Necrotizing gingivitis and stomatitis.
- Severe periodontitis.
- Vitamin C deficiency.
- Agranulocytosis.
- Neutropenia.
- Leukemia.
- Thrombocytopenic purpura.
- Infectious mononucleosis.

Laboratory Tests Complete blood count and bone marrow aspiration and histopathologic examination.

Treatment Good oral hygiene, topical oral antiseptics. Systemic treatment must be left to hematologists.

Thrombocytopenia

Definition Thrombocytopenia is a hematological disorder characterized by a profound decrease in platelets in the peripheral blood.

Etiology It may be *idiopathic* due to a primary failure of the bone marrow to generate platelets or *secondary* due to a myelotoxic drug, virus and HIV infections, leukemias and other autoimmune diseases, malignancies, radiation, etc.

Gingival Involvement Common. Non-dental biofilm-related lesions.

Other Sites of Involvement Other mucosa (conjunctiva, nose, gastrointestinal, urinary), skin.

Clinical Features
- Gingival bleeding, spontaneous and/or prolonged is a constant early feature (Fig. 32.11). There is no evidence that thrombocytopenia increases susceptibility to periodontal disease.
- Petechiae, ecchymoses, and hematomas may occur in oral mucosa (Fig. 32.12).
- Bleeding episodes from gastrointestinal and urinary tracts and epistaxis are common. Purpuric skin rash and occasionally bleeding occur (Fig. 32.13).
- The breadth and the severity of the manifestations are related to the extent of platelet reduction.
- Clinical diagnosis should be confirmed by laboratory tests.

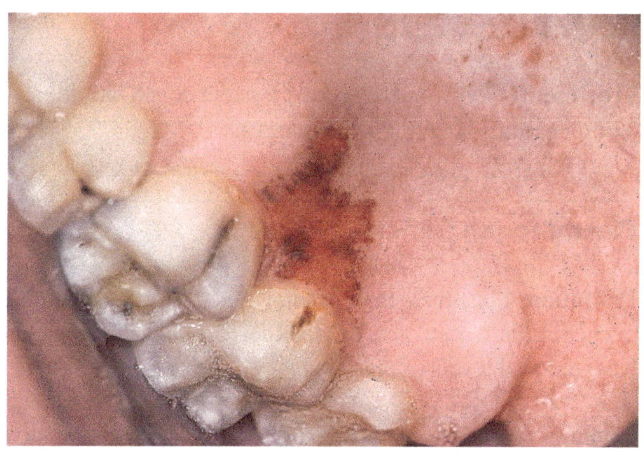

Fig. 32.11 Thrombocytopenia, ecchymoses on the gingiva and palate

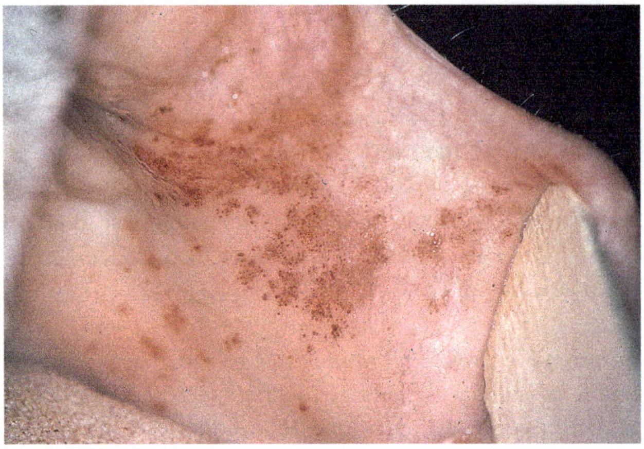

Fig. 32.12 Thrombocytopenia, ecchymoses and petechiaes on the buccal mucosa

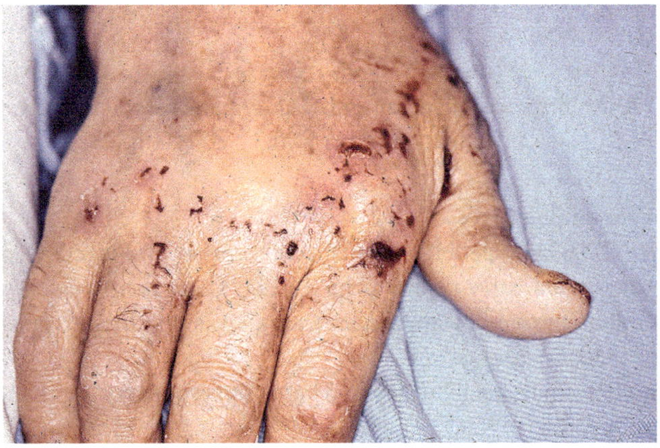

Fig. 32.13 Thrombocytopenia, purpuric skin rash

Differential Diagnosis
- Leukemia.
- Aplastic anemia.
- Agranulocytosis.

Laboratory Tests Complete blood count and bone marrow aspiration.

Treatment Good oral hygiene. Systemic and etiological treatment must be left to hematologists.

Plasminogen Deficiency Type I

Definition Plasminogen deficiency type I, or hypoplasminogenemia, is a rare genetic disorder in which individuals have reduced levels of plasminogen.

Etiology Genetic. An autosomal recessive disorder that affects clot formation and hemostasis.

Gingival Involvement Common. Non-dental biofilm-induced lesions due to plasminogen deficiency.

Other Sites of Involvement Eyes, nose, larynx, cervix.

Clinical Features
- In health, body fluid fibrinolytic activity clears fibrin deposits, but plasminogen deficiency leads to accumulation and deposition of fibrin in the form of nodules and plaques mainly on the mucosae. Surprisingly, there is a rare tendency to thrombosis.
- Generalized painful ulcerated gingival swelling covered with white-yellow membranes since late childhood (Fig. 32.14). Gingival enlargement is more severe and is typically seen in the interdental papillae (Fig. 32.15). Progressive alveolar bone loss and early loss of teeth may occur.
- The conjunctiva is most commonly affected by recurrent, fibrin-rich chronic membranous lesions of wood-like consistency *(ligneous conjunctivitis)*.

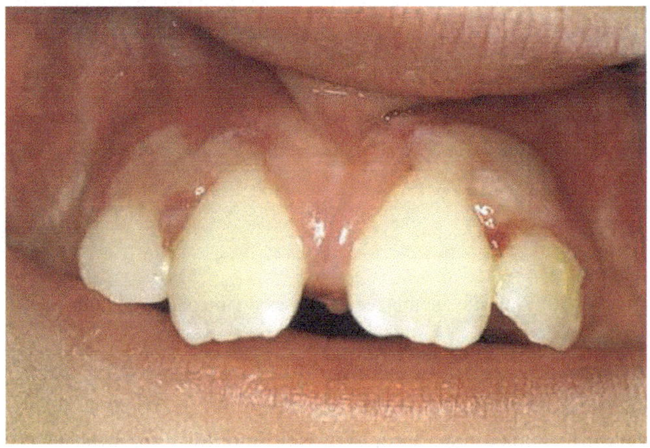

Fig. 32.14 Plasminogen deficiency type I, gingival ulcerations

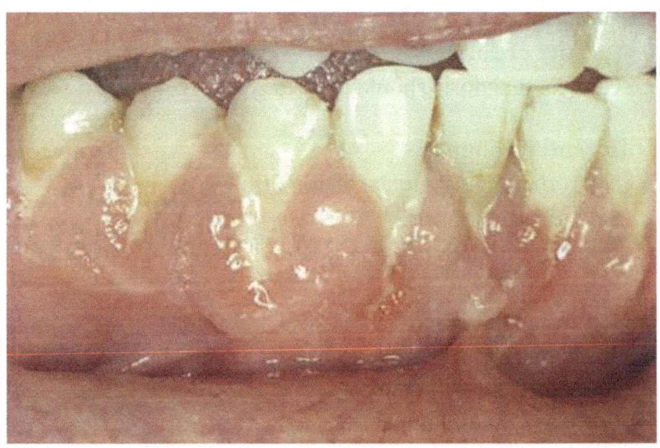

Fig. 32.15 Plasminogen deficiency type I, severe gingival enlargement and minor ulcerations

- Occasionally, lesions in the larynx and vocal cords occur causing hoarseness.
- Clinical diagnosis should always be confirmed by laboratory tests.

Differential Diagnosis
- Hereditary gingival fibromatosis and related disorders.
- Juvenile hyaline fibromatosis.
- Lipoid proteinosis.
- Amyloidosis.
- Mucopolysaccharidosis I-H(Hurler syndrome).
- Leukemias.

Laboratory Tests Histopathologic examination, plasminogen concentration.

Treatment Topical heparin or intravenous infusion with a purified plasminogen concentrate.

Polycythemia Vera

Definition Polycythemia vera is an acquired myeloproliferative bone marrow disorder characterized by overproduction of all three hematopoietic cell lines, most prominently the red blood cells. This leads to an elevated volume of red blood cells in the peripheral blood.

Etiology The exact etiology is unknown. However, a mutation in JAK2 gene has been demonstrated in 95% of cases and is almost certainly involved in the pathogenesis.

Gingival Involvement Common. Non-dental biofilm-induced gingivitis.

Other Sites of Involvement Oral mucosa, skin, eyes, spleen, respiratory system, gastrointestinal tract.

Clinical Features
- The main clinical signs and symptoms are headache, dizziness, tinnitus, fatigue, visual disturbances, epistaxis, dyspnea, and generalized pruritus. The spleen is enlarged and palpable in 75% of cases.
- Clinically, the gingiva is usually deep red in color, sometimes enlarged, and is usually bleeding (Fig. 32.16). The oral mucosa is commonly deep red, associated with petechiae, ecchymoses, and hematomas. The gingival and oral lesions are not pathognomonic.
- Thrombosis is the most common complication and the major cause of morbidity and death.
- Over time, the disease may turn into acute or chronic leukemia. Polycythemia vera is more common in males (60%) older than 60 years of age.
- Clinical diagnosis should be confirmed by laboratory tests.

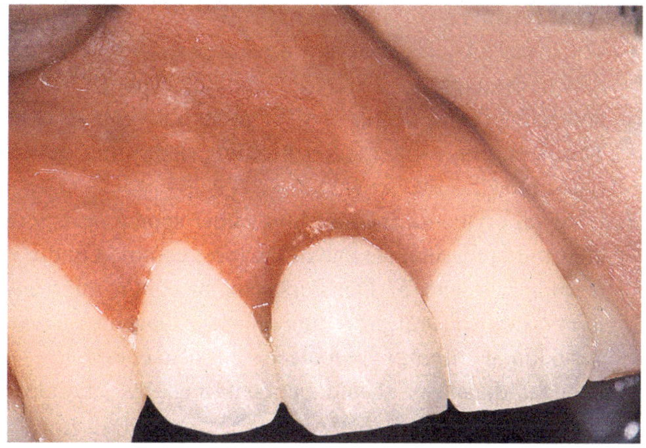

Fig. 32.16 Polycythemia vera, deep red hemorrhagic gingiva

Differential Diagnosis
- Thrombocytopenia.
- Secondary polycythemia from other causes.
- Other myeloproliferative disorders.

Laboratory Tests The hallmark of polycythemia vera is an increase in hematocrit; greater than 54% in men and greater than 51% in women. The white blood count is elevated to 10–20,000/mL and the platelet count greater than 1 million/mL. The bone marrow is also hypercellular. The final diagnosis should be confirmed with the detection of JAK2 mutation.

Treatment The treatment of choice is phlebotomy and must be performed by a hematologist. Alternatively, myelosuppressive therapy may be given.

Von Willebrand Disease

Definition Von Willebrand disease is the most common inherited bleeding disorder with 30–100 cases per 1,000,000 in the general population.

Etiology Genetic. It is transmitted via an autosomal dominant trait (types I and II) and an autosomal recessive trait (type III). The responsible geneVWF, which is located on chromosome 12, makes a blood clotting protein called von Willebrand factor that promotes platelet aggregation and prolongs the half-life of factor VIII protecting it from proteolytic degradation.

Gingival Involvement Relatively common. Non-dental biofilm-induced gingival lesions.

Other Sites of Involvement Oral and other mucosae, skin, internal organs.

Clinical Features

- The disease is classified into three types: (a) type I (75–80%); (b) type II (15–20%); and (c) type III (rare), depending on the degree of VWF reduction.
- The main clinical feature is bleeding depending on the type of the disease.
- Gingival erythema and bleeding, either spontaneously or after mild pressure, are one of the most common findings (Figs. 32.17 and 32.18). Persistent bleeding, after any minor surgical oral procedure (biopsy, tooth extraction, periodontal probing). Skin bleeding is also common.
- Clinical diagnosis should be confirmed by laboratory tests.

Differential Diagnosis

- Hemophilia.
- Other clotting disorders.
- Antithrombotic therapy.

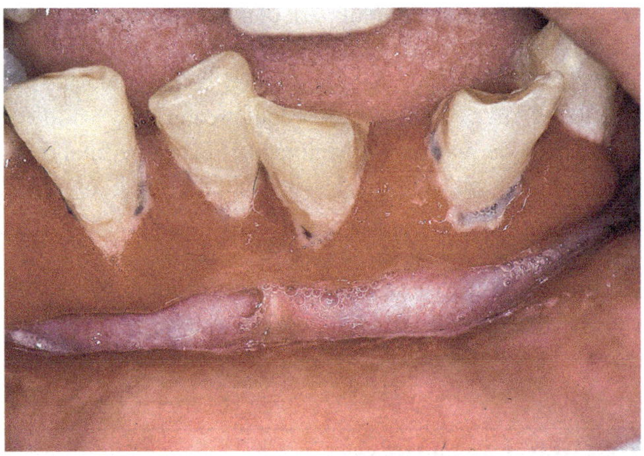

Fig. 32.17 Von Willebrand disease, severe gingivitis with erythema

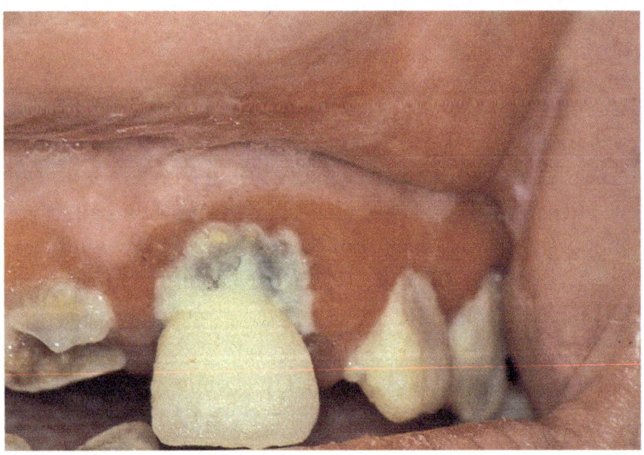

Fig. 32.18 Von Willebrand disease, gingivitis with severe erythema on the upper gingiva

Laboratory Tests Factor VIII level and activity test should be performed. A vWF activity-ristocetin cofactor is also useful. Clotting time tests and an activated partial thromboplastin time test are useful.

Treatment The treatment is the responsibility of the hematologist.

Myelodysplastic Syndromes

Definition Myelodysplastic syndromes are a heterogenous group of acquired clonal disorders of hematopoietic stem cells, leading to refractory anemias often associated with thrombocytopenia, neutropenia, and monocytosis. Older individuals are more often affected.

Etiology The etiology remains unknown. The disorders may be developed secondary to radiotherapy and chemotherapy. However, in most cases the disorders are idiopathic.

Classification Myelodysplastic syndromes are classified by WHO into seven groups depending on cell line criteria in the peripheral blood and the bone marrow as well as on clinical features.

Gingival Involvement Rare. Non-dental biofilm-related lesions.

Other Sites of Involvement Oral mucosa, other mucosae, skin, and other systems.

Clinical Features

- Gingival lesions may appear as chronic, localized swelling and/or ulcerations associated with bleeding (Figs. 32.19 and 32.20).

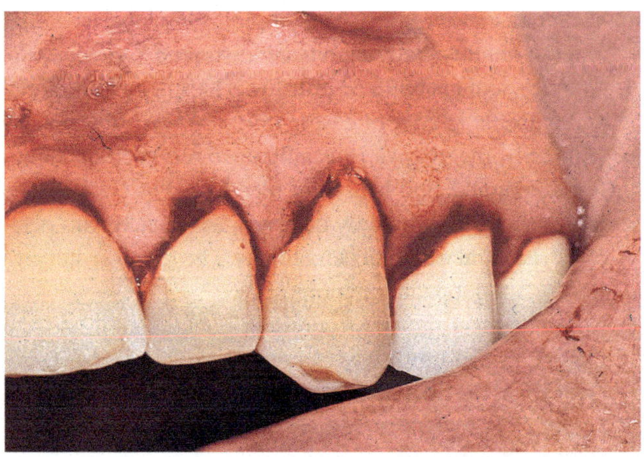

Fig. 32.19 Myelodysplastic syndrome, gingival bleeding

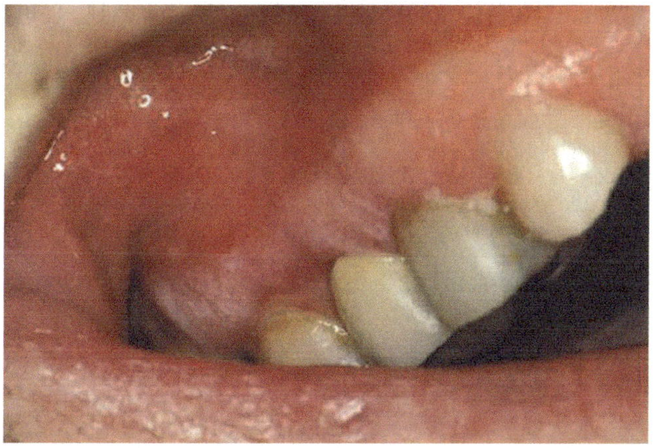

Fig. 32.20 Myelodysplastic syndrome, gingival ulcerations

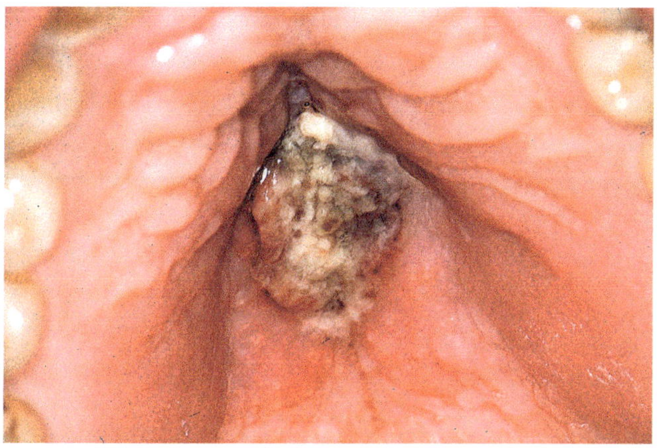

Fig. 32.21 Myelodysplastic syndrome, palatal necrotic ulceration

- Oral lesions appear as persistent and recurrent painful ulcerations and bleedings (Fig. 32.21). Less often, oral candidiasis may develop.
- Anemia, multiple bacterial infections, and hemorrhage are the main features of the disease due to neutropenia and thrombocytopenia. Splenomegaly and lymphadenopathy may be present.
- Malaise, fatigue, fever, and muscular weakness are common systemic symptoms.
- Clinical diagnosis should be confirmed by laboratory tests.

Differential Diagnosis
- Necrotizing gingivitis.
- Leukemias.
- Agranulocytosis.
- Neutropenia.
- Aplasticanemia.
- Thrombocytopenia.
- Non-Hodgkin lymphoma.
- Multiple myeloma.
- Sweet syndrome.
- Langerhans cell histiocytosis.

Laboratory Tests Complete blood count, bone marrow aspiration, and histopathologic examination.

Treatment Good oral hygiene, topical oral antiseptics. Systemic treatment must be left to hematologists.

References

1. Halai H, Somani C, Donos N, Nibali L. Periodontal status of children with primary immunodeficiencies: a systematic review. Clin Oral Investig. 2020;24(6):1939–51. https://doi.org/10.1007/s00784-019-03055-z. Epub 2019 Oct 18
2. Goultschin J, Attal U, Goldstein M, et al. The relationship between peripheral levels of leukocytes and neutrophils and periodontal disease status in a patient with congenital neutropenia. J Periodontol. 2000;71(9):1499–505. https://doi.org/10.1902/jop.2000.71.9.1499. PMID: 11022781
3. Tözüm TF, Berker E, Ersoy F, et al. The relationship between periodontal status and peripheral levels of neutrophils in two consanguineous siblings with severe congenital neutropenia: case reports. Quintessence Int. 2003;34(3):221–6. PMID: 12731605
4. Rezaei N, Moin M, Pourpak Z, et al. The clinical, immunohematological, and molecular study of Iranian patients with severe congenital neutropenia. J Clin Immunol. 2007;27:525–33.
5. Chen Y, Fang L, Yang X. Cyclic neutropenia presenting as recurrent oral ulcers and periodontitis. J Clin Pediatr Dent. 2013;37(3):307–8. https://doi.org/10.17796/jcpd.37.3.n8k0111177074828. PMID: 23855177
6. Arora R, Sharma A, Dimri D, Sharma H. Methimazole-induced neutropenic gingival ulcerations and necrosis in a middle-aged female: a case report with clinical management. J Midlife Health. 2018;9(2):106–9. https://doi.org/10.4103/jmh.JMH_18_18. PMID: 29962811; PMCID: PMC6006798
7. Scully C, Mac Fadyen E, Campbell A. Oral manifestations in cyclic neutropenia. Br J Oral Surg. 1982;20:96–101.
8. Grein Cavalcanti L, Fuentes Araújo RL, Bonfim C, Torres-Pereira CC. Oral manifestations compatible with chronic graft-versus-host disease in patients with Fanconi anemia. Biol Blood Marrow Transplant. 2015;21(2):275–80. https://doi.org/10.1016/j.bbmt.2014.10.009. Epub 2014 Oct 12. PMID: 25316110
9. Tewari S, Tewari S, Sharma RK, et al. Necrotizing stomatitis: a possible periodontal manifestation of deferiprone-induced agranulocytosis. Oral Surg Oral Med Oral Pathol Oral Radiol Endod. 2009;108(4):e13–9. https://doi.org/10.1016/j.tripleo.2009.06.021. PMID: 19778731
10. Brennan MT, Sankar V, Baccaglini L, et al. Oral manifestations in patients with aplastic anemia. Oral Surg Oral Med Oral Pathol Oral Radiol Endod. 2001;92:503–8.
11. Sepulveda E, Brethauer U, Rojas J, Le Fort P. Oral manifestations of aplastic anemia in children. J Am Dent Assoc. 2006;137:474–8.
12. Adeyemo TA, Adeyemo WL, Adediran A, et al. Orofacial manifestation of hematological disorders: hemato-oncologic and immuno-deficiency disorders. Indian J Dent Res. 2011;22(5):688–97. https://doi.org/10.4103/0970-9290.93458. PMID: 22406715
13. Magister MJ, Crist H, Oberman BS. Rapid progression of necrotic lesion of the mandibular gingiva in a pancytopenic patient. Invasive necrotizing fungal gingivitis. JAMA Otolaryngol Head Neck Surg. 2015;141(10):937–8. https://doi.org/10.1001/jamaoto.2015.1733. PMID: 26379226
14. Chi AC, Prichard E, Richardson MS, et al. Pseudomembranous disease (ligneous inflammation) of the female genital tract, peritoneum, gingiva, and paranasal sinuses associated with plasminogen deficiency. Ann Diagn Pathol. 2009;13(2):132–9. https://doi.

org/10.1016/j.anndiagpath.2008.02.005. Epub 2008 Jun 12. PMID: 19302964
15. Silva GB, Bariani C, Mendonca EF, Batista AC. Clinical manifestations due to severe plasminogen deficiency: a case report. J Dent Child (Chic). 2006;73:179–82.
16. Hassan FW, Mohd N. Periodontal management in a primary polycythemia rubra vera patient: a case report. Spec Care Dentist. 2021;41(1):92–7. https://doi.org/10.1111/scd.12537. Epub 2020 Oct 30. PMID: 33125720
17. Rassoulzadegan M, Ala F, Jazebi M, et al. Molecular and clinical profile of type 2 von Willebrand disease in Iran: a thirteen-year experience. Int J Hematol. 2020;111(4):535–43. https://doi.org/10.1007/s12185-019-02814-8. Epub 2020 Jan 14. PMID: 31939074
18. Castaman G, Linari S. Diagnosis and treatment of von Willebrand disease and rare bleeding disorders. J Clin Med. 2017;6(4):45. https://doi.org/10.3390/jcm6040045. PMID: 28394285; PMCID: PMC5406777
19. Ziv O, Ragni MV. Bleeding manifestations in males with von Willebrand disease. Haemophilia. 2004;10:162–8.
20. Pereira CM, Gasparetto PF, Coracin FL, et al. Severe gingival bleeding in a myelodysplastic patient: management and outcome. J Periodontol. 2004;75(3):483–6. https://doi.org/10.1902/jop.2004.75.3.483. PMID: 15088888

Mucocutaneous Diseases

33

Contents

Erythema Multiforme

Definition Erythema multiforme is an acute mucocutaneous disease that occurs most frequently in young males.

Etiology Several factors have been implicated in the etiology of erythema multiforme, including drugs (sulphonamides, penicillin, barbiturates, nonsteroidal anti-inflammatory drugs, phenytoin, and others), *herpes simplex virus,* and *Mycoplasma pneumoniae* infection. However, in more than 50% of cases, a causative factor cannot be found.

Classification Two main forms of the disease are recognized:

(a) *Erythema multiforme minor* with distinct skin lesions with or without mucosal involvement; and (b). *Erythema multiforme major*, which almost invariably involves the oral mucosa, other mucosae and the skin.

Gingival Involvement Relatively common. Non-dental biofilm-induced lesions with no attachment loss.

Other Sites of Involvement Oral mucosa (lips, buccal mucosa, tongue, palate), about 20–30% in the minor form and almost invariably there in the major form of the disease. Other mucosae (conjunctiva, genitalia). Skin is very often affected in a symmetrical pattern (palms, soles, back of the hands and feet, neck, trunk).

G. Laskaris et al., *Periodontal Manifestations of Local and Systemic Diseases*, https://doi.org/10.1007/978-3-031-10828-0_33

Clinical Features

- Gingival lesions may appear as diffuse erythema, sometimes mimicking *desquamative gingivitis* or localized or diffuse painful erosions covered by a whitish pseudomembrane (Figs. 33.1 and 33.2).
- Oral lesions appear as small vesicles that soon rupture, creating extensive painful erosions covered by pseudomembranes and hemorrhagic crusts (Fig. 33.3).
- Photophobia, conjunctivitis, keratitis, uveitis, and panophthalmitis may also occur.
- Skin lesions present as erythematous maculopapules, usually creating the characteristic *"target or iris lesions"* (Fig. 33.4). Less often, purpuric plaques and bullous formation may appear, usually in association with target lesions.
- Fever, coughing, difficulty in swallowing, malaise, arthralgias, and atypical pneumonia occur in the major form of the disease. The disease recurs in 20–30% of cases.
- Diagnosis is primarily based on clinical criteria but should be confirmed by laboratory tests.

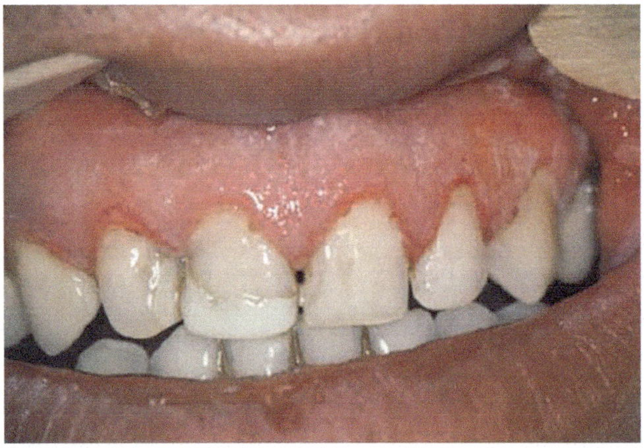

Fig. 33.1 Erythema multiforme, early lesions on the gingiva presenting as desquamative gingivitis

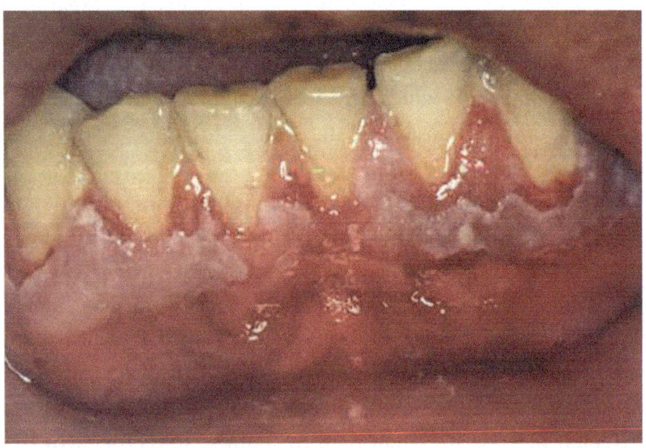

Fig. 33.2 Erythema multiforme, erythema and erosions on the gingiva mimicking desquamative gingivitis

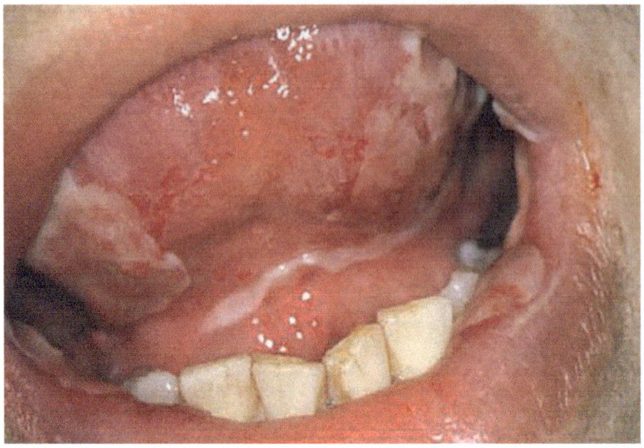

Fig. 33.3 Erythema multiforme, extensive erosions of the tongue and lower lip

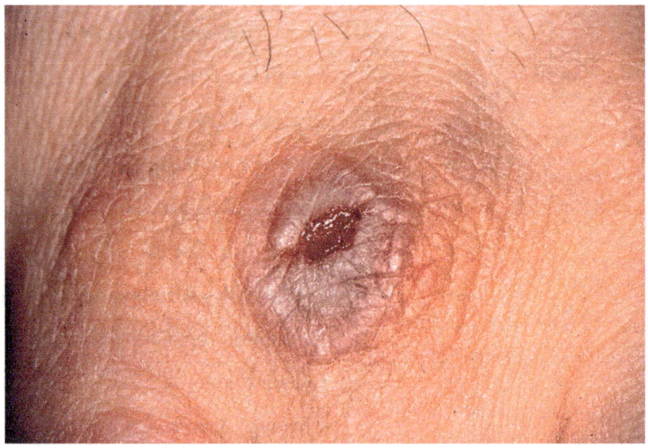

Fig. 33.4 Erythema multiforme, skin lesion forming typical "target lesion"

Differential Diagnosis

- Primary herpetic gingivostomatitis.
- Herpetiform ulcers.
- Kawasaki disease.
- Mucous membrane pemphigoid.
- Bullous pemphigoid.
- Linear IgA disease.
- Pemphigoid gestationis.
- Pemphigus.

Laboratory Tests Histopathologic examination, direct immunofluorescence.

Treatment Systemic corticosteroids. Aciclovir, valaciclovir, or other new antivirals may be helpful in the management of patients with recurrent erythema multiforme.

Stevens-Johnson Syndrome

Definition Stevens-Johnson syndrome is a relatively rare, acute and severe mucocutaneous disease, unrelated to erythema multiforme and is considered as a milder form of toxic epidermal necrolysis.

Etiology It is nearly always drug-related in the form of immune complex-mediated hypersensitivity.

Gingival Involvement Relatively common. Non-dental biofilm-induced gingival lesions.

Other Sites of Involvement Oral, ocular, and genital mucosae (>90–95%), pharynx, larynx, esophagus, respiratory system, and skin.

Clinical Features

- Gingival lesions are characterized by erythema and multiple painful nonspecific erosions covered by whitish or hemorrhagic pseudomembranes (Fig. 33.5). In some areas, the gingival lesions may mimic *desquamative gingivitis.*
- The oral cavity is almost always involved with extensive formation of vesicles or bullae that rupture quickly leaving extensive and painful erosions. The lips, buccal mucosa, palate, tongue, and floor of the mouth are more commonly affected (Fig. 33.6). Similar severe erosions appear on other mucosae (Fig. 33.7).
- Skin lesions are variable in both extent and gravity. They start as epidermal, erythematous, red, or purpuric macules that tend to coalesce (Fig. 33.8). As lesions progress toward full-thickness necrosis of the epidermis, they soon detach from the dermis. Finally, the skin resembles *wet cigarette paper* as it is pulled away by trauma, often revealing large areas of bleeding dermis, which is referred to as *"scalding."* The *Nikolsky sign* may be positive.
- Prodromal early symptoms include fever, cough, fatigue, malaise, sore throat, arthralgia, myalgia, diarrhea, and photophobia. They usually precede mucosal and skin manifestations by 1–3 days.
- The diagnosis is mainly based on the history and the clinical features.

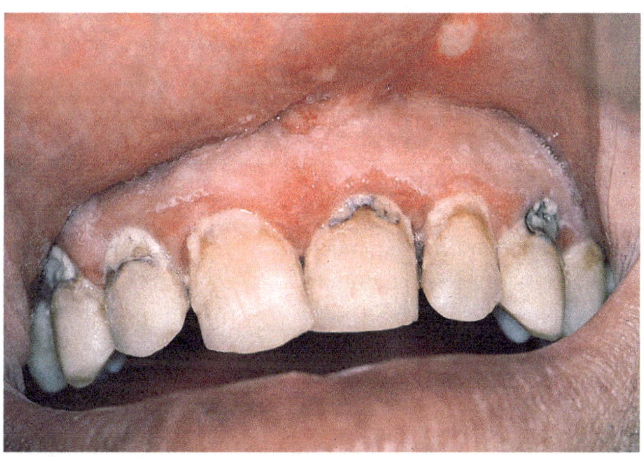

Fig. 33.5 Stevens-Johnson syndrome, hemorrhagic, erythematous gingiva covered with pseudomembranes

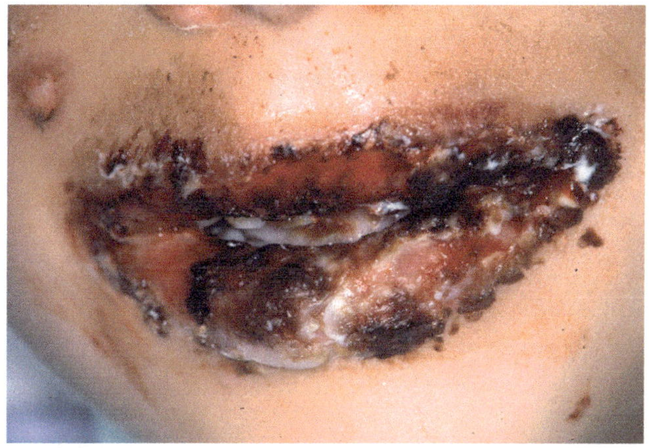

Fig. 33.6 Stevens-Johnson syndrome, severe crusted ulcerations on the lips of an 8 years-old-child

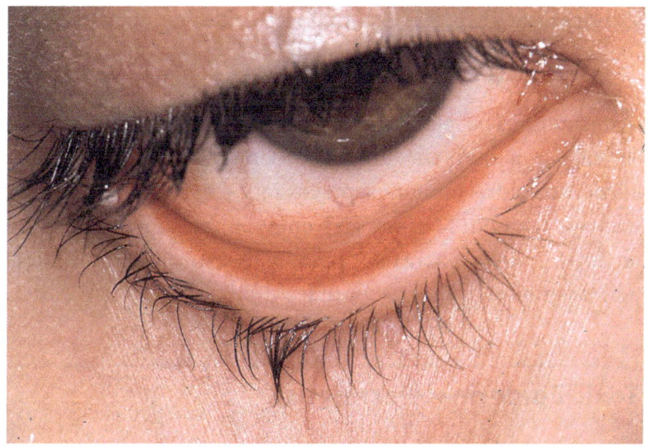

Fig. 33.7 Stevens-Johnson syndrome, conjunctivitis

Differential Diagnosis

- Erythema multiforme.
- Toxic epidermal necrolysis.
- Paraneoplastic pemphigus.
- Graft-Versus-Host Disease (acute form).
- Sweet syndrome.

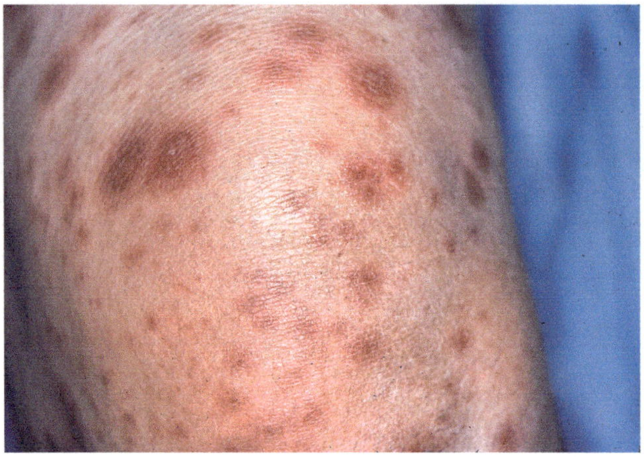

Fig. 33.8 Stevens-Johnson syndrome, multiple red macules and target-like lesions on the skin

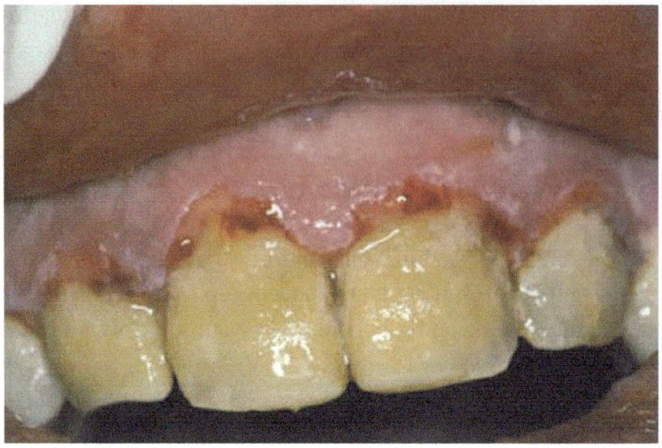

Fig. 33.9 Toxic epidermal necrolysis, early lesions presenting as erythema and erosions on the gingiva

Laboratory Tests Histopathologic examination, direct and indirect immunofluorescence.

Treatment The patient should be referred to the hospital (intensive or burn care unit) as soon as possible. Systemic corticosteroids, immunosuppressants, thalidomide, Tumor necrosis factor α(TNF-α), TNF antagonists (infliximab, etanercept), plasmapheresis, hemodialysis, and parenteral administration of Ig have been used.

Toxic Epidermal Necrolysis

Definition Toxic epidermal necrolysis or Lyell disease is a rare and severe exfoliative mucocutaneous disease with high mortality.

Etiology Drug-induced reaction (sulphonamides, antibiotics, nonsteroidal anti-inflammatory agents, anticonvulsants).

Gingival Involvement Common. Non-dental biofilm-induced lesions with no attachment loss.

Other Sites of Involvement Oral mucosa (lips, buccal mucosa, tongue, palate), other mucosae (conjunctiva, oropharynx, genitalia, anus), skin (widespread skin detachment involving more than 30% of the body surface).

Clinical Features

- The disease usually commences with a cough, sore throat, burning eyes, low fever, and malaise followed by skin and mucous membrane lesions within1–2 days.
- Gingival lesions appear as dense inflammation with blister formation leading to painful and widespread erosions (Fig. 33.9).

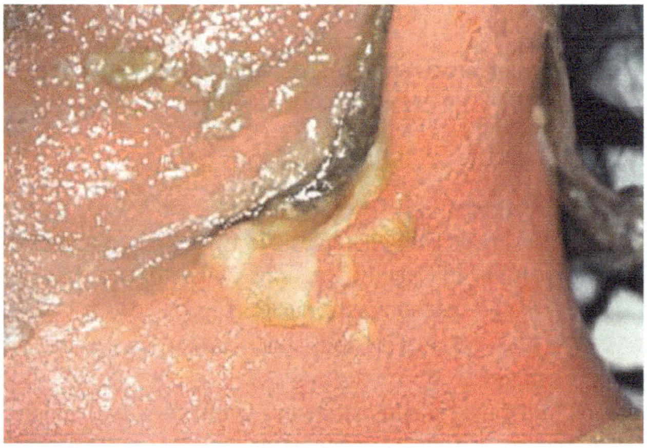

Fig. 33.10 Toxic epidermal necrolysis, sheet-like loss of the epidermis

- Oral lesions are characterized by diffuse erythema, blistering, and painful erosions seen anywhere in the oral cavity.
- Skin lesions appear as a sheet-like loss of epidermis (Fig. 33.10). The epidermis is raised by flaccid blisters, which spread on application of pressure. *Nikolsky sign* is positive.
- Diagnosis is usually based on clinical criteria but should be confirmed by laboratory tests.

Differential Diagnosis

- Necrotizing gingivitis.
- Erythema multiforme major.
- Stevens-Johnson syndrome.
- Pemphigus.
- Sweet syndrome.
- Staphylococcal scalded skin syndrome.

Laboratory Tests Histopathologic examination, direct immunofluorescence.

Treatment Patients must be admitted to a critical care unit as soon as possible, where disease management will be provided by a multidisciplinary team of specialists.

Pemphigus Vulgaris

Definition Pemphigus is a severe chronic mucocutaneous bullous disease.

Etiology Autoimmune. Autoantibodies against desmoglein 3 and desmoglein 1 are responsible for oral and skin lesions, respectively.

Classification Pemphigus is classified into three major types: (a) *pemphigus vulgaris*; (b) *pemphigus foliaceus*; and (c) *paraneoplastic pemphigus* with five major clinical subtypes. Pemphigus vulgaris is the most common and severe form of the disease accounting for 90–95% of all cases. Using clinical criteria, pemphigus vulgaris is classified into three subtypes: (a) the *mucosal dominant* type with mucosal lesions and limited cutaneous involvement; (b) the *mucocutaneous* type involving both the mucosa and epidermis; and (c) the *cutaneous type* with skin lesions only.

Gingival Involvement Common, approximately 30–40% of cases. Non-dental biofilm-induced lesions with no attachment loss.

Other Sites of Involvement Oral mucosa (soft palate, buccal, tongue, floor of the mouth, lips), very common in 75–90% of cases. Other mucosae (conjunctiva, nose, genital, rectal, larynx, pharynx, esophagus). Skin common.

Clinical Features

- Gingival lesions may appear either in the form of *desquamative gingivitis*, usually localized or as multiple painful erosions on an erythematous base.
- Rarely, gingival lesions may be the only site of involvement (Figs. 33.11, 33.12, and 33.13).
- Oral lesions present as erythema, bullous formation, and painful erosions (Fig. 33.14).
- Skin lesions present as bullous formation that soon rupture, leaving painful erosions with a tendency to enlarge centrifugally as the epidermis strips off at the edges (Fig. 33.15). The erosions quickly become partially covered with crusts without the tendency to heal. Eventually, after healing skin pigmentation remains with no scarring. The most commonly affected areas of the skin are the trunk, axillae, genital areas, umbilicus, scalp, periocular areas, and ears. The *Nikolsky sign* is positive.
- Clinical diagnosis should always be confirmed by laboratory tests.

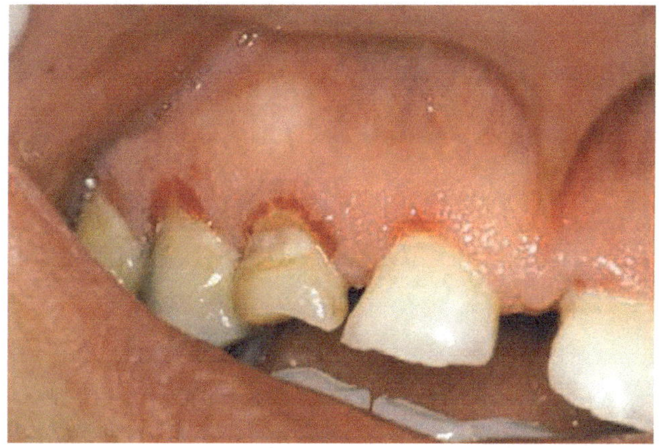

Fig. 33.11 Pemphigus vulgaris, early lesions on the gingiva

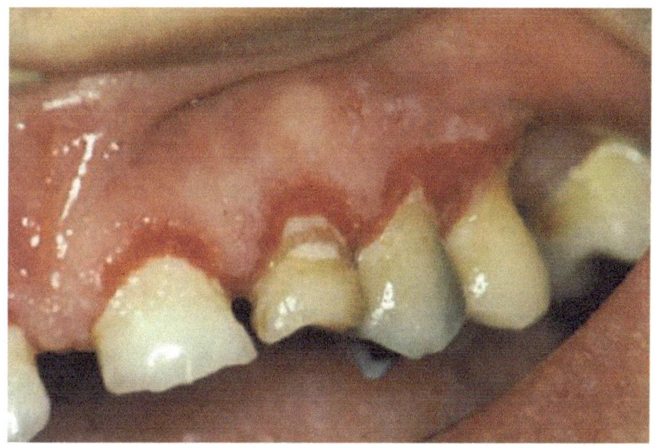

Fig. 33.12 Pemphigus vulgaris, erythema and erosions on the gingiva presenting as desquamative gingivitis

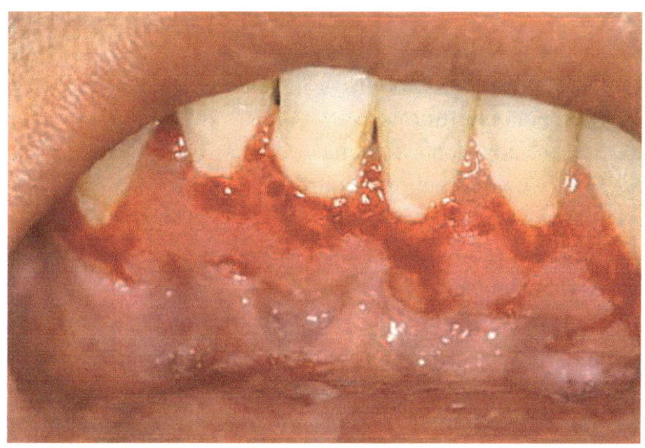

Fig. 33.13 Pemphigus vulgaris, multiple erosions on the gingiva and the alveolar mucosa

Differential Diagnosis

- Mucous membrane pemphigoid.
- Bullous pemphigoid.
- Pemphigoid gestationis.

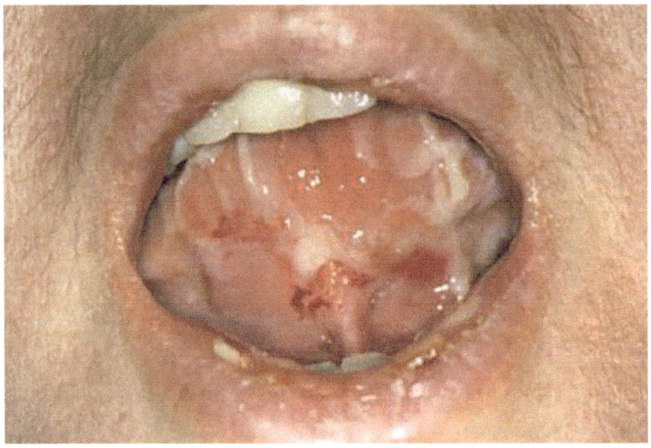

Fig. 33.14 Pemphigus vulgaris, extensive chronic erosions on the tongue and lower lip

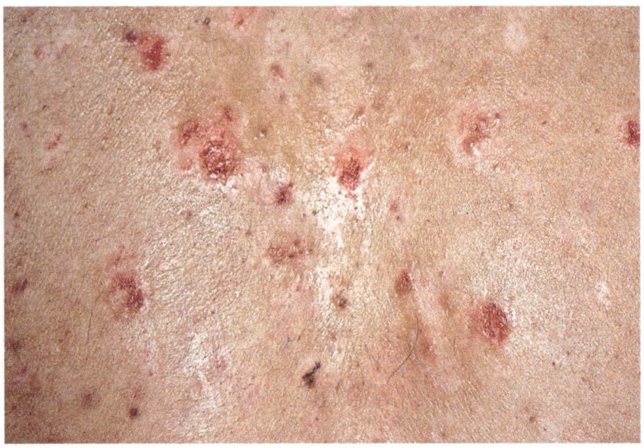

Fig. 33.15 Pemphigus vulgaris, erupted bullae and erosions on the skin

- Linear IgA disease.
- Dermatitis herpetiformis.
- Erythema multiforme.
- Stevens-Johnson syndrome.
- Epidermolysis bullosa acquisita.
- Lichen planus, erosive type.
- Herpetic gingivostomatitis.
- Aphthous ulcers.

Laboratory Tests Histopathologic examination, direct and indirect immunofluorescence, Tzanck smear test. Detection of anti-desmoglein 3 and 1 antibodies by enzyme-linked immunosorbent assay (ELISA). Immunoprecipitation and immunoblot may be used.

Treatment High doses of systemic corticosteroids is the treatment of choice. Azathioprine, cyclosporine, cyclophosphamide, mycophenolate mofetil or acid, monoclonal antibodies (Rituximab) as adjuvant treatment, almost exclusively in combination with corticosteroids. Plasmapheresis.

Mucous Membrane Pemphigoid

Definition Mucous membrane pemphigoid is a chronic autoimmune bullous disease that primarily affects mucous membranes and rarely the skin.

Etiology Autoimmune. The disorder should not be considered as a single clinical entity, but rather as a heterogeneous group of diseases *(disease phenotype)* with clinical and antigenic heterogeneity.

Classification Four variants are currently recognized based on the clinical expression and the antigenic target.

Gingival Involvement Very common, approximately 60% of cases. Non-dental biofilm-induced lesions with no attachment loss.

Other Sites of Involvement Oral mucosa (soft palate, buccal mucosa, tongue, lips) in 90–95% of cases. Involvement of other mucosae (ocular, nose, genitalia, pharynx, larynx, anus) and skin (5%).

Clinical Features

- The disease affects more frequently females than males (1.5–2:1), usually during the fifth to sixth decade of life.
- Frequently, the disease affects exclusively the gingiva in the form of *desquamative gingivitis* (erythema, edema, desquamation of the epithelium, or bullous formation after pressure of the gingiva) (Figs. 33.16, 33.17, and 33.18).
- Oral lesions present as erythematous plaques and bullae that quickly rupture leaving painful erosions (Fig. 33.19).
- Lesions usually recur and persist for a long time, leading occasionally to atrophy or scarring (except gingiva).

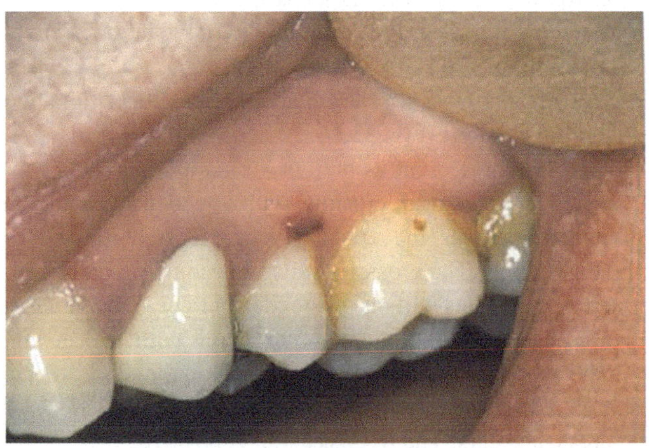

Fig. 33.16 Mucous membrane pemphigoid, early small hemorrhagic bulla on the gingiva

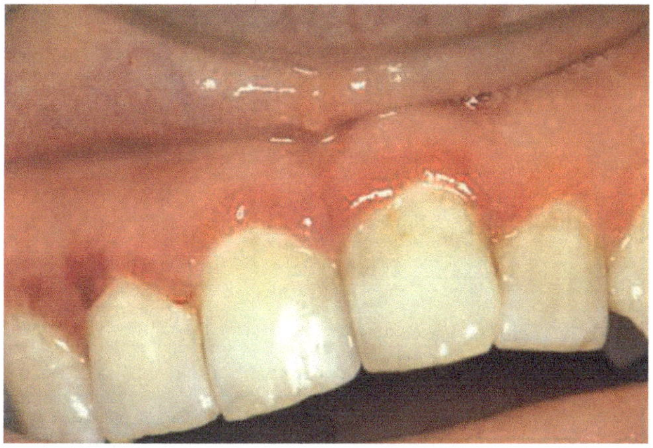

Fig. 33.17 Mucous membrane pemphigoid, typical desquamative gingivitis

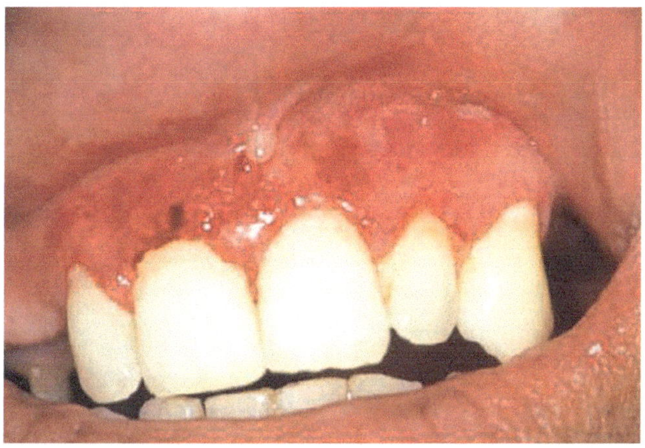

Fig. 33.18 Mucous membrane pemphigoid, desquamative gingivitis

- Ocular lesions consist of conjunctivitis, symblepharon, trichiasis, dryness, and opacity of the cornea, occasionally leading to complete blindness (Fig. 33.20).
- Skin lesions consist of bullae, usually on the scalp and neck and may heal with scarring.
- Clinical diagnosis should be confirmed by laboratory tests.

Differential Diagnosis
- Bullous pemphigoid.
- Pemphigus.
- Linear IgA disease.
- Erythema multiforme.
- Epidermolysis bullosa acquisita.
- Chronic ulcerative stomatitis.
- Lichen planus (mainly erosive and bullous type).
- Angina bullosa hemorrhagica.
- Plasma cell gingivitis.
- Herpetic gingivostomatitis.

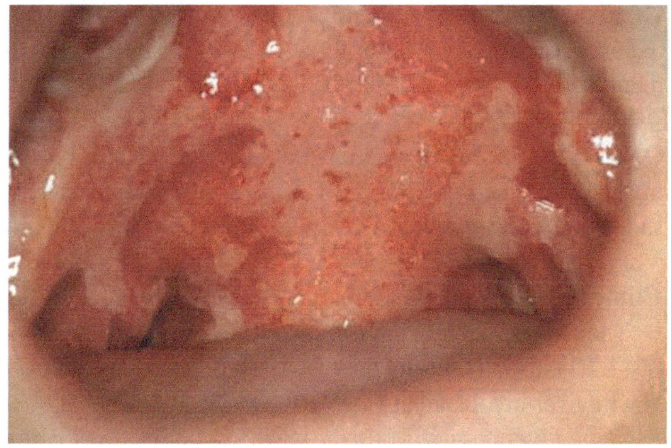

Fig. 33.19 Mucous membrane pemphigoid, extensive erosions on the palate

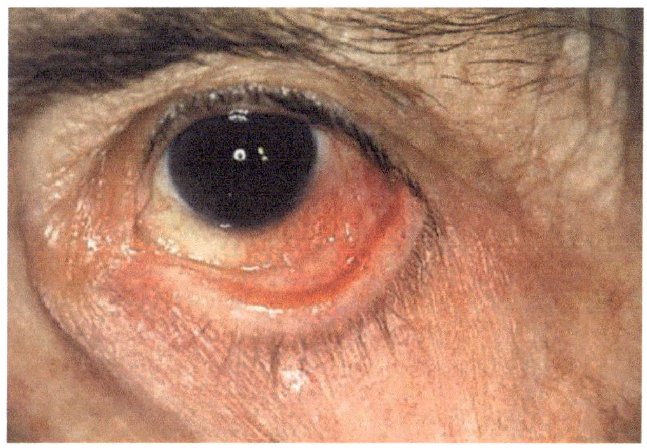

Fig. 33.20 Mucous membrane pemphigoid, conjunctivitis and symblepharon

Laboratory Tests Histopathologic examination, direct and indirect immunofluorescence, immunoelectron microscopy, immunochemical examinations.

Treatment Topical or systemic corticosteroids depending on disease activity. Immunosuppressive treatment (azathioprine, cyclophosphamide, mycophenolate mofetil, and dapsone) only in severe and persistent cases, always as adjuvant to corticosteroid therapy.

Bullous Pemphigoid

Definition Bullous pemphigoid is the most common chronic autoimmune bullous disease that primarily affects the skin and less often the mucous membranes.

Etiology Autoimmune.

Gingival Involvement Relatively common, about 10–15% of cases. Non-dental biofilm-induced lesions with no attachment loss.

Other Sites of Involvement Oral mucosa (palate, buccal mucosa, tongue, lips), about 30–40% of cases. Other mucosae (conjunctiva, esophagus, vagina, anus) and skin, always.

Clinical Features

- The disease affects more frequently females than males (1.7:1), usually during the fifth to sixth decade of life.
- Gingival involvement is usually seen in the form of *desquamative gingivitis* or as a localized bullous formation that ruptures quickly, leaving painful erosions (Figs. 33.21, 33.22, and 33.23).
- Localized or widespread lesions may also appear in the oral and other mucosae (conjunctivae, esophagus, vagina, anus).
- Skin lesions usually begin as a nonspecific generalized rash (pruritic, erythematous urticarial-like plaques). Ultimately, tense bullae develop, isolated or in clusters, that rupture leaving superficial ulcerations without a tendency to extend peripherally. (Fig. 33.24). The *Nikolsky sign* is negative.
- The eruption is mostly located on both the extremities and the trunk in a symmetrical pattern.
- The disease has a chronic course with exacerbations and remissions. Prognosis is good.
- Clinical diagnosis should be confirmed by laboratory tests.

Differential Diagnosis

- Mucous membrane pemphigoid.
- Lichen planus.
- Desquamative gingivitis.
- Linear IgA disease.
- Pemphigoid gestationis.
- Epidermolysis bullosa acquisita.
- Pemphigus.
- Dermatitis herpetiformis.
- Plasma cell gingivitis.

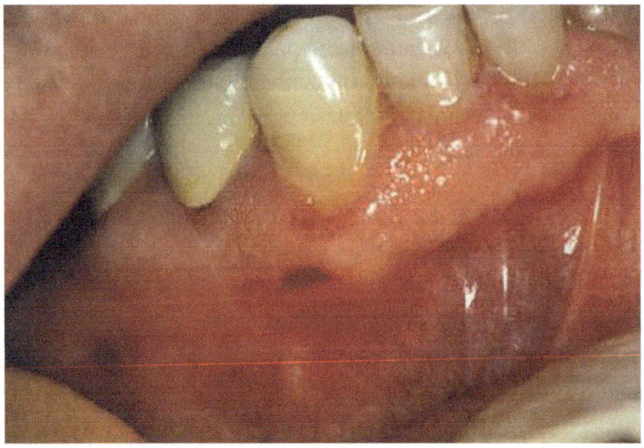

Fig. 33.21 Bullous pemphigoid, slight erythema on the gingiva and small hemorrhagic bulla

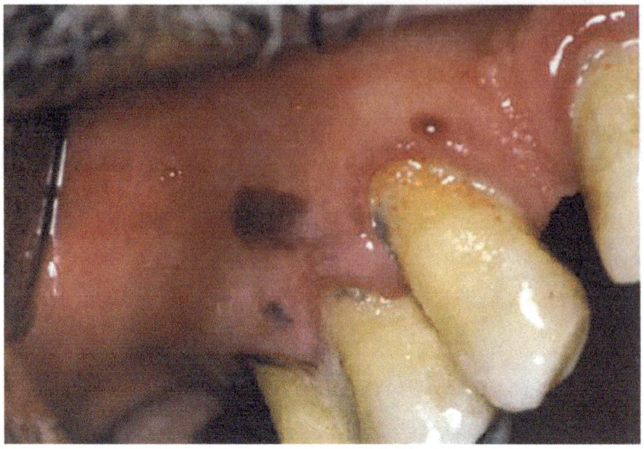

Fig. 33.22 Bullous pemphigoid, multiple hemorrhagic bullae on the gingiva

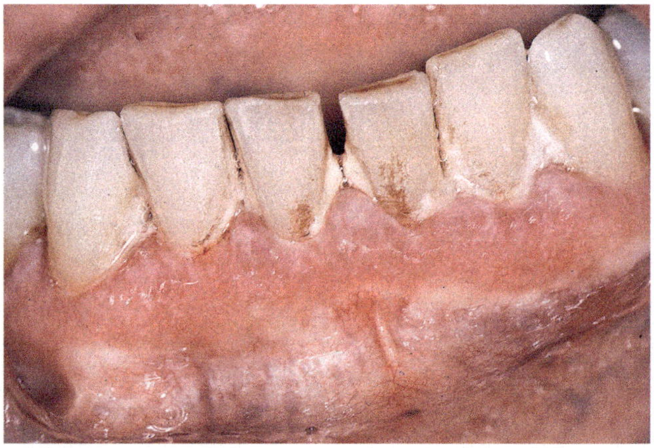

Fig. 33.23 Bullous pemphigoid, lesions on the gingiva presenting as desquamative gingivitis

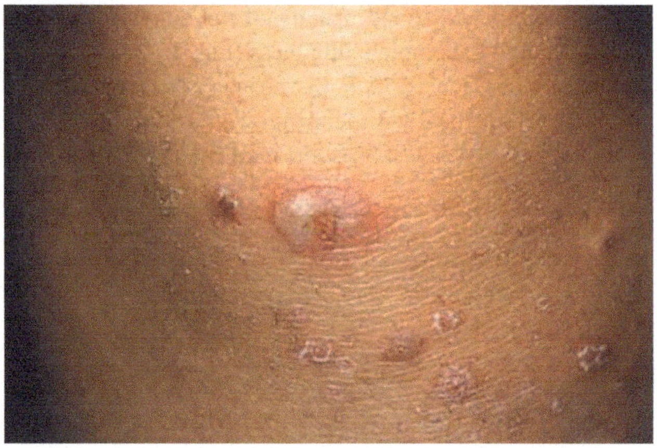

Fig. 33.24 Bullous pemphigoid, small bullae on the skin

Laboratory Tests Histopathologic examination, direct and indirect immunofluorescence, and ELISA testing.

Treatment Topical and/or systemic corticosteroids. Immunosuppressives as adjuvant therapy.

Pemphigoid Gestationis

Definition Pemphigoid gestationis, or herpes gestationis, is a rare autoimmune bullous dermatosis of pregnancy and the immediate postpartum characterized by a self-limiting and sometimes recurrent period. It usually resolves within 3–4 months after delivery.

Etiology Autoimmune.

Gingival Involvement Rare. Non-dental biofilm-induced lesions with no attachment loss.

Other Sites of Involvement Oral mucosa (buccal mucosa, tongue, palate), rare. Skin (abdomen, chest, back, face, extremities, palms, soles), always.

Clinical Features

- Gingival lesions may appear as localized hemorrhagic bullae that quickly rupture leaving painful erosions (Fig. 33.25).
- Multiple bullae that quickly rupture also appear in oral cavity that leave nondiagnostic painful erosions. Oral lesions always follow skin lesions and quickly retreat.
- Skin manifestations are characterized by intensely pruritic, urticarial-like plaques with an abrupt onset. The plaques then evolve into vesicles and small tense bullae, which coalesce to occupy extensive areas on the trunk, abdomen, axillae, extremities, and face (Fig. 33.26). The eruptions usually appear during the second and third trimester of pregnancy or immediately postpartum and resolve within 3–4 months after delivery.
- Rarely, the disease may arise in association with trophoblastic malignancy.
- Clinical diagnosis should be confirmed by laboratory tests.

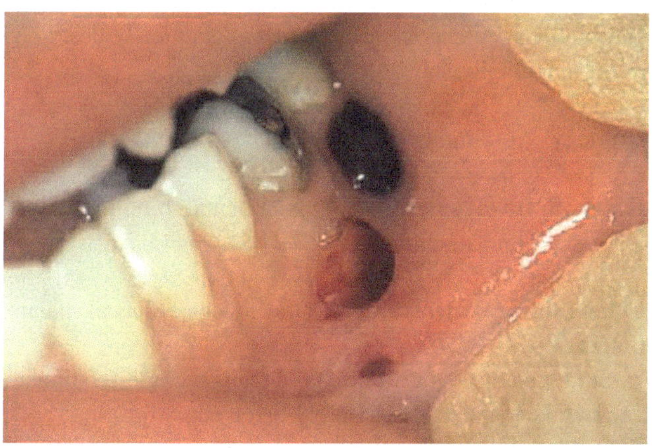

Fig. 33.25 Pemphigoid gestationis, hemorrhagic bullae on the gingiva

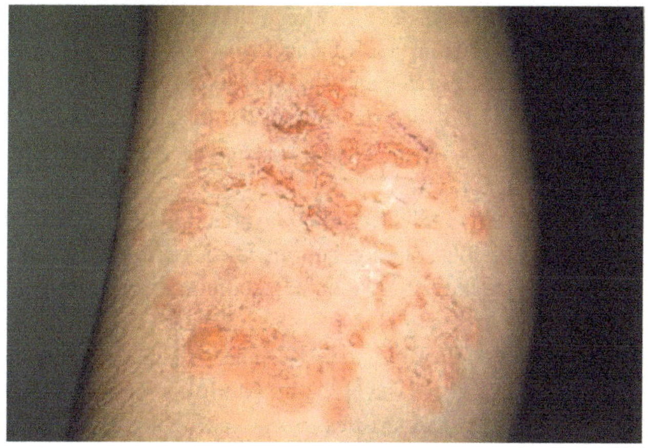

Fig. 33.26 Pemphigoid gestationis, multiple vesicles on the skin

Differential Diagnosis

- Bullous pemphigoid.
- Linear IgA disease.
- Pemphigus.
- Mucous membrane pemphigoid.
- Erythema multiforme (bullous type).
- Dermatitis herpetiformis.

Laboratory Tests Histopathologic examination, direct and indirect immunofluorescence. Immunoelectron microscopy, immunoblotting, and ELISA testing.

Treatment Systemic corticosteroids. Azathioprine, dapsone, cyclosporine, intravenous immunoglobulin (IVIg), methotrexate, and others may also be used as adjuvant therapy.

Linear IgA Disease

Definition Linear IgA disease is a rare, chronic, autoimmune subepidermal blistering disease characterized by linear IgA deposits along the basement membrane zone of the epidermis/epithelium.

Etiology Autoimmune, of unknown etiology.

Gingival Involvement Rare. Non-dental biofilm-induced gingivitis with no attachment loss.

Other Sites of Involvement Oral mucosa (25–30%), other mucosae (rare), skin (100%).

Clinical Features

- Depending on the age of onset, two groups are recognized: (a) *adult type*; and (b) *childhood type*. Depending on the region of IgA deposition, the disease is classified into two types: (a) the *lamina lucida type*; and (b) the *sub-lamina lucida type*.
- Clinically, the affected gingiva is red with superficial painful erosions. Rarely, bullous lesions are present. The features are not pathognomonic, sometimes presenting as *desquamative gingivitis* (Figs. 33.27 and 33.28). In the remainder of the oral cavity vesicles or bullae are developed, which rapidly evolve into painful erosions without any specific characteristics.
- Skin lesions are characterized by a sudden onset of vesicles and bullae on the face, trunk, buttocks, and extremities in a symmetrical pattern (Fig. 33.29). They tend to have a herpetiform or annular pattern.
- Clinical diagnosis should be confirmed by laboratory tests.

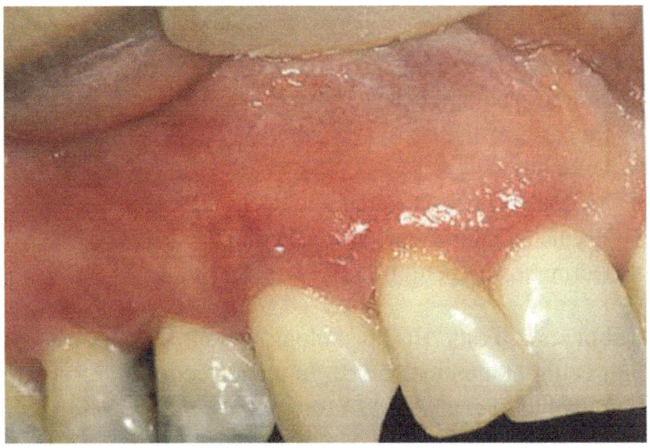

Fig. 33.27 Linear IgA disease, gingival lesions presenting as desquamative gingivitis

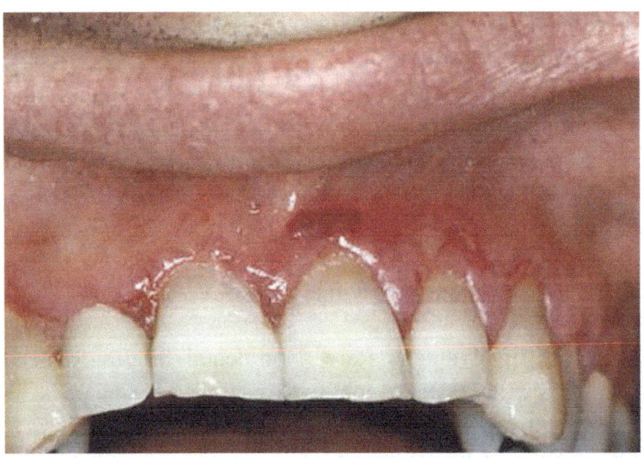

Fig. 33.28 Linear IgA disease, erythema and bulla formation in the form of desquamative gingivitis

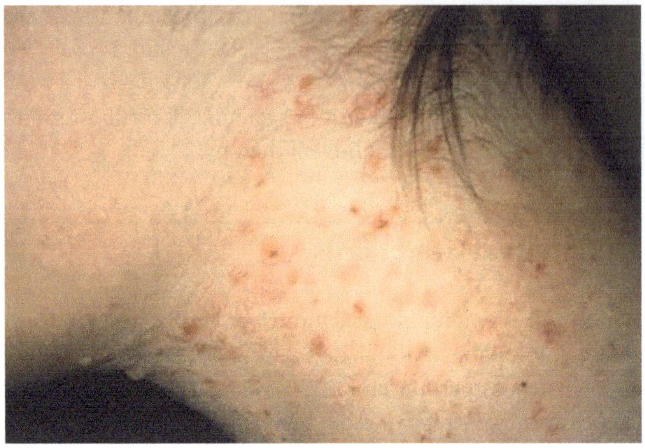

Fig. 33.29 Linear IgA disease, small vesicles on the skin

Differential Diagnosis

- Bullous pemphigoid.
- Mucous membrane pemphigoid.
- Dermatitis herpetiformis.
- Pemphigus.
- Epidermolysis bullosa aquisita.
- Erythema multiforme.
- Stevens-Johnson syndrome.

Laboratory Tests Histopathologic examination, direct and indirect immunofluorescence, immunoelectron microscopy.

Treatment The treatment of choice is dapsone, usually in combination with systemic prednisolone. Alternative treatments are sulfapyridine, colchicine, antibiotics, immunosuppressive drugs. For the gingival lesions supportive treatment is recommended.

Epidermolysis Bullosa Acquisita

Definition Epidermolysis bullosa acquisita is a rare and chronic mucocutaneous disease that is classically described as mechanobullous disorder.

Etiology Autoimmune.

Gingival Involvement Rare. Non-dental biofilm-induced lesions with no attachment loss.

Other Sites of Involvement Oral mucosa (buccal, palate, tongue, lips).

Skin, usually over the joints. Other mucosae (conjunctival, nasal, esophageal) are rarely involved.

Clinical Features

- Gingival involvement may appear either in the form of *desquamative gingivitis* or as localized bullous forma-

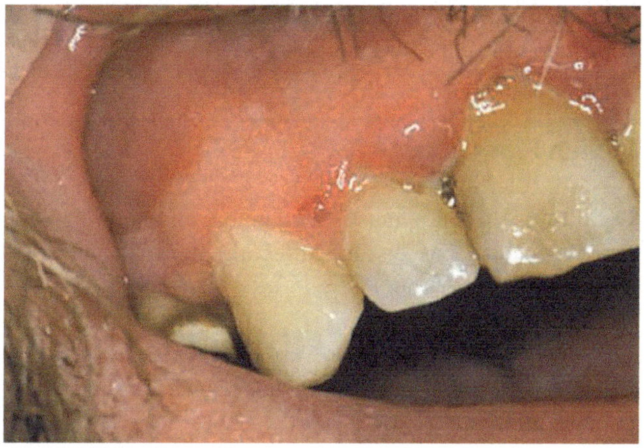

Fig. 33.30 Epidermolysis bullosa acquisita, erythema and small vesicle on the gingiva in the form of desquamative gingivitis

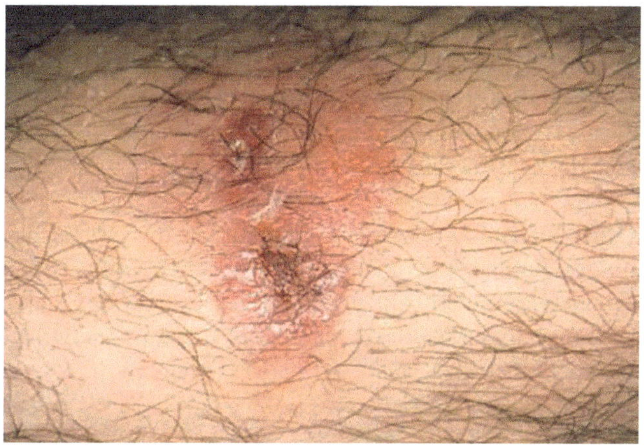

Fig. 33.31 Epidermolysis bullosa acquisita, erythema and scarring on the skin

tions that rupture leaving quickly nonspecific painful erosions (Fig. 33.30).

- Localized and, rarely, widespread bullae and erosions may develop, particularly in friction-associated areas of the oral mucosa.
- Skin lesions are characterized by hemorrhagic bullae, which are developed spontaneously or after mild trauma. The rupture of bullae leaves ulcers that may heal with scarring (Fig. 33.31). Milia, atrophic areas, hyperpigmentation, and nail dystrophy may occur.
- Clinical diagnosis should be confirmed by laboratory tests.

Differential Diagnosis

- Mucous membrane pemphigoid.
- Bullous pemphigoid.
- Systemic lupus erythematosus, bullous type.
- Porphyria cutanea tarda.
- Linear IgA disease.
- Pemphigus.
- Genetic epidermolysis bullosa.

Laboratory Tests Histopathologic examination, direct and indirect immunofluorescence. Immunoelectron microscopy.

Treatment Local and systemic corticosteroids. Dapsone, azathioprine. Mycophenolate mofetil. Recently, IVIgs and intravenous infusion of anti-CD20 antibodies (rituximab) have been used. Avoid trauma.

Dermatitis Herpetiformis

Definition Dermatitis herpetiformis or Duhring-Brocq disease is a rare, chronic and recurrent vesiculopapular dermatosis.

Etiology Autoimmune. A strong association with HLA-B8, HLA-A1, HLA-DR3, HLA-Dw_3, HLA-Dw_2 has been found. Gluten hypersensitivity plays an important role in pathogenesis.

Gingival Involvement Rare. Non-dental biofilm-induced gingival lesions with no attachment loss.

Other Sites of Involvement Oral mucosa (palate, tongue, buccal mucosa, lips) approximately 5–10%. Skin (in a symmetrical distribution of the extensor surfaces of the elbows, knees, shoulders, buttocks, posterior neck, scale) always.

Clinical Features

- The disease is more common between 20 and 50 years of age and males are more frequently affected than females (ratio1.5 vs. 2:1).
- Gingival and other oral lesions appear as localized whitish maculopapular lesions, erythema and formation of bullae that soon rapture, leaving nonspecific painful erosions (Figs. 33.32 and 33.33). The oral lesions usually follow the skin eruption.

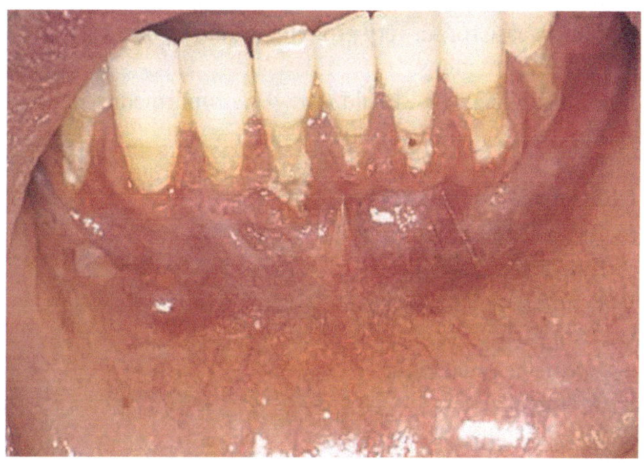

Fig. 33.32 Dermatitis herpetiformis, erythema and erosions on the gingiva and small bulla on the labial mucosa

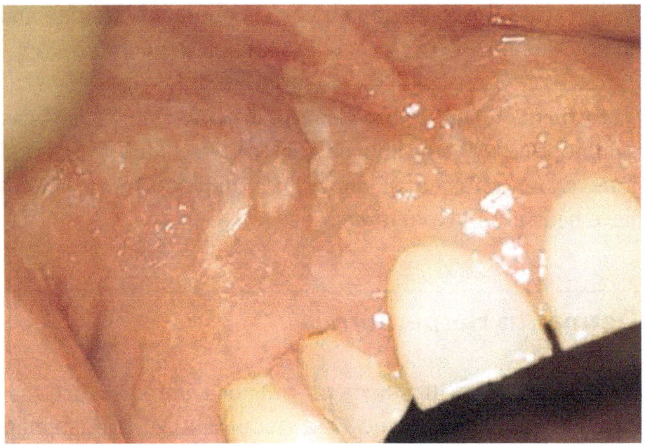

Fig. 33.33 Dermatitis herpetiformis, whitish maculopapular lesions and vesicles on the gingiva and the alveolar mucosa

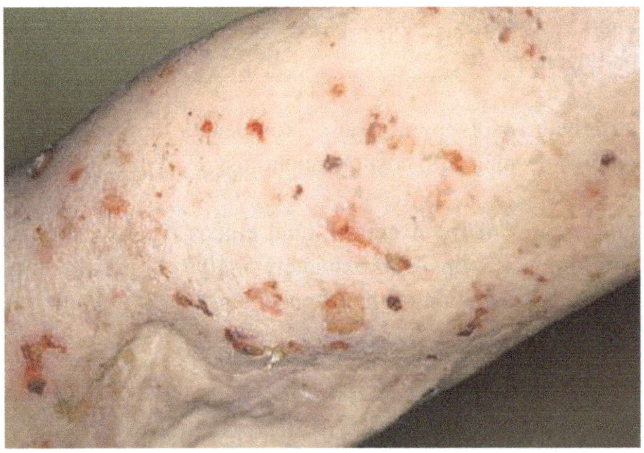

Fig. 33.34 Dermatitis herpetiformis, group of vesicles and erosions on the skin, in a herpes-like pattern

- Skin lesions appear as erythematous papules or plaques accompanied by severe burning and pruritus as well as by small vesicles coalescing in groups that mimic herpes (Fig. 33.34). Elbows, knees, scapular region, glutes, neck, trunk, and scalp are most commonly affected.
- The disease runs a very prolonged course with remissions and exacerbations.
- Clinical diagnosis should always be confirmed by laboratory tests.

Differential Diagnosis
- Bullous pemphigoid.
- Linear IgA disease.
- Pemphigoid gestationis.
- Pemphigus.
- Erythema muhiforme.
- Aphthous ulcers.
- Herpetic gingivostomatitis.

Laboratory Tests Histopathologic examination, direct and indirect immunofluorescence.

Treatment Gluten-free diet. Dapsone and sulphapyridine, corticosteroids in persistent cases.

Lichen Planus

Definition Lichen planus is a common, chronic inflammatory mucocutaneous disease, affecting approximately 0.5–2.5% of the population.

Etiology Autoinflammatory. Current evidence suggests that there is a local cell-mediated immune response with a T lymphocyte infiltrate.

Classification Seven clinical forms of oral lichen planus have been described: (a) *Papular*; (b) *Reticular*; (c) *Erosive*; (d) *Atrophic*; (e) *Hypertrophic (plaque-like)*; (f) *Bullous*; and (g) *Pigmented*.

Gingival Involvement Common(approximately 30–40% of cases). Non-dental biofilm-induced lesions with no attachment loss.

Other Sites of Involvement Oral mucosa (buccal, tongue, lips, palate) in approximately 50–70% of cases, usually in a symmetrical pattern. Other mucosae (vulva, vagina, penis). Skin (usually on the flexor surfaces of forearms and wrists, the back, the sacral area, and nails), commonly in a symmetrical pattern.

Clinical Features
- Females are affected more often than males, usually between 40 and 60 years of age.
- Most patients with oral lichen planus present with a combination of various clinical forms. Polygonal white papules and lines are the basic clinical features of the disease.
- Frequently, the disease affects the gingiva and, occasionally, can be the initial or the only sign of oral involvement. Clinically, gingival lesions may appear in the form of *desquamative gingivitis* (Figs. 33.35, 33.36, and 33.37). White papules and lines, erosions, or atrophy may also occur (Fig. 33.38).
- In oral mucosa, small white papules occur that usually coalesce and form lines *(Wickham's striae)* and network of lines (Fig. 33.39). Annular distribution of the papules, painful erosions, atrophic or hypertrophic areas, bullous or pigmented lines may also be seen depending on the clinical form.
- Skin lesions appear as small, red or violaceous flat, polygonal, shiny, and pruritic papules.
- Lichen planus may follow a course of remissions and exacerbations.
- Diagnosis is mainly based on clinical criteria, but laboratory tests may be supportive.

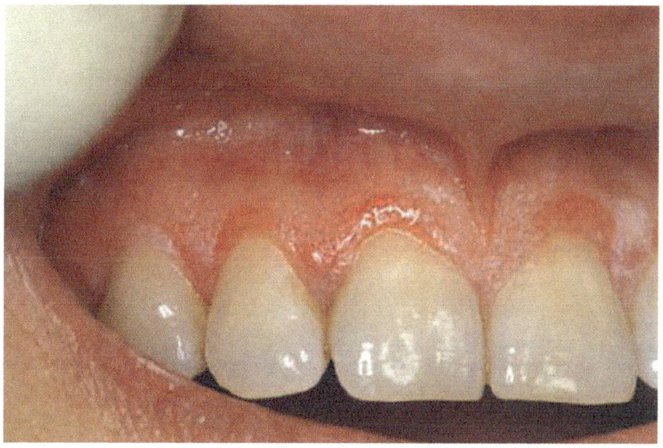

Fig. 33.35 Lichen planus, erythema and white lines on the gingiva in the form of desquamative gingivitis

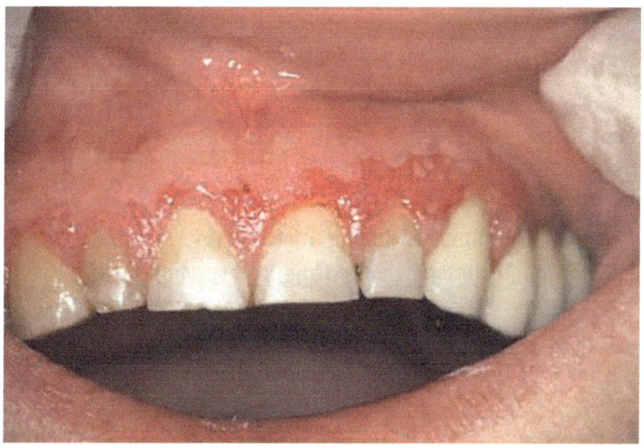

Fig. 33.36 Lichen planus, typical lesions of desquamative gingivitis

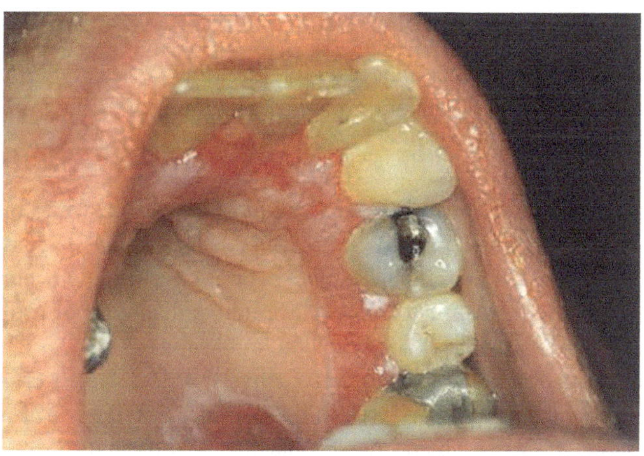

Fig. 33.37 Lichen planus, diffuse erythema on the gingiva and palate

Differential Diagnosis
- Mucous membrane pemphigoid.
- Chronic ulcerative stomatitis.
- Discoid lupus erythematosus.
- Cinnamon contact stomatitis.
- Candidiasis.

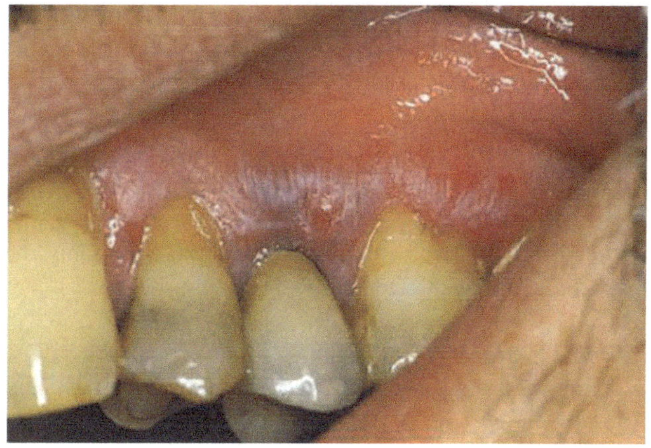

Fig. 33.38 Lichen planus, characteristic papules and lines on the gingiva

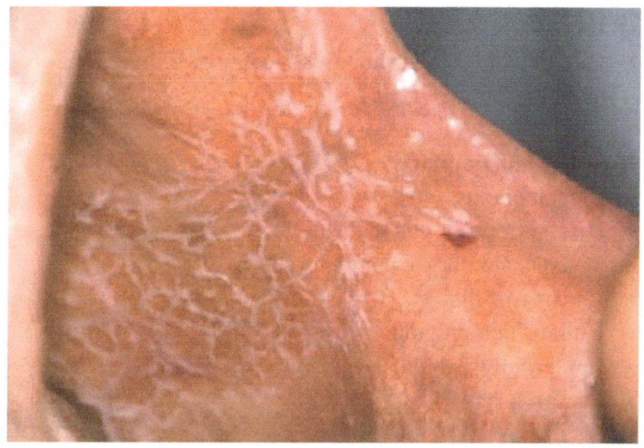

Fig. 33.39 Lichen planus, typical "Wickham striae" on the buccal mucosa

- Lichenoid reaction to dental materials or drugs.
- Graft-Versus-Host Disease.
- Plasma cell gingivitis.

Laboratory Tests Histopathologic examination, direct immunofluorescence.

Treatment Good oral hygiene. Avoid pressure/irritation to the gingiva. Topical corticosteroids in an adhesive base. Systemic corticosteroids in extremely painful lesions. Dapsone, cyclosporine, tacrolimus, and azathioprine may also be used in persistent cases.

Chronic Ulcerative Stomatitis

Definition Chronic ulcerative stomatitis is a rare autoimmune disease that resembles, clinically and histopathologically, lichen planus and lupus erythematosus, but possesses a unique immunofluorescent pattern.

Etiology Autoimmune. Circulating and tissue-bound autoantibodies against Delta Np63α protein are the pathogenic agents of disease.

Gingival Involvement Common. Non-dental biofilm-induced gingival lesions with no attachment loss.

Other Sites of Involvement Oral mucosa, commonly the buccal mucosa and the tongue.

Clinical Features

- Gingival lesions usually appear in the form of *desquamative gingivitis* or as localized and painful erythema and erosions (Fig. 33.40).
- Oral lesions appear as painful erosions usually associated with white reticular lesions identical to those seen in oral lichen planus and discoid lupus erythematosus (Fig. 33.41).
- Clinical diagnosis should be confirmed by laboratory tests.

Differential Diagnosis

- Lichen planus.
- Discoid lupus erythematosus.
- Mucous membrane pemphigoid.
- Linear IgA disease.
- Bullous pemphigoid.
- Epidermolysis bullosa aquisita.
- Pemphigus.

Laboratory Tests Histopathologic examination, direct and indirect immunofluorescence.

Treatment Systemic or local corticosteroids are the drugs of choice. Hydroxychloroquine sulfate (Plaquenil) and other antimalarial agents. Patients should avoid inducing gingival trauma with a hard toothbrush.

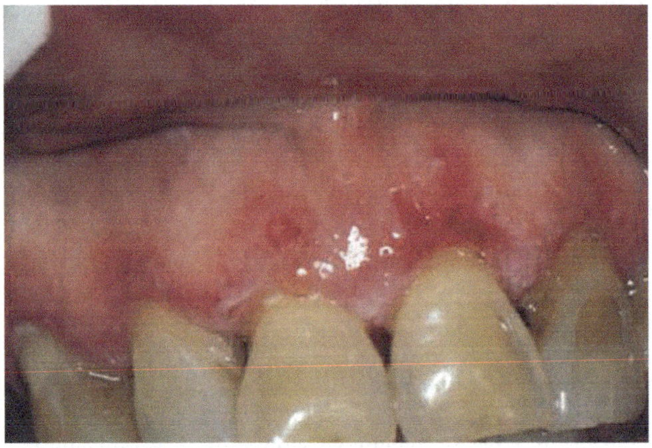

Fig. 33.40 Chronic ulcerative stomatitis, erythema and erosions on the gingiva in the form of desquamative gingivitis

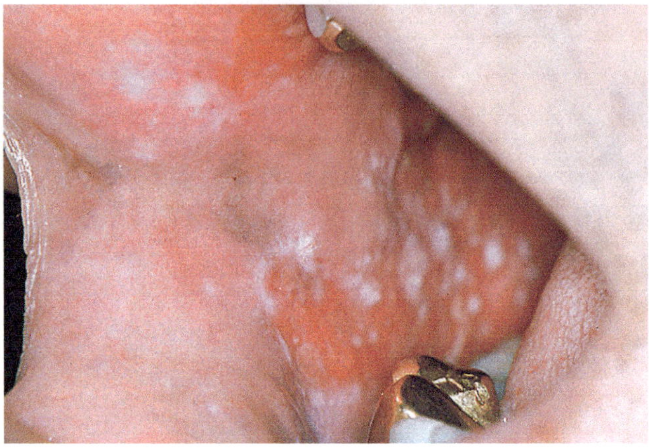

Fig. 33.41 Chronic ulcerative stomatitis, erosions and white lesions on the buccal mucosa

Psoriasis

Definition Psoriasis is a common, chronic and recurrent inflammatory skin disease.

Etiology Immune-mediated mechanism, combined with genetic, environmental, and drug predisposing facts.

Gingival Involvement Very rare. Non-dental biofilm-induced lesions with no attachment loss.

Other Sites of Involvement Oral mucosa (tongue. Buccal mucosa. lips), rare (approximately 2–4%). Skin (elbows, knees, scalp, lumbar area, nails), always.

Clinical Features

- Gingival lesions may resemble *desquamative gingivitis*; however, desquamation of the epithelium after pressure does not occur (Fig. 33.42). This pattern is an exceptional phenomenon.
- Oral lesions may appear as atypical erythema, white or greyish plaques, and, more often, as circinate lesions mimicking geographic tongue. Oral lesions usually occur following skin involvement. Definitive diagnosis of psoriasis cannot be made based on oral lesions.
- Skin lesions are characterized by well-demarcated erythematous plaques with silvery scales on the surface (Fig. 33.43). The lesions are usually asymptomatic.
- Clinical diagnosis should be confirmed by laboratory tests.

Differential Diagnosis

- Geographic tongue and stomatitis.
- Cinnamon contact stomatitis.
- Candidiasis.

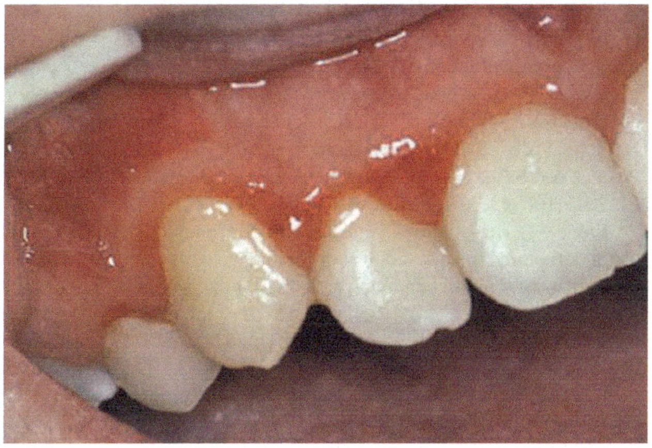

Fig. 33.42 Psoriasis, unusual involvement on the gingiva in the form of desquamative gingivitis

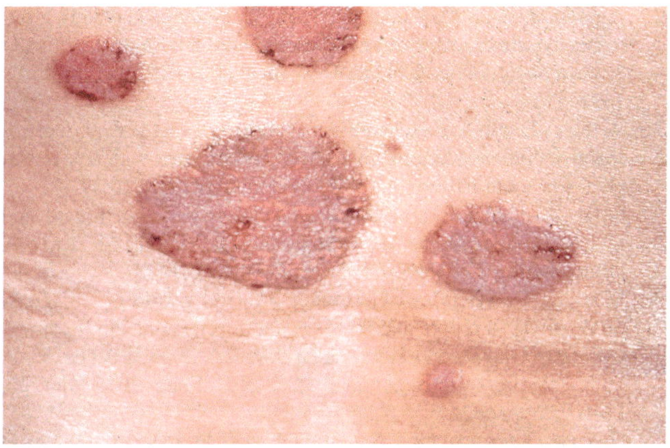

Fig. 33.43 Psoriasis, multiple skin erythematous plaques

- Plasma cell gingivitis.
- Linear gingival erythema.
- Granulomatous gingivitis.
- Lichen planus.
- Mucous membrane pemphigoid.
- Reiter syndrome.

Laboratory Tests Histopathologic examination.

Treatment Gingival lesions should be treated with good oral hygiene and topical corticosteroids. The treatment of skin lesions must be left to dermatologists.

References

1. Chan LS, Ahmed AR, Anhalt GJ, et al. The first international consensus on mucous membrane pemphigoid: definition, diagnostic criteria, pathogenic factors, medical treatment, and prognostic indicators. Arch Dermatol. 2002;138(3):370–9. https://doi.org/10.1001/archderm.138.3.370.
2. Zoghaib S, Kechichian E, Souaid K, et al. Triggers, clinical manifestations, and management of pediatric erythema multiforme: a systematic review. J Am Acad Dermatol. 2019;81(3):813–22. https://doi.org/10.1016/j.jaad.2019.02.057. Epub 2019 Jul 19. PMID: 31331726
3. Du Y, Wang F, Liu T, et al. Recurrent oral erythema multiforme: a case series report and review of the literature. Oral Surg Oral Med Oral Pathol Oral Radiol. 2020;129(4):e224–9. https://doi.org/10.1016/j.oooo.2019.11.013. Epub 2019 Nov 28. PMID: 31926837
4. Barea-Jiménez N, Calero J, Molina-Negrón D, López Del-Valle LM. Treatment for oral lesions in pediatric patients with Stevens-Johnson's syndrome: a case report and literature review. Int J Paediatr Dent. 2020;30(4):489–96. https://doi.org/10.1111/ipd.12615. Epub 2020 Jan 24. PMID: 31923328
5. Adams L, Creamer D. Controlling oral hemorrhages in Steven-Johnson syndrome/toxic epidermal necrolysis. J Am Acad Dermatol. 2020;82(1):e3–4. https://doi.org/10.1016/j.jaad.2019.06.1299. Epub 2019 Jul 3. PMID: 31279017
6. Sultan AS, Villa A, Saavedra AP, et al. Oral mucous membrane pemphigoid and pemphigus vulgaris-a retrospective two-center cohort study. Oral Dis. 2017;23(4):498–504. https://doi.org/10.1111/odi.12639. Epub 2017 Feb 22. PMID: 28084005
7. Javali MA, Zainab H. Pemphigus vulgaris presenting as gingival involvement. Indian Dermatol Online J. 2012;3(3):202–4. https://doi.org/10.4103/2229-5178.101821. PMID: 23189256; PMCID: PMC3505431
8. Rath SK, Reenesh M. Gingival pemphigus vulgaris preceding cutaneous lesion: a rare case report. J Indian Soc Periodontol. 2012;16(4):588–91. https://doi.org/10.4103/0972-124X.106922. PMID: 23493851; PMCID: PMC3590732
9. Scully C, Laskaris G. Mucocutaneous disorders. Periodontol. 2000;1998(18):81–94. https://doi.org/10.1111/j.1600-0757.1998.tb00140.x. PMID: 10200714
10. Alessi SS, Nico MM, Fernandes JD, Lourenço SV. Reflectance confocal microscopy as a new tool in the in vivo evaluation of desquamative gingivitis: patterns in mucous membrane pemphigoid, pemphigus vulgaris and oral lichen planus. Br J Dermatol. 2013;168(2):257–64. https://doi.org/10.1111/bjd.12021. Epub 2012 Nov 20. PMID: 22924499
11. Laskaris G. Oral pemphigus vulgaris: an immunofluorescent study of fifty-eight cases. Oral Surg Oral Med Oral Pathol. 1981;51(6):626–31. https://doi.org/10.1016/s0030-4220(81)80013-8. PMID: 6942362
12. Laskaris G, Stoufi E. Oral pemphigus vulgaris in a 6-year-old girl. Oral Surg Oral Med Oral Pathol. 1990;69(5):609–13. https://doi.org/10.1016/0030-4220(90)90245-n. PMID: 2185451
13. Ohki M, Kikuchi S. Nasal, oral, and pharyngolaryngeal manifestations of pemphigus vulgaris: endoscopic ororhinolaryngologic examination. Ear Nose Throat J. 2017;96(3):120–7. https://doi.org/10.1177/014556131709600311. PMID: 28346642
14. Arduino PG, Broccoletti R, Carbone M, et al. Describing the gingival involvement in a sample of 182 Italian predominantly oral mucous membrane pemphigoid patients: a retrospective series. Med Oral Patol Oral Cir Bucal. 2017;22(2):e149–52. https://doi.org/10.4317/medoral.21431. PMID: 28160581; PMCID: PMC5359700
15. Kavlakova L, Bachurska S. Topical occlusive corticosteroid therapy for the treatment of gingival manifestation of mucous membrane pemphigoid–a case report. Folia Med (Plovdiv). 2020;62(4):866–70. https://doi.org/10.3897/folmed.62.e51339. PMID: 33415936
16. Sklavounou A, Laskaris G. Childhood cicatricial pemphigoid with exclusive gingival involvement. Int J Oral Maxillofac Surg. 1990a;19(4):197–9. https://doi.org/10.1016/s0901-5027(05)80388-1. PMID: 2120357

17. Laskaris G, Sklavounou A, Stratigos J. Bullous pemphigoid, cicatricial pemphigoid, and pemphigus vulgaris. A comparative clinical survey of 278 cases. Oral Surg Oral Med Oral Pathol. 1982a;54(6):656–62. https://doi.org/10.1016/0030-4220(82)90080-9. PMID: 6760033
18. Laskaris G, Angelopoulos A. Cicatricial pemphigoid: direct and indirect immunofluorescent studies. Oral Surg Oral Med Oral Pathol. 1981;51(1):48–54. https://doi.org/10.1016/0030-4220(81)90125-0. PMID: 7007955
19. Laskaris G, Nicolis G. Immunopathology of oral mucosa in bullous pemphigoid. Oral Surg Oral Med Oral Pathol. 1980;50(4):340–5. https://doi.org/10.1016/0030-4220(80)90419-3. PMID: 7005803
20. Ohki M, Kikuchi S, Ohata A, Baba Y, et al. Features of oral, pharyngeal, and laryngeal lesions in bullous pemphigoid. Ear Nose Throat J. 2016;95(10–11):E1–5. PMID: 27792825
21. Bagan J, Jiménez Y, Murillo J, Bagan L. Oral mucous membrane pemphigoid: a clinical study of 100 low-risk cases. Oral Dis. 2018;24(1–2):132–4. https://doi.org/10.1111/odi.12744. PMID: 29480624
22. Gagari E, Laskaris G. Pemphigoid gestationis with oral manifestations: case report and review of the literature. Balkan J Stomatol. 2010;14:31–6.
23. Leuci S, Gurcan HM, Ahmed AR. Serological studies in bullous pemphigoid: a literature review of antibody titers at presentation and in clinical remission. Acta Derm Venereol. 2010;90:115–21.
24. Laskaris G, Triantafyllou A, Economopoulou P. Gingival manifestations of childhood cicatricial pemphigoid. Oral Surg Oral Med Oral Pathol. 1988;66(3):349–52. https://doi.org/10.1016/0030-4220(88)90244-7. PMID: 3050709
25. Sklavounou A, Laskaris G. Frequency of desquamative gingivitis in skin diseases. Oral Surg Oral Med Oral Pathol. 1983;56(2):141–4. https://doi.org/10.1016/0030-4220(83)90278-5. PMID: 6578475
26. Suresh L, Neiders ME. Definitive and differential diagnosis of desquamative gingivitis through direct immunofluorescence studies. J Periodontol. 2012;83(10):1270–8. https://doi.org/10.1902/jop.2012.110627. Epub 2012 Jan 20. PMID: 22264207
27. Joseph TI, Sathyan P, Goma Kumar KU. Linear IgA dermatosis adult variant with oral manifestation: a rare case report. J Oral Maxillofac Pathol. 2015;19(1):83–7. https://doi.org/10.4103/0973-029X.157207. PMID: 26097313; PMCID: PMC4451675
28. Eguia del Valle A, Aguirre Urizar JM, Martinez SA. Oral manifestations caused by the linear IgA disease. Med Oral. 2004;9:39–44.
29. Nishida E, Nishio E, Murashima H, et al. Case of epidermolysis bullosa acquisita with concomitant anti-laminin-332 antibodies. J Dermatol. 2018;45(4):472–4. https://doi.org/10.1111/1346-8138.14169. Epub 2017 Dec 4. PMID: 29205468
30. Economopoulou P, Laskaris G. Dermatitis herpetiformis: oral lesions as an early manifestation. Oral Surg Oral Med Oral Pathol. 1986;62:77–80.
31. Sehgal VN, Syed NH, Aggarwal A, Sehgal S. Oral lichen planus: a cross-sectional/descriptive study of 33 patients. Skin Med. 2017;15(5):333–7. PMID: 29139359
32. Stone SJ, Heasman PA, Staines KS, McCracken GI. The impact of structured plaque control for patients with gingival manifestations of oral lichen planus: a randomized controlled study. J Clin Periodontol. 2015;42(4):356–62. https://doi.org/10.1111/jcpe.12385. Epub 2015 Apr 10. PMID: 25728699
33. Laskaris G, Sklavounou A, Angelopoulos A. Direct immunofluorescence in oral lichen planus. Oral Surg Oral Med Oral Pathol. 1982b;53(5):483–7. https://doi.org/10.1016/0030-4220(82)90461-3. PMID: 7048185
34. Sklavounou AD, Laskaris G, Angelopoulos AP. Serum immunoglobulins and complement (C'3) in oral lichen planus. Oral Surg Oral Med Oral Pathol. 1983;55(1):47–51. https://doi.org/10.1016/0030-4220(83)90304-3. PMID: 6402750
35. Ingafou M, Leao JC, Porter SR, Scully C. Oral lichen planus: a retrospective study of 690 British patients. Oral Dis. 2006;12(5):463–8. https://doi.org/10.1111/j.1601-0825.2005.01221.x. PMID: 16910916
36. Bermejo-Fenoll A, Sanchez-Siles M, Lopez-Jornet P, et al. A retrospective clinicopathological study of 550 patients with oral lichen planus in south-eastern Spain. J Oral Pathol Med. 2010;39:491–6.
37. Sklavounou A, Laskaris G. Oral psoriasis: report of a case and review of the literature. Dermatologica. 1990b;180(3):157–9. https://doi.org/10.1159/000248018. PMID: 2187720
38. Mattsson U, Warfvinge G, Jontell M. Oral psoriasis-a diagnostic dilemma: a report of two cases and a review of the literature. Oral Surg Oral Med Oral Pathol Oral Radiol. 2015;120(4):e183–9. https://doi.org/10.1016/j.oooo.2015.03.005. Epub 2015 Mar 26. PMID: 25944682
39. Ganzetti G, Campanati A, Santarelli A, et al. Periodontal disease: an oral manifestation of psoriasis or an occasional finding? Drug Dev Res. 2014;75(Suppl 1):S46–9. https://doi.org/10.1002/ddr.21194. PMID: 25381976
40. Laskaris G, Satriano RA. Drug-induced blistering oral lesions. Clin Dermatol. 1993;11(4):545–50. https://doi.org/10.1016/0738-081x(93)90164-8. PMID: 8124645

Paraneoplastic Mucocutaneous Diseases

34

Contents

Paraneoplastic mucocutaneous disorders is a small group of diseases that present with cutaneous, oral, and other mucosal manifestations. Only a few of them may develop gingival lesions as well. These lesions themselves are not malignant, but they are linked with solid or hematologic malignancies. The criteria used to associate a mucocutaneous disorder and malignancy (*Curth's postulates*) are the following: (a) *concurrent onset*; (b) *parallel course*; (c) *uniform type of malignancy*; (d) *statistical association;* and (e) *genetic linkage.*

Malignant Acanthosis Nigricans

Definition The most common paraneoplastic disease that can affect the skin and mucosae. Malignant acanthosis nigricans is a form of acanthosis nigricans that is strongly associated with an internal malignancy, usually adenocarcinoma of the stomach, and less commonly with Non-Hodgkin lymphoma or other malignancies.

Etiology It is obscure, although a cytokine-like peptide produced by the malignant tumor may stimulate the epidermal and mucosal cells causing hyperplasia.

Gingival Involvement Relatively rare. Non-dental biofilm-induced gingival lesions.

Other Sites of Involvement Oral mucosa, relatively common (30–40%), other mucosae (conjunctiva, anus, vagina, pharynx, esophagus), rare. Skin, always.

Clinical Features

- Gingival lesions present as a multiple papillomatous overgrowth of normal color that may cover the crowns of the teeth (Fig. 34.1).
- Oral lesions also present as diffuse velvety papillary lesions of normal color, particularly on the lips, commis-

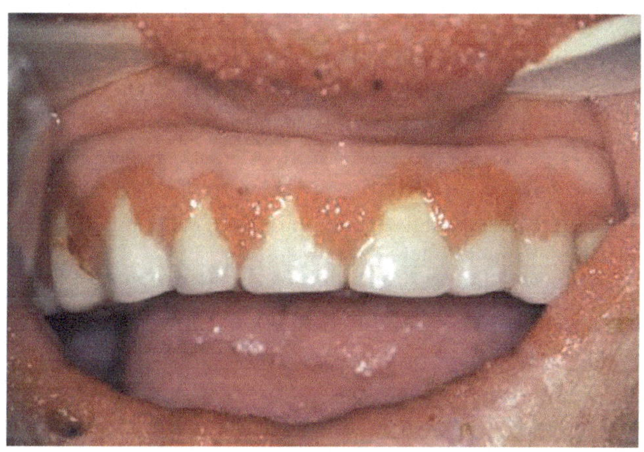

Fig. 34.1 Malignant acanthosis nigricans, generalized papillomatous overgrowths on the gingiva

G. Laskaris et al., *Periodontal Manifestations of Local and Systemic Diseases*, https://doi.org/10.1007/978-3-031-10828-0_34

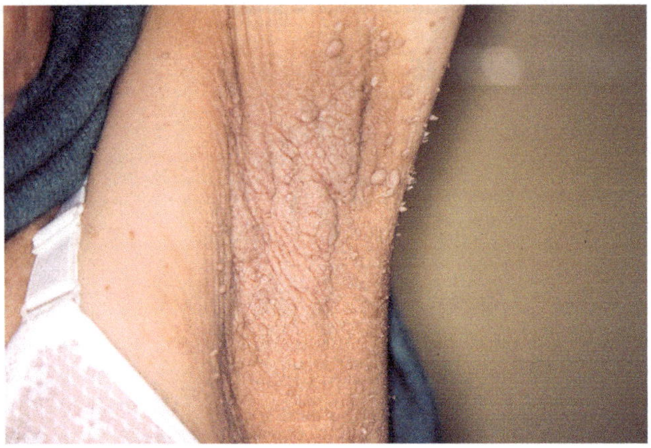

Fig. 34.2 Malignant acanthosis nigricans, brown papillary growths on the axilla of a patient with stomach adenocarcinoma

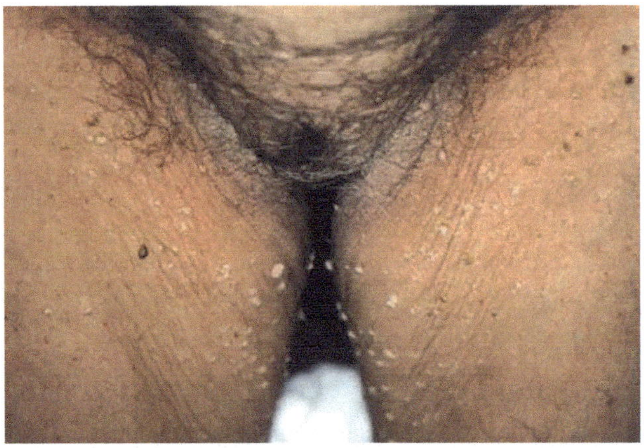

Fig. 34.3 Malignant acanthosis nigricans, brownish papillary overgrowths on the skin

sures, tongue, and palate. Similar lesions may occur in other mucosae.
- Skin lesions appear as brownish or black, asymptomatic, papillary and rough growths, usually on the axillae, the inguinal area, neck, palms, and soles (Figs. 34.2 and 34.3). The mucocutaneous lesions are benign but are important as they represent a marker for internal malignancy.
- Diagnosis is usually based on clinical criteria but should be confirmed by laboratory tests.

Differential Diagnosis
- Familial acanthosis nigricans.
- Darier disease.
- Pemphigus vegetans.
- Cowden syndrome.
- Goltz syndrome.
- Multiple papillomas.
- Lipoid proteinosis.

Laboratory Tests Histopathologic examination. Other tests for identification of primary malignancy.

Treatment The mucocutaneous lesions may resolve when the malignancy is treated. Dental biofilm control and occasionally gingivectomy for the gingival overgrowths.

Paraneoplastic Pemphigus

Definition Paraneoplastic pemphigus is a unique and rare variant in the pemphigus group, which is commonly associated with non-Hodgkin lymphoma, chronic lymphocytic leukemia, Castleman disease, thymoma, and sarcomas. Paraneoplastic pemphigus has specific clinical, histopathologic, and immunologic characteristics that differ from those of pemphigus vulgaris.

Etiology Autoimmune. Autoantibodies against desmoplakins I and II are specific markers for paraneoplastic pemphigus.

Gingival Involvement Common. Non-dental biofilm-induced gingival lesions.

Other Sites of Involvement Oral mucosa, always. Other mucosae (conjunctiva, pharynx, esophagus, penis, and vagina), relatively common. Skin, always.

Clinical Features
- Gingival lesions present as painful, generalized, and persistent erosions identical to those seen in pemphigus vulgaris (Figs. 34.4 and 34.5).
- Oral lesions present as early, multiple, severe, and treatment-resistant erosions on the lips, buccal mucosa,

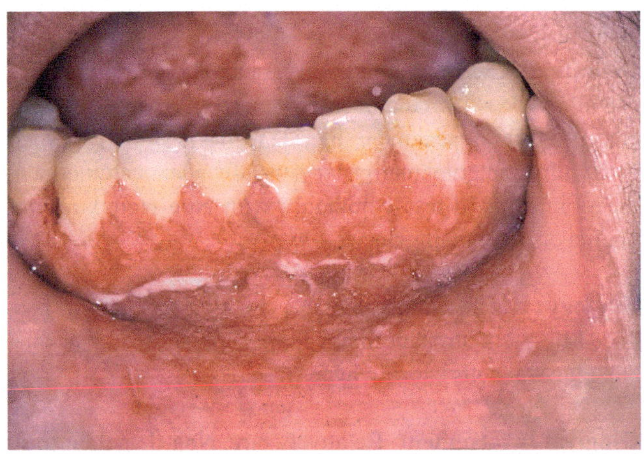

Fig. 34.4 Paraneoplastic pemphigus, generalized gingival erosions of a patient with pemphigus associated with myelocytic leukemia

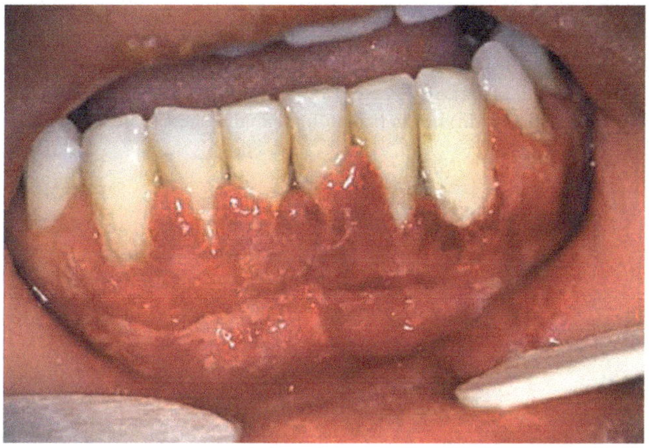

Fig. 34.5 Paraneoplastic pemphigus, erythema and erosions on the gingiva of a patient with pemphigus associated with chronic lymphocytic leukemia

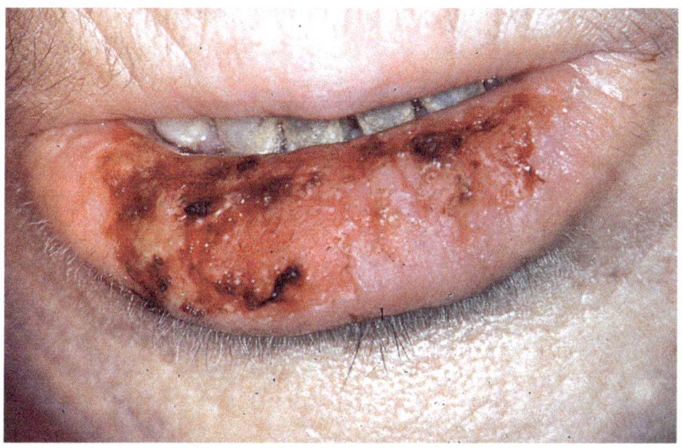

Fig. 34.6 Paraneoplastic pemphigus, severe erosions on the lips of a patient with underlying myelocytic leukemia

tongue, palate, usually extending to the oropharynx and esophagus causing severe sore throat (Fig. 34.6). Persistent bilateral conjunctival erosions and edema are common. In some cases, ocular lesions result in scarring and adhesions.

- Skin lesions are polymorphous and include bullae, erythematous and/or verrucous papules or plaques mimicking the *"target-like"* lesions seen in erythema multiforme. *Nikolskysign* is positive.
- Clinical diagnosis should be confirmed by laboratory tests.

Differential Diagnosis
- Pemphigus vulgaris.
- Bullous pemphigoid.
- Mucous membrane pemphigoid.
- Linear IgA disease.
- Erythema multiforme.
- Stevens-Johnson syndrome.
- Graft-Versus-Host-Disease.
- Persistent HSV infection.
- Lichenplanus (erosivetype).

Laboratory Tests Histopathologic examination. Direct and indirect immunofluorescence, immunoprecipitation study. Characteristically, IgG autoantibodies react against multiple antigenic targets such as desmoglein 1 and 3, desmoplakins I and II, envoplakin, periplakin, plectin, and bullous pemphigoid antigen 1 (BPAG1). Identification of primary malignancy.

Treatment Systemic corticosteroids alone or in combination with immunosuppressive drugs. Treatment of the underlying malignancy is necessary. Skin lesions are more responsive to treatment than mucosal lesions.

Anti-Laminin 5 Mucous Membrane Pemphigoid (see p. 200)

Mucous membrane pemphigoid patients with anti-laminin 5 autoantibodies have a relatively low risk to develop mainly adenocarcinomas.

Dermatitis Herpetiformis (see p. 205)

In cases of dermatitis herpetiformis associated with gluten-sensitive enteropathy patients, present a low risk to develop a non-Hodgkin T cell lymphoma.

References

1. Laskaris GC, Papavasiliou SS, Bovopoulou OD, Nicolis GD. Association of oral pemphigus with chronic lymphocytic leukemia. Oral Surg Oral Med Oral Pathol. 1980;50(3):244–9. https://doi.org/10.1016/0030-4220(80)90378-3. PMID: 6931999
2. Pentenero M, Carrozzo M, Pagano M, Gandolfo S. Oral acanthosis nigricans, tripe palms and sign of leser-trélat in a patient with gastric adenocarcinoma. Int J Dermatol. 2004;43(7):530–2. https://doi.org/10.1111/j.1365-4632.2004.02159.x. PMID: 15230897
3. Paolino G, Didona D, Magliulo G, et al. Paraneoplastic pemphigus: insight into the autoimmune pathogenesis, clinical features and therapy. Int J Mol Sci. 2017;18(12):2532. https://doi.org/10.3390/ijms18122532. PMID: 29186863; PMCID: PMC5751135
4. Kaplan I, Hodak E, Ackerman L, et al. Neoplasms associated with paraneoplastic pemphigus: a review with emphasis on non-hematologic malignancy and oral mucosal manifestations. Oral Oncol. 2004;40(6):553–62. https://doi.org/10.1016/j.oraloncology.2003.09.020. PMID: 15063382
5. Lu T, Song B, Pu H, et al. Paraneoplastic pemphigus and myasthenia gravis as the first manifestations of a rare case of pancreatic follicular dendritic cell sarcoma: CT findings and review of literature. BMC Gastroenterol. 2019;19(1):92. https://doi.org/10.1186/s12876-019-1008-y. PMID: 31200650; PMCID: PMC6570917

6. Benoit S, Schmidt E, Sitaru C, et al. Schleimhautpemphigoid mit Autoantikörpern gegen Laminin 5 [Anti-laminin 5 mucous membrane pemphigoid]. J Dtsch Dermatol Ges. 2006;4(1):41–4. https://doi.org/10.1111/j.1610-0387.2005.05826.x. PMID: 16503930
7. Sklavounou A, Laskaris G. Paraneoplastic pemphigus: a review. Oral Oncol. 1998;34:437–40.
8. Steele HA, George BJ. Mucocutaneous paraneoplastic syndromes associated with hematologic malignancies. Oncology. 2011;25:1076–83.
9. Zappasodi P, Forno C, Corso A, Lazzarino M. Mucocutaneous paraneoplastic syndromes in hematologic malignancies. Int J Dermatol. 2006;45:14–22.

35 Autoimmune and Autoinflammatory Diseases

Contents

Lupus Erythematosus

Definition Lupus erythematosus is a chronic inflammatory autoimmune disease with a variable spectrum of clinical forms.

Etiology It is thought that a genetically susceptible autoimmune mechanism, triggered by environmental factors, is responsible for the pathogenesis of the disease.

Classification The disease is classified into two major forms: (a) *Discoid*; and (b) *Systemic*.

Gingival Involvement Relatively rare. Non-dental biofilm-induced gingival lesions.

Other Sites of Involvement Oral mucosa (15–25% in discoid form and 30–45% in systemic form), other mucosae (conjunctiva, nose, genitals), skin, other organ systems (kidneys, cardiovascular system, nervous system, joints).

Clinical Features

- Gingival lesions may appear either as localized erythema, usually associated with erosions that may occasionally mimic *desquamative gingivitis* (Figs. 35.1 and 35.2). Less frequently, lupus erythematosus may present as a nonspecific painful ulceration surrounded by whitish spots or lines.
- Oral lesions appear as well-defined atrophic red plaques usually surrounded by a sharp elevated border of radiating whitish striae. Erosions, atrophy, telangiectasias, white plaques, and xerostomia may also occur (Fig. 35.3).
- Skin lesions are characterized by flat or slightly elevated erythematous papules and plaques with scaling and follicular hyperkeratosis (Fig. 35.4).
- Many patients in both forms develop the classic *"butterfly rash"* on the face.
- Systemic lupus erythematosus is characterized by a broad spectrum of clinical and laboratory diagnostic criteria.

G. Laskaris et al., *Periodontal Manifestations of Local and Systemic Diseases*, https://doi.org/10.1007/978-3-031-10828-0_35

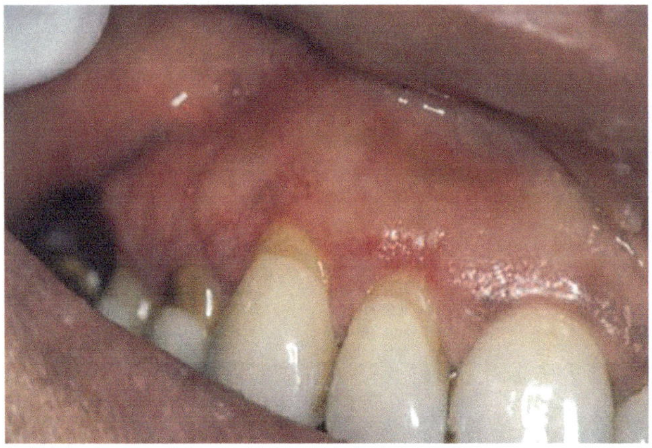

Fig. 35.1 Lupus erythematosus, irregular erythema and erosions as early lesions on the gingiva

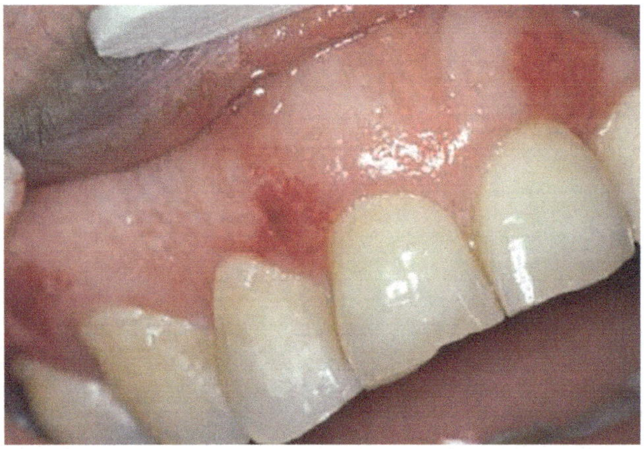

Fig. 35.2 Lupus erythematosus, localized erosions on the gingiva

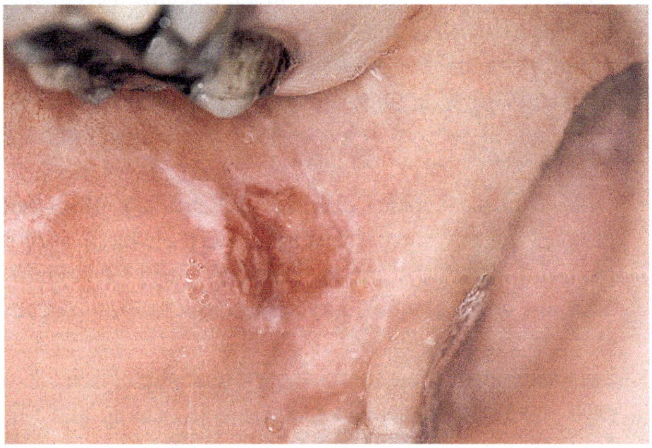

Fig. 35.3 Lupus erythematosus, erosion with peripheral radiating striae on the buccal mucosa

- Constitutional symptoms include fatigue, malaise, fever, and weight loss associated with arthralgia and myalgia.
- Clinical diagnosis should be confirmed by laboratory tests.

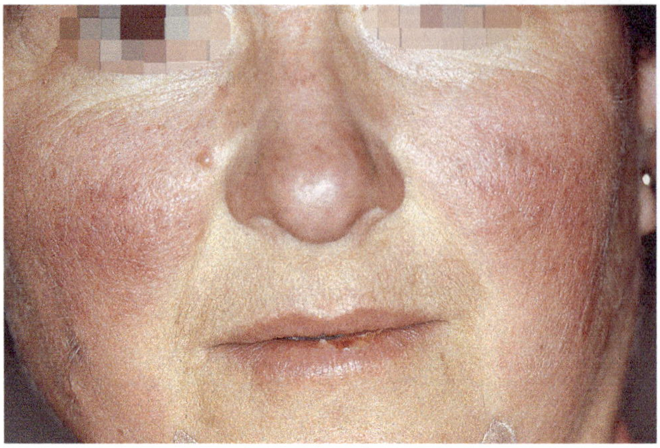

Fig. 35.4 Lupus erythematosus, skin lesions presenting with erythematous papules in the "butterfly rash pattern"

Differential Diagnosis
- Lichen planus.
- Graft-Versus-Host Disease.
- Mixed connective tissue disease.
- Mucous membrane pemphigoid.
- Bullous pemphigoid.
- Linear IgA disease.
- Pemphigus.

Laboratory Tests Histopathologic examination of oral and skin lesions, direct and indirect immunofluorescence.

Treatment Good dental biofilm control. Topical corticosteroids. Systemic corticosteroids, antimalarials. The treatment of systemic lupus erythematosus should be left to specialists.

Sjögren Syndrome

Definition Sjögren syndrome is a relatively common, multisystemic, and chronic autoimmune exocrinopathy that predominantly involves lacrimal, salivary, and other exocrine glands.

Etiology Genetic factors, viral infection, and autoimmunity may be involved in the pathogenesis.

Classification Two forms are recognized: (a) *primary* (sicca syndrome) with mainly oral and eye disorders; and (b) *secondary*, if it coexists with other autoimmune diseases, usually rheumatoid arthritis.

Gingival Involvement Rare. Dental biofilm-induced gingival lesions modified by systemic factors.

Other Sites of Involvement Salivary glands, lacrimal glands, and other exocrine glands. Several organs and systems.

Clinical Features

- Chronic gingivitis, localized or generalized, due to xerostomia and/or Candida infection may occur (Fig. 35.5). Rarely, increased alveolar bone loss may also be seen.
- Xerostomia is the hallmark of the disease. The oral mucosa is reddish, dry, smooth, and shiny (Fig. 35.6). Oral soreness, discomfort, and dysphagia are common symptoms. Candidiasis, angular cheilitis, and dental caries are relatively common. Recurrent swelling of parotid and other major salivary glands may occur.
- The ocular manifestations are characterized by dryness of the eyes, keratoconjunctivitis sicca, and more severe lesions as the disease progresses (Fig. 35.7). *Schirmer* test and *Rose Bengal* dye test should be performed by an ophthalmologist.
- Vaginal dryness may occur.
- In the secondary form of the disease, clinical manifestations depend on the associated autoimmune diseases.
- There is an increased risk of B cell non-Hodgkin lymphoma development.
- Clinical diagnosis should be confirmed by laboratory tests.

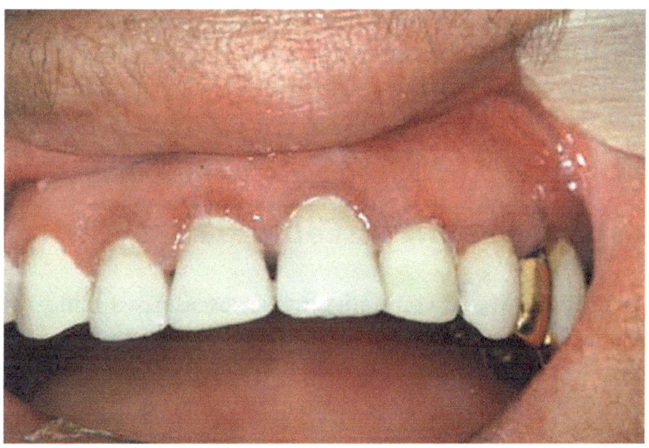

Fig. 35.5 Sjögren syndrome, generalized gingivitis

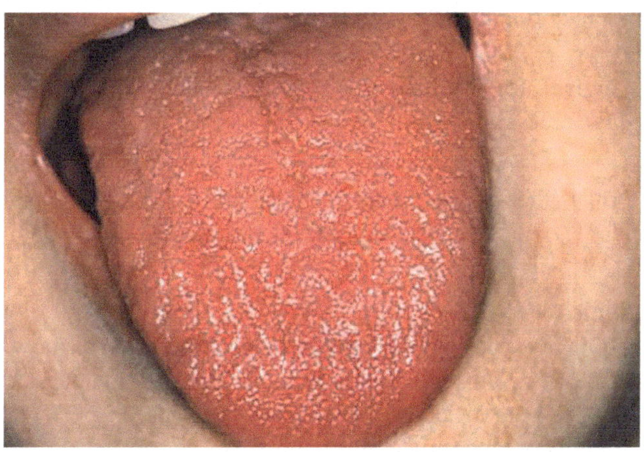

Fig. 35.6 Sjögren syndrome, dry, reddish and shiny dorsum of the tongue

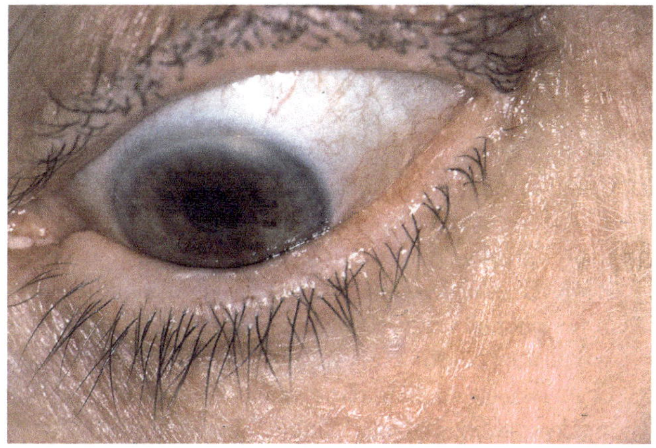

Fig. 35.7 Sjögren syndrome, keratoconjunctivitis sicca

Differential Diagnosis

- Graft-Versus-Host Disease.
- Amyloidosis.
- Sialosis.
- Xerostomia due to drugs and radiation.
- Mikulicz syndrome.
- Heerfordt syndrome.
- Systemic sclerosis.
- Mixed connective tissue disease.

Laboratory Tests Histopathologic examination of the minor salivary glands. Serological tests: antinuclear antibodies (ANA), anti-SSA/Ro and anti-SSB/La antibodies, rheumatoid factor (RF).

Treatment Good dental biofilm control. Saliva and tear substitutes. Systemic pilocarpine hydrochloride or systemic cevimeline hydrochloride. Antimalarial drugs, corticosteroids, and immunosuppressants, that should be left to specialists.

Systemic Sclerosis

Definition Systemic sclerosis is a chronic, multisystemic autoimmune connective tissue disorder that causes inflammation with a broad spectrum of manifestations.

Etiology An autoimmune pathogenesis may be involved. *In vitro* studies suggest that the products of the autoimmune reaction may influence the behavior of fibroblasts and endothelial cells leading to the overproduction of connective tissue by fibroblasts.

Gingival Involvement Rare. Non-dental biofilm-induced gingival lesions.

Other Sites of Involvement Oral mucosa (relatively common), skin (always), viscera (esophagus, intestinal tract, kidney, lungs, heart, skeletal muscles).

Clinical Features

- Gingival lesions are minor and are characterized by pallor of free and attached gingiva, gingival regression, and very rarely greater evidence of periodontitis (Fig. 35.8). However, other studies revealed no significant differences in periodontal status between systemic sclerosis patients and healthy controls.
- Oral lesions include:xerostomia, thin and pale oral mucosa, short and hard lingual frenulum, atrophy of tongue papillae, microglossia, microstomia, limited mouth opening, perioral radial folds (Fig. 35.9). Difficulty in swallowing and dysphagia are also common.
- Dental radiographs show a diffuse widening of the periodontal ligament space, approximately in 10–20% of patients.
- Skin lesions are characterized initially by edema but, as the disease progresses, the skin becomes thin, hard, inelastic, and pale. Facial skin involvement results in the characteristic *mask-like facies*. Skin ulcers, telangiectasias, and Raynaud phenomenon are also common. CREST syndrome (Calcinosis cutis, Raynaud phenomenon, Esophageal dysmotility, Sclerodactyly, Telangiectasia) is a clinical limited variant of systemic sclerosis.
- Visceral involvement usually leads to organ failure.
- Clinical diagnosis should be confirmed by laboratory tests.

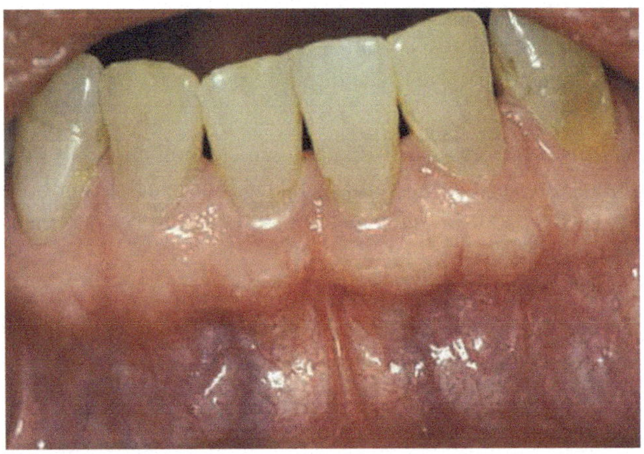

Fig. 35.8 Systemic sclerosis, pallor and thin gingiva

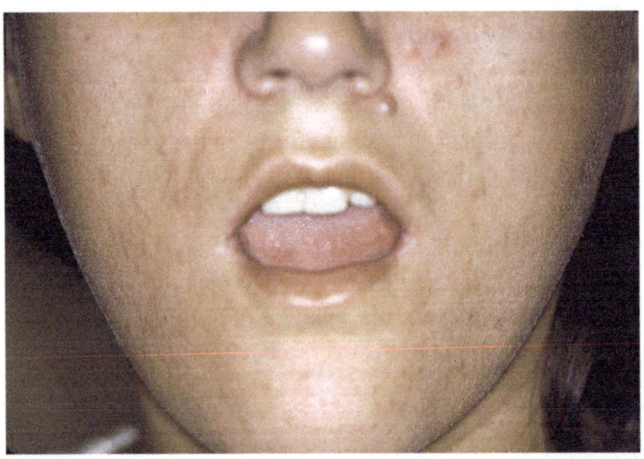

Fig. 35.9 Systemic sclerosis, mouth opening stenosis

Differential Diagnosis

- Oral submucous fibrosis.
- Graft-Versus-Host Disease.
- Mixed connective tissue disease.
- Epidermolysis bullosa.
- Lipoid proteinosis.
- Mucous membrane pemphigoid.

Laboratory Tests Histopathologic and immunological examinations.

Treatment Good oral hygiene. Systemic treatment includes antimalarials, corticosteroids, immunosuppressive drugs, D-penicillamine, colchicine, and monoclonal antibodies, that should be left to specialists.

Mixed Connective Tissue Disease

Definition Mixed connective tissue disease is a multisystemic disorder characterized by the simultaneous clinical manifestations mainly seen in lupus erythematosus, systemic sclerosis,polymyositis, and rheumatoid arthritis.

Etiology The cause and pathogenesis remain obscure. Autoimmune response to nuclear U1RNP antigen plays an essential role in pathogenesis.

Gingival Involvement Rare. Non-dental biofilm-induced gingival lesions.

Other Sites of Involvement Oral mucosa, skin, skeletal muscles, lymph nodes, and several other organs.

Clinical Features

- Gingival lesions may appear as localized or diffuse erythema and/or nonspecific irregular erosions identical to those seen in lupus erythematosus patients (Fig. 35.10). Periodontal destruction is impossible.
- Oral lesions are characterized by nonspecific erythema, edema, erosions, and xerostomia (Fig. 35.11).

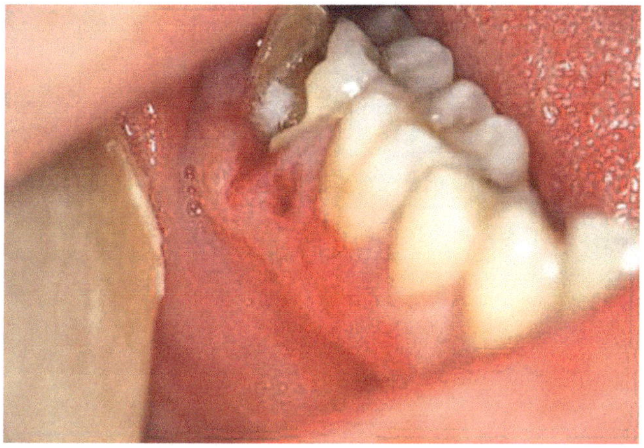

Fig. 35.10 Mixed connective tissue disease, irregular erosions on the gingiva

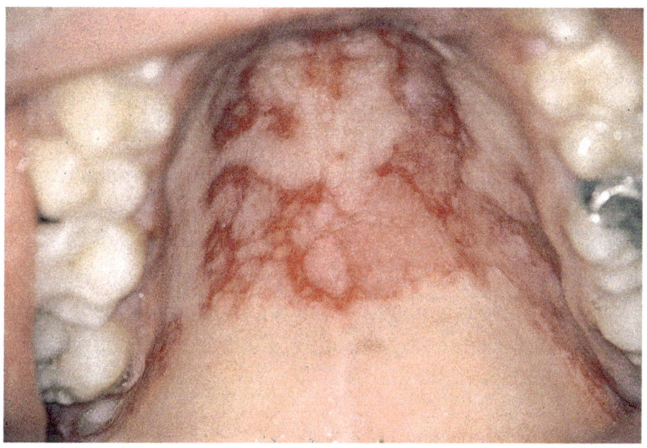

Fig. 35.11 Mixed connective tissue disease, erythema and erosions on the palate

- Skin and other manifestations are those seen in systemic lupus erythematosus, systemic scleroderma, and polymyositis (Fig. 35.12).
- Clinical diagnosis should be confirmed by laboratory tests.

Differential Diagnosis
- Systemic lupus erythematosus.
- Systemic sclerosis.
- Polymyositis.
- Dermatomyositis.
- Other connective tissue diseases.

Laboratory Tests High titers of anti-ribonucleoprotein antibodies (anti-RNP) is the most diagnostic laboratory finding. Other serological tests specific for the group of diseases included. Histopathologic examination.

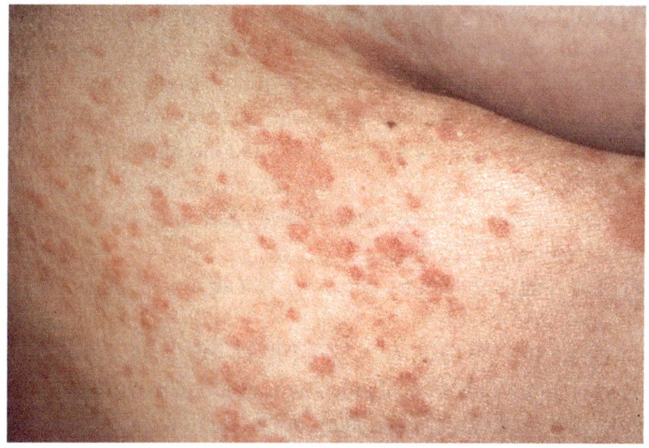

Fig. 35.12 Mixed connective tissue disease, skin pruritic rash on the skin

Treatment Good oral hygiene, topical corticosteroids. Systemic treatment includes corticosteroids, immunosuppressive drugs, and antimalarials, and should be left to specialists.

Dermatomyositis

Definition Dermatomyositis is an autoimmune connective tissue inflammatory disorder, characterized by symmetric extensor inflammatory myopathies and skin eruptions.

Etiology Autoimmune. Autoantigens activate a humoral immune reaction with complement deposition in capillaries causing inflammation, necrosis, and ischemia, in association with genetic and other factors such as infections, drugs, and malignancies.

Gingival Involvement Rare. Non-dental biofilm-induced gingivitis.

Other Sites of Involvement Oral mucosa (relatively rare), skin, and muscles (common).

Classification The disease is classified into two main forms, based on the age of onset: *juvenile* and *adult.*

Clinical Features
- The disease most commonly affects females than males, ratio 2:1, usually over 40 years of age and less commonly children and adolescents.
- Clinically, progressive symmetrical muscle weakness is the first and most important manifestation in the majority of cases, usually associated by myalgia, malaise, and fever.

- Poikiloderma (hyperpigmentation, hypopigmentation, telangiectasias, and epidermal atrophy) is the important clinical sign of cutaneous eruption characterized by a pink-violet color and classical distribution around the eyes *heliotrope sign* (Fig. 35.13) and the nail fold changes (*telangiectasias*), *Gottron's papules and signs*. The chest, neck, upper back, elbows, knees, and knuckles are also commonly affected (Fig. 35.14).
- The gingival lesions appear as localized or generalized not specific deep erythema, edema, and ulcerations (Fig. 35.15). Erythema, painful edema, and ulcers may develop on the buccal mucosa, tongue, palate, and uvula.
- Adult dermatomyositis may be associated, in 30% of the cases, with internal malignancy (colon, ovarian, breast, lung, pancreatic, female genital tract carcinomas, and non-Hodgkin lymphoma) and other systemic diseases (autoimmune arthritis, pulmonary, renal, cardiac, and other).
- The diagnosis of dermatomyositis is based on clinical and laboratory criteria.

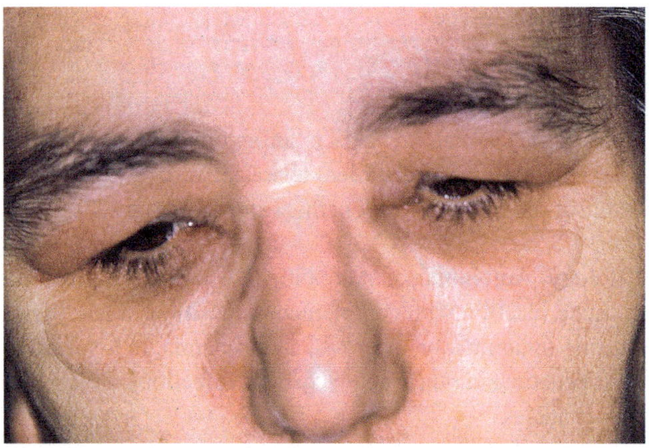

Fig. 35.13 Dermatomyositis, violet lesions around the eyes and the skin of the face

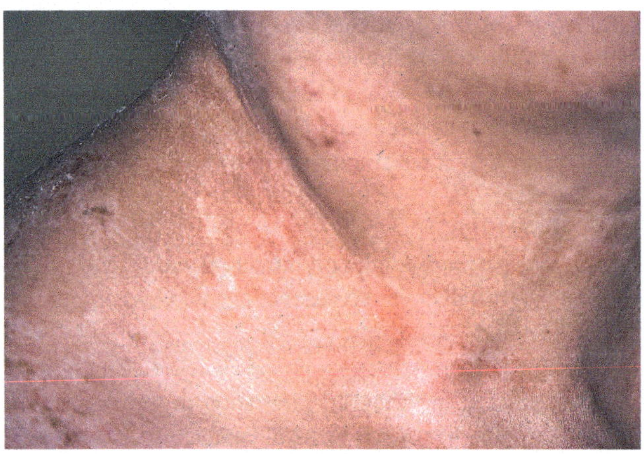

Fig. 35.14 Dermatomyositis, neck cutaneous lesions, hypopigmentation, atrophy and teleangiectasias

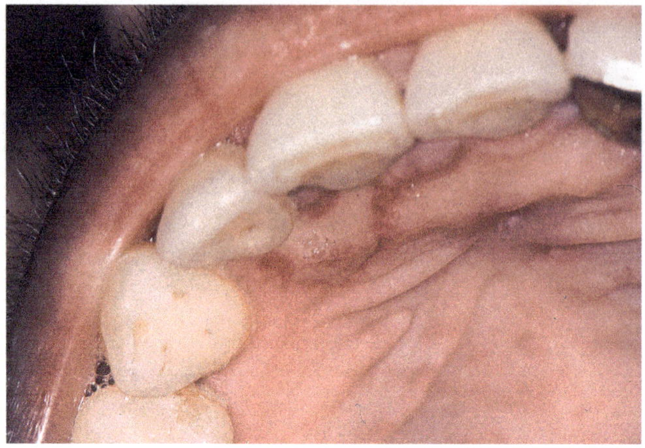

Fig. 35.15 Dermatomyositis, edematous ulcerations on the palatal gingiva

Differential Diagnosis
- Sarcoidosis.
- Scleroderma.
- Systemic lupus erythematosus.
- Psoriasis.
- Various oral diseases associated with erythema and non-specific ulcerations.

Laboratory Tests Histopathologic examination of oral, skin, and muscle lesions. Serum muscle enzyme determination, serum immunologic testing. Pulmonary function tests, CT, MRI, electromyography.

Treatment High level of oral hygiene and symptomatic treatment of gingivitis. First line of systemic treatment is corticosteroids usually in association with other immunosuppressives (azathioprine, cyclophosphamide, mycophenolate mofetil, methotrexate, tacrolimus, rituximab, infliximab, and others), but it must be handled by the Specialists.

Graft-Versus-Host Disease

Definition Graft-Versus-Host Disease (GVHD) is a complex multisystemic disorder due to immune reaction between the transplanted T lymphocytes and the patient's normal tissues.

Etiology Autoimmune**.** The disease occurs in recipients of allogeneic bone marrow transplants that are used to treat life-threatening diseases of the blood or bone marrow.

Classification Two forms of the disorder are recognized: (a) *acute*, which is typically observed within 100 days of transplantation; and (b) *chronic*, which develops more than 100 days after transplantation.

Gingival Involvement Rare. Non-dental biofilm-induced gingival lesions.

Other Sites of Involvement Oral mucosa (40–80%), skin, gastrointestinal tract, liver, lungs, eyes.

Clinical Features

- Gingival lesions are not specific and are characterized by diffuse or localized erythema usually associated with a fine, reticular network of white striae and/or erosions similar to those seen in lichen planus (Fig. 35.16). The condition occasionally mimics *desquamative gingivitis*.
- Oral lesions appear as diffuse erythema, lichenoid pattern, and painful ulcerations (Figs. 35.17 and 35.18). Atrophy of the oral mucosa, a burning sensation, and xerostomia are common. Oral and gingival lesions are more common in the chronic form of the disorder.

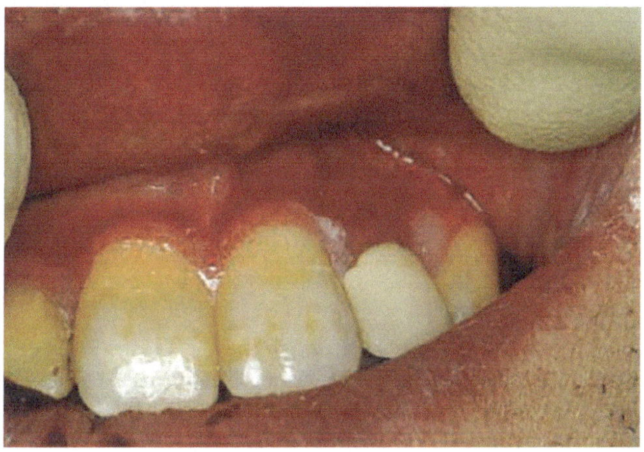

Fig. 35.16 Graft-versus-host disease, diffuse erythema on the gingiva and small erosion

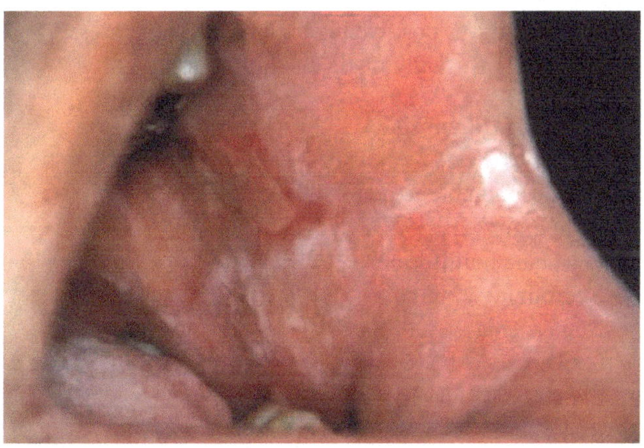

Fig. 35.17 Graft-versus-host disease, lichenoid lesions on the buccal mucosa

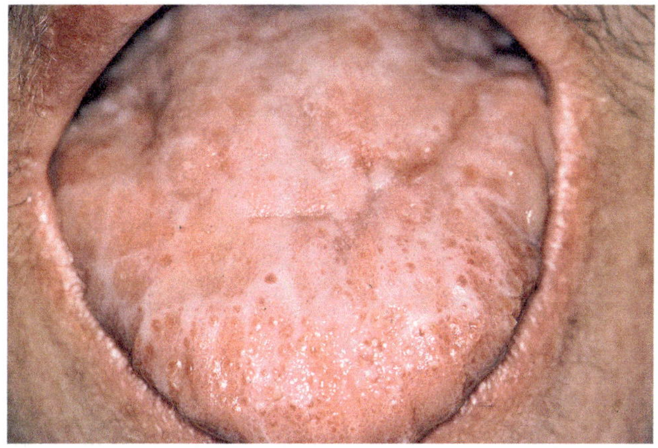

Fig. 35.18 Graft-versus-host disease, erythema, and erosions with lichenoid appearance

- Skin lesions range from mild rash with hyperpigmentation to lesions that may resemble systemic sclerosis and lichen planus.
- Other signs and symptoms are nausea, vomiting, abdominal pain, diarrhea, and liver dysfunction.
- Diagnosis is usually based on clinical criteria and less on laboratory tests.

Differential Diagnosis

- Lichen planus.
- Lupus erythematosus.
- Systemic sclerosis.
- Sjögren syndrome.
- Dermatomyositis.
- Drug reactions.
- Leukemia.

Laboratory Tests Histopathologic examination. Increased salivary sodium concentration.

Treatment Good dental biofilm control, topical corticosteroids. Systemic corticosteroids, immunosuppressive drugs, thalidomide, should be left to the specialists.

Adamandiades-Behçet Disease

Definition Adamandiades–Behçet disease is a chronic multisystemic and polysymptomatic inflammatory disorder that affects more commonly certain ethnic groups (Japanese, Turkish, Greek, and other Mediterranean origins).

Etiology The exact etiology remains obscure. Autoinflammatory disorder. Genetic, immunological factors, and viral infection may be involved in the pathogenesis of the disease.

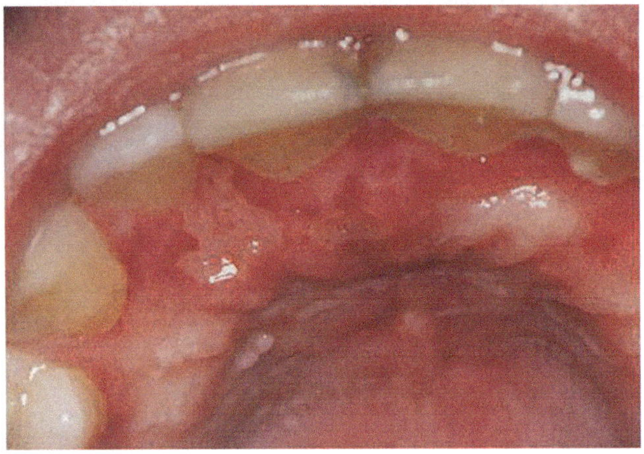

Fig. 35.19 Adamandiades-Behçet disease, aphthous ulcers on the maxillary gingiva

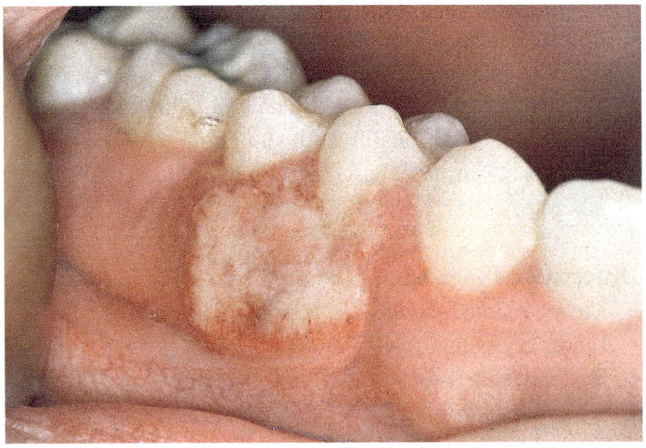

Fig. 35.20 Adamandiades-Behçet disease, major aphthous ulcer on the mandibular gingiva

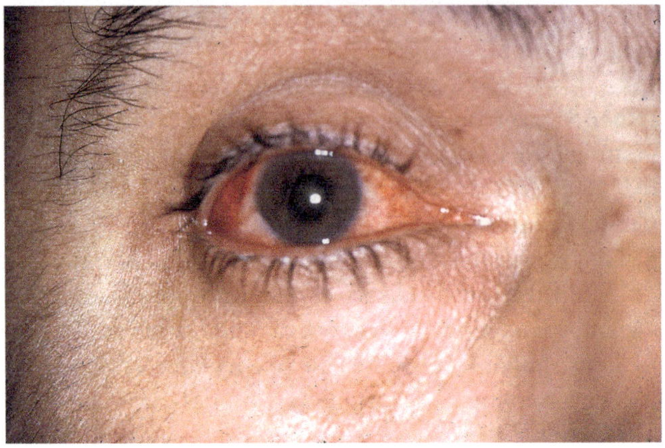

Fig. 35.21 Adamandiades-Behçet disease, conjunctivitis and iridocyclitis

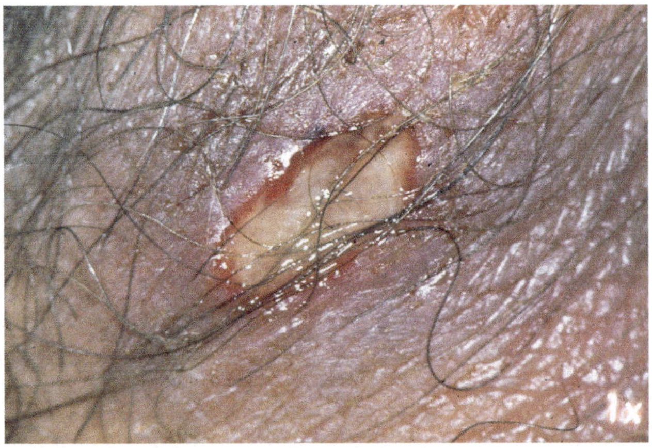

Fig. 35.22 Adamandiades-Behçet disease, skin ulceration aphthous - like on the scotrum

Gingival Involvement Rare. Non-dental biofilm-induced gingival lesions.

Other Sites of Involvement Oral mucosa (very common), other mucosae (eyes, genitalia, intestinal), skin, joints, cardiovascular systems, lungs, and central nervous system.

Clinical Features

- The main oral manifestations of Adamandiades-Behçetdise use are recurrent aphthous ulcerations (minor, major, herpetiform, or atypical).
- Painful aphthous ulcers, usually minor or atypical, may rarely develop on the attached gingiva (Figs. 35.19 and 35.20).
- Conjunctivitis, iritis, iridocyclitis with hypopyon, and uveitis are the most frequent eye manifestations (Fig. 35.21).
- Skin lesions present as genital round ulcerations on the scrotum, penis, or vulva (Fig. 35.22). Folliculitis, papules, pustules, nodular erythema, and less often necrotic lesions are common cutaneous lesions.
- Vascular, intestinal, joint, and neurological involvement may occur.
- Pathergy test is positive in about 60–70% of cases.
- Diagnosis is usually made on clinical criteria.

Differential Diagnosis

- Aphthous ulcers.
- Mucous membrane pemphigoid.
- Pemphigus.
- Erythema multiforme.
- Necrotizing gingivitis.
- Neutropenia.
- Leukemia.
- Langerhans cell histiocytosis.
- Reiter disease.

Laboratory Tests Histopathologic examinations and serologic tests may be supportive.

Treatment Corticosteroids topically. Systemic corticosteroids, immunosuppressive drugs, thalidomide, and colchicines are the drugs of choice and should be left to specialists.

PFAPA Syndrome

Definition PFAPA (periodic fever, aphthous stomatitis, pharyngitis, and cervical adenitis) syndrome is a rare recurrent disorder that mainly affects children and rarely adolescents or adults.

Etiology Unknown. An autoinflammatory mechanism is possible, reflecting excess release of interleukin 1β production.

Gingival Involvement Very rare.

Other Sites of Involvement Soft palate, uvula, pharynx, cervical lymph nodes.

Clinical Features

- The classical clinical frame of the disease includes (a) periodic fever (38–39 °C) lasting 4–6 days; (b) aphthous-like ulcerations of the oral mucosa; (c) pharyngitis and tonsillitis; and (d) cervical bilateral lymphadenitis. Headache, abdominal pain, and arthralgia may occur.
- Clinically, oral lesions present as painful, large, atypical aphthous-like ulcerations mainly on the ovula, tonsils, and soft palate, which may uncommonly involve the palatal gingival tissue as well (Fig. 35.23). The disease usually recurs every 4–8 weeks for 1–2 years and then resolves spontaneously.
- Diagnosis is mainly based on medical history and clinical features.

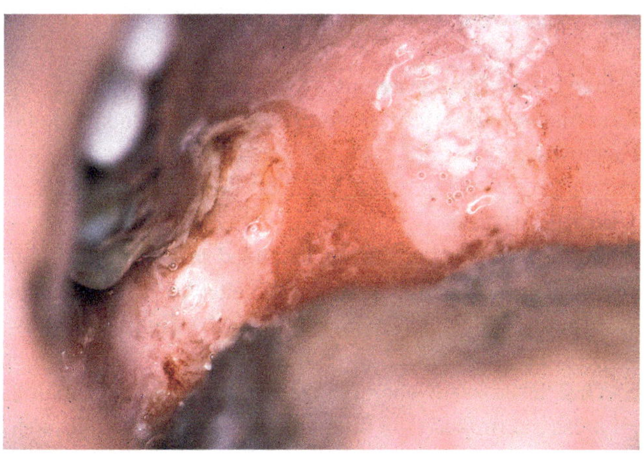

Fig. 35.23 PFAPA syndrome, major aphthous ulcers on the gingiva and the palate

Differential Diagnosis

- Aphthous ulcers.
- Adamandiades-Behçetdisease.
- Hand-foot and mouth disease.
- Mediterranean fever.
- Congenital neutropenia.
- Cyclic neutropenia.
- Leukemia.

Laboratory Tests There are not any specific tests.

Treatment First-line treatment is cimetidine that has immunomodulatory effects for week and second-line treatment is systemic prednisolone in low doses 15–20 mg/day for 7–10 days.

Wegener Granulomatosis

Definition Wegener granulomatosis or granulomatosis with polyangiitis is a relatively rare necrotizing granulomatous vasculitis of the upper and lower respiratory system that may affect almost all organ systems.

Etiology The exact etiology is unknown. However, genetic and environmental factors may be involved in the pathogenesis. A cell-mediated immune response to a microbial agent or an abnormal immune reaction to an unknown antigen may be the cause.

Classification The disease is classified into two forms: (a) *Generalized;* and (b) *Localized.*

Gingival Involvement Relatively rare, non-dental biofilm-related gingivitis.

Other Sites of Involvement Oral mucosa and skin (30–40%). Upper and lower respiratory tract(>90%), nasal, tracheal, sinus, ear, and renal (>60–70%). Rarely, ocular, cardiac, gastrointestinal, and musculoskeletal systems.

Clinical Features

- The hallmark clinical features include granulomatous inflammation of the upper and/or lower respiratory tract with necrotizing vasculitis, necrotizing glomerulonephritis, palpable skin purpura and necrotic skin, and oral lesions.
- A characteristic feature is the gingival manifestation of the disease that presents either as red papillary granulomatous hyperplasia with multiple hemorrhagic and friable projections *(strawberry gingiva)* or as irregular ulcerations (Figs. 35.24 and 35.25).

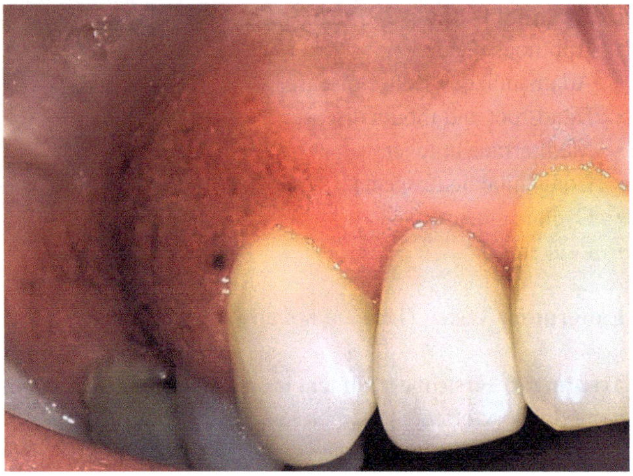

Fig. 35.24 Wegener granulomatosis, localized "strawberry—like gingivitis" on the maxillary gingiva

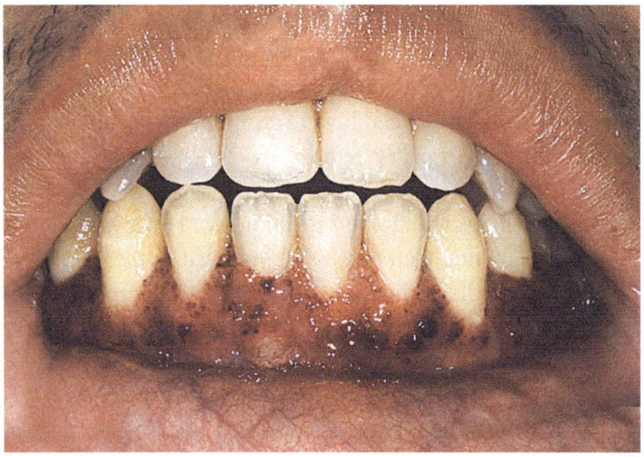

Fig. 35.25 Wegener granulomatosis, generalized "strawberry—like gingivitis" on the mandibular gingiva

- Oral lesions present as solitary or multiple inflammatory ulcers on the tongue, buccal mucosa, and palate (Fig. 35.26).
- Other affected organs may present several signs and symptoms.
- Clinical diagnosis should be confirmed by laboratory tests.

Differential Diagnosis

- Non-Hodgkin lymphoma.
- Nasal natural killer (NK)-T cell lymphoma.
- Systemic mycoses.
- Necrotizing sialadeno metaplasia.
- Chung-Strauss syndrome.
- other ANCA-associated vasculities.

Laboratory Tests

Histopathologic examination, ESR and C-reactive protein, C-ANCA with anti-PR3 specificity (positive 80–90% in generalized form), chest CT scan.

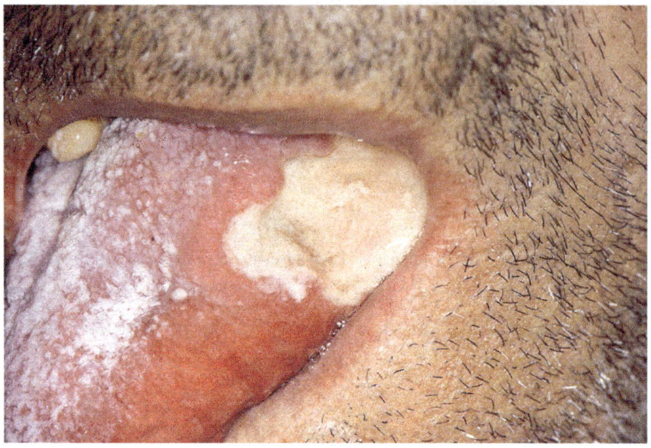

Fig. 35.26 Wegener granulomatosis, inflammatory ulcer on the tongue

Treatment

Systemic prednisolone in conjunction with cyclophosphamide is the treatment of choice. Alternatively, prednisolone with rituximab or with azathioprine may be effective and should be left to specialists.

Reiter Disease

Definition

Reiter disease or reactive arthritis is an uncommon multisystemic disorder that may be triggered by an infectious agent in a genetically susceptible individual.

Etiology

Autoinflammatory. The exact etiology remains unknown, although the pathogenesis is mediated by an immunological mechanism.

Gingival Involvement

Rare. Non-dental biofilm-induced gingival lesions.

Other Sites of Involvement

Oral mucosa (20–40%), genitals, eyes, skin, joints, skeletal, cardiovascular system.

Clinical Features

- Gingival lesions appear as localized or generalized nonspecific erythema, usually on the attached gingiva, occasionally associated with superficial, slightly sensitive erosions (Figs. 35.27 and 35.28).
- Oral lesions are characterized by diffuse erythematous areas intermixed with thin whitish dots or lines and superficial erosions. Localized loss of the tongue filiform papillae in the form of geographic tongue may occur (Fig. 35.29).
- Skin manifestations appear as macular, vesicular or pustular, psoriasiform lesions, and keratoderma (Fig. 35.30).

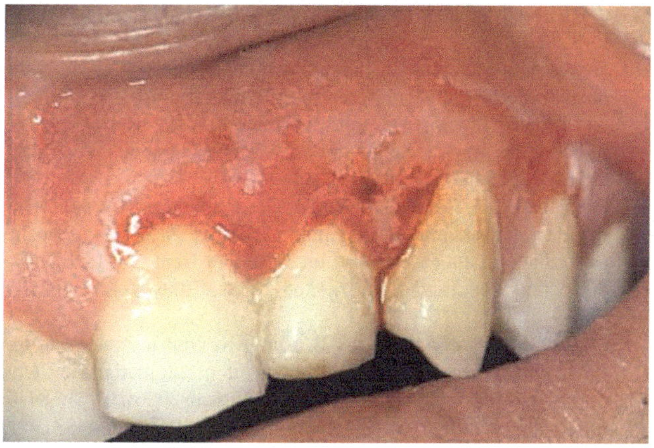

Fig. 35.27 Reiter disease, diffuse deep erythema and erosions on the upper gingiva

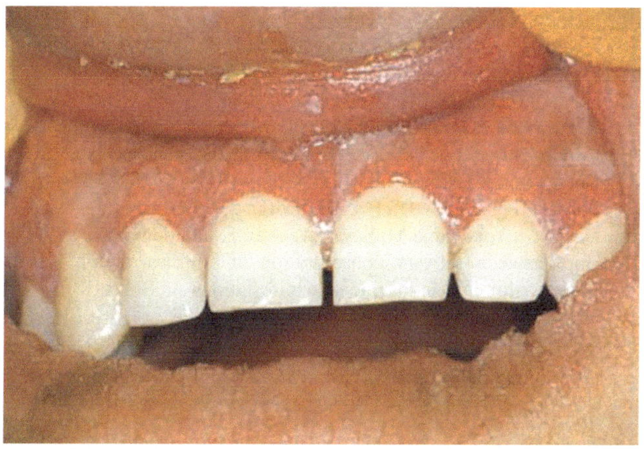

Fig. 35.28 Reiter disease, erythema and edema on the upper gingiva

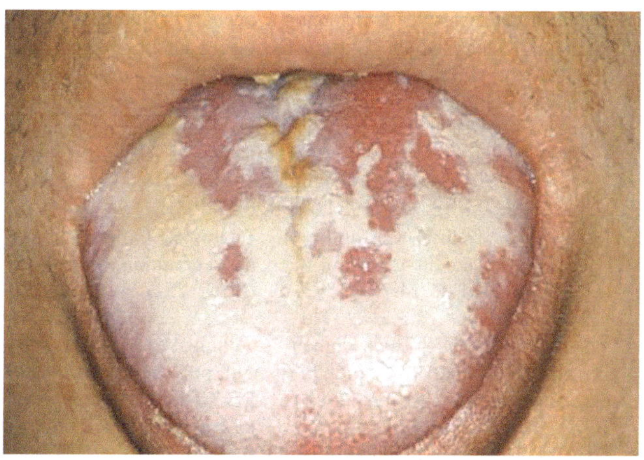

Fig. 35.29 Reiter disease, localized loss of the filiform papillae on the dorsum of the tongue

- Other manifestations include conjunctivitis, cyclic balanitis, non-gonococcal urethritis, prostatitis, cervicitis, and nail disturbances.

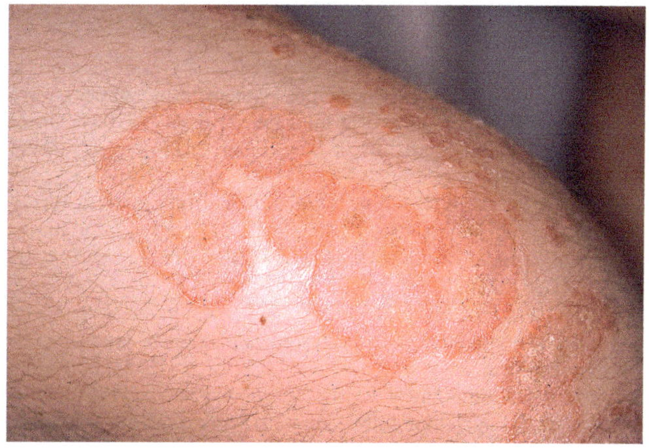

Fig. 35.30 Reiter disease, psoriasiform lesions on the skin

- The most characteristic feature of the disease is "symmetric" arthritis affecting the same joints on both sides of the body.
- Clinical diagnosis should be confirmed by laboratory tests.

Differential Diagnosis
- Adamandiades-Behçetdisease.
- Erythema multiforme.
- Geographic stomatitis.
- Psoriasis.
- Sneddon-Wilkinson disease.
- Drugeruption.

Laboratory Tests
Histopathologic examination. Blood and serological tests, HLA antigens, synovial fluid analysis.

Treatment
Nonsteroidal anti-inflammatory drugs, salicylates, and systemic corticosteroids, that should be left to specialists.

References

1. Pessoa L, Aleti G, Choudhury S, et al. Host-microbial Interactions in systemic lupus erythematosus and periodontitis. Front Immunol. 2019;10:2602. https://doi.org/10.3389/fimmu.2019.02602. PMID: 31781106; PMCID: PMC6861327
2. Menzies S, O'Shea F, Galvin S, Wynne B. Oral manifestations of lupus erythematosus. Ir J Med Sci. 2018;187(1):91–3. https://doi.org/10.1007/s11845-017-1622-z. Epub 2017 May 3. PMID: 28470356
3. Saccucci M, Di Carlo G, Bossù M, et al. Autoimmune diseases and their manifestations on oral cavity: diagnosis and clinical management. J Immunol Res. 2018;2018:6061825. https://doi.org/10.1155/2018/6061825. PMID: 29977929; PMCID: PMC5994274
4. Benli M, Batool F, Stutz C, et al. Orofacial manifestations and dental management of systemic lupus erythematosus: a review. Oral

Dis. 2021;27(2):151–67. https://doi.org/10.1111/odi.13271. Epub 2020 Mar 3. PMID: 31886584

5. Calderaro DC, Ferreira GA, de Mendonça SM, et al. Is there an association between systemic lupus erythematosus and periodontal disease? Rev Bras Reumatol Engl Ed. 2016;56(3):280–4. https://doi.org/10.1016/j.rbre.2015.08.003. Epub 2015 Sep 8. PMID: 27267648
6. Kranti K, Seshan H, Juliet J. Discoid lupus erythematosus involving gingiva. J Indian Soc Periodontol. 2012;16(1):126–8. https://doi.org/10.4103/0972-124X.94621. PMID: 22628979; PMCID: PMC3357022
7. Crincoli V, Di Comite M, Guerrieri M, et al. Orofacial manifestations and temporomandibular disorders of Sjögren syndrome: An observational study. Int J Med Sci. 2018;15(5):475–83. https://doi.org/10.7150/ijms.23044. PMID: 29559836; PMCID: PMC5859770
8. Serrano J, Lopez-Pintor RM, Gonzalez-Serrano J, et al. Oral lesions in Sjogren's syndrome: a systematic review. Med Oral Patol Oral Cir Bucal. 2018;23(4):e391–400. https://doi.org/10.4317/medoral.22286. PMID: 29924754; PMCID: PMC6051685
9. Savioli C, Ribeiro AC, Fabri GM, et al. Persistent periodontal disease hampers anti-tumor necrosis factor treatment response in rheumatoid arthritis. J Clin Rheumatol. 2012;18(4):180–4. https://doi.org/10.1097/RHU.0b013e31825828be. PMID: 22647860
10. Kaushal S, Singh AK, Lal N, et al. Effect of periodontal therapy on disease activity in patients of rheumatoid arthritis with chronic periodontitis. J Oral Biol Craniofac Res. 2019;9(2):128–32. https://doi.org/10.1016/j.jobcr.2019.02.002. Epub 2019 Feb 2. PMID: 30834192; PMCID: PMC6384305
11. Aliko A, Alushi A, Tafaj A, Lela F. Oral mucosa involvement in rheumatoid arthritis, systemic lupus erythematosus and systemic sclerosis. Int Dent J. 2010;60:353–8.
12. Smirani R, Truchetet ME, Poursac N, et al. Impact of systemic sclerosis oral manifestations on patients' health-related quality of life: a systematic review. J Oral Pathol Med. 2018;47(9):808–15. https://doi.org/10.1111/jop.12739. Epub 2018 Jul 5. PMID: 29855076
13. Selifanova EI, Makeeva MK, Turkina AY, Esayan MS. Stomatologicheskiĭ status patsientov s sistemnoĭ sklerodermieĭ [Oral health in patients with systemic sclerosis]. Stomatologiia (Mosk). 2019;98(3):104–8. https://doi.org/10.17116/stomat201998031104. PMID: 31322605
14. Alhendi FJ, Werth VP, Sollecito TP, Stoopler ET. Systemic sclerosis: update for oral health care providers. Spec Care Dentist. 2020;40(5):418–30. https://doi.org/10.1111/scd.12492. Epub 2020 Jul 6. PMID: 33448431
15. Marton K, Hermann P, Danko K, et al. Evaluation of oral manifestations and masticatory force in patients with polymyositis and dermatomyositis. J Oral Pathol Med. 2005;34:164–9.
16. Porter S, Scully C. Connective tissue disorders and the mouth. Dent Update. 2008;35:294–6.
17. Gonzales TS, Coleman GC. Periodontal manifestations of collagen vascular disorders. Periodontol 2000;1999(21):94 105. https://doi.org/10.1111/j.1600-0757.1999.tb00170.x. PMID: 10551177
18. Shikino K, Hanazawa N, Noda K, Ikusaka M. Gingival telangiectases due to dermatomyositis. J Gen Fam Med. 2020;22(1):49–50. https://doi.org/10.1002/jgf2.365. PMID: 33457157; PMCID: PMC7796783
19. Bernet LL, Lewis MA, Rieger KE, et al. Ovoid palatal patch in dermatomyositis: a novel finding associated with anti-TIF1γ (p155) antibodies. JAMA Dermatol. 2016;152(9):1049–51. https://doi.org/10.1001/jamadermatol.2016.1429. PMID: 27224238; PMCID: PMC5224833
20. Hattori Y, Matsuyama K, Takahashi T, et al. Anti-MDA5 antibody-positive dermatomyositis presenting with cellulitis-like erythema on the mandible as an initial symptom. Case Rep Dermatol. 2018;10(2):110–4. https://doi.org/10.1159/000488077. PMID: 29867431; PMCID: PMC5981633
21. Gonçalves LM, Bezerra-Júnior JR, Gordón-Núñez MA, et al. Oral manifestations as important symptoms for juvenile dermatomyositis early diagnosis: a case report. Int J Paediatr Dent. 2011;21(1):77–80. https://doi.org/10.1111/j.1365-263X.2010.01074.x. PMID: 20659183
22. Healy CM, Tobin AM, Kirby B, Flint SR. Oral lesions as an initial manifestation of dermatomyositis with occult malignancy. Oral Surg Oral Med Oral Pathol Oral Radiol Endod. 2006;101(2):184–7. https://doi.org/10.1016/j.tripleo.2005.08.030. PMID: 16448919
23. Haverman TM, Raber-Durlacher JE, Raghoebar II, et al. Oral chronic graft-versus-host disease: what the general dental practitioner needs to know. J Am Dent Assoc. 2020;151(11):846–56. https://doi.org/10.1016/j.adaj.2020.08.001. PMID: 33121606
24. Elad S, Aljitawi O, Zadik Y. Oral graft-versus-host disease: a pictorial review and a guide for dental practitioners. Int Dent J. 2020;71(1):9–20. https://doi.org/10.1111/idj.12584. Epub ahead of print. PMID: 32594516
25. Cantarini L, Vitale A, Bersani G, et al. PFAPA syndrome and Behçet's disease: a comparison of two medical entities based on the clinical interviews performed by three different specialists. Clin Rheumatol. 2016;35(2):501–5. https://doi.org/10.1007/s10067-015-2890-5. Epub 2015 Feb 10. PMID: 25665824
26. Doino M, Yokoyama M, Sasaki Y, et al. Evaluation of the relationship between salivary concentration of anti-heat shock protein immunoglobulin and clinical manifestations of Behçet's disease. Scand J Rheumatol. 2017;46(5):381–7. https://doi.org/10.1080/03009742.2016.1249942. Epub 2017 Feb 14. PMID: 28276957
27. Stratigos AJ, Laskaris G, Stratigos JD. Behçet's disease. Semin Neurol. 1992;12(4):346–57. https://doi.org/10.1055/s--2008-1041191. PMID: 1485044
28. Stoopler ET, Mirfarsi S, Alawi F, Sollecito TP. Recalcitrant gingival lesions in a patient previously iagnosed with Behçet's disease. Compend Contin Educ Dent. 2019;40(1):46–8. PMID: 30601021
29. Apoita-Sanz M, Blanco-Jauset P, Polis-Yanes C, et al. Granulomatosis with poliangeitis (Wegener's Granulomatosis): orofacial manifestations. Systematic review and case report. Oral Health Prev Dent. 2020;18(1):929–43. https://doi.org/10.3290/j.ohpd.a45433. PMID: 33215484
30. Fonseca FP, Benites BM, Ferrari A, et al. Gingival granulomatosis with polyangiitis (Wegener's granulomatosis) as a primary manifestation of the disease. Aust Dent J. 2017;62(1):102–6. https://doi.org/10.1111/adj.12441. Epub 2016 Dec 23. PMID: 27439744
31. Aravena V, Beltrán V, Cantín M, Fuentes R. Gingival hyperplasia being the first sign of Wegener's granulomatosis. Int J Clin Exp Med. 2014;7(8):2373–6. PMID: 25232440; PMCID: PMC4161600
32. Hanisch M, Fröhlich LF, Kleinheinz J. Gingival hyperplasia as first sign of recurrence of granulomatosis with polyangiitis (Wegener's granulomatosis): case report and review of the literature. BMC Oral Health. 2016;17(1):33. https://doi.org/10.1186/s12903-016-0262-4. PMID: 27485511; PMCID: PMC4969735

Orofacial Granulomatosis

36

Contents

Introduction

"*Orofacial granulomatosis*" is a general term proposed in 1985 by Wiesenfeld et al. to describe a group of noninfectious and non-necrotizing granulomatous disorders affecting the mouth, lips, and face. Local disorders, such as cheilitis granulomatosa, granulomatous gingivitis, and systemic diseases together with orofacial manifestations, such as Melkersson-Rosenthal syndrome, Crohn's disease, and sarcoidosis, belong to the group.

The precise etiology remains unclear. However, the prevailing view is that chronic antigenic stimulation, resulting in a cell-mediated hypersensitivity to foodstuffs, flavoring agents, products of dental hygiene, foreign materials, and others, is responsible. The most common systemic disorders which are classified in the orofacial granulomatosis group will be described in the following pages.

Melkersson-Rosenthal Syndrome

Definition Melkersson-Rosenthal syndrome is a clinical variant of orofacial granulomatosis. It consists of a triad of *(a) recurrent facial and lip swelling; (b) facial nerve paralysis; and (c) fissured tongue.*

Etiology Unknown.

Gingival Involvement Rare. Non-dental biofilm-induced gingival lesions.

Other Sites of Involvement Oral mucosa, lips, facial.

Clinical Features

- The disease affects both sexes equally and usually young individuals.
- Gingival lesions present as irregular, edematous swelling, slightly erythematous, affecting mainly the anterior interdental papillae as well as the free and attached gingiva (Figs. 36.1, 36.2, and 36.3).
- Granulomatous cheilitis, which presents as a diffuse recurrent swelling of the lips, is the cardinal feature of the syndrome. It is usually the first sign (Fig. 36.4). After a long period of attacks, the swelling persists and may become permanent. Buccal, palatal, and lingual swelling may also occur.
- Fissured tongue is present in about 50% of patients.
- Facial nerve palsy is present in 20–30% of cases and is frequently associated with facial edema. It may be the first sign and is usually unilateral.
- Diagnosis is based on clinical and laboratory criteria.

Differential Diagnosis

- Angioedema.
- Cheilitis glandularis.

G. Laskaris et al., *Periodontal Manifestations of Local and Systemic Diseases*, https://doi.org/10.1007/978-3-031-10828-0_36

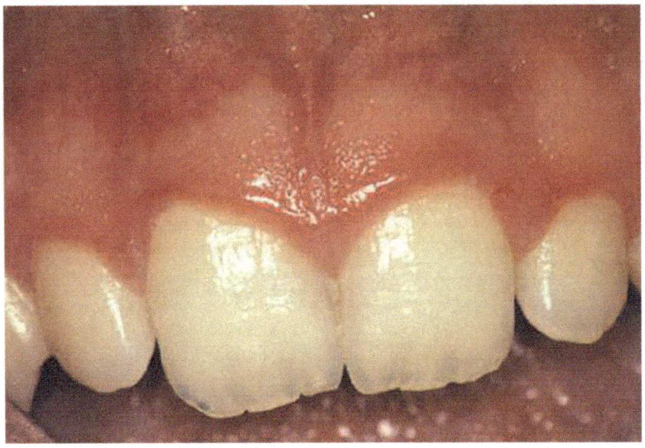

Fig. 36.1 Melkersson-Rosenthal syndrome, early gingival lesions mimicking gingivitis

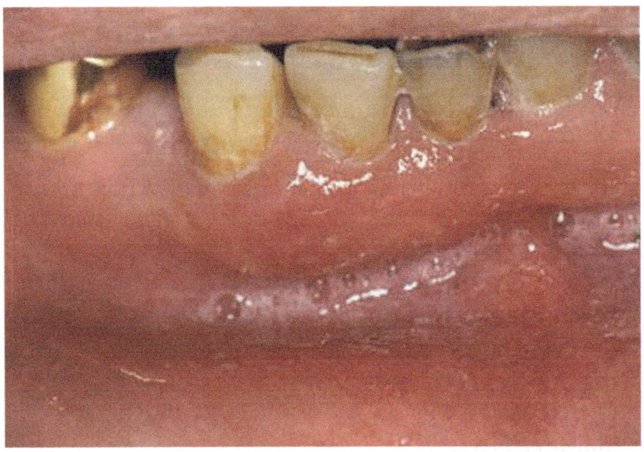

Fig. 36.2 Melkersson-Rosenthal syndrome, localized gingival swelling

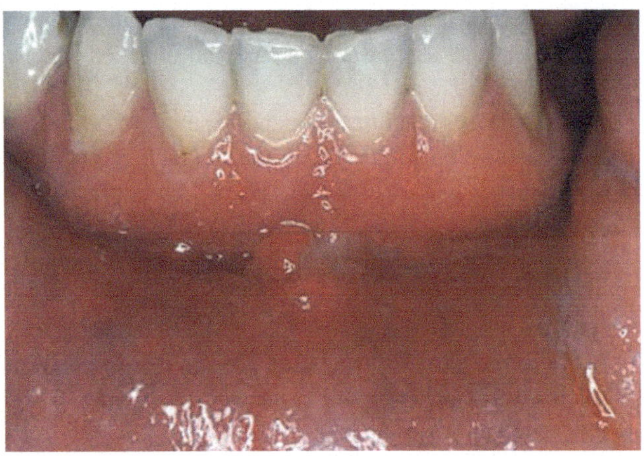

Fig. 36.3 Melkersson-Rosenthal syndrome, diffuse gingival and labial swelling

- Crohn's disease.
- Sarcoidosis.
- Amyloidosis.

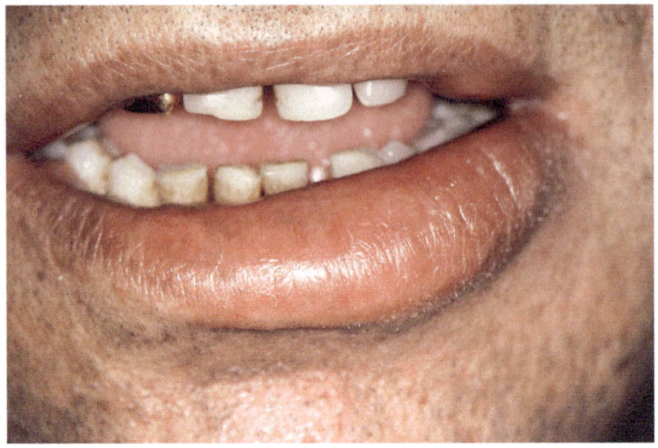

Fig. 36.4 Melkersson-Rosenthal syndrome, granulomatous cheilitis

Laboratory Tests Histopathologic examination of oral lesions, allergy tests.

Treatment Dental biofilm control and surgical excision of the hyperplastic gingival lesions. Topical or systemic corticosteroids along with systemic administration of tetracyclines or metronidazole. If facial nerve palsy is present, neurological consultation should be carried out.

Crohn Disease

Definition Crohn disease is a chronic granulomatous inflammatory disease that may affect any part of the gastrointestinal tract, from the oral cavity to the anus.

Etiology Unknown. A hereditary susceptibility is possible. An immune-mediated mechanism against microbial antigens may be involved in the pathogenesis.

Gingival Involvement Relative common. Non-dental biofilm-induced gingival lesions.

Other Sites of Involvements Oral mucosa, gastrointestinal tract, skin, eyes, joints.

Clinical Features

- Gingival lesions present as erythematous and edematous gingival enlargement, which may be localized or generalized, usually affecting the anterior gingiva (Figs. 36.5, 36.6, and 36.7). Rarely, gingival involvement may be the presenting feature.
- Oral lesions may manifest as diffuse granulomatous lip swelling, and nodular or diffuse swelling of the tongue, soft palate, and buccal mucosa, resulting in a cobblestone pattern. Mucosal folds and tags, lip fissures, aphthous or aphthous-like ulcerations, soft tissue granulomas, metal-

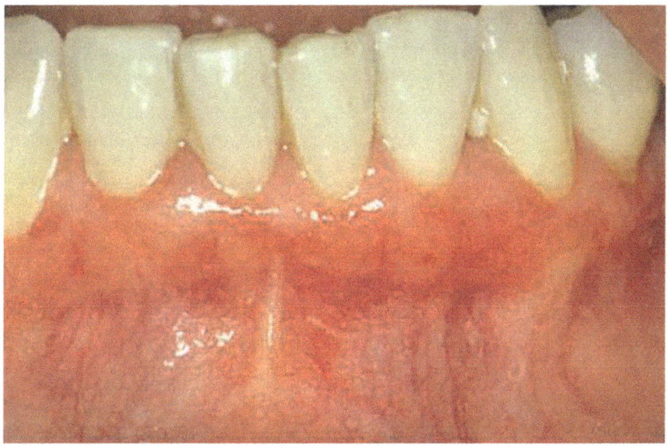

Fig. 36.5 Crohn disease, localized gingival swelling

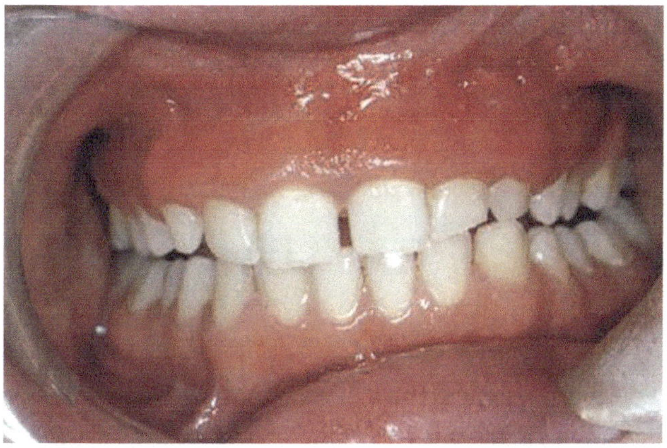

Fig. 36.6 Crohn disease, generalized swelling on the upper gingiva

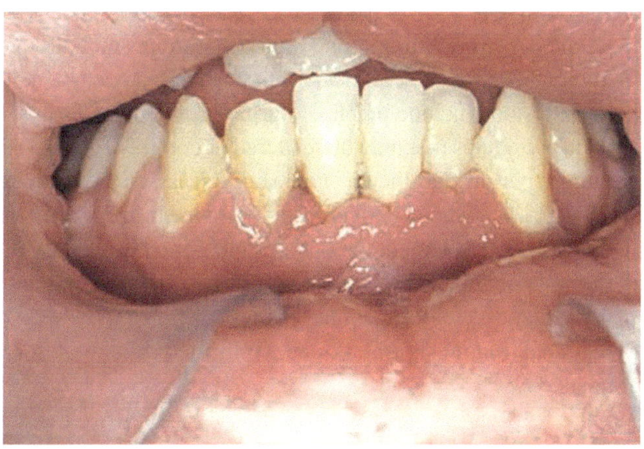

Fig. 36.7 Crohn disease, edematous swelling of the lower gingiva and lips

lic dysgeusia, and persistent lymph node enlargement may occur (Fig. 36.8).

- The gastrointestinal signs and symptoms include abdominal discomfort, diarrhea, vomiting, anorexia, weight loss,

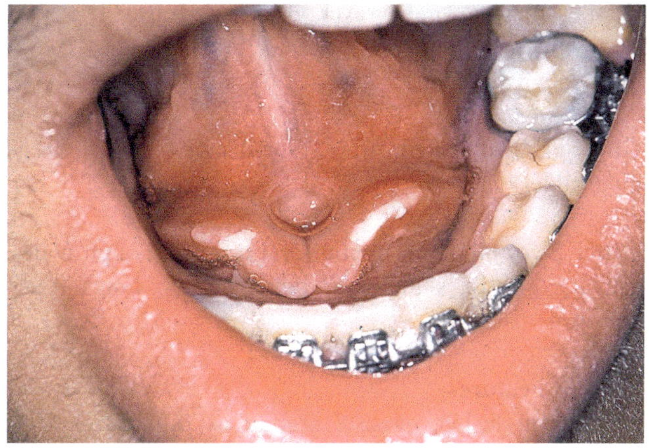

Fig. 36.8 Crohn disease, erythema, edema and vegetative ulcerated lesions on the floor of the mouth

low-grade fever, and rectal bleeding. These signs and symptoms may persist for many years with periods of exacerbation and remission.

- Extra-intestinal manifestations include arthritis, ankylosing spondylitis, and uveitis.
- Clinical diagnosis should be confirmed by laboratory tests.

Differential Diagnosis

- Melkersson-Rosenthal syndrome.
- Sarcoidosis.
- Ulcerative colitis.
- Celiac disease.
- Pyostomatitis vegetans.
- Cheilitis glandularis.
- Contact hypersensitivity reactions.
- Idiopathic orofacial disorder.

Laboratory Tests Histopathologic examination of oral and gut lesions. Colonoscopy, bowel radiology. Immunologic test for perinuclear antineutrophil cytoplasmic antibodies (P-ANCA).

Treatment Good oral hygiene. Topical corticosteroids for oral lesions. Systemic corticosteroids, sulfasalazine, azathioprine, cyclosporine, metronidazole, tetracycline, and antitumor necrosis factor for gut lesions.

Sarcoidosis

Definition Sarcoidosis is a chronic multisystemic granulomatous disease usually affecting one or multiple organs or tissues.

Etiology Unknown. However, the disease is usually associated with depressed cell-mediated immunity and B cell hyperactivity.

Gingival Involvement Rare. Non-dental biofilm-induced gingival lesions.

Other Sites of Involvement Oral mucosa, lymph nodes, salivary glands, skin, eyes, bone, nerves, lungs, liver, spleen.

Clinical Features

- Gingival lesions usually present as diffuse erythema extending to alveolar mucosa (Fig. 36.9). The affected gingiva is slightly edematous and sensitive, and occasionally may be the initial sign of sarcoidosis (Fig. 36.10).
- Oral lesions present as painless, solitary or multiple, red nodules that may rarely ulcerate. Lip and, less often, buccal and tongue swelling may occur (Fig. 36.11). Salivary gland swelling (minor and major), temporomandibular dysfunction, and facial nerve palsy may also occur.

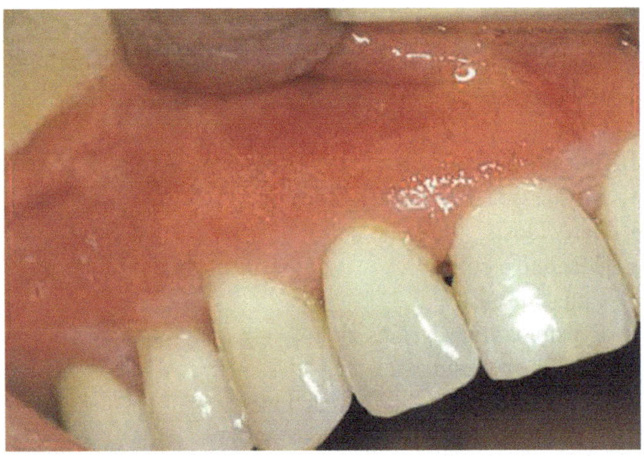

Fig. 36.9 Sarcoidosis, diffuse erythema and slight edema on the gingiva

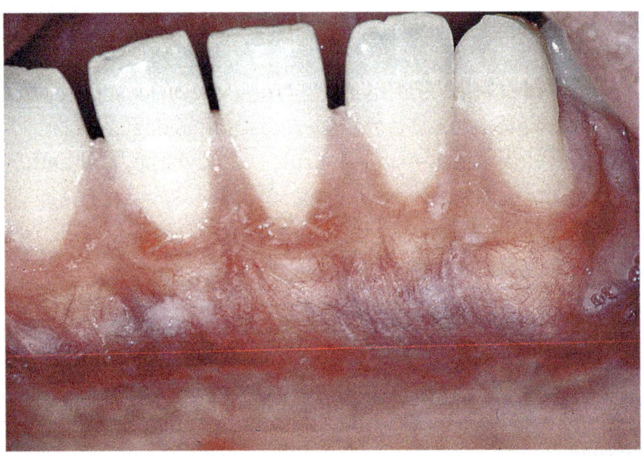

Fig. 36.10 Sarcoidosis, granulomatous gingivitis

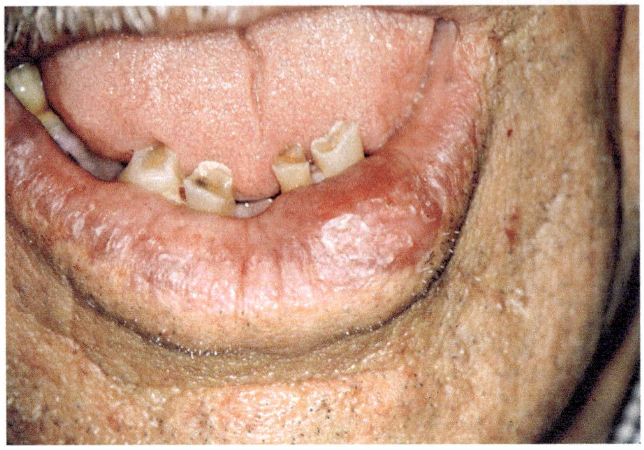

Fig. 36.11 Sarcoidosis, lip nodular swelling

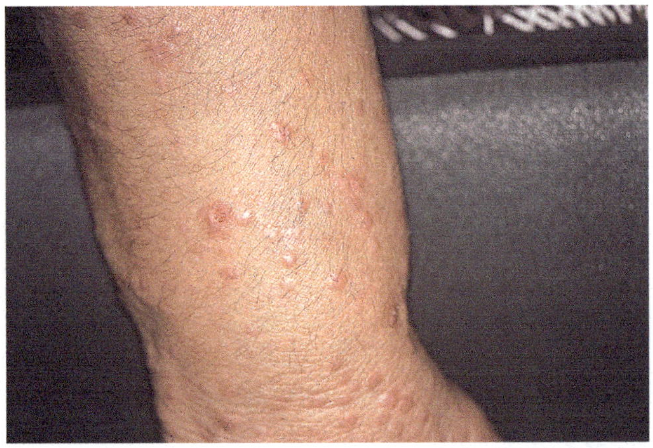

Fig. 36.12 Sarcoidosis, skin purple macules and papules

- Skin lesions include painless, purple-brown macules, papules or nodules that may be scattered or confluent as well as lupus pernio, erythema nodosum, scars, and plaques (Fig. 36.12). The skin manifestations appear in 25–30% of cases and may remain the only lesions for a long time.
- Lymphadenopathy, liver and spleen enlargement, and lung disturbances are common.
- Clinical diagnosis should be confirmed by laboratory tests.

Differential Diagnosis

- Crohn disease.
- Tuberculosis.
- Amyloidosis.
- Melkersson-Rosenthal syndrome.

Laboratory Tests Histopathologic and serologic examinations. Serum levels of angiotensin-converting enzyme (SACE), chest radiography, gallium scan.

Treatment Good oral hygiene and topical corticosteroids for gingival lesions. Corticosteroids, hydroxychloroquine, allopurinol, immunosuppressants, and biologic agents for systemic manifestations.

Pyostomatitis Vegetans

Definition Pyostomatitis vegetans is a relatively rare, pustular disorder of the mouth associated with inflammatory bowel diseases, particularly ulcerative colitis, and Crohn's disease.

Etiology Unknown. It is believed that immunologic and bacterial factors play a role in pathogenesis.

Gingival Involvement Common. Non-dental biofilm-induced gingival lesions.

Other Sites of Involvement Oral mucosa (buccal, labial, mucolabial and mucobuccal folds, soft palate, ventral tongue), skin (pyodermatitis vegetans is the equivalent of oral lesions).

Clinical Features

- Gingival lesions present as diffuse erythema and multiple, painless, yellow-white vegetative mucosal folds, which consist of pustular microabscesses in a linear pattern that coalesce (Figs. 36.13 and 36.14) The pustules then rupture, leaving painful shallow *"snail track"* ulcerations (Fig. 36.15).
- Similar lesions may be present in other mucosal sites.
- Rarely, similar lesions may be present on the skin (*pyodermatitis vegetans* and *pyoderma gangrenosum).*
- Clinical diagnosis should be confirmed by laboratory tests.

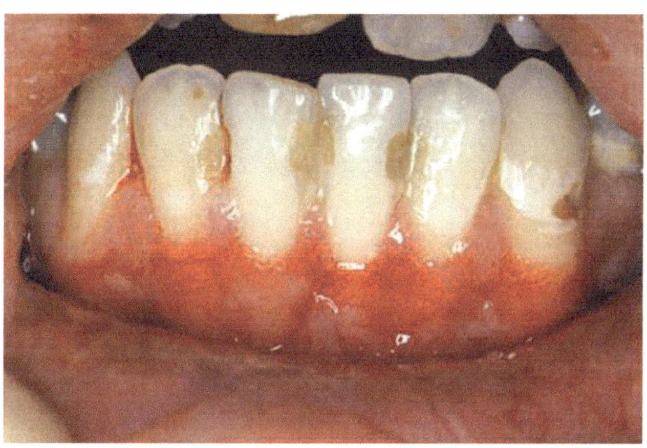

Fig. 36.13 Pyostomatitis vegetans, early lesions on the gingiva presenting with erythema and edema

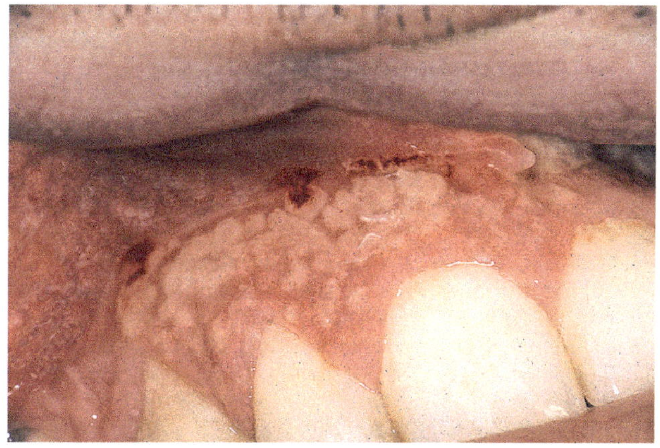

Fig. 36.14 Pyostomatitis vegetans, erythema and multiple pustular microabscesses on the upper gingiva

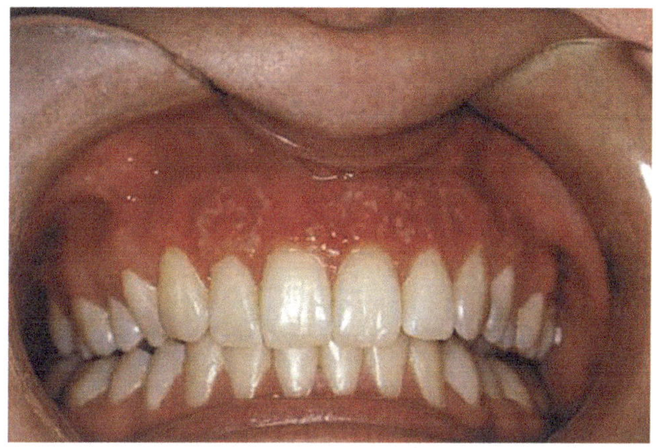

Fig. 36.15 Pyostomatitis vegetans, erythema and multiple pustular microabscesses on the upper gingiva

Differential Diagnosis

- Pemphigus vegetans.
- Dermatitis herpetiformis.
- Wegener granulomatosis.

Laboratory Tests Histopathologic examination and direct immunofluorescence to rule out chronic bullous oral diseases.

Treatment Systemic corticosteroids, sulfasalazine, azathioprine, dapsone. Spontaneous remission of oral lesions may occur when bowel lesions subside.

References

1. Mignogna MD, Fedele S, Lo Russo L, Lo ML. Orofacial granulomatosis with gingival onset. J Clin Periodontol. 2001;28(7):692–6. https://doi.org/10.1034/j.1600-051x.2001.028007692.x.
2. Bansal S, Garg A, Khurana R, Bansal A. Primary orofacial granulomatous involvement of lip and gingiva only: a diagnostic chal-

lenge. J Indian Soc Periodontol. 2020;24(6):575–8. https://doi.org/10.4103/jisp.jisp_18_20. Epub 2020 Nov 14. PMID: 33424177; PMCID: PMC7781253

3. Ozgursoy OB, Karatayli Ozgursoy S, Tulunay O, Kemal O, et al. Melkersson-Rosenthal syndrome revisited as a misdiagnosed disease. Am J Otolaryngol. 2009;30:33–7.
4. Sciubba JJ, Said-Al-Naief N. Orofacial granulomatosis: presentation, pathology and management of 13 cases. J Oral Pathol Med. 2003;32:576–85.
5. Guandalini S, Assiri A. Celiac disease: a review. JAMA Pediatr. 2014;168(3):272–8. https://doi.org/10.1001/jamapediatrics.2013.3858. PMID: 24395055
6. Capodiferro S, Maiorano E, Limongelli L, et al. Cheilitis and gingivitis as first signs of Crohn's disease in a pediatric patient. Clin Case Rep. 2019;7(2):387–8. https://doi.org/10.1002/ccr3.1975. PMID: 30847214; PMCID: PMC6389475
7. Favia G, Limongelli L, Tempesta A, et al. Oral lesions as first clinical manifestations of Crohn's disease in paediatric patients: a report on 8 cases. Eur J Paediatr Dent. 2020;21(1):66–9. https://doi.org/10.23804/ejpd.2020.21.01.13. PMID: 32183532
8. Vavricka SR, Manser CN, Hediger S, et al. Periodontitis and gingivitis in inflammatory bowel disease: a case-control study. Inflamm Bowel Dis. 2013;19(13):2768–77. https://doi.org/10.1097/01.MIB.0000438356.84263.3b. PMID: 24216685
9. Antunes KB, Miranda AM, Carvalho SR, et al. Sarcoidosis presenting as gingival erosion in a patient under long-term clinical control. J Periodontol. 2008;79(3):556–61. https://doi.org/10.1902/jop.2008.070139. PMID: 18315440
10. Tripathi P, Aggarwal J, Chopra D, et al. Sarcoidosis presenting as isolated gingival enlargement: a rare case entity. J Clin Diagn Res. 2014;8(11):ZD25–6. https://doi.org/10.7860/JCDR/2014/9888.5194. Epub 2014 Nov 20. PMID: 25584337; PMCID: PMC4290337
11. Thrash B, et al. Cutaneous manifestations of gastrointestinal disease: part II. J Am Acad Dermatol. 2013;68(2):211.e1–33. https://doi.org/10.1016/j.jaad.2012.10.036. PMID: 23317981
12. Atarbashi-Moghadam S, Lotfi A, Atarbashi-Moghadam F. Pyostomatitis Vegetans: a clue for diagnosis of silent Crohn's disease. J Clin Diagn Res. 2016;10(12):ZD12–3. https://doi.org/10.7860/JCDR/2016/22573.9032. Epub 2016 Dec 1. PMID: 28209014; PMCID: PMC5296587

Metabolic Diseases

37

Contents

Porphyrias

Definition The porphyrias are a group of genetic disorders that are characterized by a deficiency of one of the eight enzymes of the porphyrin-heme biosynthetic pathway.

Etiology Genetic. It is inherited as an autosomal dominant and recessive trait.

Classification Classically, porphyrias are subdivided into *erythropoietic* and *hepatic* forms. Recently, a new classification has been proposed: *acute* and *non-acute* or *cutaneous* and *non-cutaneous* forms.

Gingival Involvement Uncommon. Non-dental biofilm-induced gingival lesions.

Other Sites of Involvement Oral mucosa (rare), skin (common), internal organs.

Clinical Features

- Gingival involvement occur only in erythropoietic protoporphyria and porphyria cutanea tarda. Gingival lesions present as diffuse erythema of free and attached vestibular gingiva, occasionally mimicking *desquamative gingivitis* (Fig. 37.1).
- Oral lesions present as diffuse erythema, atrophy, vesicles, and ulcerations especially on the lips.
- Skin lesions appear mainly on the sun-exposed areas and are characterized by photosensitivity, erythema, fragility, vesicles, ulcerations, scar formation, and hypertrichosis (Fig. 37.2).
- Clinical diagnosis should be confirmed by laboratory tests.

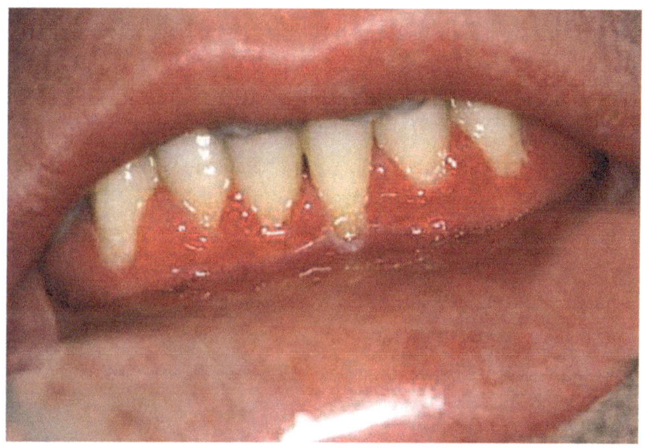

Fig. 37.1 Porphyria cutanea tarda, diffuse erythema on the lower gingiva mimicking desquamative gingivitis

Differential Diagnosis

- Desquamative gingivitis.
- Epidermolysis bullosa.
- Mucous membrane pemphigoid.
- Pellagra.

Laboratory Tests Histopathologic examination of oral and skin lesions. Biochemical tests (erythrocyte, urine, fecal), photobiological tests, and direct immunofluorescence.

G. Laskaris et al., *Periodontal Manifestations of Local and Systemic Diseases*, https://doi.org/10.1007/978-3-031-10828-0_37

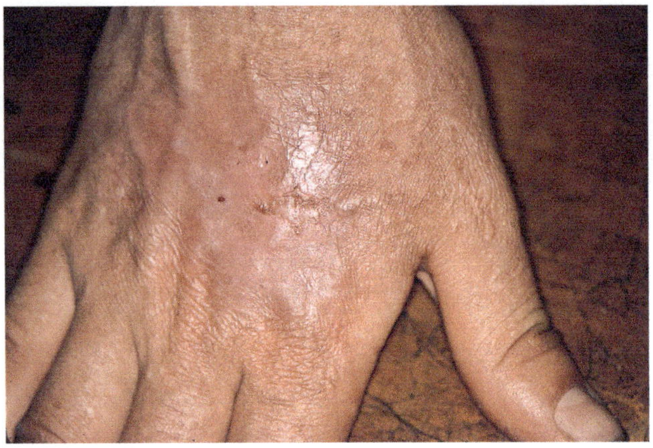

Fig. 37.2 Porphyria, skin scarring and atrophy

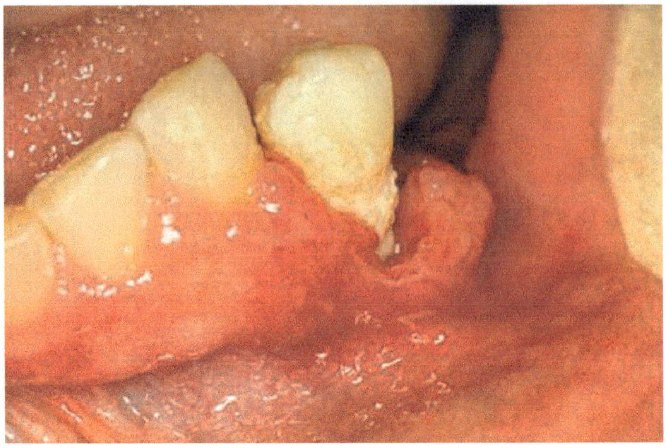

Fig. 37.3 Amyloidosis, localized irregular enlargement of the gingiva

Treatment Dental biofilm control. Systemic therapy must be left to specialists.

Amyloidosis

Definition Amyloidosis is a relatively rare metabolic disorder characterized by the extracellular deposition of an amorphous proteinaceous substance known as amyloid.

Etiology Unknown.

Classification

1. *Systemic* (generalized) forms: (a). primary systemic (AL); (b). secondary systemic (AA); (c). hemodialysis-related; and (d). hereditary.
2. *Localized* forms: (a). cutaneous; (b). endocrine; and (c). cerebral.

Gingival Involvement Relatively rare. Non-dental plaque-induced gingival lesions.

Other Sites of Involvement Oral mucosa (tongue, lips, buccal) common, particularly in primary systemic form. Skin, gastrointestinal tract, joints, skeletal muscles, heart, kidneys, and rarely other organs.

Clinical Features

- Gingival lesions usually present as localized and painless nodules or diffuse swelling with characteristic reddish color (Figs. 37.3 and 37.4).
- The most common oral mucosal manifestations are petechiae, ecchymoses, nodules, hemorrhagic bullae, ulcers, macroglossia, minor and major salivary gland enlargements, xerostomia, and regional lymph node swelling (Figs. 37.5 and 37.6.). Oral lesions may be the early presenting signs of the disease.

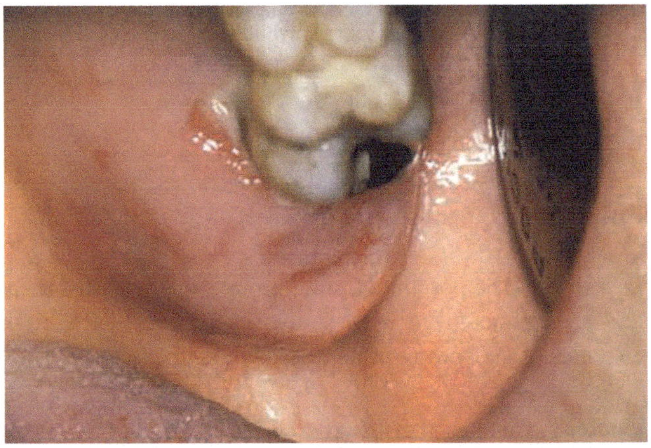

Fig. 37.4 Amyloidosis, gingival swelling on the maxillary gingiva

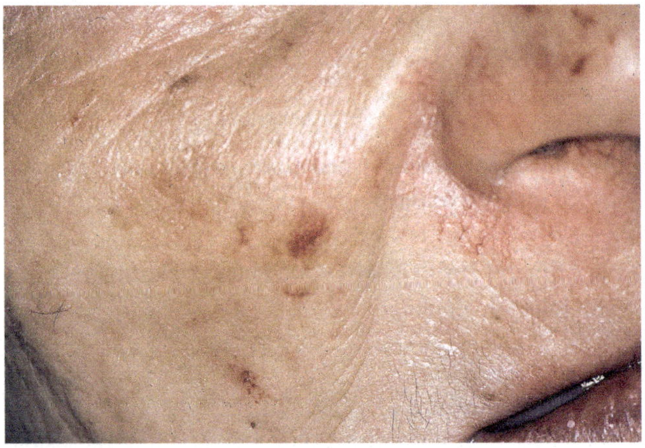

Fig. 37.5 Amyloidosis, petechiae and ecchymoses on the skin

- The most common skin lesions are purpura, petechiae, papules, nodules, bullae, ulcers, and alopecia.
- Common presenting symptoms are weakness, fatigue, weight loss, edema, dyspnea, hoarseness, bleeding, pain, carpal tunnel syndrome.

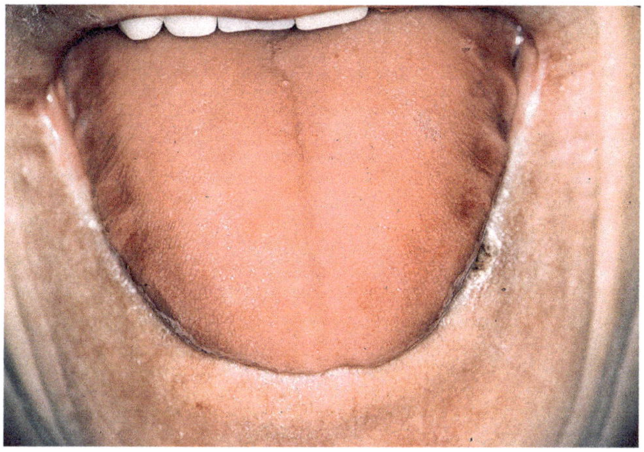

Fig. 37.6 Amyloidosis, macroglossia due to amyloid deposition

- About 20–30% of cases of primary systemic amyloidosis are associated with multiple myeloma. The prognosis is unfavorable.
- Clinical diagnosis should be confirmed by laboratory tests.

Differential Diagnosis

- Soft tissue, gingival plasmacytoma.
- Sarcoidosis.
- Crohn's disease.
- Benign and malignant neoplasms.
- Macroglossia due to other causes.

Laboratory Tests Histopathologic examination with special stains (e.g., Congo red, methyl violet, thioflavin-T). Serum and urine electrophoresis, immunohistochemical techniques.

Treatment Symptomatic treatment of gingival and oral lesions. Systemic treatment must be left to specialists and includes corticosteroids, colchicines, melphalan, chlorambucil, dimethyl sulfoxide, and autologous hematopoietic stem cell transplantation.

References

1. Gilhuus-Moe O, Koppang HS. Oral manifestations of porphyria. Oral Surg Oral Med Oral Pathol. 1972;33(6):926–33. https://doi.org/10.1016/0030-4220(72)90184-3.
2. Kooijman MM, Brand HS. Oral aspects of porphyria. Int Dent J. 2005;55(2):61–6. https://doi.org/10.1111/j.1875-595x.2005.tb00035.x. PMID: 15880959
3. Dissanayaka DWVN, Bandara HMMR, Sabesan T, et al. Case report: oral manifestations of systemic amyloidosis, an aid to diagnosis of multiple myeloma-report of two cases. Braz J Otorhinolaryngol. 2020;88(1):S1808–8694. https://doi.org/10.1016/j.bjorl.2020.11.011. Epub ahead of print. PMID: 33408060
4. Elad S, Czerninski R, Fischman S, et al. Exceptional oral manifestations of amyloid light chain protein (al) systemic amyloidosis. Amyloid. 2010;17:27–31.
5. Viggor SF, Frezzini C, Farthing PM, et al. Amyloidosis: an unusual case of persistent oral ulceration. Oral Surg Oral Med Oral Pathol Oral Radiol Endod. 2009;108:e46–50.

Endocrine Diseases

38

Contents

Diabetes Mellitus

Definition Diabetes mellitus is a chronic, systemic, heterogeneous group of carbohydrate metabolism, protein, and fat disorders that are strongly associated with microvascular and macrovascular complications.

Etiology Multifactorial. It is due to insufficient secretion of insulin from the pancreas or tissue resistance to the action of insulin, or a combination of both.

Classification Two main forms of diabetes mellitus are recognized:

a. *Type 1, insulin-dependent* (children onset).
b. *Type 2, non-insulin-dependent* (adult onset).

There are also other *"specific types"* of the disease.

Gingival and Periodontal Involvement Common, in both types 1 and 2. Dental biofilm-induced gingivitis and periodontitis, while diabetes mellitus is an important modifying factor.

Other Sites of Involvement Oral mucosa, relatively rare. Many organs and systems.

Clinical Features

- The clinical features of gingivitis are particularly associated with uncontrolled diabetes mellitus and are characterized by the presence of dental biofilm at the gingival margin, erythema, edema, bleeding upon probing, increased gingival exudates, and the absence of attachment and alveolar bone loss (Figs. 38.1 and 38.2). The gingival inflammation is usually reversible after the control of diabetic state. In uncontrolled diabetes mellitus patients, periodontitis with attachment loss and alveolar bone loss may develop. However, diabetes mellitus-associated periodontitis is not a distinct disease.
- Recent data do not support a particular pathophysiologic relation in patients with diabetes mellitus and periodontal disease. Diabetes mellitus may alter the occurrence, severity, and treatment response of periodontitis.

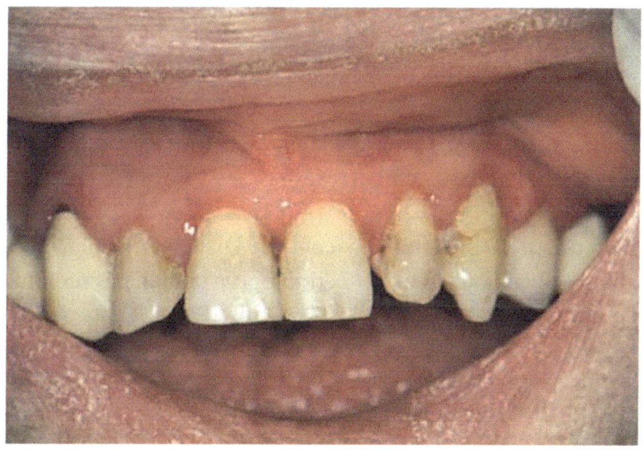

Fig. 38.1 Diabetes mellitus, early periodontitis

G. Laskaris et al., *Periodontal Manifestations of Local and Systemic Diseases*, https://doi.org/10.1007/978-3-031-10828-0_38

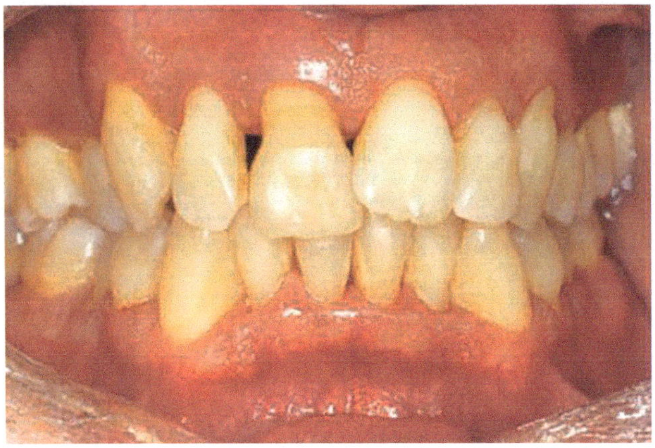

Fig. 38.2 Diabetes mellitus, severe periodontitis

- The oral mucosa manifestations are not specific and include xerostomia, superficial erosions, retardation of wound healing, burning mouth, taste disturbances, candidiasis. Salivary gland swelling (*sialosis*) may occur.
- Clinical diagnosis should be confirmed by laboratory tests.

Differential Diagnosis

- Dental biofilm-induced gingivitis.
- Sex hormone-associatedgingivitis.

Laboratory Tests Blood examination for plasma glucose levels. Oral glucose tolerance test.

Treatment Dental biofilm control. Diabetes management should be conducted by endocrinologists or diabetes mellitus specialists.

Addison Disease

Definition Addison disease is a rare, acquired dysfunction of adrenal glands characterized by insufficient secretion of glucocorticoids and mineralocorticoids.

Etiology Destruction of the adrenal cortex due to infection, autoimmunity, infiltration by a tumor, hemorrhage, or infarction. The levels of ACTH and melanocyte-stimulating hormone (MSH) are elevated, causing increased hyperpigmentation of the skin and oral mucosa.

Gingival Involvement Relatively common. Non-dental biofilm-induced gingival lesions.

Other Sites of Involvement Oral mucosa (buccal, palate, lips), skin.

Clinical Features

- Gingival lesions present as multiple melanotic macules or irregular plaques (Figs. 38.3 and 38.4).

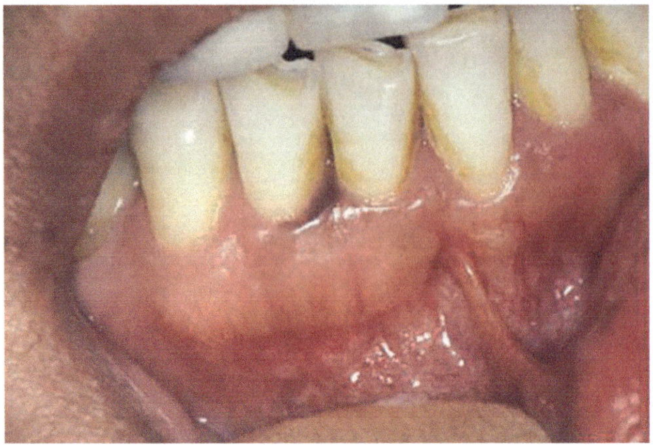

Fig. 38.3 Addison disease, early melanotic macule on the interdental papilla

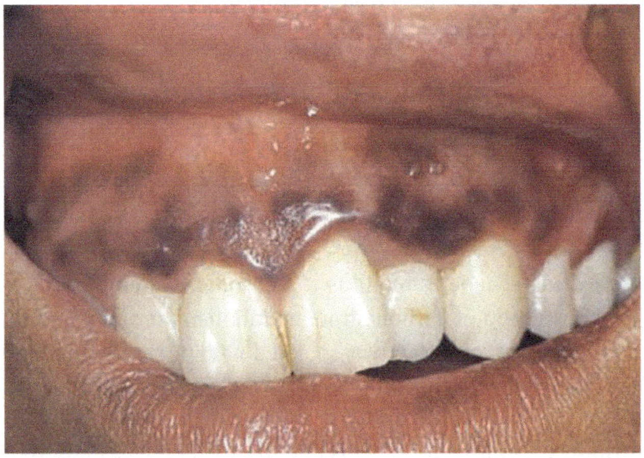

Fig. 38.4 Addison disease, generalized pigmentation on the gingiva and the alveolar mucosa

- Similar lesions appear in other areas of oral mucosa. The oral manifestations are usually early and have a high diagnostic value.
- Skin lesions present as diffuse bronze to grey hyperpigmentation, particularly on sun-exposed skin.
- Malaise, weakness, nausea, vomiting, and weight loss are common.
- Clinical diagnosis should be confirmed by laboratory tests.

Differential Diagnosis

- Normal gingival melanosis (racial).
- Smoking melanosis.
- Drug-induced hyperpigmentation.
- Amalgam tattoo.
- Melanocytic nevi.
- Malignant melanoma.

Laboratory Tests ACTH measurement, ACTH stimulation, and assay of plasma cortisol.

Treatment No treatment is needed for gingival and oral lesions. Systemic treatment must be left to specialists.

Sex Steroid Hormones

Definition Sex steroid hormones (androgens, estrogens, and progestins) may influence the periodontal tissue, and particularly the gingiva, and they are associated with an exaggerated inflammatory response in these tissues.

Etiology Dental biofilm-induced gingivitis modified by sex steroid hormones.

Classification Four forms of gingival disorders may be developed: *(a) puberty-associated gingivitis; (b) menstrual cycle-associated gingivitis; (c) pregnancy-associated gingivitis;* and *(d) oral contraceptive-associated gingivitis.*

Gingival Involvement Common. Dental biofilm-induced gingivitis modified by sex steroid hormones.

Other Sites of Involvement Oral mucosa, skin, nails, hair.

Clinical Features

- All four forms of gingivitis display a similar clinical pattern. The clinical features include the presence of dental biofilm at the gingival margin, redness, and edema of the gingiva, bleeding upon probing, loss of attachment, and alveolar bone loss (Figs. 38.5, 38.6, and 38.7). The lesions can resolve following puberty, ovulation, parturition, and discontinuation of oral contraceptives.
- Diagnosis is based on clinical criteria and laboratory tests.

Differential Diagnosis

- Dental biofilm-induced gingivitis.
- Diabetes mellitus-associated gingivitis.

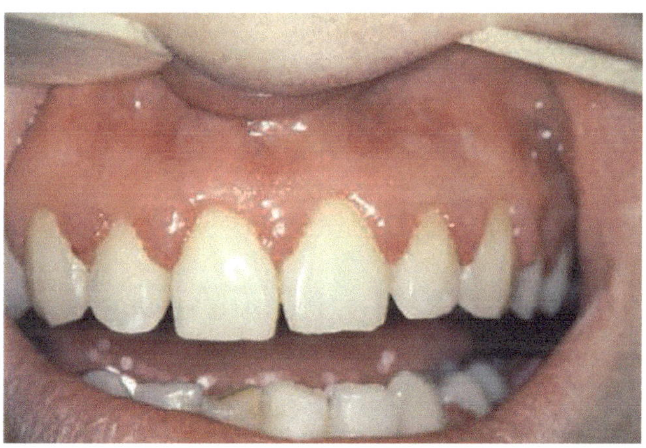

Fig. 38.5 Sex steroid hormones disorder, early pregnancy-associated gingivitis

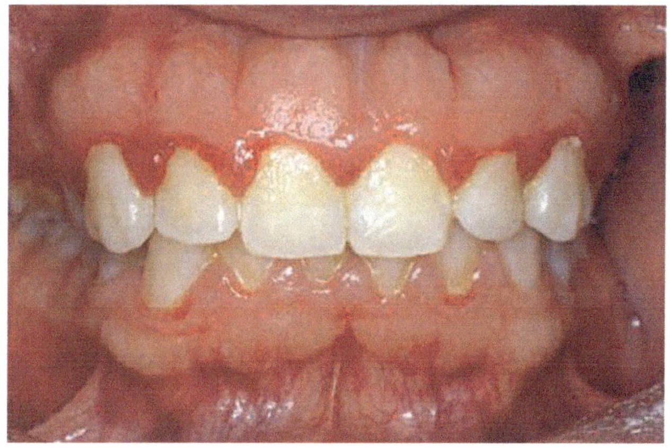

Fig. 38.6 Sex steroid hormones disorder, pregnancy-associated gingivitis

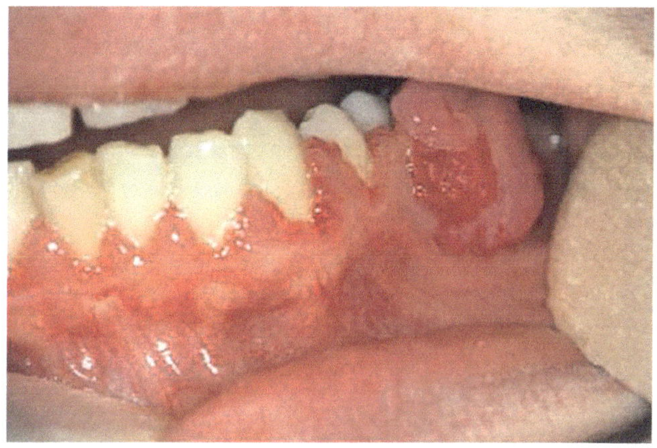

Fig. 38.7 Sex steroid hormones disorder, severe pregnancy-associated gingivitis and pyogenic granulomas

Laboratory Tests Sex hormone measurement.

Treatment Dental biofilm control. Hormonal balance of sex steroid hormones will be restored by specialists.

References

1. Kathiresan TS, Masthan KMK, Sarangarajan R, et al. A study of diabetes associated oral manifestations. J Pharm Bioallied Sci. 2017;9(Suppl 1):S211–6. https://doi.org/10.4103/jpbs.JPBS_157_17. PMID: 29284966; PMCID: PMC5731015
2. Sadeghi R, Taleghani F, Mohammadi S, Zohri Z. The effect of diabetes mellitus type I on periodontal and dental status. J Clin Diagn Res. 2017;11(7):ZC14–7. https://doi.org/10.7860/JCDR/2017/25742.10153. Epub 2017 Jul 1. PMID: 28893034; PMCID: PMC5583944
3. Sarkar SB, Sarkar S, Ghosh S, Bandyopadhyay S. Addison's disease. Contemp Clin Dent. 2012;3(4):484–6. https://doi.org/10.4103/0976-237X.107450. PMID: 23633816; PMCID: PMC3636818
4. Balan U, Gonsalves N, Jose M, Girish KL. Symptomatic changes of oral mucosa during normal hormonal turnover in healthy young menstruating women. J Contemp Dent Pract. 2012;13(2):178–81. https://doi.org/10.5005/jp-journals-10024-1117. PMID: 22665744

Vitamin Deficiencies

39

Contents

Scurvy

Definition Scurvy is a rare vitamin C deficiency that is usually limited to individuals, whose diets are poor in fresh fruits and vegetables.

Etiology Vitamin C (ascorbic acid) deficiency leads to impairment of peptidyl hydroxylation of procollagen and a reduction in collagen formation and secretion by connective tissue. This deficiency leads to capillary fragility that correlates with hemorrhagic features and poor healing of wounds.

Gingival Involvement Common. Non-dental biofilm-induced gingival lesions modified by vitamin C deficiency.

Other Sites of Involvement Oral mucosa, skin, hair, nails, muscles, joints

Clinical Features

- Gingival lesions, which are present early, are common and cause generalized swelling and redness of the interdental and marginal gingiva (Fig. 39.1). Spontaneous gingival hemorrhage and ulcers are also common. Periodontal bone loss and tooth mobility may also occur.
- Oral mucosal petechiae, hemorrhages, ecchymoses, and delayed wound healing are commonly seen as well as enamel hypoplasia of developing teeth.

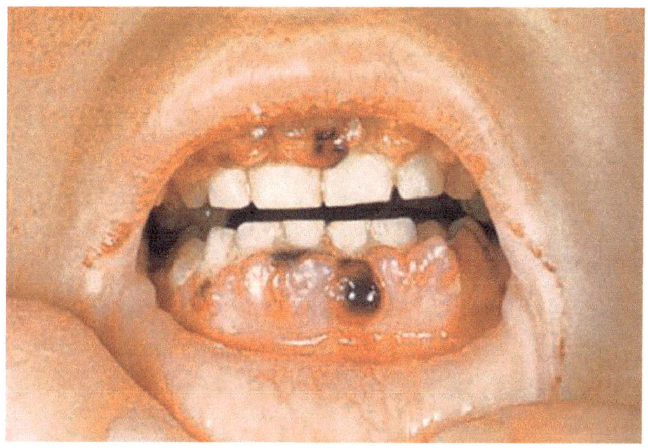

Fig 39.1 Scurvy, generalized gingival swelling associated with hemorrhages

- Hemorrhages, ecchymoses of the skin, nail beds, muscles, and joints are common.
- Severe to moderate anemia is common. Melena, hematuria, and orbital hemorrhage may occur.
- Retrobulbar, subarachnoid, and intracerebral hemorrhage may also occur. Delayed treatment can cause malaise and weakness.
- Diagnosis is mainly based on clinical criteria, but it should be confirmred by laboratory tests.

Differential Diagnosis

- Necrotizing gingivitis
- Herpetic gingivostomatitis

G. Laskaris et al., *Periodontal Manifestations of Local and Systemic Diseases*, https://doi.org/10.1007/978-3-031-10828-0_39

- Agranulocytosis
- Leukemia
- Thrombocytopenic purpura

Laboratory Tests Platelet and plasma ascorbic acid levels are reduced.

Treatment Ascorbic acid orally 1–2 g/d. Diet rich in fresh fruits and vegetables. Dental biofilm control.

References

1. Pflipsen M, Zenchenko Y. Nutrition for oral health and oral manifestations of poor nutrition and unhealthy habits. Gen Dent. 2017;65(6):36–43.
2. Firth N, Marvan E. Oral lesions in scurvy. Aust Dent J. 2001;46(4):298–300. https://doi.org/10.1111/j.1834-7819.2001.tb00294.x. PMID: 11838878
3. Brand AJ, Lieberman MB, Hajishengallis E. Severe gingivitis associated with ascorbic acid-deficiency in a pediatric patient. J Dent Child (Chic). 2019;86(2):125–8. PMID: 31395119

Part V

Potentially Malignant Disorders Affecting Periodontal Tissues

Potentially Malignant Disorders

40

Contents

Leukoplakia

Definition Leukoplakia is the most common potentially malignant disorder of the oral mucosa. It is defined as a white patch or plaque that cannot be rubbed off and cannot be characterized as any other condition or disease. It is a clinical term without a specific histopathologic basis. Leukoplakia is characterized by biological heterogeneity since some lesions have a risk of malignant transformation to squamous cell carcinoma and others do not.

Etiology The exact etiology remains unknown. Smoking, alcohol consumption, and HPV are the main environmental causative factors.

Classification Clinically, leukoplakia is classified into two main groups: a. homogeneous (low risk); and b. nonhomogeneous (high risk), which is subdivided into speckled or nodular, verrucous and proliferative verrucous forms.

Gingival Involvement Relatively common. Unrelated to dental biofilm-induced gingival lesions.

Other Sites of Involvement Buccal mucosa, commissures, floor of the mouth, lips, palate, alveolar mucosa.

Clinical Features

- *Homogeneous leukoplakia*(almost 95% of cases) clinically appears as a white, thin and flat, painless plaque, which cannot be scraped off and is attached to oral mucosa (Figs. 40.1, 40.2 and 40.3). It has a lowrisk of malignant transformation.
- *Speckled leukoplakia* (2–3%) clinically presents as a red area with multiple, small white macules and is often infected by *candida albicans.* It has a high risk of malignant transformation (Fig. 40.4).
- *Verrucous leukoplakia* (0.2–1%) clinically appears as an exophytic, irregular, wrinkled, or corrugated white plaque (Figs. 40.5 and 40.6). It has a relatively high risk of malignant transformation.
- *Proliferative verrucous leukoplakia* (0.1–0.5%) is a rare variant of verrucous form, which is clinically characterized by multifocal locations, a tendency to recur after surgical excision and has a high risk of malignant transformation.

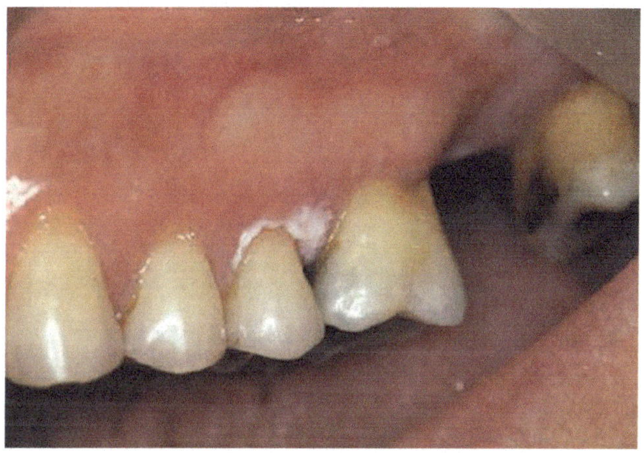

Fig. 40.1 Gingival Leukoplakia, early homogeneous type

G. Laskaris et al., *Periodontal Manifestations of Local and Systemic Diseases*, https://doi.org/10.1007/978-3-031-10828-0_40

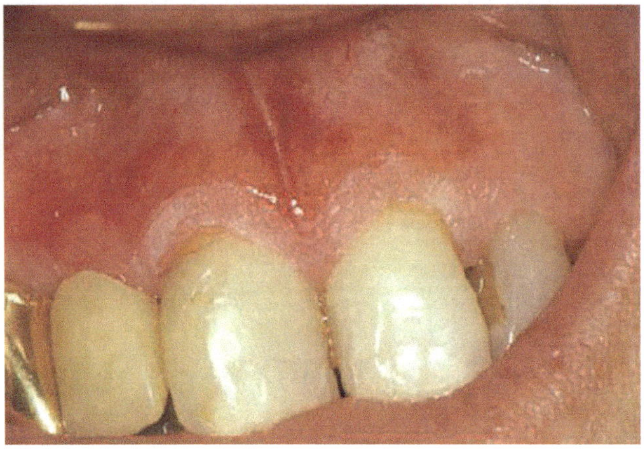

Fig. 40.2 Gingival Leukoplakia, homogeneous type

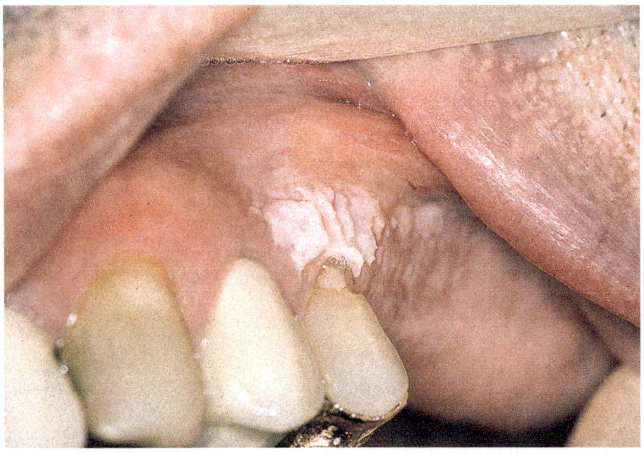

Fig. 40.3 Gingival leukoplakia, homogeneous type

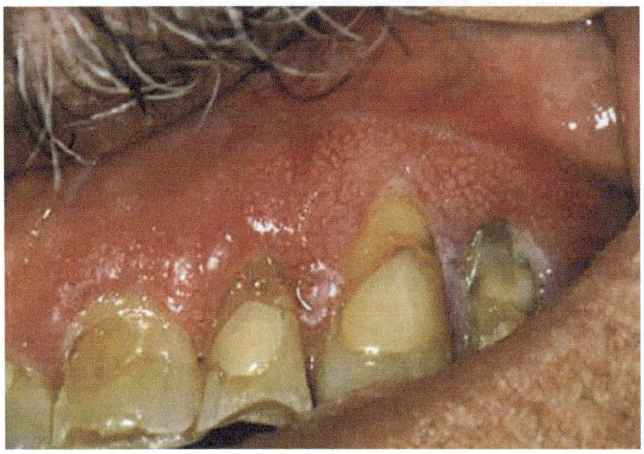

Fig. 40.4 Gingival leukoplakia, speckled type

- The size may vary from a few millimeters to several centimeters. The total risk of malignant transformation of leukoplakia in 5 years is 3–6%.
- Gingival lesions of leukoplakia have a low risk of malignant transformation. Leukoplakic lesions on the lateral border and ventral surface of the tongue as well as in the floor of the mouth are of high risk, particularly in smokers.
- The risk of malignant transformation in leukoplakia lesions must be exclusively supported by histopathologic criteria.
- Clinical diagnosis should be confirmed by laboratory tests.

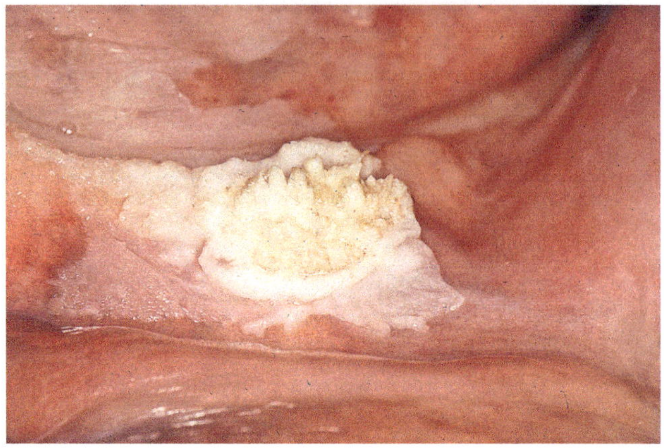

Fig. 40.5 Gingival leukoplakia, verrucous type exophytic plaque surrounded by homogeneous leukoplakia

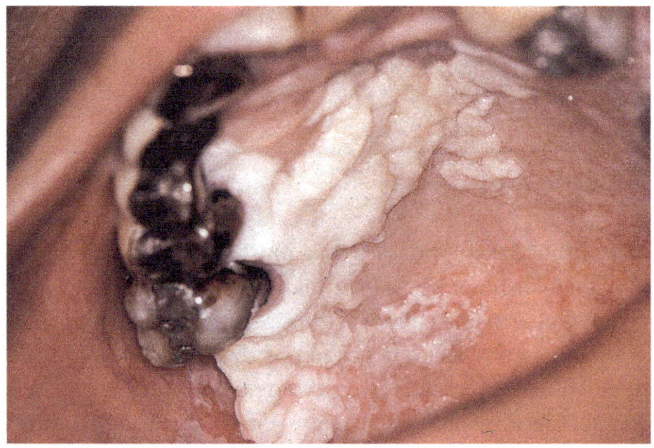

Fig. 40.6 Verrucous leukoplakia on the palate and the palatal gingiva

Differential Diagnosis

- Friction keratosis
- Lichen planus
- Discoid lupus erythematosus
- Candidiasis
- Hairy leukoplakia
- Uremic stomatitis
- Cinnamon contact stomatitis
- Early squamous cell carcinoma
- Chemical burn
- Leukoedema
- Genetic syndromes

Laboratory Tests Histopathologic examination (*low-moderate-high* epithelial dysplasia or carcinoma in *situ)*. Molecular examination (p53 gene, loss of heterozygosity, DNA ploidy analysis, etc.), presence of high-risk HPV types (16,18).

Treatment The treatment of choice is surgical excision and alternatively electrosurgery, cryosurgery, and lasers. Smoking and alcohol consumption cessation is necessary. The patient should be followed up every 6 months for 3–5 years after treatment.

Erythroplakia

Definition Oral erythroplakia is a clinical term for a non-specific fiery red patch that is adherent and cannot be attributed to a specific lesion or disease.

Etiology The exact etiology remains unknown, although tobacco and alcohol may be involved.

Gingival Involvement Rare. Unrelated to dental biofilm-induced gingival lesions.

Other Sites of Involvement Soft palate, buccal mucosa, floor of the mouth, tongue. Glans penis mucosa (common).

Clinical Features

- Clinically, it appears as an asymptomatic *Erythroplakia*, red patch with a smooth or granular surface, which may be flat or slightly elevated (Figs. 40.7 and 40.8). Small white or deep red spots or macules can develop inside the lesion.
- Oral erythroplakia is the most dangerous potentially malignant disorder of oral mucosa. In more than 90% of cases, severe epithelial dysplasia or carcinoma in situ is confirmed histologically at the time of diagnosis.
- Without treatment, the great majority of erythroplakia will undergo malignant transformation.
- Clinical diagnosis should be confirmed histopathologically.

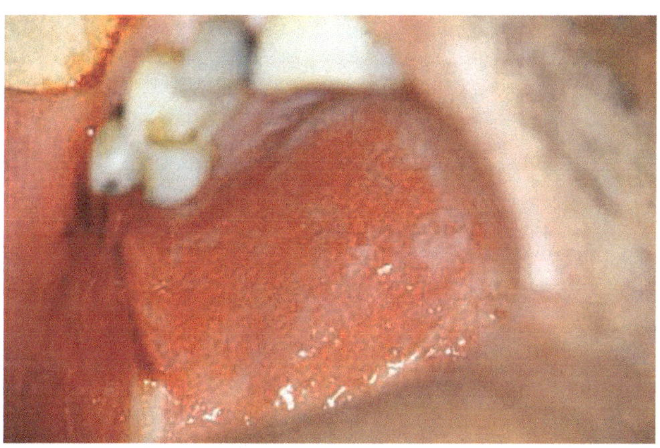

Fig. 40.7 Erythroplakia, velvet-like red lesions on the gingiva, alveolar mucosa and palate

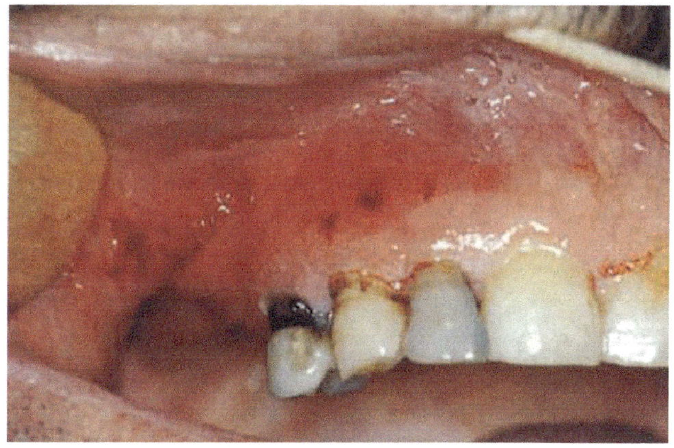

Fig. 40.8 Erythroplakia on the labial gingiva and alveolar mucosa

Differential Diagnosis

- Erythematous candidiasis
- Lichen planus, erosive type
- Discoid lupus erythematosus
- Desquamative gingivitis
- Plasmacell gingivitis or stomatitis
- Cinnamon contact stomatitis
- Soft tissue plasmacytoma
- Reiter syndrome (Reactive arthritis)

Laboratory Tests Histopathologic examination.

Treatment Surgical excision is the treatment of choice.

References

1. Anderson A, Ishak N. Marked variation in malignant transformation rates of oral leukoplakia. Evid Based Dent. 2015;16(4):102–3. https://doi.org/10.1038/sj.ebd.6401128.
2. van der Waal I, Reichart PA. Oral proliferative verrucous leukoplakia revisited. Oral Oncol. 2008;44(8):719–21. https://doi.org/10.1016/j.oraloncology.2007.09.010. Epub 2007 Dec 3. PMID: 18061520
3. Torrejon-Moya A, Jané-Salas E, López-López J. Clinical manifestations of oral proliferative verrucous leukoplakia: a systematic review. J Oral Pathol Med. 2020;49(5):404–8. https://doi.org/10.1111/jop.12999. Epub 2020 Feb 9. PMID: 31990082
4. Dionne KR, Warnakulasuriya S, Zain RB, Cheong SC. Potentially malignant disorders of the oral cavity: current practice and future directions in the clinic and laboratory. Int J Cancer. 2015;136(3):503–15. https://doi.org/10.1002/ijc.28754. Epub 2014 Feb 11. PMID: 24482244
5. Upadhyaya JD, Fitzpatrick SG, Islam MN, et al. Marginal linear gingival leukoplakia progressing to "ring around the collar"-an ominous sign of proliferative verrucous leukoplakia. J Periodontol.

2020;92(2):273–85. https://doi.org/10.1002/JPER.19-0621. Epub ahead of print. PMID: 32725623
6. Gambino A, Carbone M, Broccoletti R, et al. A report on the clinical-pathological correlations of 788 gingival lesion. Med Oral Patol Oral Cir Bucal. 2017;22(6):e686–93. https://doi.org/10.4317/medoral.21845. Epub ahead of print
7. Vail M, Robinson S, Condon H. Recognition of oral potentially malignant disorders and transformation to oral cancer. JAAPA. 2020;33(11):14–8. https://doi.org/10.1097/01.JAA.0000718268.52634.59. Epub ahead of print. PMID: 33048859.
8. Reichart PA, Philipsen HP. Oral erythroplakia–a review. Oral Oncol. 2005;41:551–61.
9. Zhang X, Li C, Song Y, Reichart PA. Oral leukoplakia in China: a review. Oral Maxillofac Surg. 2010;14:195–202.

Part VI

Tumors Affecting Periodontal Tissues

Benign Tumors

41

Contents

Fibroma

Definition Fibroma is the most common benign intraoral tumor that originates from the connective tissue.

Etiology Chronic local irritation. In most cases, it is not a true neoplasm but a reactive hyperplasia of fibrous connective tissue.

Gingival Involvement Relatively common. Non-dental biofilm-induced gingival lesion.

Other Sites of Involvement Buccal mucosa, tongue, lips, palate.

Clinical Features

- Clinically, fibroma appears as a well-circumscribed, usually sessile or pandiculated, asymptomatic nodule, with smooth surface of normal color and firm consistency (Figs. 41.1 and 41.2). Not uncommonly, the surface has a whitish color and is rarely ulcerated due to mechanical irritation.

G. Laskaris et al., *Periodontal Manifestations of Local and Systemic Diseases*, https://doi.org/10.1007/978-3-031-10828-0_41

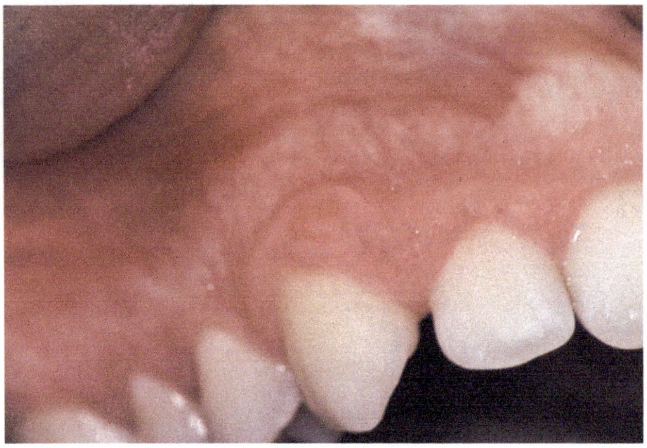

Fig. 41.1 Fibroma, small, smooth nodule on the gingiva of the canine

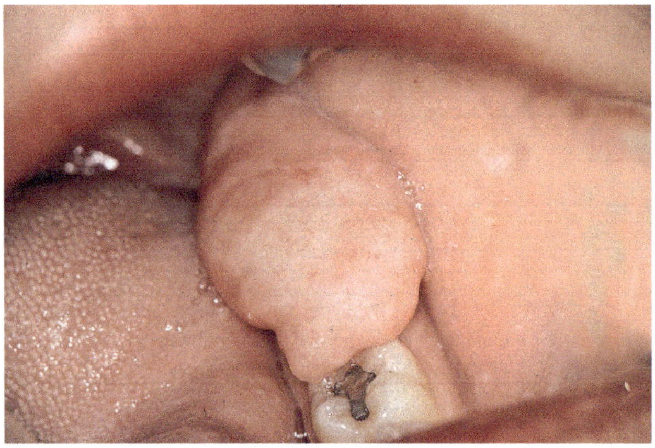

Fig. 41.2 Fibroma, smooth lobulated nodule on the gingiva of the retromolar area

- Fibroma is usually solitary and the size varies from a few mm to several cm. It affects almost equally both sexes most commonly between 40 and 60 years of age.
- Clinical diagnosis should be confirmed histologically.

Differential Diagnosis

- Peripheral ossifying fibroma
- Giant cell fibroma
- Neurofibroma
- Schwannoma
- Lipoma
- Myxoma
- Fibrous histiocytoma
- Oral focal mucinosis

Laboratory Test Histopathologic examination.

Treatment Conservative surgical excision.

Giant Cell Fibroma

Definition Giant cell fibroma is a connective tissue tumor with distinct clinical and histopathologic features.

Etiology Unknown. It is not associated with chronic irritation or trauma.

Gingival Involvement Common, over 50% of all cases. Non-dental biofilm-induced gingival lesion.

Other Sites of Involvement Tongue, palate, and buccal mucosa.

Clinical Features

- Clinically, the gingival lesion appears as a painless, well-circumscribed, usually pedunculated, or less often sessile tumor of normal color and slightly papillary surface, commonly less than 1 cm in size (Figs. 41.3 and 41.4). The mandibular gingival is more often affected than the maxillary.

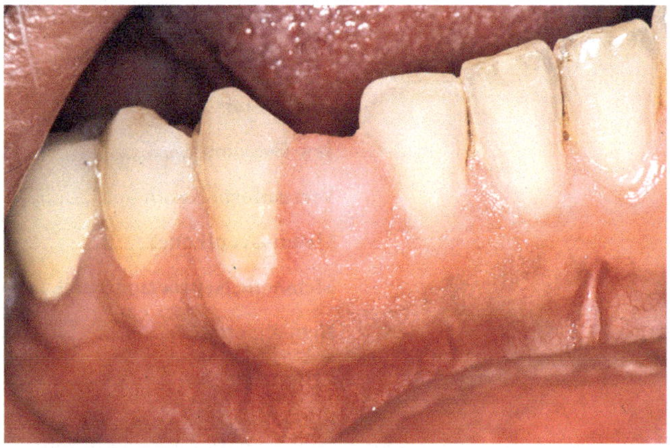

Fig. 41.3 Giant cell fibroma, normal color tumor on the mandibular gingiva, misplacing the teeth

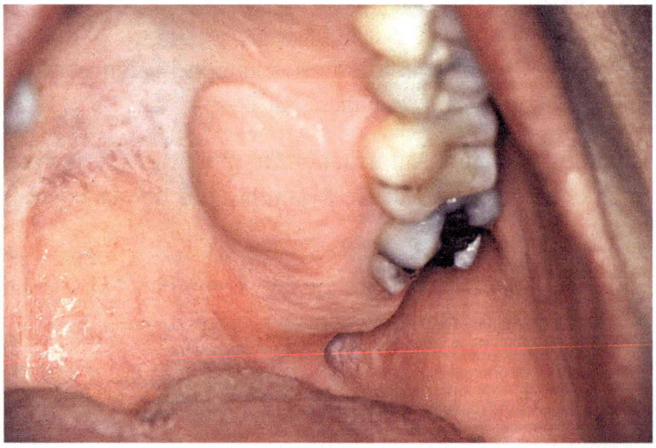

Fig. 41.4 Giant cell fibroma, sessile tumor on the palate extending to the gingiva

- It affects, almost equally, both sexes and usually occurs during the first three decades of life.
- Clinical diagnosis should be confirmed histologically.

Differential Diagnosis
- Fibroma
- Neurofibroma
- Peripheral ossifying fibroma
- Schwannoma
- Fibrous histiocytoma

Laboratory Tests Histopathologic examination with a characteristic pattern.

Treatment Conservative surgical excision.

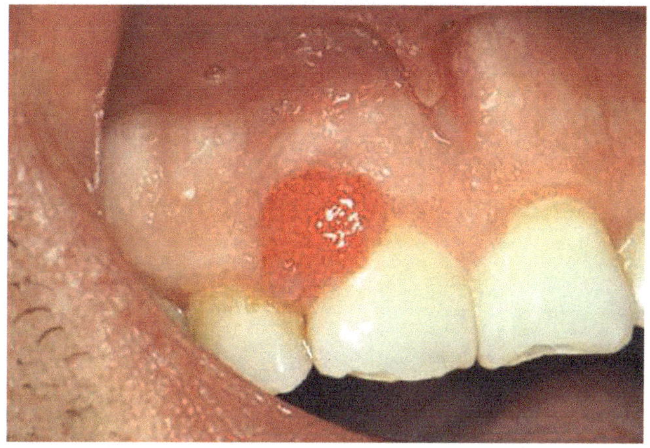

Fig. 41.5 Peripheral ossifying fibroma, erythematous growth on the gingiva

Peripheral Ossifying Fibroma

Definition The peripheral ossifying fibroma is a relatively common benign tumor that occurs exclusively on the gingiva.

Etiology Unknown. The exact histogenesis is unclear, but it is believed to derive from either the periodontal membrane or the periosteum.

Gingival Involvement Exclusively. Unrelated to the dental-biofilm lesion.

Other Sites of Involvement None.

Clinical Features
- Clinically, it presents as a circumscribed gingival growth, sessile or pedunculated, which is covered by normal mucosa (Figs. 41.5, 41.6 and 41.7). However, commonly the surface can be erythematous or even ulcerated due to mechanical irritation (Fig. 41.8).
- The tumor equally affects the maxilla and mandible, usually in the incisor-cuspid region.
- Clinical diagnosis should be confirmed by laboratory tests.

Differential Diagnosis
- Abscesses
- Exostoses
- Fibroma
- Giant cell tumor
- Pyogenic granuloma
- Peripheral odontogenic tumors

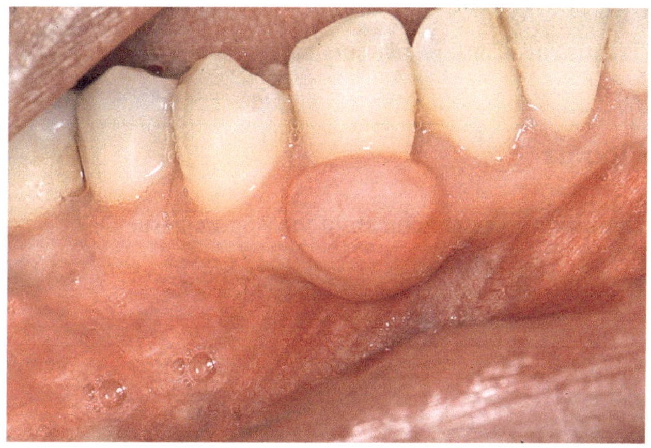

Fig. 41.6 Peripheral ossifying fibroma, nodule covered with normal mucosa on the gingiva

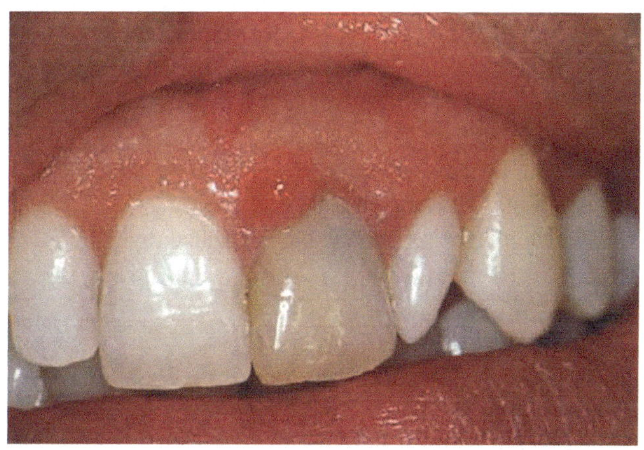

Fig. 41.7 Peripheral ossifying fibroma, tumor on the gingiva

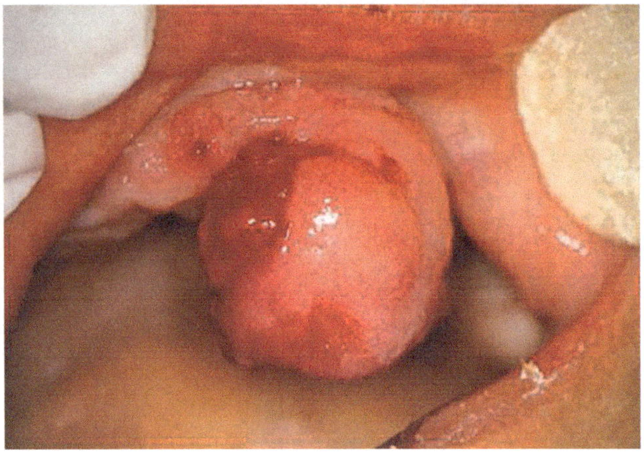

Fig. 41.8 Peripheral ossifying fibroma, large lesion on the edentulous alveolar mucosa

Laboratory Tests Histopathologic examination, radiography.

Treatment Conservative surgical excision.

Lipoma

Definition A benign tumor of the adipose tissue.

Etiology Unclear.

Gingival Involvement Rare.Unrelated lesion to dental biofilm.

Other Sites of Involvement Oral mucosa, other mucosae, skin.

Clinical Features

- Clinically, oral lipoma presents as a well-demarcated, painless tumor, usually sessile, of yellow or pink-yellow color. It is covered by a thin mucosal layer with visible blood capillaries. On palpation, it is usually soft and occasionally fluctuant.
- Gingival lesions may rarely develop on the attached gingiva. (Figs. 41.9 and 41.10).
- Clinical diagnosis should be confirmed by laboratory tests.

Differential Diagnosis

- Abscesses
- Fibroma
- Peripheral ossifying fibroma
- Cysts
- Giant cell tumor
- Pyogenic granuloma
- Oral focal mucinosis

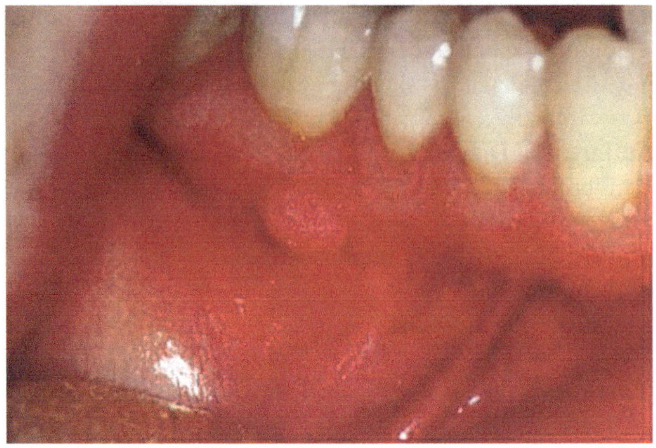

Fig. 41.9 Lipoma, presenting as swelling on the attached gingiva

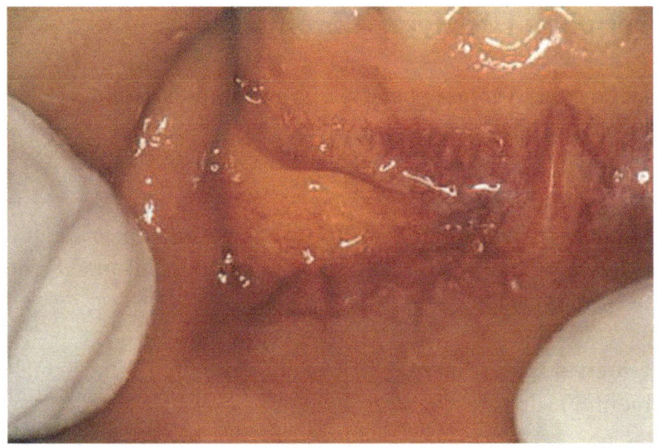

Fig. 41.10 Lipoma, swelling at the labial-gingival fold of the mandible

Laboratory Tests Histopathologic examination.

Treatment Conservative surgical excision.

Neurofibroma

Definition Neurofibroma is a benign tumor of a peripheral nerve (axon, cylinder, Schwann cells, and fibrous connective tissue), arranged in a variety of patterns.

Etiology Unknown.

Gingival Involvement Rare. Unrelated to dental biofilm lesion.

Other Sites of Involvement Oral mucosa, other mucosae, skin. It may be solitary or multiple as part of neurofibromatosis.

Clinical Features

- Clinically, oral neurofibroma presents as a slowly developing, well-circumscribed, usually pedunculated and painless tumor of relatively firm consistency that is covered by normal mucosa. The size varies from several mm to several cm.
- Gingival neurofibroma is rare and commonly develops on the attached gingiva (Fig. 41.11).
- Skin lesions present as solitary or multiple nodules, which can be a manifestation of several types of Neurofibromatosis (Fig. 41.12).
- Clinical diagnosis should be confirmed by laboratory tests.

Differential Diagnosis

- Schwannoma
- Fibroma
- Cysts
- Giant cell tumor
- Pyogenic granuloma
- Abscesses

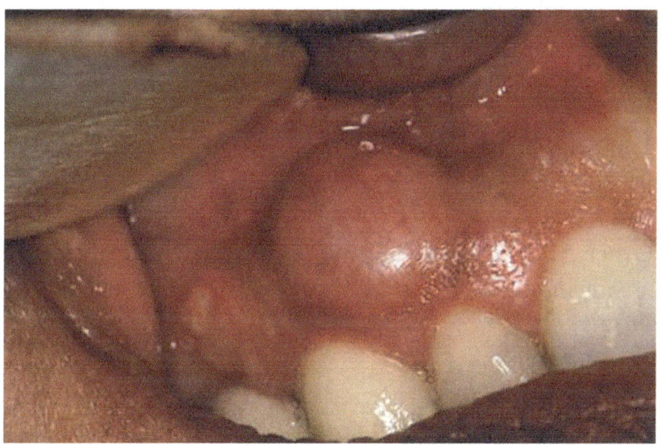

Fig. 41.11 Neurofibroma, tumor on the gingiva covered by normal mucosa

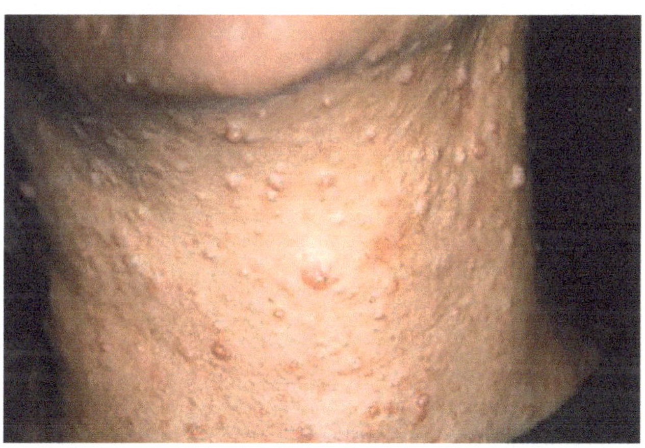

Fig. 41.12 Neurofibromatosis (Von Recklinghausen disease), multiple skin neurofibromas

Laboratory Tests Histopathologic and immunohistochemical examinations.

Treatment Conservative surgical excision.

Schwannoma

Definition Schwannoma or neurilemmoma is a relatively rare, benign tumor of the nervous tissue that derives from the *Schwann cells.*

Etiology Unknown.

Gingival Involvement Rare. Gingival lesion unrelated to dental biofilm.

Other Sites of Involvement Tongue (common), buccal mucosa, palate, floor of the mouth, lips, jaws, skin of the head and neck (common). The tumor may be solitary or part of neurofibromatosis type-2.

Clinical Features

- Clinically, gingival and oral schwannoma presents as a slowly growing, well-circumscribed, solitary, firm, and usually painless tumor that is covered by normal mucosa (Fig. 41.13). The size ranges from 0.5 to 2 cm in diameter.
- The clinical features are not diagnostic, and the diagnosis should be confirmed by laboratory tests.

Differential Diagnosis

- Neurofibroma
- Leiomyoma
- Fibrous histiocytoma
- Granular cell tumor

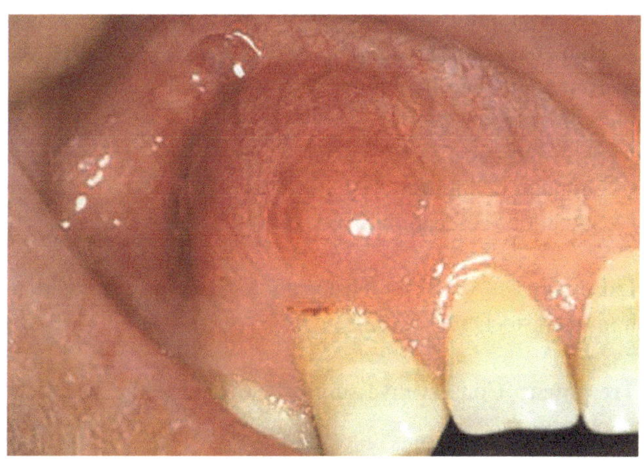

Fig. 41.13 Schwannoma, swelling on the gingiva

- Fibroma
- Peripheral ossifying fibroma

Laboratory Tests Histopathologic and immunohistochemical examination.

Treatment Conservative surgical excision.

Leiomyoma

Definition Leiomyoma is a benign tumor which originates from smooth muscle tissue.

Etiology Unknown.

Classification Three main types are recognized: a. *solid*, b. *vascular*, c. *epithelioid*.

Gingival Involvement Rare.

Other Sites of Involvement Gastrointestinal tract, uterus, skin and oral mucosa (rare).

Clinical Features

- Oral leiomyoma affects equally males and females usually over the age of 30 years.
- Oral leiomyoma originates from the smooth muscles of blood vessels or the circumvallate papillae of the tongue.
- Clinically, it presents as a slow-developing, usually painless, firm, well-circumscribed nodule of normal or red-brown color (Fig. 41.14). The tumor may rarely be ulcerated.
- The most common affected oral sites are the tongue, buccal mucosa, palate, and lips.
- Clinical diagnosis should be confirmed by laboratory tests.

Differential Diagnosis

- Hemangioma
- Hemangiopericytoma
- Hemangioendothelioma
- Neurofibroma
- Schwannoma
- Granular cell tumor
- Squamous cell carcinoma

Laboratory Tests Histopathologic examination, immunohistochemistry.

Treatment Conservative surgical excision is the treatment of choice.

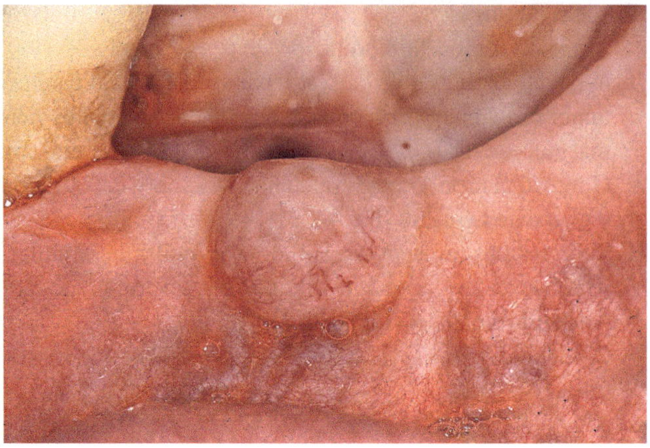

Fig. 41.14 Leiomyoma, ulcerated redish nodule on the alveolar mucosa

Soft Tissue Chondroma

Definition A benign tumor of cartilage tissue that may exceedingly rarely develop in the oral soft tissues.

Etiology Unclear.

Gingival Involvement Rare. Unrelated to dental biofilm lesion.

Other Sites of Involvement Usually presents as a lesion arising in the jaw, sometimes only revealed coincidentally by imaging.

Clinical Features

- The tumor is rare in the jaws, rarely may present as a swelling involving the gingiva.
- Chondromas are typically found in the elderly in the anterior maxilla, mandibular symphysis, and the coronoid and condylar processes. Clinically, the gingival lesions form slow-growing, painless masses covered by normal mucosa (Fig. 41.15).
- Multiple enchondromas are seen in the Ollier syndrome, but oral tumors are a rare feature of this condition.
- Clinical diagnosis should be confirmed by laboratory tests.

Differential Diagnosis

- Abscesses
- Fibroma
- Giant cell tumor
- Pyogenic granuloma
- Peripheral ossifying fibroma

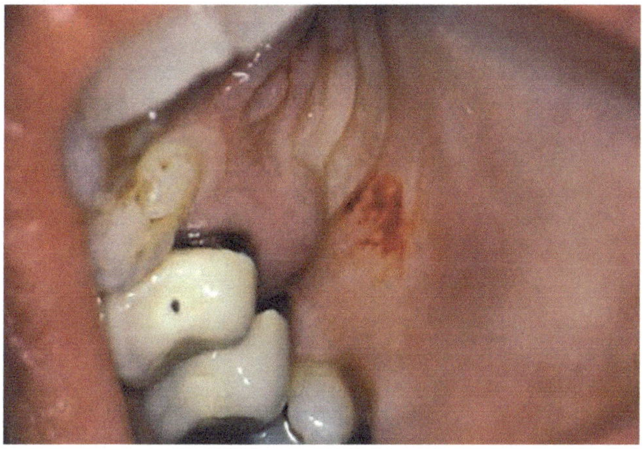

Fig. 41.15 Soft tissue chondroma, swelling on the gingiva of the palate

Laboratory Tests Histopathologic examination, radiography.

Treatment Conservativesurgical excision.

Jaw Osteoma

Definition Osteoma is a benign tumor composed of mature compact or cancellous bone, unrelated to jaws tori.

Etiology Unknown.

Gingival Involvement Almost never. However, peripheral osteoma of the jaws at the alveolar ridge may form localized gingival swelling.

Other Sites of Involvement Craniofacial skeleton.

Clinical Features

- Clinically, alveolar bone osteoma presents as painless and well-circumscribed hard enlargement covered by thin, smooth normal mucosa. The size ranges from 0.5 to 1 cm in diameter (Fig. 41.16).
- The neighboring gingival tissue is usually normal, although the color may be pale.
- Clinical diagnosis should be confirmed by laboratory tests.

Differential Diagnosis

- Torus mandibularis
- Multiple buccal jaws exostoses
- Gardner syndrome

Laboratory Tests Histopathologic examination, panoramic radiography.

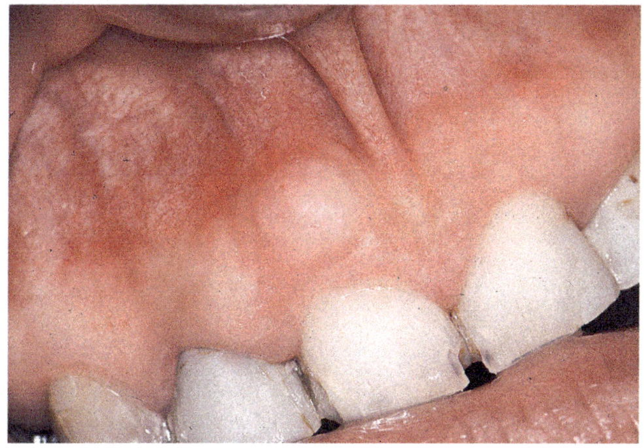

Fig. 41.16 Osteoma, tumor covered with normal mucosa on the upper gingiva

Treatment Conservative surgical excision.

Verruciform Xanthoma

Definition Verruciform xanthoma is a rare benign lesion of the oral mucosa with characteristic histopathologic pattern.

Etiology Unknown. Non-dental biofilm-induced gingival lesion.

Gingival Involvement The gingiva and the alveolar mucosa are the most commonly affected.

Other Sites of Involvement Buccal mucosa, tongue, palate, floor of the mouth, lips.

Clinical Features

- Clinically, gingival lesion appears as a painless, sessile, well-demarcated, and usually slightly elevated lesion with a papillary surface and normal or whitish-yellowish color (Figs. 41.17 and 41.18). The size ranges from 0.2 to 2.0 cm in diameter.
- The lesion is not associated with any other systemic metabolic disease.
- Clinical diagnosis should be confirmed by laboratory tests.

Differential Diagnosis

- Papilloma
- Condyloma accuminatum
- Verruca vulgaris
- Sialadenoma papilliferum
- Verrucous leukoplakia
- Early verrucous carcinoma

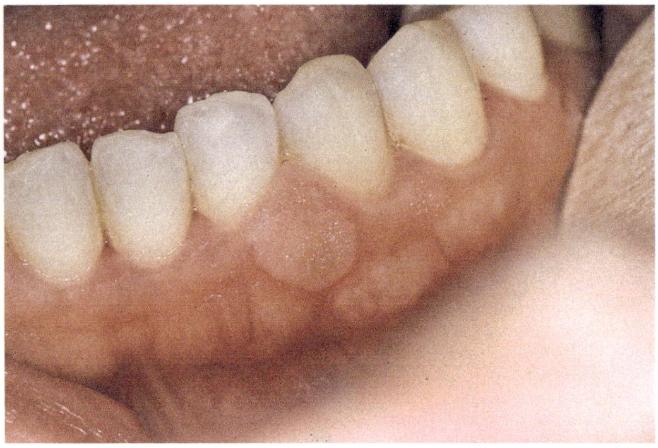

Fig. 41.17 Verruciform xanthoma, papillary nodule on the gingiva

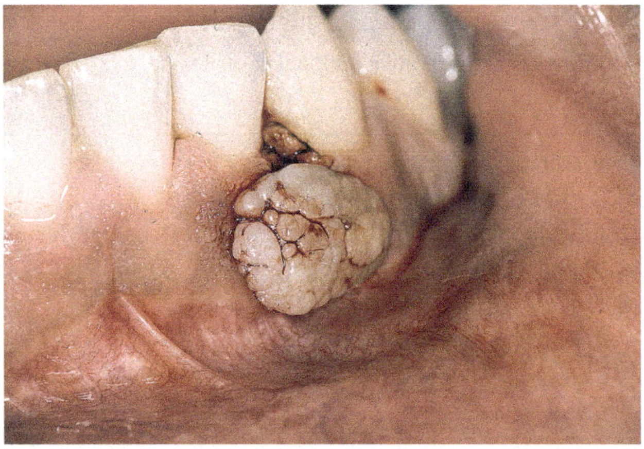

Fig. 41.18 Verruciform xanthoma, large papillary white nodule on the gingiva

Laboratory Tests Histopathologic and immunohistochemical examination.

Treatment Conservative surgical excision.

Melanoacanthoma

Definition Melanoacanthoma is a benign, acquired pigmentary disorder due to an increased number of dendritic melanocytes and melanin production.

Etiology Unknown.

Gingival Involvement Rare. Non-dental biofilm-induced gingival lesion.

Other Sites of Involvement Skin (common), oral mucosa, (palate, lips) (rare).

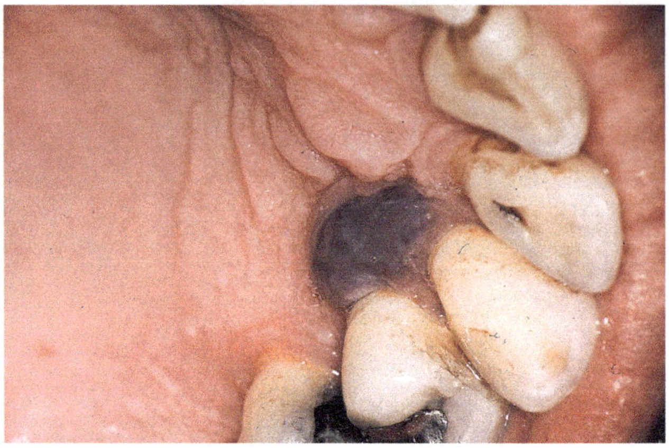

Fig. 41.19 Melanoacanthoma, black tumor on the palatal gingiva

Clinical Features
- Clinically, gingival and oral melanoacanthoma appears as a flat or slightly elevated macule or plaque of black or brown-black color (Fig. 41.19). The size varies from 1 to 3 cm.
- Clinical diagnosis should be confirmed by laboratory tests.

Differential Diagnosis
- Melanocytic nevi
- Lendigosimplex
- Ephelides
- Malignant melanoma
- Amalgam tattoo
- Drug-induced melanosis

Laboratory Tests Histopathologic and histochemical examination.

Treatment Conservative surgical excision.

Melanotic Neuroectodermal Tumor of Infancy

Definition Melanotic neuroectodermal tumor of infancy is a rare benign tumor of neural crest origin, with a propensity to develop in tooth-bearing areas that usually appears during the first 2 years of life.

Etiology Unknown.

Gingival Involvement None. Bone, alveolar mucosa, or gingival swelling usually at the anterior part of the maxilla is the main feature (70–75%).

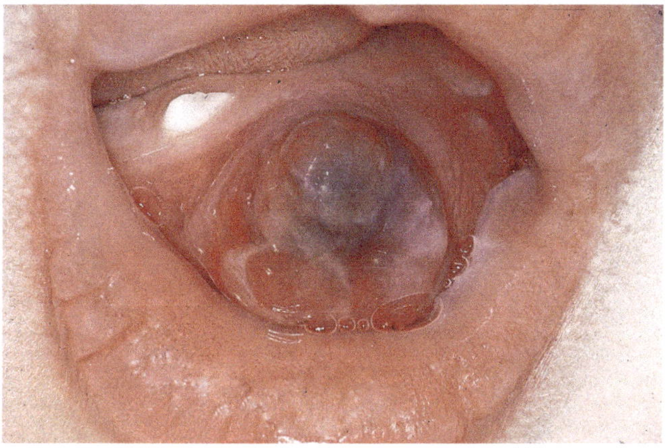

Fig. 41.20 Melanotic neuroectodermal tumor of infancy, red-blue irregular mass on the mandible

Other Sites of Involvement Skull, brain, epididymis, testicles, mandible.

Clinical Features

- Clinically, oral tumor appears as a rapidly growing painless mass of red brown-brown or normal color, which is usually covered by normal mucosa (Fig. 41.20). The tumor potentially destroys the underlying bone and may provoke displacement of teeth. This, in association with rapid development, mimics a malignancy.
- Clinical diagnosis should be confirmed by laboratory tests.

Differential Diagnosis

- Granular cell tumor of infancy
- Osteosarcoma
- Chondrosarcoma
- Ewing sarcoma
- Neuroblastoma
- Odontogenic tumors
- Eruption cyst

Laboratory Tests Histopathologic and immunohistochemical examination. Dental scan tomography. Increased level of vanillymandelic acid in urine.

Treatment Conservative surgical removal or curettage.

Hemangioma

Definition Hemangioma is a benign vascular tissue tumor classified in the spectrum of vascular malformations that develop during infancy and childhood.

Etiology Developmental disorder due to endothelial cell proliferation.

Gingival Involvement Relatively common.

Other Sites of Involvement Oral mucosa (lips, tongue, palate) common, jaws rare, skin common.

Classification Three forms are recognized: a. *Superficial*or *capillary*, b.*deep* or *cavernous,* and c. *mixed.*

Clinical Features

- Clinically gingival superficial hemangioma consists of multiple, small capillaries that present as flat or slightly elevated painless bright red macule or plaque (Fig. 41.21). The deep form consists of large vascular blood-filled spaces and clinically presents as an elevated asymptomatic red or brown-red color (Fig. 41.22).
- The size varies between a few to several centimeters.
- A characteristic clinical sign is branching with pressure.
- Diagnosis is mainly based on the history and the clinical features.

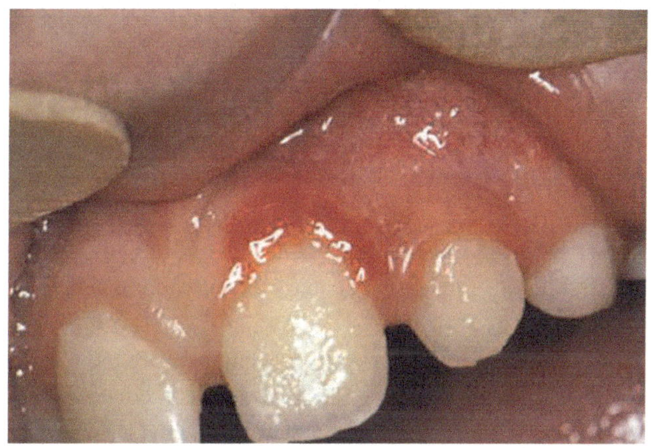

Fig. 41.21 Hemangioma, red elevated lesion on the gingiva of a central incisor

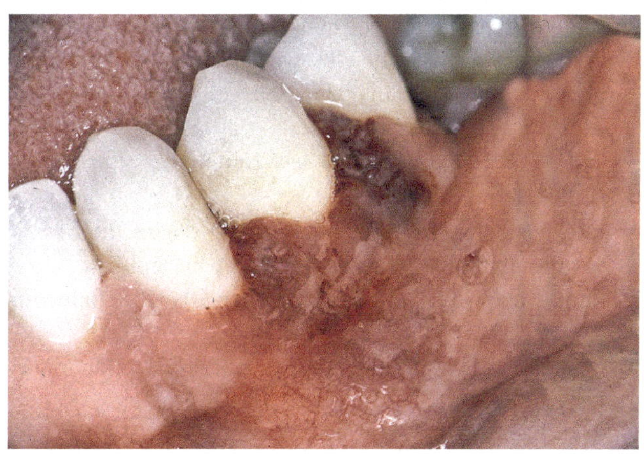

Fig. 41.22 Hemangioma, red-blue colored elevated plaque on the gingiva

Differential Diagnosis

- Localized juvenile spongiotic gingival hyperplasia
- Vascular malformations
- Pyogenic granuloma
- Lymphangioma
- Leiomyoma
- Angiosarcoma
- Kaposi sarcoma
- Genetic syndromes associated with vascular anomalies

Laboratory Tests Histopathologic examination. However, during biopsy precautions should be taken for the danger of bleeding.

Treatment Surgical excision, laser, cryotherapy for small lesions. Embolization and sclerotherapy for major lesions.

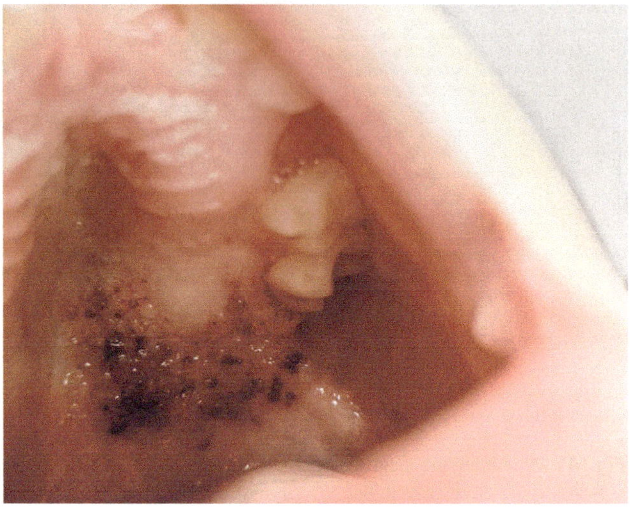

Fig. 41.23 Lymphangioma on the gingiva expanding to the palate

Lymphangioma

Definition Lymphangioma is a benign developmental disorder of the lymphatic system.

Etiology Developmental malformation.

Gingival Involvement Rare.

Other Sites of Involvement Oral mucosa (tongue, buccal mucosa, floor of the mouth, palate, lips) common, skin.

Classification Four forms of lymphangioma are recognized a. *Microcystic* or *capillary,* b.*macrocystic*or *cavernous,* c. *mixed* or *micro-macrocystic,* and d. the *cystic hygroma,* a specific type of macrocystic form.

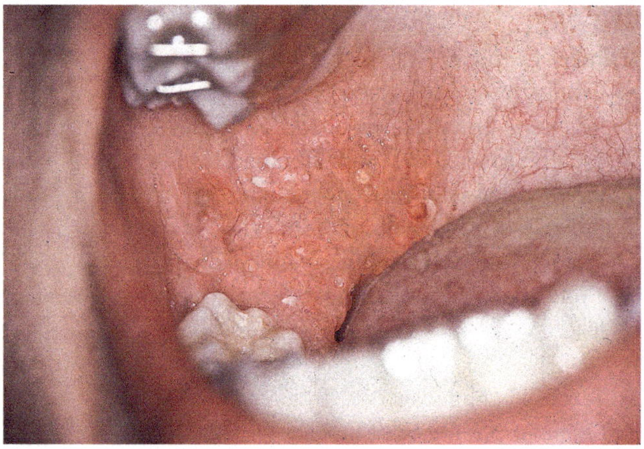

Fig. 41.24 Lymphangioma on the gingiva extended to the palate and retromolar area

Clinical Features

- Clinically gingival lymphangioma presents as multiple small, soft asymptomatic nodules resembling a small cyst or vesicle, with a yellow-brown or red color, if the lymphatic spaces contain red blood cells (Fig. 41.23 and 41.24).
- The size ranges from a few millimeters to several centimeters.
- Extensive oral lymphangiomas on the tongue, floor of the mouth and palate may cause mild pain and discomfort during chewing and speech, particularly after infection (Fig. 41.25).
- Clinical diagnosis should be confirmed by laboratory tests.

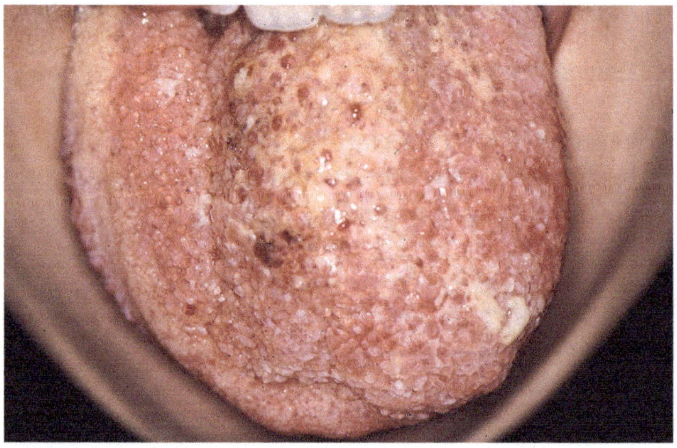

Fig. 41.25 Lymphangioma, multiple lesions on the dorsum of the tongue

Differential Diagnosis

- Hemangioma
- Vascular malformation
- Vesicular and bullous lesions on the gingiva
- Acquired lymphangiectasia
- Papillary hyperplasia of the palate
- Lymphoepithelial cysts
- Median rhomboid glossitis

Laboratory Tests Histopathologic examination, MRI, CT scan for large lesions.

Treatment Conservative surgical excision or laser for small lesions. Large lymphangiomas should be referred to specialized oral surgeons.

References

1. Bawazir M, Islam MN, Cohen DM, et al. Gingival fibroma: an emerging distinct gingival lesion with well-defined histopathology. Head Neck Pathol. 2021;15(3):917–22. https://doi.org/10.1007/s12105-021-01315-7. Epub ahead of print
2. Garg R, Margabandhu M, Paul A, Babu K. Gingival fibroma versus verrucous leukoplakia - a clinical dilemma. J Indian Soc Periodontol. 2016;20(6):635–7. https://doi.org/10.4103/jisp.jisp_200_16. PMID: 29238146; PMCID: PMC5713089
3. Kuo RCWY, CheKruse-Losler Bn HM, Sun A, et al. Clinicopathological study of oral giant cell fibromas. J Formos Med Assoc. 2009;108:725.
4. daSilva FC, Piazzetta CM, Torres-Pereira CC, et al. Gingival proliferative lesions in children and adolescents in Brazil: a 15-year-period cross-sectional study. J Indian Soc Periodontol. 2016;20(1):63–6. https://doi.org/10.4103/0972-124X.168493. PMID: 27041840; PMCID: PMC4795138
5. Franco-Barrera MJ, Zavala-Cerna MG, Fernández-Tamayo R, et al. An update on peripheral ossifying fibroma: case report and literature review. Oral Maxillofac Surg. 2016;20(1):1–7. https://doi.org/10.1007/s10006-015-0535-0. Epub 2015 Nov 10. Erratum in: Oral Maxillofac Surg. 2017 Mar;21(1):105. PMID: 26556782
6. Furlong MA, Fanburg-Smith JC, Childers EL. Lipoma of the oral and maxillofacial region: site and subclassification of 125 cases. Oral Surg Oral Med Oral Pathol Oral Radiol Endod. 2004;98:441–50.
7. Schafer DR, Glass SH. A guide to yellow oral mucosal entities: etiology and pathology. Head Neck Pathol. 2019;13(1):33–46. https://doi.org/10.1007/s12105-018-0977-4. Epub 2019 Jan 31. PMID: 30693453; PMCID: PMC6405798
8. Fontana S, Menutti L, Borrego F, et al. Neurofibroma solitario intrabuccal. Reporte de un caso de manifestación poco frecuente [Isolated neurofibroma of oral cavity. An unusual manifestation case report.]. Rev Fac Cien Med Univ Nac Cordoba. 2020;77(1):45–8. https://doi.org/10.31053/1853.0605.v77.n1.25244. PMID: 32238258
9. Kubota S, Imai T, Iwai S, et al. Gingival neurofibroma with teardrop-shaped defects of the interdental alveolar bone: an unusual oral manifestation of Neurofibromatosis type 1. J Craniofac Surg. 2019;30(3):e205–7. https://doi.org/10.1097/SCS.0000000000005094. PMID: 30444769
10. Kumar M, Rao M, Elhence P, et al. Schwannoma of head-and-neck region: a clinical chameleon–report of two cases occurring at rare sites with unusual clinical manifestations. J Oral Maxillofac Pathol. 2020;24(1):164–7. https://doi.org/10.4103/jomfp.JOMFP_13_20. Epub 2020 May 8. PMID: 32508467; PMCID: PMC7269292
11. Sanchis JM, Navarro CM, Bagán JV, et al. Intraoral schwannomas: presentation of a series of 12 cases. J Clin Exp Dent. 2013;5(4):e192–6. https://doi.org/10.4317/jced.51176. PMID: 24455080; PMCID: PMC3892247
12. Gianluca S, Marini R, Tonoli F, Cristalli MP. Leiomyoma of oral cavity: case report and literature review. Ann Stomatol (Roma). 2011;2(1–2):9–12. Epub 2011 Jul 18. PMID: 22238716; PMCID: PMC3254389
13. Veeresh M, Sudhakara M, Girish G, Naik C. Leiomyoma: a rare tumor in the head and neck and oral cavity: report of 3 cases with review. J Oral Maxillofac Pathol. 2013;17(2):281–7. https://doi.org/10.4103/0973-029X.119770. PMID: 24250094; PMCID: PMC3830242
14. Kim Y, Moses M, Zegarelli DJ, Yoon AJ. Cartilage choristoma (soft tissue chondroma): a rare presentation in the lower lip. J Clin Pediatr Dent. 2009;33:253–4.
15. Tosios K, Laskaris G, Eveson J, Scully C. Benign cartilaginous tumor of the gingiva. A case report. Int J Oral Maxillofac Surg. 1993;22(4):231–3. https://doi.org/10.1016/s0901-5027(05)80642-3. PMID: 8409565
16. Ostrofsky M, Morkel JA, Titinchi F. Osteoma of the mandibular condyle: a rare case report and review of the literature. J Stomatol Oral Maxillofac Surg. 2019;120(6):584–7. https://doi.org/10.1016/j.jormas.2019.01.013. Epub 2019 Jan 25. PMID: 30685345
17. Jones AC, Prihoda TJ, Kacher JE, et al. Osteoblastoma of the maxilla and mandible: a report of 24 cases, review of the literature, and discussion of its relationship to osteoid osteoma of the jaws. Oral Surg Oral Med Oral Pathol Oral Radiol Endod. 2006;102(5):639–50. https://doi.org/10.1016/j.tripleo.2005.09.004. Epub 2006 Apr 17. PMID: 17052641
18. Hu JA, Li Y, Li S. Verruciform xanthoma of the oral cavity: Clinicopathological study relating to pathogenesis: report of three cases. APMIS. 2005;113:629–34.
19. Philipsen HPRP, Takata T, Ogawa I. Verruciform xanthoma–biological profile of 282 oral lesions based on a literature survey with nine new cases from Japan. Oral Oncol. 2003;39:325.
20. Tandon A, Srivastava A, Jaiswal R, Bordoloi B. A rare case of oral melanoacanthoma. J Oral Maxillofac Pathol. 2018;22(3):410–2. https://doi.org/10.4103/jomfp.JOMFP_96_18. PMID: 30651689; PMCID: PMC6306582
21. Soles BS, Wilson A, Lucas DR, Heider A. Melanotic neuroectodermal tumor of infancy. Arch Pathol Lab Med. 2018;142(11):1358–63. https://doi.org/10.5858/arpa.2018-0241-RA. PMID: 30407852
22. Yu Q, Wang WX. Camrelizumab (SHR-1210) leading to reactive capillary hemangioma in the gingiva: a case report. World J Clin Cases. 2020;8(3):624–9. https://doi.org/10.12998/wjcc.v8.i3.624. PMID: 32110675; PMCID: PMC7031842
23. Havle AD, Shedge SA, Dalvi RG. Lobular capillary hemangioma of the palate–a case report. Iran J Otorhinolaryngol. 2019;31(107):399–402. https://doi.org/10.22038/ijorl.2019.38928.2285. PMID: 31857986; PMCID: PMC6914325
24. Müller S. Update from the 4th edition of the World Health Organization of head and neck Tumours: Tumours of the oral cavity and mobile tongue. Head Neck Pathol. 2017;11(1):33–40. https://doi.org/10.1007/s12105-017-0792-3. Epub 2017 Feb 28. PMID: 28247230; PMCID: PMC5340733
25. Corrêa PH, Nunes LC, Johann AC, et al. Prevalence of oral hemangioma, vascular malformation and varix in a Brazilian population. Braz Oral Res. 2007;21(1):40–5. https://doi.org/10.1590/s1806-83242007000100007. PMID: 17384854
26. Barrón-Peña A, Martínez-Borras MA, Benítez-Cárdenas O, et al. Management of the oral hemangiomas in infants and children: scoping review. Med Oral Patol Oral Cir Bucal. 2020;25(2):e252–61. https://doi.org/10.4317/medoral.23329. PMID: 31967983; PMCID: PMC7103441.
27. Pugalagiri P, Muller S, Cox DP, et al. Lymphangioma-like Kaposi sarcoma of the oral mucosa. Oral Surg Oral Med Oral

Pathol Oral Radiol. 2013;116(1):84–90. https://doi.org/10.1016/j.oooo.2013.04.007. PMID: 23768875

28. Devi A, Narwal A, Yadav AB, et al. Classical cases of lymphangioma–as multiple vesicular eruptions. J Clin Diagn Res. 2016;10(6):ZD22–3. https://doi.org/10.7860/JCDR/2016/18043.8046. Epub 2016 Jun 1. PMID: 27504428; PMCID: PMC4963788
29. Babu DB, Kumar BR, Boinepally NH, Gannepalli A. A case of intraoral lymphangioma circumscripta–A diagnostic dilemma. J Clin Diagn Res. 2015;9(10):ZD11–3. https://doi.org/10.7860/JCDR/2015/14741.6629. Epub 2015 Oct 1. PMID: 26557627; PMCID: PMC4625346
30. Motahhary P, Sarrafpour B, Abdirad A. Bilateral symmetrical lymphangiomas of the gingiva: case report. Diagn Pathol. 2006;1:9. https://doi.org/10.1186/1746-1596-1-9. PMID: 16759365; PMCID: PMC1479837

Malignant Tumors

42

Contents

Oral malignant tumors (neoplasms) may occur usually as *primary* lesions of periodontal tissues or, rarely, as *secondary* metastatic neoplasms from primary lesions of other organs.

Surface Epithelium

Squamous Cell Carcinoma

Definition Squamous cell carcinoma is the most common malignant tumor of the oral cavity, accounting for 90–95% of oral malignancies.

Etiology Multifactorial (extrinsic and intrinsic factors). The most important factors are: smoking (over 90% of the patients are smokers), alcohol consumption, chemicals, HPV (mainly types 16, 18, 33, 53), sunlight exposure (lips), malnutrition, iron deficiency anemia, immunodeficiency, and genetics. The hallmarks of human cancer share some common properties such as: sustained proliferation, escape from apoptosis, and genomic instability.

Gingival Involvement Relatively rare (8–10%). Non-dental biofilm-induced gingival lesion.

Other Sites of Involvement Tongue (over 50%), lower lip, buccal mucosa, floor of the mouth, palate, alveolar mucosa.

Clinical Features

- The disease appears equally among males and females, commonly over 40 years of age.
- Oral squamous cell carcinoma presents with great clinical polymorphism. In the *early stage*, it appears as an asymptomatic white or red or mixed color plaque, small nodule, or erosion. In *advanced stage,* it appears as a superficial or deep ulcer with irregular vegetating surface and elevated hard border, or as an exophytic, usually ulcerated, irregular mostly painful mass, or as an endophytic process, indurated on palpation.
- Gingival lesions usually present as white or red plaques or tumors with elevated nodular surface, mimicking a reactive tumor or severe periodontitis (Figs. 42.1, 42.2, 42.3). In *advanced stage*, the gingival carcinoma often destroys the underlying bone and causes increased probing depths and tooth mobility (Figs. 42.4, 42.5). The mandibular gin-

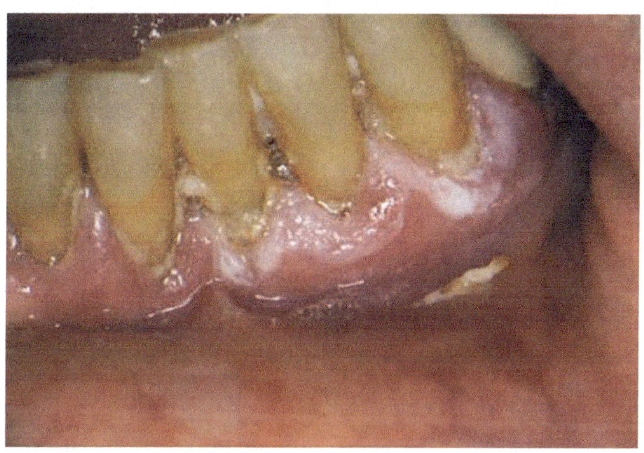

Fig. 42.1 Squamous cell carcinoma, early lesion on the anterior gingiva of the mandible

G. Laskaris et al., *Periodontal Manifestations of Local and Systemic Diseases*, https://doi.org/10.1007/978-3-031-10828-0_42

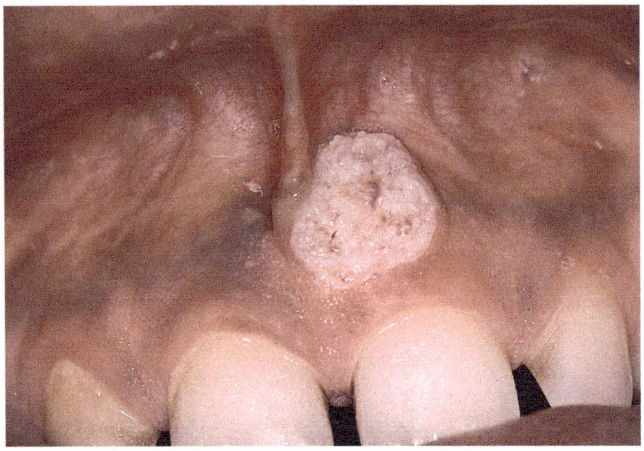

Fig. 42.2 Early squamous cell carcinoma on the gingiva

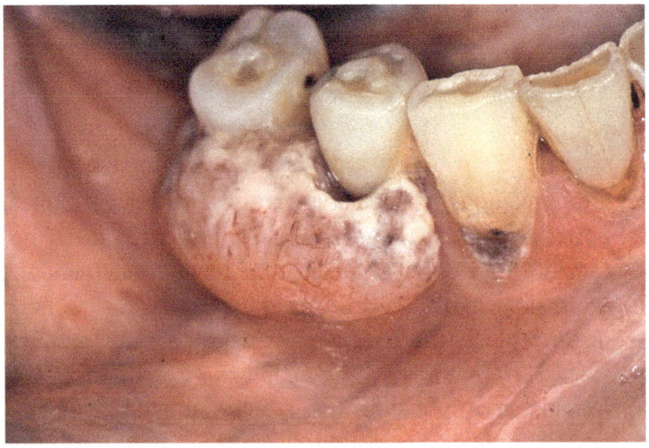

Fig. 42.3 Squamous cell carcinoma on the gingiva presenting as exophytic mass

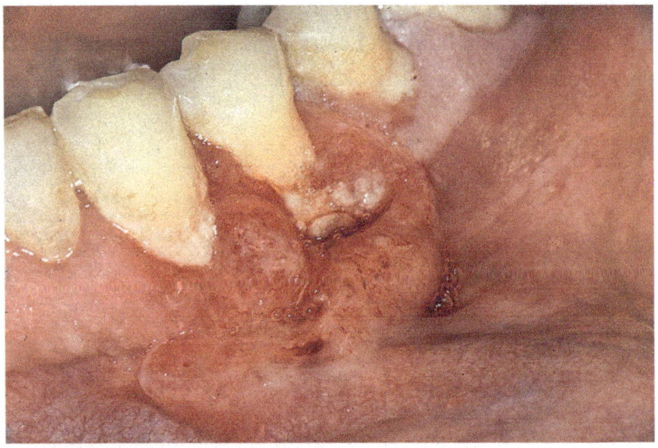

Fig. 42.4 Squamous cell carcinoma, large ulcerated tumor on the gingiva, advanced stage

gival and the retromolar region are more frequently affected.

- Metastases to the regional cervical lymph nodes are common.

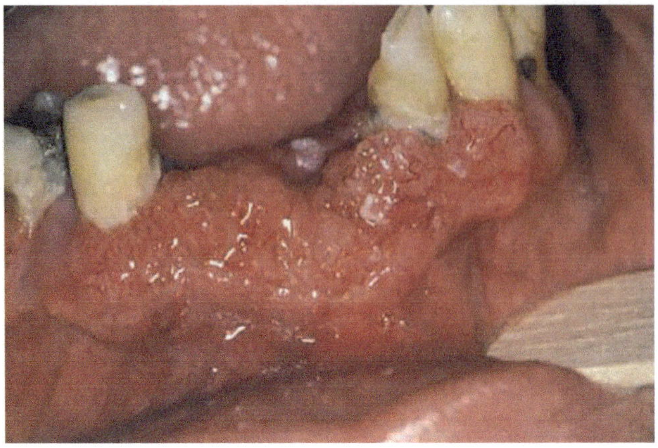

Fig. 42.5 Squamous cell carcinoma on the mandibular gingiva, advanced stage

- Periodontists and general dentists should suspect gingival carcinoma, if a lesion persists for more than 10–15 days, in the absence of a clear etiologic factor. In such cases, a biopsy and histopathologic examination are necessary.

Differential Diagnosis
- Severe localized, with rapid rate of progression periodontitis
- Leukoplakia
- Erythroplakia
- Traumatic ulcer
- Aphthous ulcer
- Reactive tumors
- Wegener granulomatosis
- Non-Hodgkin lymphoma
- Leukemia
- Tuberculous ulcer
- Drug-induced ulceration
- Any atypical gingival lesion that persists over 10–15 days.

Laboratory Tests Histopathologic and immunohistochemical examination. Molecular detection of HPV types.

Treatment Radical surgical excision with or without radiotherapy and/or chemotherapy. Targeted therapy with monoclonal antibodies has been recently used.

Verrucous Carcinoma

Definition Verrucous carcinoma is a low-grade variant of squamous cell carcinoma with good biologic behavior and prognosis.

Etiology Smoking, human papilloma virus (HPV), mainly types 16, 18, and 33.

Gingival Involvement Relatively common. Non-dental biofilm-related lesions.

Other Sites of Involvement Alveolar mucosa, buccal mucosa, palate, floor of the mouth. Other mucosa (larynx, pharynx, vagina, anus), skin.

Clinical Features

- Clinically, gingival verrucous carcinoma presents as a slow-growing, painless, exophytic mass with a characteristic cauliflower-like whitish surface (Figs. 42.6, 42.7, 42.8). The size ranges from 1 to several centimeters if left untreated. It develops more commonly in males than females (2:1), usually older than 60 years of age.
- It rarely metastasizes and has a characteristic histopathologic pattern. If untreated for a long time, it may transform into squamous cell carcinoma.
- Clinical diagnosis should be confirmed by laboratory tests.

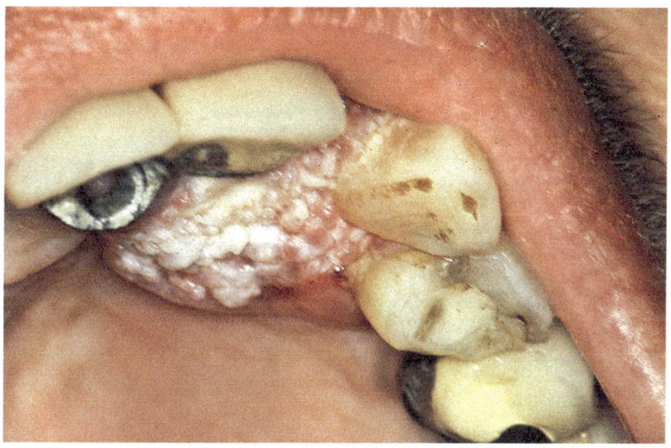

Fig. 42.6 Verrucous carcinoma, tumor with cauliflower appearance on the palatal gingiva

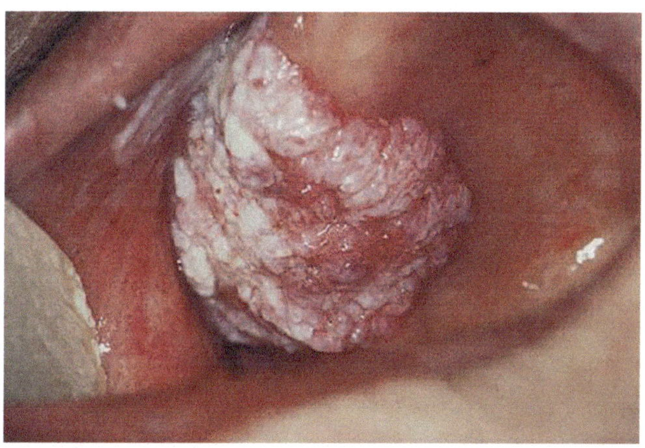

Fig. 42.7 Verrucous carcinoma, large tumor on edentulous gingiva

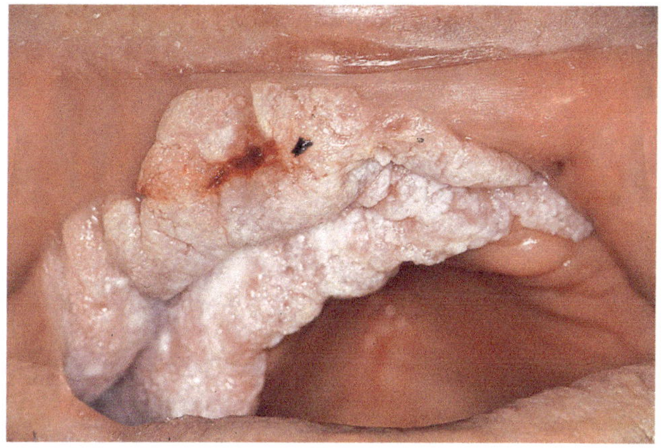

Fig. 42.8 Verrucous carcinoma, extensive large tumor on the alveolar mucosa

Differential Diagnosis

- Verrucous leukoplakia
- Verrucous hyperplasia
- Papilloma
- Squamous cell carcinoma
- Verruciform xanthoma
- White sponge nevous

Laboratory Tests Histopathologic and molecular examination.

Treatment Surgical excision is the treatment of choice. Radiotherapy and/or chemotherapy only when surgery is not indicated in advanced cases.

Mesenchyme

Malignant Fibrous Histiocytoma

Definition Maligant fibrous histiocytoma is one of the most common soft tissue sarcomas in adults, but it is very rare in the head and neck area as well as in oral cavity. It derives from fibroblasts and histiocytes.

Etiology Unknown.

Gingival Involvement Very rare. Unrelated to dental biofilm lesions.

Other Sites of Involvement Skin and other connective soft tissue organs, mouth (rare).

Clinical Features

- Clinically, gingival tumor presents as a rapidly growing painless or painful exophytic mass of deep red-brown

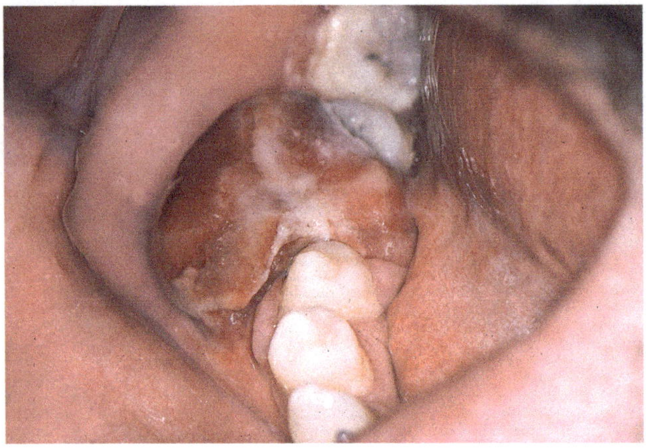

Fig. 42.9 Malignant fibrous histiocytoma, exophytic reddish mass on the gingiva

color with or without ulceration (Fig. 42.9). The size ranges from 2 to 5 cm.
- The clinical features are not characteristic, and clinical diagnosis should be confirmed with laboratory tests.

Differential Diagnosis
- Pyogenic granuloma
- Peripheral giant cell granuloma
- Kaposi sarcoma
- Other types of sarcomas

Laboratory Tests Histopathologic and histochemical examination.

Treatment Radical surgical excision is the treatment of choice. Radiotherapy and chemotherapy are adjunctive therapies.

Leiomyosarcoma

Definition Leiomyosarcomais a malignant neoplasm of the smooth muscle tissue, which accounts for 4–8% of all cases of soft tissue sarcomas.

Etiology Unknown.

Gingival Involvement Rare. Unrelated to dental biofilm lesions.

Other Sites of Involvement Oral mucosa (rare), gastrointestinal tract, uterus, skin.

Clinical Features
- Oral leiomyosarcoma may derive from the smooth muscle cells of the blood vessels and the circumvallate papillae of the tongue.
- Clinically, gingival leiomyosarcoma presents as a slow-growing, painless or painful, raised firm mass with a smooth red surface that may or may not be ulcerated (Figs. 42.10, 42.11).
- Oral leiomyosarcoma is more common in females, usually over 50 years of age.
- Clinical diagnosis should be confirmed with laboratory tests.

Differential Diagnosis
- Leiomyoma
- Pyogenic granuloma
- Peripheral giant cell granuloma
- Peripheral gingival fibroma
- Angiosarcoma
- Kaposi sarcoma
- Squamous cell carcinoma

Laboratory Tests Histopathologic and histochemical examination.

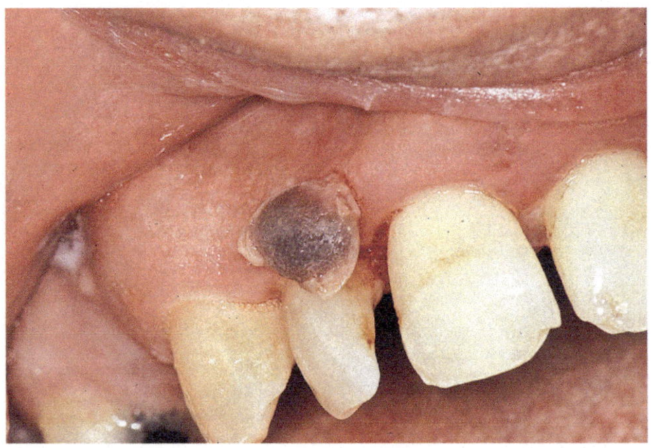

Fig. 42.10 Leiomyosarcoma on the gingiva, small red smooth tumor

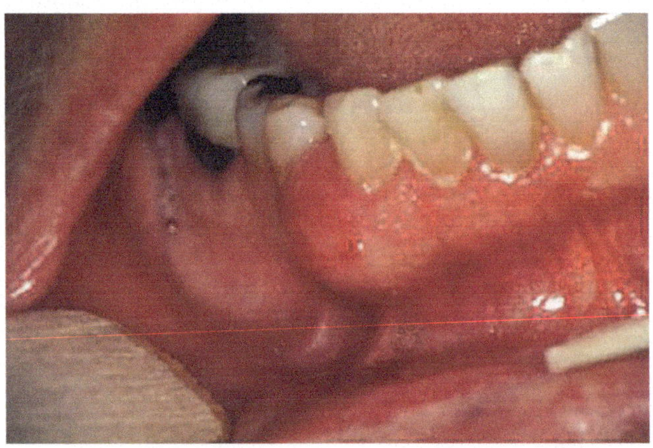

Fig. 42.11 Leiomyosarcoma, swelling on the mandibular gingiva

Treatment Radical surgical excision with or without adjunctive radiotherapy and/or chemotherapy.

Angiosarcoma

Definition Angiosarcoma is a rare malignant neoplasm originating from the endothelial cells of the blood or lymph vessel wall, that primarily occurs in adults.

Etiology Unknown.

Gingival Involvement Very rare.

Other Sites of Involvement Oral mucosa (rare), skin and superficial soft tissue (common).

Clinical Features

- Cutaneous angiosarcoma has a predilection for female patients over 50 years of age, manifested more commonly on the face, scalp, and forehead.
- Clinically, it appears as an elevated firm mass with a violaceous or brown-red color with or without ulceration, that bleeds easily.
- Gingival and oral mucosa lesions present as a nonspecific deep red nodule or plaque that increases centrifugally and soon ulcerates (Figs. 42.12, 42.13).
- The prognosis is usually poor.
- The clinical diagnosis should be confirmed by laboratory tests.

Differential Diagnosis

- Kaposi sarcoma
- Malignant fibrous histiocytoma
- Hemangioma
- Leiomyoma

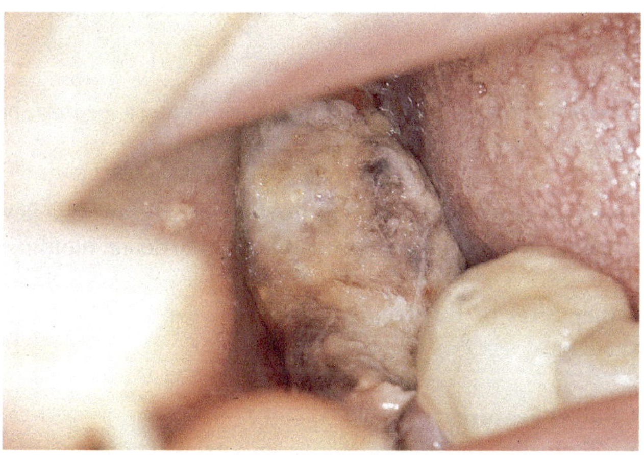

Fig. 42.12 Angiosarcoma, brown-red ulcerated mass on the gingiva and alveolar mucosa of the mandible

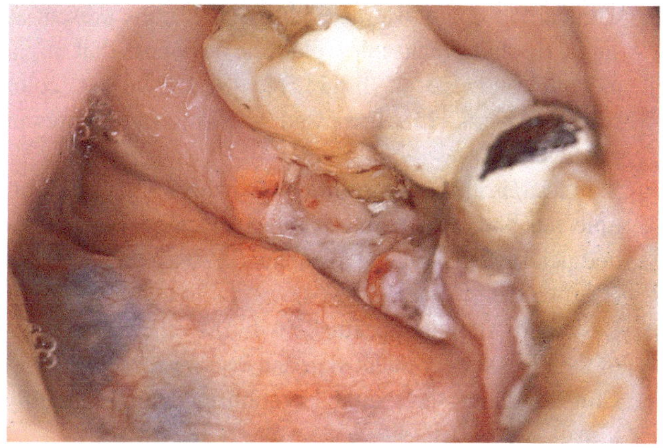

Fig. 42.13 Angiosarcoma, ulcerated irregular mass on the alveolar mucosa and the gingiva

- Leiomyosarcoma
- Peripheral giant cell granuloma
- Pyogenic granuloma

Laboratory Tests Histopathologic and immunohistochemical examination.

Treatment Radical surgical excision is the treatment of choice, usually followed by palliative radiotherapy.

Kaposi Sarcoma

Definition Kaposi sarcoma is a vascular neoplasm described by Moritz Kaposi in 1872, which derives from endothelial cells and predominantly affects the skin.

Etiology The main etiologic factor is human herpes virus-type 8 (HHV-8).

Classification Four clinical types are recognized: a. *classic; b. African endemic; c. iatrogenic (immunosupression-related);* and *d.epidemic (AIDS-related).*

Gingival Involvement Relatively rare. Non-dental biofilm-related lesions.

Other Sites of Involvement Skin (common), oral and other mucosae (rare), viscera.

Clinical Features

- The classic Kaposi sarcoma primarily affects males usually over 60 years of age. It is more common on the Balkan peninsula as well as in individuals of Mediterranean and Jewish descent. The disease mainly affects the skin and rarely the oral and other mucosae and viscera.

- Clinically, the gingival and other oral lesions present as single or multiple macules, plaques, or tumors that might ulcerate and are of bright red or brown-red color (Figs. 42.14, 42.15). The palate and gingiva are sites of predilection.
- Skin lesions also appear as slow-growing solitary or multiple red or brown-purple painless macules, plaques, or nodules, usually on the feet, hand, nose, and the ears (Fig. 42.16).
- Lesions of similar appearance with the other three types of the disease may affect skin and oral mucosa.
- Clinical diagnosis should be confirmed by laboratory tests.

Differential Diagnosis

- Pyogenic granuloma
- Peripheral giant cell granuloma
- Bacillary angiomatosis
- Pigmented nevi
- Amalgam tattoo

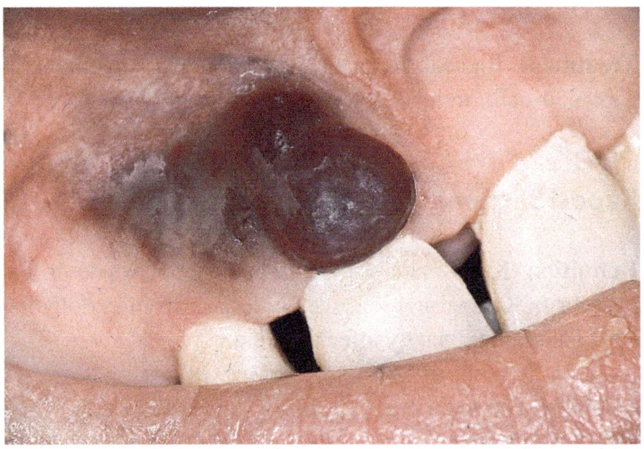

Fig. 42.14 Kaposi sarcoma, brown-red tumor on the gingiva

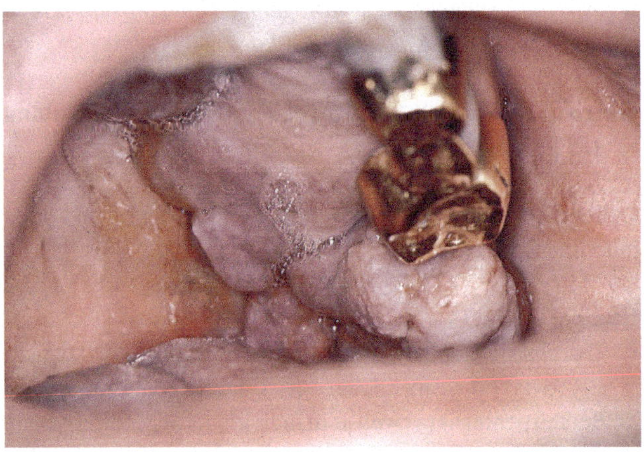

Fig. 42.15 Kaposi sarcoma, extensive red masses on the gingiva of an AIDS patient

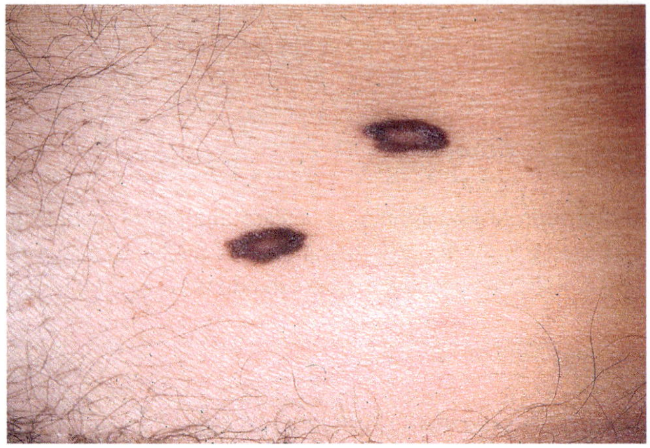

Fig. 42.16 Kaposi sarcoma, two red plaques on the skin

- Angiosarcoma
- Leiomyosarcoma
- Malignant melanoma
- Non-Hodgkin lymphoma

Laboratory Tests Histopathologic and immunohistochemical examinations. PCR to detect HHV-8 genome.

Treatment Chemotherapy with or without radiotherapy is the treatment of choice. For localized lesions, surgical excision, laser, cryotherapy, or photodynamic therapy are recommended.

Osteosarcoma

Definition Osteosarcoma is the most common malignancy of mesenchymal cells that have the capability to produce bone.

Etiology Unknown. Risk factors are radiation for other lesions, drugs, Paget disease of bone, hereditary retinoblastoma, and genetics.

Classification It is classified into three forms: a. *central*; b. *juxtacortical;* and c. *extraskeletal*.

Gingival Involvement Very rare, but may present as a jaw swelling involving the gingival, unrelated to dental biofilm.

Other Sites of Involvement Jaws (6–7%), long bones of skeleton.

Clinical Features

- Clinically, oral osteosarcoma appears as a hard enlargement of jaw bones that increases rapidly. The most common clinical symptoms include pain and swelling,

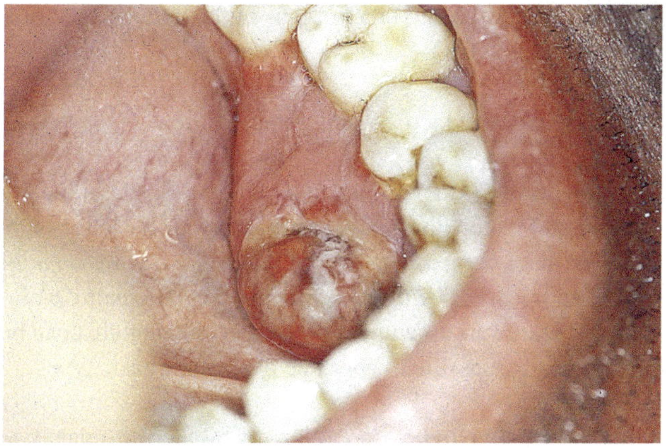

Fig. 42.17 Osteosarcoma, irregular ulcerated gingival mass

osteolytic expanding disorder in the jaw, followed by gingival enlargement, and tooth mobility (Fig. 42.17).

- Following the osseous destruction, the tumor may present as a soft exophytic mass usually ulcerated on the gingiva.
- The mandible and maxilla are equally affected.
- Clinical diagnosis should be confirmed by laboratory tests.

Differential Diagnosis

- Chondrosarcoma
- Ewing sarcoma
- Odontogenic tumor
- Squamous cell carcinoma
- Pyogenic granuloma
- Peripheral or central giant cell granuloma

Laboratory Tests Histopathologic examination. Panoramic x-ray, CT scan.

Treatment Surgical excision and chemotherapy are the treatment options.

Chondrosarcoma

Definition Chondrosarcoma is a malignant cartilage-forming neoplasm.

Etiology Unknown.

Classification a. *Primary* that develops de novo; and b. *Secondary* that develops from a preexisting benign cartilage tumor.

Gingival Involvement Very rare, but may occasionally present as gingival swelling unrelated to dental biofilm.

Other Sites of Involvement Jaws (rare), skeleton bones.

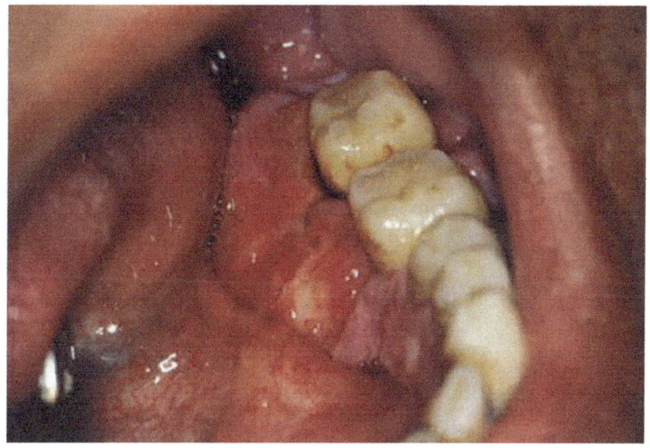

Fig. 42.18 Chondrosarcoma, large tumor on the gingiva of the mandible

Clinical Features

- It accounts for 8–10% of all primary bone tumors. The tumor is rare in the head and neck area (1–3%) and exceedingly rare in the jaws (0.5–1%).
- Clinically, it presents as a painless swelling on the gingiva that may cause osteolytic expanding lesions in the jaw and loosening of the teeth (Fig. 42.18). Occasionally, a large, red, lobulated, and ulcerated soft mass may present around gingiva.
- Clinical diagnosis must be confirmed by laboratory tests.

Differential Diagnosis

- Osteosarcoma
- Ewing sarcoma
- Squamous cell carcinoma
- Malignant fibrous histiocytoma
- Pyogenic granuloma
- Peripheral giant cell granuloma
- Odontogenic tumors

Laboratory Tests Histopathologic examination. Radiographic, CT, and MRI examination.

Treatment Radical surgical excision in combination with chemotherapy and/or radiotherapy.

Ewing Sarcoma

Definition Ewing sarcoma is a primary malignant neoplasm of undifferentiated mesenchymal small round cells.

Etiology Unknown.

Gingival Involvement Very rare but may present as a secondary swelling involving gingiva, unrelated to dental biofilm.

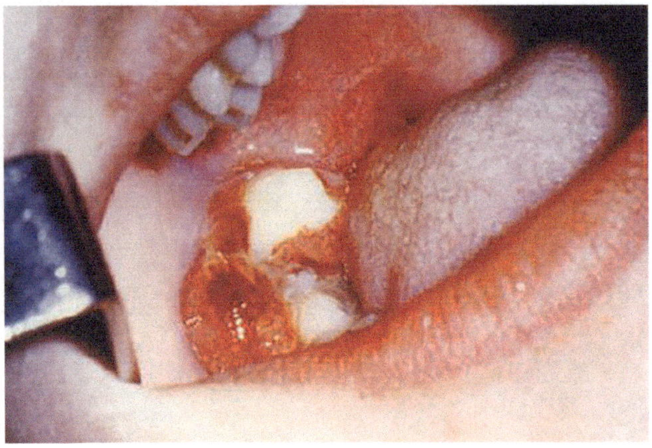

Fig. 42.19 Ewing sarcoma, enlargement on the gingiva of the mandible

Other Sites of Involvement Jaws (rare), lung, bones, pelvis, and ribs.

Clinical Features

- The tumor mainly affects children, adolescents, and young adults.
- Clinically, the jaw lesions present as a painful swelling that progresses to osseous destruction. There are teeth mobility and paresthesia. The tumor often penetrates the cortex, resulting in a soft red mass, ulcerated or not, mimicking gingival hyperplasia, and originating from the affected area of the bone (Fig. 42.19). The mandible is more commonly affected than the maxilla.
- Clinical diagnosis should be confirmed by laboratory tests.

Differential Diagnosis

- Osteosarcoma
- Chondrosarcoma
- Neuroblastoma
- Non-Hodgkin lymphoma
- Metastatic small cell malignant neoplasms
- Squamous cell carcinoma
- Peripheral or central giant cell tumor
- Osteomyelitis
- Odontogenic tumors

Laboratory Tests Histopathologic and immunohistochemical examinations. Radiographic, CT, and MRI examinations.

Treatment Radical surgical excision with chemotherapy and/or radiotherapy.

Malignant Melanoma

Definition Malignant melanoma is an aggressive neoplasm of melanocytic origin that primarily involves the skin and rarely the mucosae and other organs of the body (where pigmented tissue exists).

Etiology Genetic factors, sunlight exposure.

Classification Skin malignant melanoma is classified by clinical and histopathologic criteria into four basic types: a. *nodular*; b. *superficial spreading;* c. *lendigomaligna melanoma;* and d. *acral lentiginous melanoma. Amelanotic melanoma* is a rare variant without pigmented element that can be histologically classified under one of the four basic types.

Gingival Involvement Rare. Non-dental biofilm-related.

Other Sites of Involvement Skin (over 97–98%), oral mucosa (mainly on the palate and gingiva 0.5–1%), other mucosae.

Clinical Features

- Clinically, gingival melanoma presents as painless, flat, or more often nodular black or brown macule or plaque with an irregular border, which grows rapidly and bleeds easily (Figs. 42.20, 42.21, 42.22). As the lesions increase in size, multiple lobulated exophytic masses develop. Ulceration may develop and the lesions are either localized or multiple.
- In oral mucosa, over 80% of melanomas occur at the hard palate, maxillary gingiva and alveolar mucosa.
- The most common clinical forms of oral melanoma are *nodular* and *superficial spreading*. It develops either *denovo* or on a preexisting benign pigmented lesion. The prognosis of patients with oral melanoma is worse than for those with skin melanoma due to delayed detection and rapid metastasis.
- Skin melanoma presents as black nodular elevation (nodular type) (Fig. 42.23) or flat black plaque that grows peripherally (superficial spreading type).

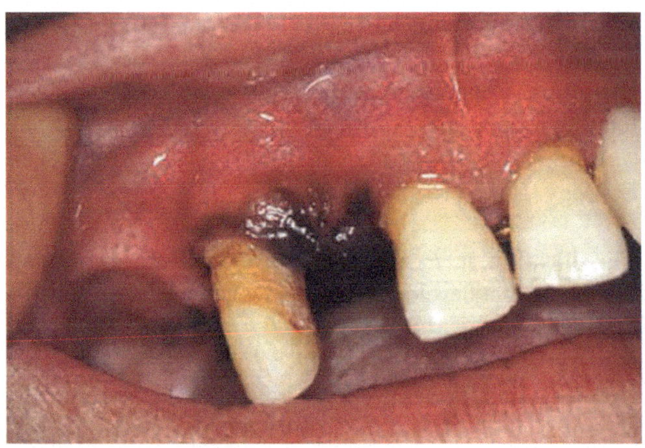

Fig. 42.20 Malignant melanoma, early nodular type

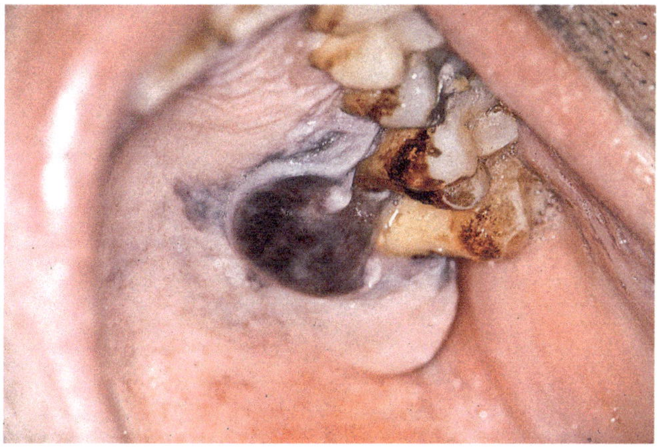

Fig. 42.21 Malignant melanoma, black irregular plaque on the palatal gingiva, nodular type

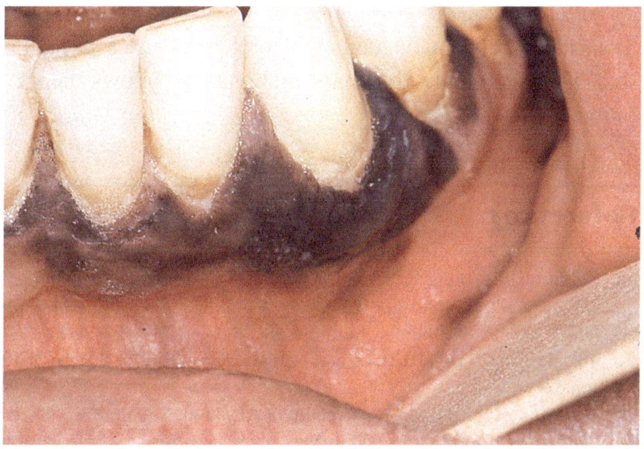

Fig. 42.22 Malignant melanoma, multiple black masses on the gingiva, superficial spreading type

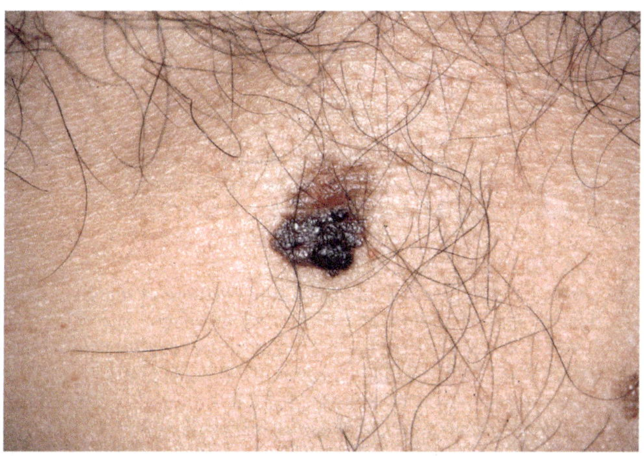

Fig. 42.23 Malignant melanoma, early, black nodular tumor on the skin

- Cells in malignant melanoma present with two growth phases: a. the *horizontal* or *radial*; and b. the *vertical* with deeper extension. Both are indicative of the form of extension and the prognosis of the neoplasm. The "ABCDE Rule" (Asymmetry, Border, Color, Diameter, Elevation) of skin melanoma can be useful for its early detection.
- Two factors determine the prognosis of skin melanoma: a. the *clinical type;* and b. the *depth of invasion determined histologically (Breslow depth* that is measured from the granular layer of the epidermis down to the deepest point of invasion*).* However, both criteria are not of practical help regarding oral melanoma.

Differential Diagnosis
- Lentigomaligna
- Pigmented nevi
- Lentigo simplex
- Ephelides
- Melanoacanthoma
- Kaposi sarcoma
- Bacillary angiomatosis
- Pyogenic granuloma
- Peripheral giant cell granuloma
- Cavernous hemangioma
- Amalgam tattoo
- Black foreign material
- Racial pigmentation
- Smoking pigmentation

Laboratory Tests Histopathologic examination (*Clark scale of infiltration, Breslow scale* of invasion depth). Immunohistochemical markers.

Treatment Radical surgical excision. Adjuvant therapy includes chemotherapy in combination with immunotherapy or molecularly targeted therapy or hormonal therapy.

Metastatic Neoplasms

Definition Metastatic neoplasms to the oral cavity are rare. Metastatic lesions may occur in the jaws and, less commonly, in the oral soft tissues.

Etiology Metastasis may occur via both hematogenous and lymphatic routes. They usually derive from carcinomas of the breast, lungs, kidney, thyroid, prostate, and gastrointestinal tract. Metastasis to the mouth may also arise from sarcomas, melanomas, and hematologic malignancies.

Gingival Involvement Rare, but it may present as a gingival swelling or periodontal destruction, unrelated to dental biofilm.

Other Sites of Involvement Jaws, tongue, palate, floor of the mouth.

Clinical Features

- Clinically, it presents as gingival swelling accompanied by pain, ulceration, tooth mobility, non-healing extraction sockets, and paresthesia or hypoesthesia (Figs. 42.24, 42.25, 42.26). Oral mucosa metastases may be asymptomatic.
- Clinical diagnosis should be confirmed by laboratory tests.

Differential Diagnosis

- Fibroma
- Peripheral ossifying fibroma
- Pyogenic granuloma
- Peripheral giant cell granuloma
- Squamous cell carcinoma
- Non-Hodgkin lymphoma
- Other neoplasms

Laboratory Tests Histopathologic and immunohistochemical examinations. Imaging studies.

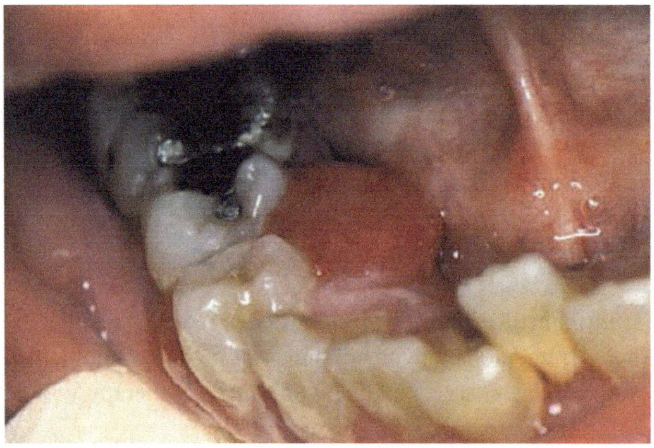

Fig. 42.24 Metastatic carcinoma, gingival metastasis from breast cancer

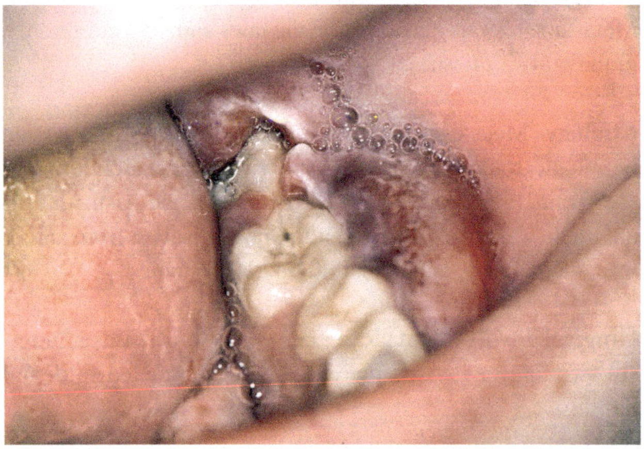

Fig. 42.25 Metastatic carcinoma, gingival metastasis from embryonal carcinoma of the rectum

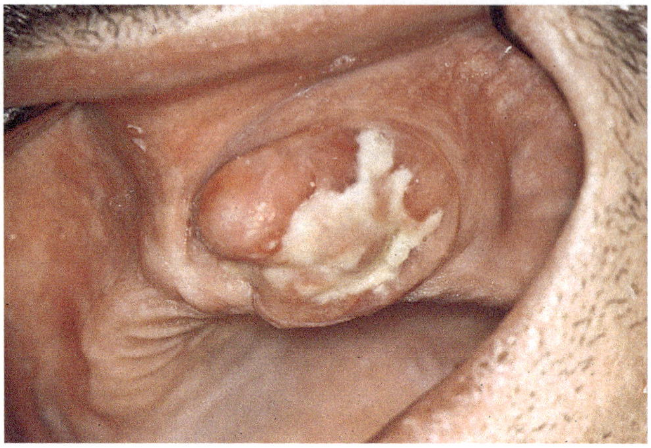

Fig. 42.26 Metastatic carcinoma, alveolar mucosa metastasis from lung carcinoma

Treatment The management of oral metastases is palliative. The treatment of primary malignancy follows the recommended protocol.

References

1. Solomon B, Young RJ, Rischin D. Head and neck squamous cell carcinoma: genomics and emerging biomarkers for immunomodulatory cancer treatments. Semin Cancer Biol. 2018;52(Pt 2):228–40. https://doi.org/10.1016/j.semcancer.2018.01.008. Epub 2018 Jan 31
2. Makridis SD, Mellado JR, Freedman AL, et al. Squamous cell carcinoma of gingiva and edentulous alveolar ridge: a clinicopathologic study. Int J Periodontics Restorative Dent. 1998;18(3):292–8. PMID: 9728112
3. Akrish S, Eskander-Hashoul L, Rachmiel A, Ben-Izhak O. Clinicopathologic analysis of verrucous hyperplasia, verrucous carcinoma and squamous cell carcinoma as part of the clinicopathologic spectrum of oral proliferative verrucous leukoplakia: a literature review and analysis. Pathol Res Pract. 2019;215(12):152670. https://doi.org/10.1016/j.prp.2019.152670. Epub 2019 Sep 25. PMID: 31630872
4. Bharanidharan R, Dineshkumar T, Raghavendhar K, Kumar AR. Squamous cell carcinoma of the gingiva: a diagnostic enigma. J Oral Maxillofac Pathol. 2015;19(2):267. https://doi.org/10.4103/0973-029X.164558. PMID: 26604512; PMCID: PMC4611944
5. Du W, Fang Q, Wu Y, et al. Oncologic outcome of marginal mandibulectomy in squamous cell carcinoma of the lower gingiva. BMC Cancer. 2019;19(1):775. https://doi.org/10.1186/s12885-019-5999-0. PMID: 31387576; PMCID: PMC6683491
6. Keshava A, Gugwad S, Baad R, Patel R. Gingival squamous cell carcinoma mimicking as a desquamative lesion. J Indian Soc Periodontol. 2016;20(1):75–8. https://doi.org/10.4103/0972-124X.164765. PMID: 27041843; PMCID: PMC4795141
7. Ramos JC, Alves FA, Kowalski LP, et al. Epidemiological profile and clinical implications of oral squamous cell carcinoma adjacent to dental implants. Oral Dis. 2020;27(7):1687–98. https://doi.org/10.1111/odi.13710. Epub ahead of print. PMID: 33140896
8. Davidova LA, Fitzpatrick SG, Bhattacharyya I, et al. Lichenoid characteristics in premalignant verrucous lesions and verrucous carcinoma of the oral cavity. Head Neck Pathol. 2019;13(4):573–9.

https://doi.org/10.1007/s12105-019-01006-4. Epub 2019 Jan 22. PMID: 30671763; PMCID: PMC6854141

9. Bagan J, Murillo-Cortes J, Leopoldo-Rodado M, et al. Oral cancer on the gingiva in patients with proliferative leukoplakia: a study of 30 cases. J Periodontol. 2019;90(10):1142–8. https://doi.org/10.1002/JPER.18-0620. Epub 2019 May 27. PMID: 31074011
10. Vijayalakshmi D, Fathima S, Ramakrishnan K, Devi M. Malignant fibrous histiocytoma of the gingiva. BMJ Case Rep. 2012;2012:bcr2012007400. https://doi.org/10.1136/bcr-2012-007400. PMID: 23257940; PMCID: PMC4544897
11. Thomas ME, Koshi R. Electron microscopy in the diagnosis of malignant fibrous histiocytoma of the lung presenting as metastasis to the maxillary gingiva. Int J Oral Maxillofac Surg. 2013;42(1):99–101. https://doi.org/10.1016/j.ijom.2012.09.019. Epub 2012 Oct 23. PMID: 23092853
12. Cassoni A, Terenzi V, Bartoli D, et al. Metastatic uterine leiomyosarcoma in the upper buccal gingiva misdiagnosed as an epulis. Case Rep Oncol Med. 2014, 2014:402342. https://doi.org/10.1155/2014/402342. Epub 2014 Oct 15. PMID: 25386373; PMCID: PMC4214049
13. Viviano M, Miracco C, Lorenzini G, et al. Gingival leiomyosarcoma in a young woman: case report and literature review. Sultan Qaboos Univ Med J. 2017;17(4):e472–6. https://doi.org/10.18295/squmj.2017.17.04.017. Epub 2018 Jan 10. PMID: 29372093; PMCID: PMC5766307
14. Komatsu Y, Miyamoto I, Ohashi Y, et al. Primary epithelioid angiosarcoma originating from the mandibular gingiva: a case report of an extremely rare oral lesion. World J Surg Oncol. 2020;18(1):260. https://doi.org/10.1186/s12957-020-01999-1. PMID: 33010804; PMCID: PMC7533036
15. Nakano Y, Sazumi Y, Mizuta Y, et al. Gingival lesion leading to a diagnosis of angiosarcoma. J Gen Fam Med. 2020;22(2):90–1. https://doi.org/10.1002/jgf2.397. PMID: 33717782; PMCID: PMC7921341
16. Wakoh M, Sasaki Y, Otonari-Yamamoto M, et al. Imaging findings in AIDS-related oral Kaposi's sarcoma. Bull Tokyo Dent Coll. 2017;58(3):145–54. https://doi.org/10.2209/tdcpublication.2016-0025. PMID: 28954949
17. Dumpala RK, Guttikonda VR, Yeluri S, Madala J. Oral metastasis of chondroblastic osteosarcoma. Contemp Clin Dent. 2012;3(3):367–9. https://doi.org/10.4103/0976-237X.103640. PMID: 23293503; PMCID: PMC3532810
18. Ferreti Bonan PR, Nogueira Dos Santos LA, Batista De-Paula AM, et al. Chondrosarcoma involving the periodontum: clinicopathological and immunohistochemical features of a case study. Minerva Stomatol. 2006;55(10):587–91.
19. Acar GO, Cansiz H, Acioglu E, et al. Chondrosarcoma of the mandible extending to the infratemporal fossa: report of two cases. Oral Maxillofac Surg. 2008;12:173–6.
20. Margaix-Muñoz M, Bagán J, Poveda-Roda R. Ewing sarcoma of the oral cavity. A review. J Clin Exp Dent. 2017;9(2):e294–301. https://doi.org/10.4317/jced.53575. PMID: 28210452; PMCID: PMC5303334
21. Aguas SC, Quarracino MC, Lence AN, Lanfranchi Tizeira HE. Primary melanoma of the oral cavity: ten cases and review of 177 cases from literature. Med Oral Patol Oral Cir Bucal. 2009;14:E265–71.
22. de Lima Morais TM, Soares CD, Wanderley AEC, et al. Oral melanomas in HIV-positive patients: report of two cases and review of the literature. Oral Oncol. 2020;101:104375. https://doi.org/10.1016/j.oraloncology.2019.07.018. Epub 2019 Jul 29. PMID: 31371241
23. Allon I, Pessing A, Kaplan I, et al. Metastatic tumors to the gingiva and the presence of teeth as a contributing factor: a literature analysis. J Periodontol. 2014;85(1):132–9. https://doi.org/10.1902/jop.2013.130118. Epub 2013 May 7. PMID: 23646853
24. Okamura T, Beppu T, Tokumaru T, et al. Cancer of the mandibular gingiva metastasizing to the small intestine. Auris Nasus Larynx. 2019;46(3):479–82. https://doi.org/10.1016/j.anl.2018.08.006. Epub 2018 Aug 28. PMID: 30170905
25. Ohnishi Y, Sugitatsu M, Watanabe M, et al. Metastasis of mesothelioma to the maxillary gingiva. Oncol Lett. 2014;8(3):1214–6. https://doi.org/10.3892/ol.2014.2273. Epub 2014 Jun 20. PMID: 25120691; PMCID: PMC4114704
26. Kaplan I, Raiser V, Shuster A, et al. Metastatic tumors in oral mucosa and jawbones: unusual primary origins and unusual oral locations. Acta Histochem. 2019;121(8):151448. https://doi.org/10.1016/j.acthis.2019.151448. Epub 2019 Sep 27. PMID: 31570205

Hematopoietic and Lymphoid Tissue Malignancies

43

Contents

These diseases may result in breakdown of periodontal tissues and occasionally may mimic the clinical features of severe periodontitis.

Leukemias

Definition Leukemias are a heterogenous group of malignant disorders of the hematopoietic system.

Etiology The etiology remains obscure, although several genetic and environmental factors play a great role in the pathogenesis.

Classification Depending on the maturation of the neoplastic cells and the clinical course, leukemias are classified into: (a) *acute;* and (b) *chronic*. Depending on the affected cell line and its origin, leukemias are subclassified into: (a) *myelogenous* or *myeloid*; (b) *lymphocytic* or *lymphoblastic*; (c) *hairy cell*; (d) *monocytic*; (e) *eosinophilic*; (f) *basophilic*; (g) *megakaryoblastic;* and (h) *erythroleukemia*.

Gingival Involvement Common. Inflammatory and gingival enlargement occasionally associated with dental biofilm-induced gingival lesions.

Other Sites of Involvement Oral mucosa, skin, lymph nodes, spleen, liver, and other internal organs.

Clinical Features

- Clinically, *localized* or more common *generalized* gingival swelling of variable severity may develop usually in acute and rarely in chronic leukemia (Figs. 43.1, 43.2, 43.3 and 43.4). It is a common, early, and characteristic finding, mainly in both monocytic and myelomonocytic types, caused by gingival infiltration of leukemic cells. Commonly, the enlarged gingival tissues bleed spontaneously and they are erythematous and inflamed to the extent of covering the crowns of teeth (Figs. 43.5, 43.6 and 43.7).
- Other common oral lesions and complications are non-specific ulcerations of oral mucosa, bleeding, oral candidiasis, herpetic infections, systemic mycosis, infections from *bacteria* and *cocci* (Fig. 43.8).

G. Laskaris et al., *Periodontal Manifestations of Local and Systemic Diseases*, https://doi.org/10.1007/978-3-031-10828-0_43

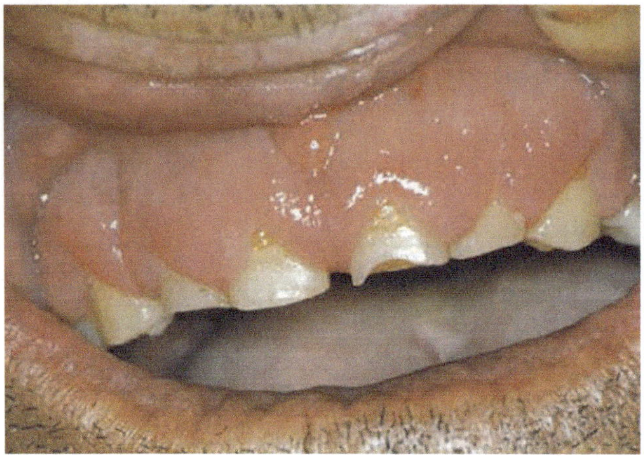

Fig. 43.1 Acute myeloblastic leukemia, early gingival enlargement

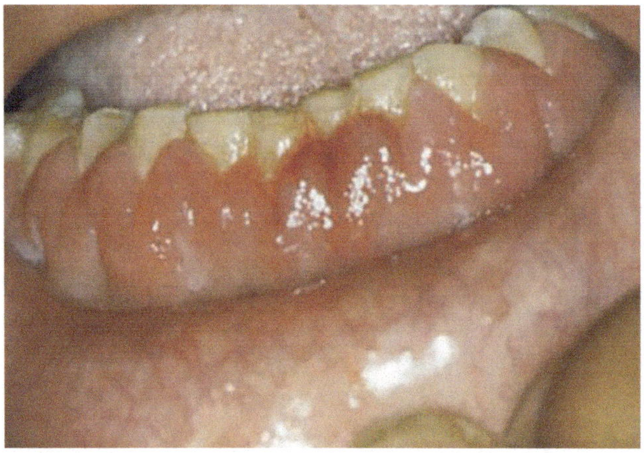

Fig. 43.2 Acute myeloblastic leukemia, severe gingival enlargement

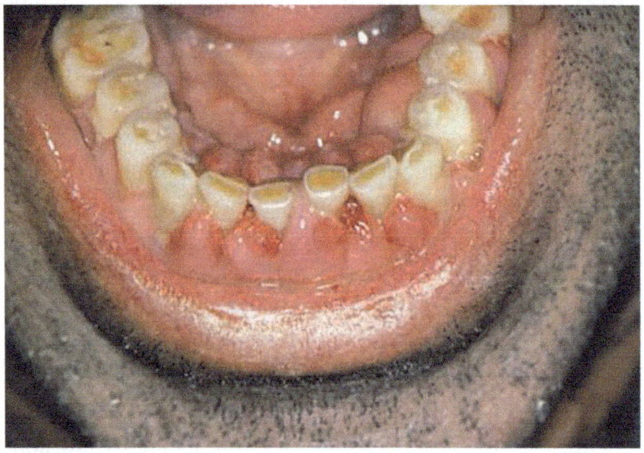

Fig. 43.3 Acute myeloblastic leukemia, severe gingival enlargement

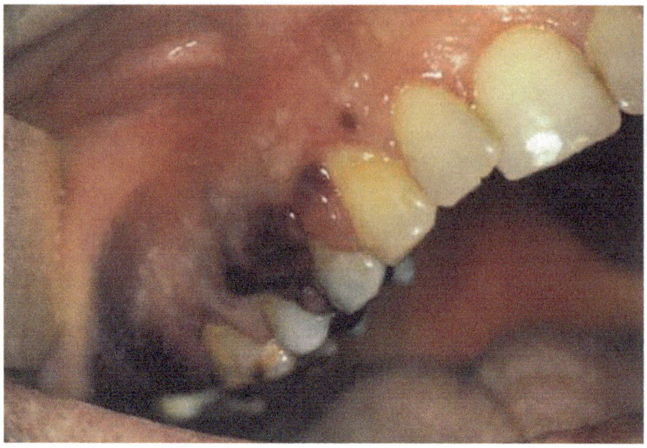

Fig. 43.4 Acute myelomonocytic leukemia, early erythematous gingival enlargement

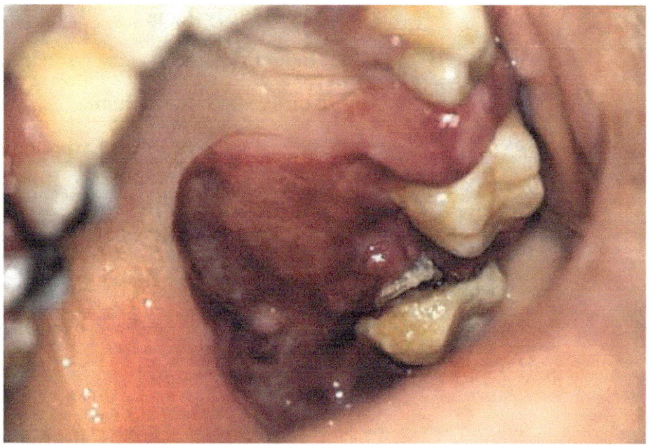

Fig. 43.5 Acute myelomonocytic leukemia, severe gingival enlargement

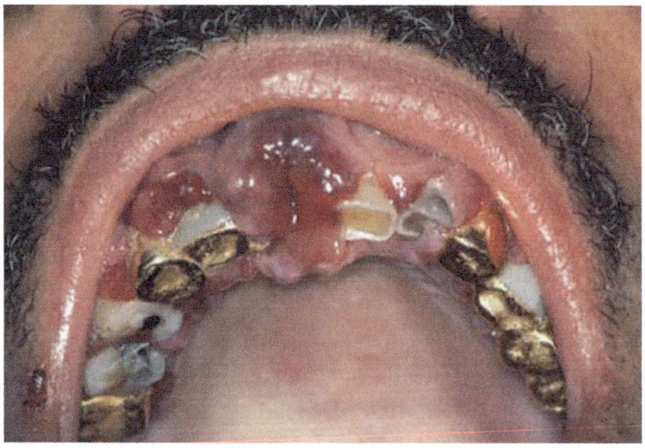

Fig. 43.6 Acute myelomonocytic leukemia, severe gingival enlargement

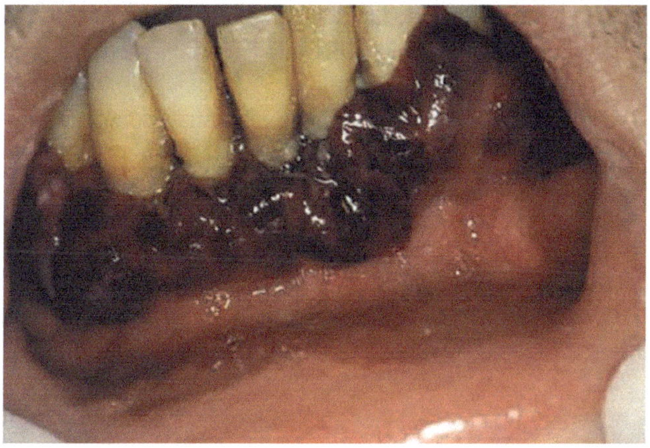

Fig. 43.7 Acute monocytic leukemia, severe erythematous gingival enlargement as a first sign of the leukemia

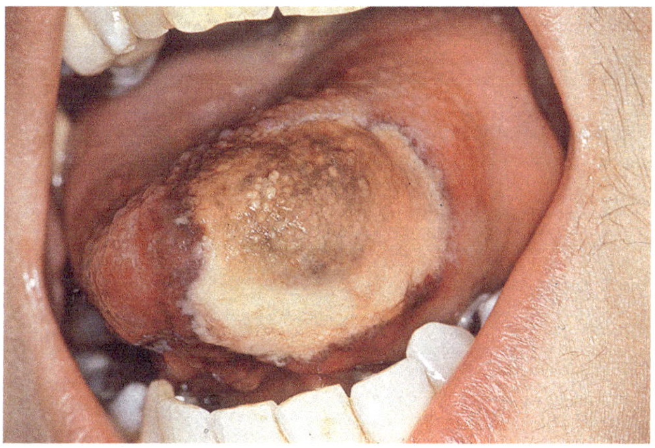

Fig. 43.8 Acute myeloblastic leukemia, nonspecific large ulceration on the tip of the tongue

- Rarely, rapid alveolar bone loss may occur, particularly in patients with preexisting periodontitis.
- Common systemic signs and symptoms are: chills, fever, headaches, fatigue, weight loss, generalized lymphadenopathy, mucosal and skin pallor, petechiae, ecchymoses, and hemorrhage.
- Clinical diagnosis should be confirmed by laboratory tests.

Differential Diagnosis

- Neutropenia
- Agranulocytosis
- Aplastic anemia
- Thrombocytopenic purpura
- Necrotizing gingivitis or periodontitis
- Drug-induced gingival enlargement
- Scurvy
- Langerhans cell histiocytosis
- Myelodysplastic syndrome

Laboratory Tests Complete blood count examination, myelogram, histopathologic examination of extramedullary tissue involved.

Treatment Good oral hygiene, topical oral antiseptics. Systemic therapy includes multiagent chemotherapy, peripheral blood stem cell or bone marrow transplantation, radiotherapy, and other medications, but these must be left to hematologists.

Soft Tissue Plasmacytoma

Definition Soft tissue plasmacytoma or solitary extramedullary plasmacytoma is an unusual monoclonal neoplasia of mucosal plasma cells, indistinguishable from those seen in multiple myeloma.

Etiology Unknown.

Classification Plasmacytoma is classified into: (a) *solitary;* and (b) *multiple*. The solitary is subclassified into: (a) *skeletal;* and (b) *extramedullary.*

Gingival Involvement Rare. Non-dental biofilm-induced gingival lesions.

Other Sites of Involvement Oral mucosa, nasopharynx, nasal cavity, paranasal sinuses, parotid, tonsils.

Clinical Features

- Clinically, oral soft tissue plasmacytoma presents as localized, painless, soft circumscribed gingival swelling with a smooth surface and normal or slightly red color that may rarely be ulcerated (Fig. 43.9). The size of the lesion varies from one to several centimeters in diameter. Periodontal destruction may rarely occur. Similar clinical features present at other oral anatomical sites (buccal mucosa, palate, tongue, floor of the mouth (Fig. 43.10).
- Several patients with oral soft tissue plasmacytoma may ultimately develop multiple myeloma.
- The disease is more common in males over 50 years of age.
- Clinical diagnosis should be confirmed by laboratory tests.

Differential Diagnosis

- Plasma cell gingivitis
- Granular cell gingivitis
- Dental and periodontal abscesses
- Non-Hodgkin lymphoma
- Multiple myeloma

Laboratory Tests Histopathologic and immunohistochemical examinations.

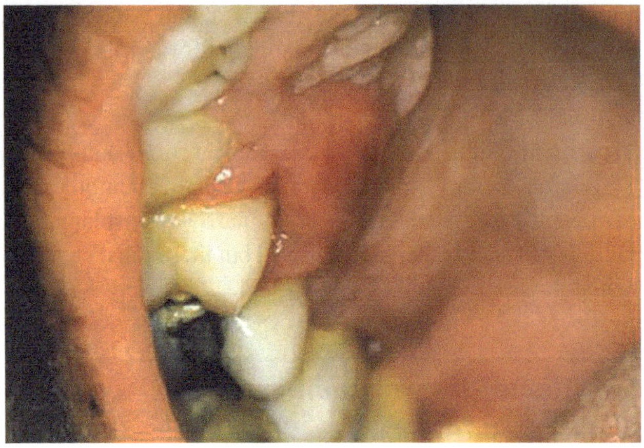

Fig. 43.9 Soft tissue plasmacytoma, localized gingival enlargement

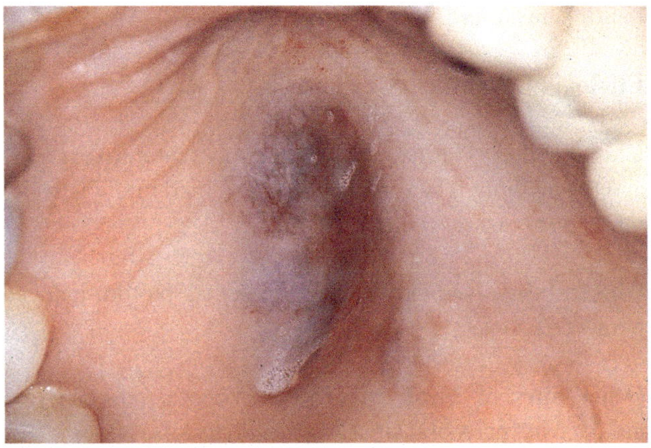

Fig. 43.10 Soft tissue plasmacytoma, ulcerated lesion on the palate

Treatment Surgical excision usually in combination with radiotherapy and chemotherapy.

Multiple Myeloma

Definition Multiple myeloma is a malignant plasma cell disorder characterized by bone marrow destruction and paraprotein formation.

Etiology Unknown.

Gingival Involvement Relatively rare. Non-dental biofilm-induced gingival lesions.

Other Sites of Involvement Oral mucosa (10–15%), jaws (25–30%), skull, spine, ribs, pelvis, clavicles, kidney.

Clinical Features

- Clinically, multiple myeloma presents with bleeding, painless, localized or generalized gingival swelling with or without ulceration. It is usually associated with alveolar bone destruction, tooth mobility, and paresthesia (Figs. 43.11, 43.12 and 43.13).
- The most common presenting signs and symptoms are osseous pain and destruction, anemia, kidney failure, neurological and visual disturbances, infections, and

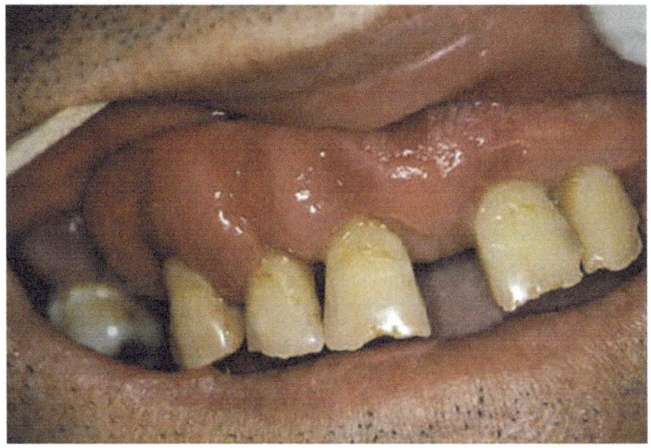

Fig. 43.11 Multiple myeloma, localized severe gingival enlargement

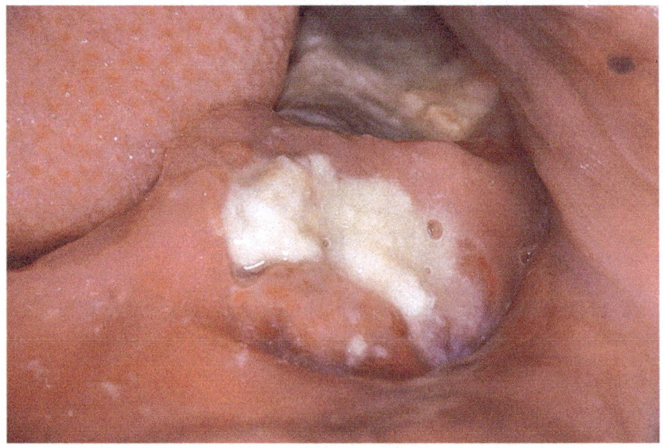

Fig. 43.12 Multiple myeloma, large ulceration of the alveolar mucosa of the mandible

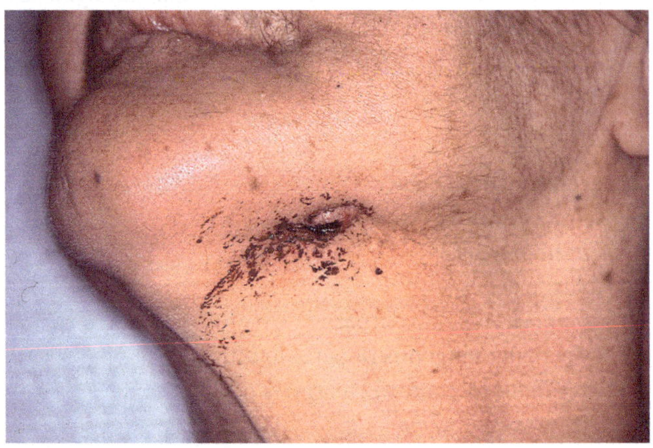

Fig. 43.13 Multiple myeloma, bone destruction and extraoral fistula formation

alterations in mental status. In about 10–20% of cases, multiple myeloma coexists with primary systemic amyloidosis. The disease usually involves individuals over 50 years of age.
- Clinical diagnosis should be confirmed by laboratory tests.

Differential Diagnosis
- Necrotizing periodontitis
- Leukemia
- Neutropenia
- Aplastic anemia
- Monoclonal gammopathy of unknown significance (MGUS)
- Non-Hodgkin lymphoma
- Langerhans cell histiocytosis
- Osteosarcoma

Laboratory Tests Histopathologic and immunohistochemical examination, radiographic examination, MRI, CT, PET, serum, and urine protein electrophoresis.

Treatment Symptomatic for gingival and oral lesions. The systemic treatment is the responsibility of hematologist-oncologists.

Hodgkin Disease

Definition Hodgkin disease is a malignant lymphoproliferative disease characterized by the presence of the *Reed-Sternberg cells* that derive from B-lymphocytes.

Etiology The exact etiology remains unknown. Genetic and environmental factors seem to be involved in the pathogenesis.

Gingival Involvement Very rare. Non-dental biofilm-induced gingival lesions.

Other Sites of Involvement Oral mucosa (very rare), lymph nodes (always), extranodular involvement (rare).

Clinical Features
- Clinically, the gingival lesions present as soft swelling or nonspecific ulceration (Fig. 43.14). Similar lesions may rarely develop in oral mucosa.
- The most frequent presenting feature is enlargement of multiple or single cervical or other lymph nodes. Involved lymph nodes are firm, mobile, and may or may not be tender on palpation.

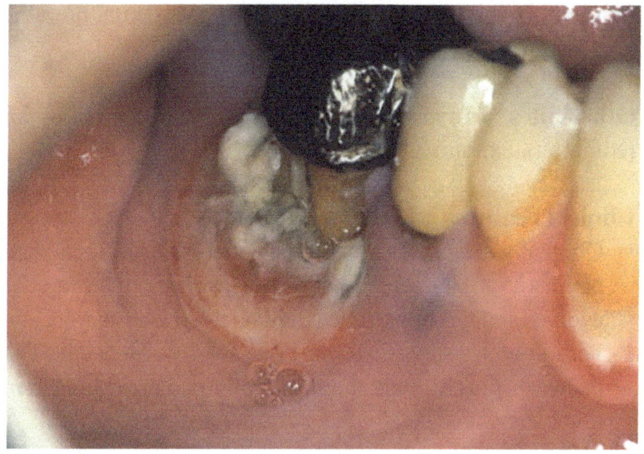

Fig. 43.14 Hodgkin disease, localized ulceration on the gingiva of a patient with AIDS

- Low-grade fever, night sweats, weight loss, anorexia, fatigue, malaise, weakness, and pruritus may occur.
- Clinical diagnosis should be confirmed by laboratory tests.

Differential Diagnosis
- Non-Hodgkin lymphoma
- Leukemia
- Plasmacytoma
- Wegener granulomatosis

Laboratory Tests Histopathologic, immunohistochemical and molecular examination.

Treatment Includes chemotherapy, radiotherapy, bone marrow transplantation administered by specialists. Symptomatic treatment for oral lesions.

Non-Hodgkin Lymphomas

Definition Non-Hodgkin Lymphomas are a heterogenous group of lymphoid tissue malignancies, which account for 70–80% of all lymphomas.

Etiology Genetic and environmental factors (viruses, medications, radiation) seem to play an important role.

Classification Based on clinical and mainly on histopathologic, immunologic, molecular, and cytogenic criteria, the non-Hodgkin lymphomas are classified into three groups: (a) *low grade*; (b) *intermediate;* and (c) *high grade.* WHO classifies them into two major groups: (a) *B cell* derived (85%); and (b) *T cell*-derived (15%). In addition, over 30 subtypes have been described.

Gingival Involvement Relatively rare. Non-dental biofilm-related lesions.

Other Sites of Involvement Oral mucosa, lymphoid organ (common), extranodal (over 40%).

Clinical Features

- Clinically, the gingival involvement presents as localized, painless, inflammatory, and soft swelling that rapidly evolves and might ulcerate (Figs. 43.15, 43.16 and 43.17). Periodontal destruction and bone loss are unusual. The posterior gingival and the retromolar pad are more often involved.
- Oral lesions present as a relatively soft, painless, reddish, or purplish in color, diffuse swelling that is commonly ulcerated. The soft palate, ovula, base of the tongue, and floor of the mouth are the sites of predilection (Fig. 43.18). The oral lesions are rarely the first and sole manifestation of the disease.

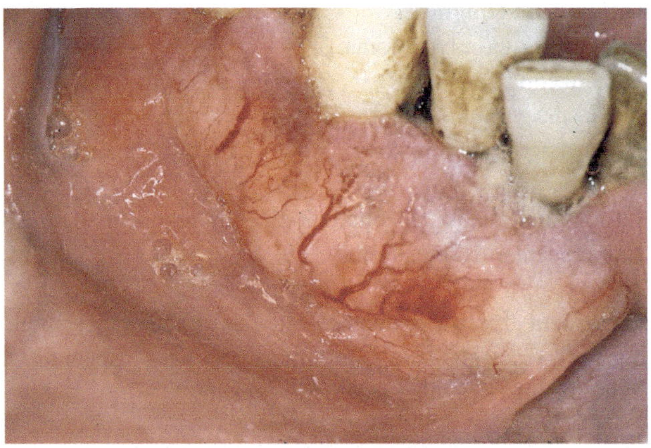

Fig. 43.15 Non- Hodgkin lymphoma, localized gingival enlargement on the mandible

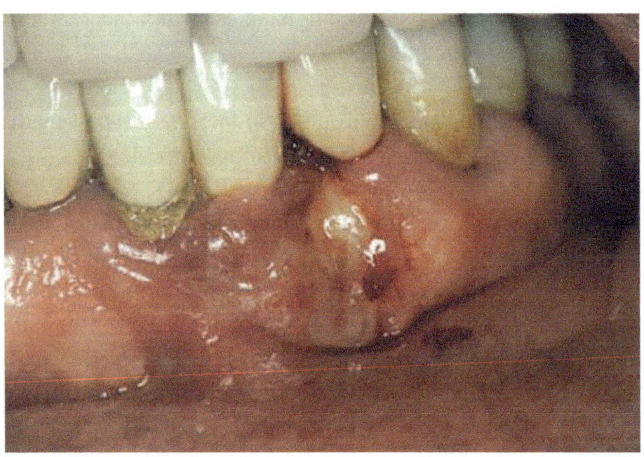

Fig. 43.16 Non- Hodgkin lymphoma, localized gingival enlargement with ulceration

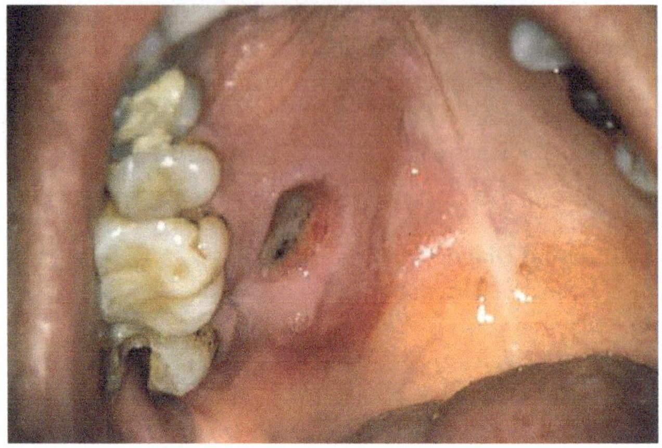

Fig. 43.17 Non- Hodgkin lymphoma, gingival and palatal enlargement (the ulceration is due to biopsy)

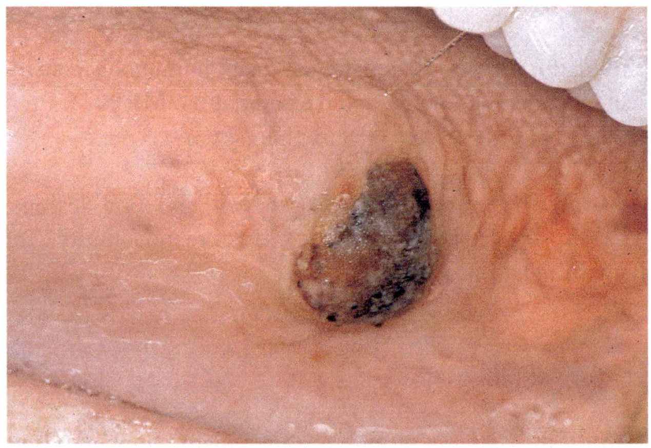

Fig. 43.18 Non-Hodgkin lymphoma, early lesion on the tongue

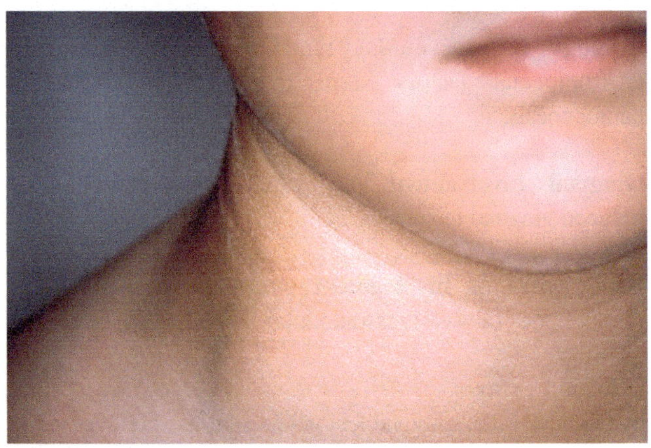

Fig. 43.19 Non-Hodgkin lymphoma, enlarged lymph node on the right side of the neck

- The hallmark clinical features include fever, night sweats, weight loss, lymphadenopathy, symptoms from the lungs, gastrointestinal tract, and skin (Fig. 43.19).
- Clinical diagnosis should be confirmed by laboratory tests.

Differential Diagnosis

- Soft tissue plasmacytoma
- Hodgkin disease
- Leukemia
- Multiple myeloma
- Wegener granulomatosis
- Squamous cell carcinoma
- Dental and periodontal abscesses

Laboratory Tests Histopathologic and immunohistochemical examination.

Treatment Chemotherapy, radiotherapy. Recently, monoclonal antibodies against the CD-20 antigen (Rituximab) of B lymphocyte membrane in combination with CHOP chemotherapy are the first-line therapy, which is administered by a hematologist/oncologist. Symptomatic therapy for oral lesions.

Extranodal NK/T Cell Lymphoma—Nasal Type

Definition Extranodal natural killer (NK)/T cell lymphoma, nasal type or angiocentric T cell lymphoma is a rare, specific, and aggressive type of non-Hodgkin lymphoma that derives from NK/T cells.

Etiology It remains unknown, although in some cases *Epstein-Barr virus* has been detected.

Gingival Involvement Rare. Non-dental biofilm-induced lesions.

Other Sites of Involvement Soft palate, nasal cavity, nasopharynx, skin.

Clinical Features

- Clinically, extranodal NK/T cell lymphoma, nasal type, initially presents with fever, weakness, nocturnal sweating, epistaxis, nasal stuffiness, foul-smelling nasal discharge, severe edema and erythema on the palate, the uvula and at the tonsil area, trismus and visual problems. As the disease progresses, deep necrotic ulcers develop, which soon spread both in-depth and peripherally (Fig. 43.20).
- The palatal gingiva may be involved. Rarely, the disease may begin from the upper gingiva with edema, erythema, and rapid necrotic ulcerations provoking catastrophic destruction of both the periodontal and surrounding tissues (Fig. 43.21).
- Oral lesions deteriorate causing major midfacial destruction of the palate, upper gingiva, nasal septum, eyes, base of the skull, and severe disfiguration of the face. Secondary infections and bleeding are common. The prognosis is unfavorable with high fatality.
- Clinical diagnosis should be confirmed by laboratory tests.

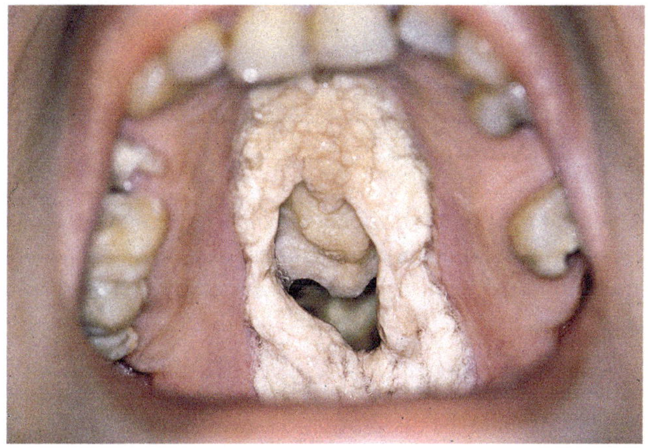

Fig. 43.20 Extranodal NK/T-cell lymphoma-nasal type. Deep necrotic ulcer with bone destruction on the palate

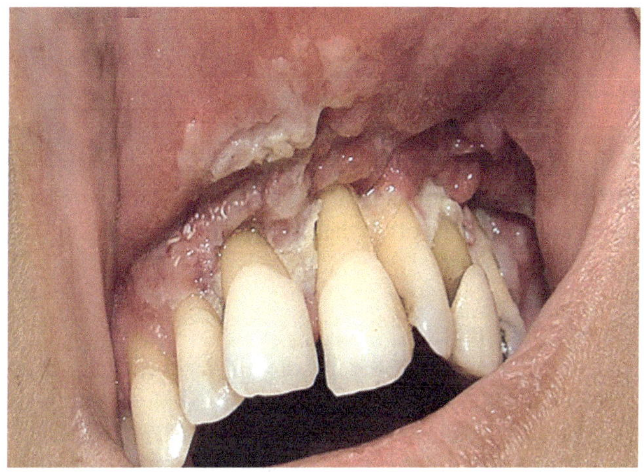

Fig. 43.21 Extranodal NK/T-cell lymphoma with unusual gingival involvement

Differential Diagnosis

- Other types of non-Hodgkin lymphoma
- Necrotizing sialadenometaplasia
- Wegener granulomatosis
- Systemic mycoses
- Salivary gland adenocarcinomas
- Florid tuberculosis
- Squamous cell carcinoma

Laboratory Tests Histopathologic and immunohistochemical examination, molecular genetic studies.

Treatment The treatment depends on the stage of the disease and the clinical status of the patient and should be left to the hematologist/oncologists in a specialized hospital. First-line treatment is usually systemic chemotherapy combined with radiation.

Burkitt Lymphoma

Definition Burkitt lymphoma is a high-grade non–Hodgkin lymphoma. It is common in Africa and rare in Western countries and usually affects children between 2 and 14 years of age.

Etiology Epstein-Barr virus, genetic, immunodeficiencies, AIDS, autoimmune diseases.

Classification Burkitt lymphoma is classified using epidemiologic and histopathologic criteria into two basic forms: (a) *the classic African or endemic;* and (b) *the non-African or sporadic.*

Gingival Involvement Rare, non-dental biofilm-induced gingival lesions.

Other Sites of Involvement Jaws (70–80%), the maxilla is twice more often involved than mandible, bone marrow, and other organs (rare).

Clinical Features

- Clinically, gingival lesions present as localized, large, ulcerated or not, painless swelling, or exophytic soft mass covered by reddish mucosa (Fig. 43.22). The tumor usually grows rapidly and may produce periodontal destruction and tooth mobility, which mimics severe periodontitis (Fig. 43.23).
- Rapidly proliferative swelling of the jaws, which may produce marked destruction of the facial bone and nerve paresis, bone pain, tenderness, and paresthesia, are the hallmark clinical features.
- Prognosis depends on the stage of the disease and clinical diagnosis should be confirmed by laboratory tests.

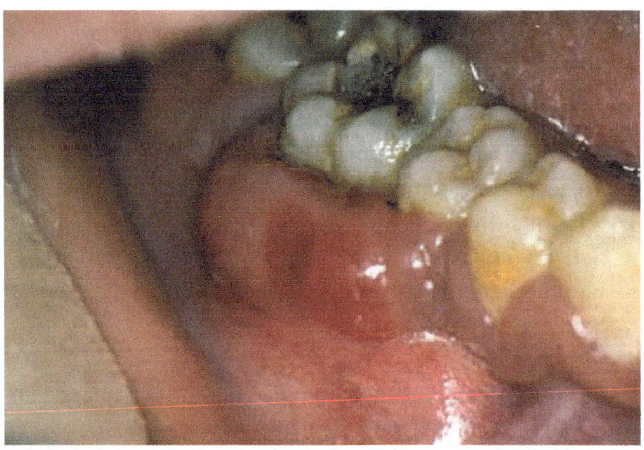

Fig. 43.22 Burkitt lymphoma, localized soft tissue tumor on the gingiva

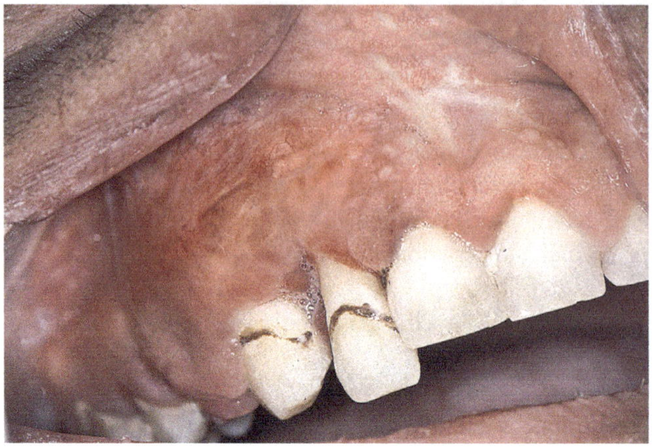

Fig. 43.23 Burkitt lymphoma, exophytic red mass on the gingiva with evident periodontal bone destruction

Differential Diagnosis

- Melanotic neuroectodermal tumor of infancy
- Cherubism
- Ewing sarcoma
- Osteosarcoma
- Chondrosarcoma
- Multiple myeloma
- Squamous cell carcinoma
- Non-Hodgkin lymphoma (other types)
- Odontogenic tumors
- Kaposi sarcoma
- Amyloidosis

Laboratory Tests Histopathologic and immunohistochemical examination. Panoramic radiography, CT, dental scan.

Treatment Treatment of choice is chemotherapy alone or in combination with radiography and surgery. Sympomatic treatment for gingival lesions.

Mycosis Fungoides

Definition Mycosis fungoides is the most common type of cutaneous T cell non-Hodgkin lymphoma with slow progress.

Etiology It remains unknown.

Classification The cutaneous lesions are classified into three stages: (a) *premycotic*; (b) *plaque;* and (c) *tumor.*

Gingival Involvement Rare, non-dental biofilm-induced lesions.

Other Sites of Involvement Oral mucosa (rare), skin (always), visceral.

Clinical Features

- Clinically, gingival lesions present as localized swellings or exophytic soft masses that may be ulcerated (Fig. 43.24). The lesions usually grow rapidly and may produce periodontal destruction and tooth mobility. Similar lesions may develop in other oral sites (Fig. 43.25). Gingival and oral lesions are usually affected during the plaque or tumor stage.
- Skin lesions on the *premycotic-patch stage* are characterized by pruritic eruption that may mimic psoriasis or eczema (Fig. 43.26) During the *plaque stage* lesions present as irregular, well-demarcated, slightly elevated, and indurated plaques. During the *tumor stage* plaque lesions develop into raised tumors that often ulcerate. Erythroderma and poikiloderma are common.
- The disease eventually affects lymph nodes and other organs, usually resulting in death (Fig. 43.27).
- Clinical diagnosis should be confirmed by laboratory tests.

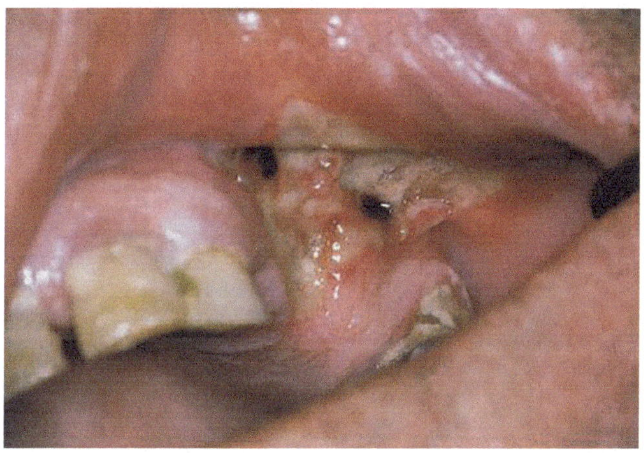

Fig. 43.24 Mycosis fungoides, irregular ulceration on the upper gingiva and alveolar mucosa

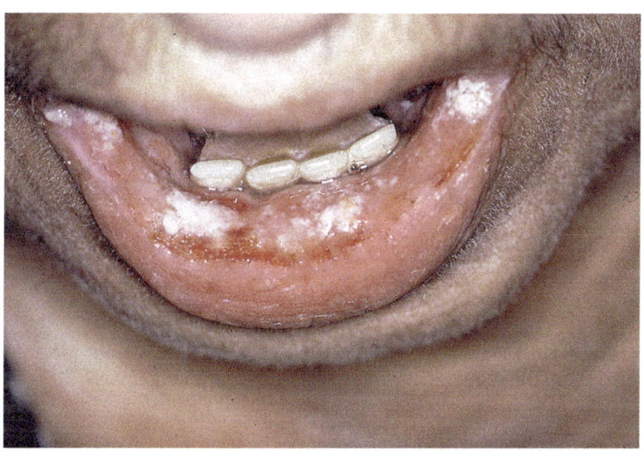

Fig. 43.25 Mycosis fungoides, extensive erosions on the lower lip

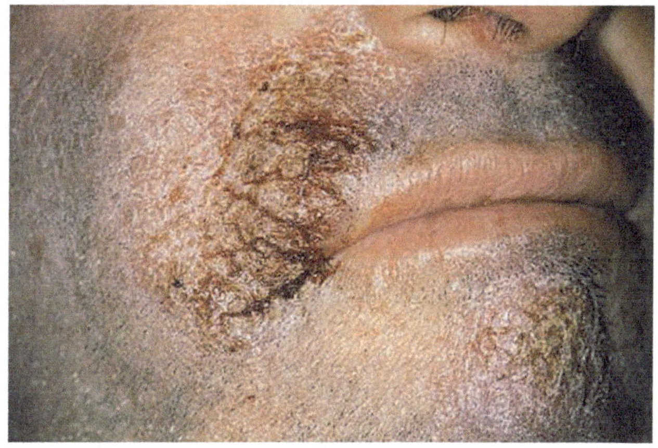

Fig. 43.26 Mycosis fungoides, perioral skin lesions

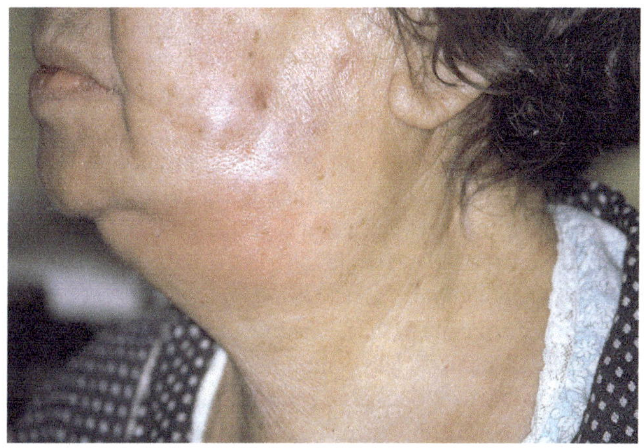

Fig. 43.27 Mycosis fungoides, submandibular lymph node enlargement

Differential Diagnosis

- Other types of Non-Hodgkin lymphomas
- Leukemia
- Myelodysplastic syndrome
- Psoriasis
- Lupus erythematosus

Laboratory Tests Histopathologic and immunohistochemical examinations.

Treatment Chemotherapy, biological response modifiers, radiotherapy. Symptomatic treatment for oral lesions.

Langerhans Cell Histiocytosis

Definition Langerhans cell histiocytosis is a clinicopathological heterogeneous group of clonal proliferative disorders characterized by dysfunction of Langerhans cells.

Etiology The cause and pathogenesis remain unclear. However, the presence of clonal CD1a and CD207 cells within the lesions indicates that the disease may be a clonal neoplastic disorder of diverse biological behavior. Recently, WHO classified Langerhans cell histiocytosis under dendritic and histiocytic cell neoplasms of the lymphatic tissue.

Classification Four major clinical forms are recognized:

(a) *Eosinophilic Granuloma:* a localized form that usually does not affect internal organs and has good prognosis. The disease most commonly affects individuals 7–15 years or older. Clinically, it is characterized mainly by solitary or multiple osseous lesions.
(b) *Hand-Schüller-Christian disease:* a chronic, multifocal form with a milder course and better prognosis. It usually presents between 2 and 6 years of age. Clinically, it is characterized by the classic triad: (a) *osteolytic* lesions; (b) *exophthalmos;* and (c) *diabetes insibitus*. Chronic otitis media and skin lesions may occur. Involvement of internal organs is less common.
(c) *Letterer-Siwe disease:* an acute multisystemic form that begins before the second year of life and has a poor prognosis. Clinically, it is characterized by fever, chills, weakness, multiple skin lesions (papules, scaly vesicles, pustules, petechiae, ecchymoses, ulcerations), enlargement of lymph nodes, involvement of internal organs, and osteolytic bone lesions.
(d) *Hashimoto-Pritzker* disease or congenital self-healing reticulohistiocytosis: a benign, self-healing clinical variant, which is limited to the skin, without oral lesions, and occurs at birth or soon after.

Gingival and Periodontal Involvement Relatively common, particularly in eosinophilic granuloma and Hand-Schüller-Christian disease. Non-dental biofilm-related gingivitis and severe periodontitis associated with osteolytic lesions in periodontal tissues and potential tooth loss.

Other Sites of Involvement Oral mucosa, jaws, bones, bone marrow, skin, visceral, lymph nodes.

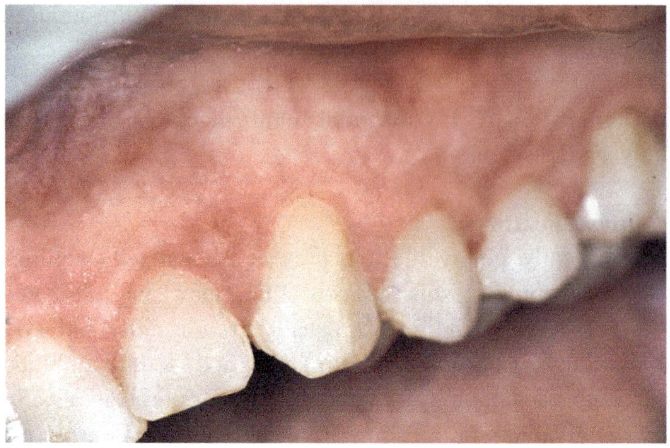

Fig. 43.28 Langerhans cell histiocytosis, early atypical gingival ulcerations of a patient with early eosinophilic granuloma

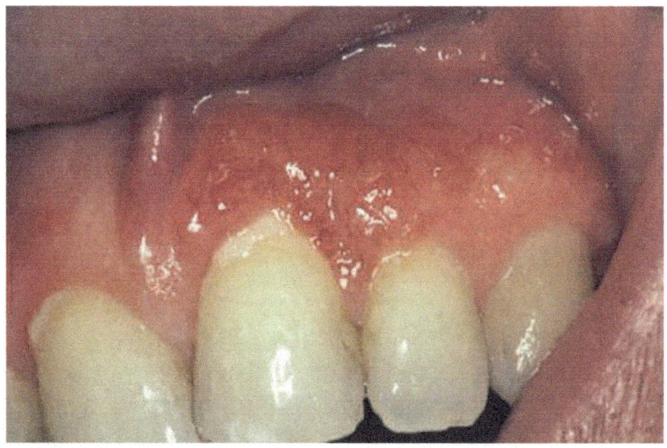

Fig. 43.29 Langerhans cell histiocytosis, localized swelling on the upper gingiva of a patient with eosinophilic granuloma

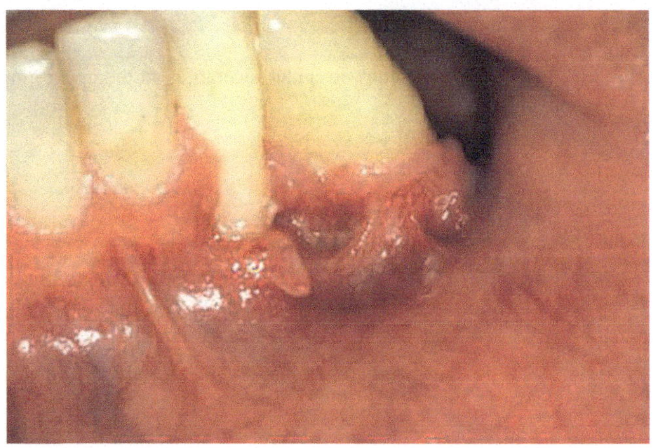

Fig. 43.30 Langerhans cell histiocytosis, localized swelling on the lower gingiva of a patient with eosinophilic granuloma

Clinical Features

- Gingival and periodontal lesions present as localized or multiple atypical ulcerations, usually associated with severe bone destruction and teeth loosening (Figs. 43.28, 43.29, 43.30, 43.31 and 43.32). Lesions may be the only manifestation for a long time, particularly in the eosinophilic granuloma.
- Oral lesions are characterized by atypical deep ulcerations, ecchymoses, edema, halitosis, taste disturbances,

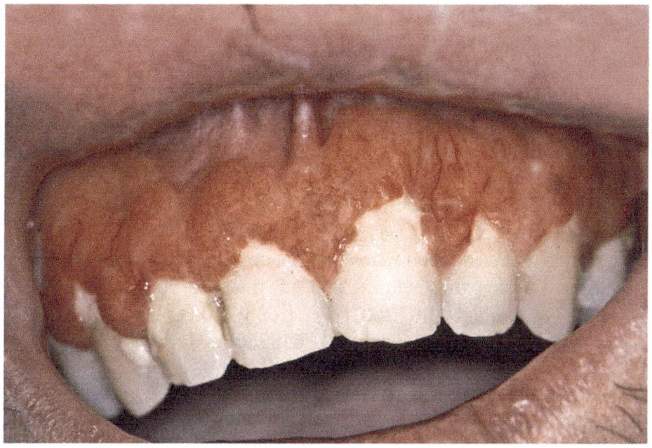

Fig. 43.31 Langerhans cell histiocytosis, marked gingival swelling of a patient with Hand-Schüller-Christian

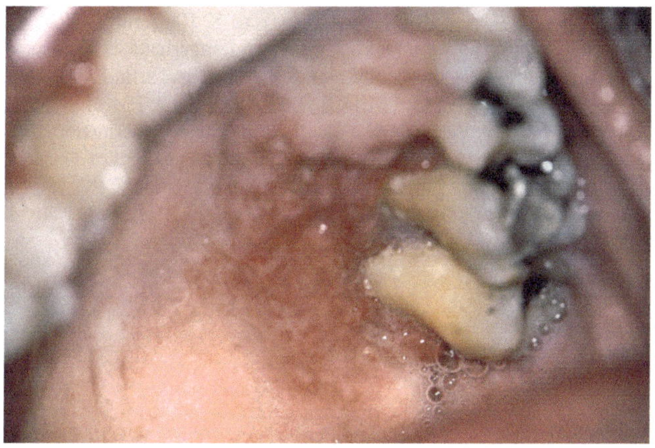

Fig. 43.32 Langerhans cell histiocytosis, ulceration on the palatal gingiva and bone destruction of a patient with Hand-Schüller-Christian

and are more common in both Hand-Schüller-Christian and Letterer-Siwe forms.
- Jawbone destruction, either solitary or multiple, is common in all three forms of the disorder.
- Clinical diagnosis should be confirmed by laboratory tests.

Differential Diagnosis
- Necrotizing gingivitis
- Severe necrotizing periodontitis
- Hypophosphatasia
- Acatalasia
- Hematological disorders
- Eosinophilic ulcer
- Leukemia
- Non-Hodgkin lymphoma
- Neoplasms

Laboratory Tests Histopathologic examination. Electron microscopy, immunohistochemical examination for CD1a and CD207 cells. Radiographic examination, CT, and MRI scans.

Treatment Dental plaque control and periodontal curettage. Surgical curettage with or without radiotherapy. Corticosteroids and chemotherapy for the systemic manifestations, should be left to specialists.

References

1. Angst PD, Dutra DA, Moreira CH, Kantorski KZ. Gingival inflammation and platelet count in patients with leukemia: preliminary results. Braz Oral Res. 2011;25:544–9.
2. Francisconi CF, Caldas RJ, Oliveira Martins LJ, et al. Leukemic oral manifestations and their management. Asian Pac J Cancer Prev. 2016;17(3):911–5. https://doi.org/10.7314/apjcp.2016.17.3.911. PMID: 27039811
3. Ishikawa S, Kato Y, Kabasawa T, et al. A case of myeloid sarcoma of the mandibular gingiva as extramedullary relapse of acute myeloid leukemia. Oral Maxillofac Surg. 2020;24(1):121–6. https://doi.org/10.1007/s10006-019-00812-y. Epub 2019 Dec 1. PMID: 31788742
4. Jin SH, Park G, Ko Y, Park JB. Myeloid sarcoma of the gingiva with myelodysplastic syndrome: a case report. Medicine (Baltimore). 2016;95(24):e3897. https://doi.org/10.1097/MD.0000000000003897. Erratum in: Medicine (Baltimore). 2016 Aug 07;95(31):e5074. PMID: 27310987; PMCID: PMC4998473
5. Arul AS, Verma S, Ahmed S, Arul AS. A clinical and fine needle aspiration cytology study of gingiva in acute leukemia. Dent Res J (Isfahan). 2012;9(1):80–5. https://doi.org/10.4103/1735-3327.92954. PMID: 22363368; PMCID: PMC3283984
6. Watson E, Wood RE, Maxymiw WG, Schimmer AD. Prevalence of oral lesions in and dental needs of patients with newly diagnosed acute leukemia. J Am Dent Assoc. 2018;149(6):470–80. https://doi.org/10.1016/j.adaj.2018.01.019. Epub 2018 Mar 30. PMID: 29606275
7. Nair SK, Faizuddin M, Jayanthi D, Malleshi SN, Venkatesh R. Extramedullary plasmacytoma of gingiva and soft tissue in neck. J Clin Diagn Res. 2014;8(11):ZD16–8. https://doi.org/10.7860/JCDR/2014/9305.5176. Epub 2014 Nov 20. PMID: 25584334; PMCID: PMC4290283
8. Moshref M, Mashhadi-Abbass F, Sargolzaei S, Nafarzadeh S. Extramedullary plasmacytoma of the gingiva. Arch Iran Med. 2007;10(1):91–3. PMID: 17198461
9. Lombardi N, Flora A, Franchini R, et al. Gingival localisation of extramedullary multiple myeloma. Lancet Oncol. 2019;20(11):e653. https://doi.org/10.1016/S1470-2045(19)30650-3. PMID: 31674324
10. Jain S, Kaur H, Kansal G, Gupta P. Multiple myeloma presenting as gingival hyperplasia. J Indian Soc Periodontol. 2013;17(3):391–3. https://doi.org/10.4103/0972-124X.115652. PMID: 24049344; PMCID: PMC3768194
11. Abdelwahed Hussein MR. Non-Hodgkin's lymphoma of the oral cavity and maxillofacial region: a pathologist viewpoint. Expert Rev Hematol. 2018;11(9):737–48. https://doi.org/10.1080/17474086.2018.1506326. Epub 2018 Aug 21. PMID: 30058399
12. Laskaris G, Stergiou G, Kittas C, Scully C. Hodgkin's disease involving the gingiva in AIDS. Eur J Cancer B Oral Oncol. 1992;28B(1):39–41. https://doi.org/10.1016/0964-1955(92)90010-x. PMID: 1422469
13. Navarro CM, Shibli JA, Ferrari RB, et al. Gingival primary extranodal non-Hodgkin's lymphoma as the first manifestation of acquired immunodeficiency syndrome. J Periodontol. 2008;79(3):562–6. https://doi.org/10.1902/jop.2008.070229. PMID: 18315441

14. Sugimoto KJ, Shimada A, Sakurai H, et al. Primary gingival diffuse large B-cell lymphoma: a case report and a review of the literature. Int J Clin Exp Pathol. 2013;7(1):418–24. PMID: 24427366; PMCID: PMC3885500
15. Tanaka J, Yoshida K, Suzuki M, Sakata Y. Hodgkin's disease of the maxillary gingiva. A case report. Int J Oral Maxillofac Surg. 1992;21(1):45–6. https://doi.org/10.1016/s0901-5027(05)80452-7. PMID: 1569365
16. Bagan JV, Carbonell F, Gómez MJ, et al. Extra-nodal B-cell non-Hodgkin's lymphomas of the head and neck: a study of 68 cases. Am J Otolaryngol. 2015;36(1):57–62. https://doi.org/10.1016/j.amjoto.2014.10.008. Epub 2014 Oct 8. PMID: 25456517
17. Patankar S, Venkatraman P, Sridharan G, Kane S. Burkitt's lymphoma of maxillary gingiva: a case report. World J Clin Cases. 2015;3(12):1011–6. https://doi.org/10.12998/wjcc.v3.i12.1011. PMID: 26677452; PMCID: PMC4677082
18. Deng D, Wang Y, Liu W, Qian Y. Oral and maxillofacial non-Hodgkin lymphomas: case report with review of literature. Medicine (Baltimore). 2017;96(35):e7890. https://doi.org/10.1097/MD.0000000000007890. PMID: 28858104; PMCID: PMC5585498
19. Meng W, Zhou Y, Zhang H, Jiang L, et al. Nasal-type NK/T-cell lymphoma with palatal ulcer as the earliest clinical manifestation: a case report with literature review. Pathol Oncol Res. 2010;16:133–7.
20. Laskaris GC, Nicolis GD, Capetanakis JP. Mycosis fungoides with oral manifestations. Oral Surg Oral Med Oral Pathol. 1978;46(1):40–2. https://doi.org/10.1016/0030-4220(78)90435-8. PMID: 277881
21. Viswanathan N, Nair RM, Nair RA. Cutaneous T cell lymphoma with multiple oral lesions. Indian J Otolaryngol Head Neck Surg. 2004;56(4):311–4. https://doi.org/10.1007/BF02974399. PMID: 23120108; PMCID: PMC3451155
22. Silva TD, Ferreira CB, Leite GB, et al. Oral manifestations of lymphoma: a systematic review. Ecancermedicalscience. 2016;10:665. https://doi.org/10.3332/ecancer.2016.665. PMID: 27594910; PMCID: PMC4990057
23. Abdull Gaffar B, Awadhi F. Oral manifestations of Langerhans cell histiocytosis with unusual histomorphologic features. Ann Diagn Pathol. 2020;47:151536. https://doi.org/10.1016/j.anndiagpath.2020.151536. Epub 2020 May 21. PMID: 32454442
24. Difloe-Geisert JC, Bernauer SA, Schneeberger N, Bornstein MM, Walter C. Periodontal manifestations of Langerhans cell histiocytosis: a systematic review. Clin Oral Investig. 2021;25(6):3341–9. https://doi.org/10.1007/s00784-021-03873-0. Epub 2021 Mar 22. PMID: 33751219; PMCID: PMC8137606.
25. Luz J, Zweifel D, Hüllner M, et al. Oral manifestation of Langerhans cell histiocytosis: a case report. BMC Oral Health. 2018;18(1):106. https://doi.org/10.1186/s12903-018-0568-5. PMID: 29884166; PMCID: PMC5994067
26. Madrigal-Martínez-Pereda C, Guerrero-Rodríguez V, Guisado-Moya B, Meniz-García C. Langerhans cell histiocytosis: literature review and descriptive analysis of oral manifestations. Med Oral Patol Oral Cir Bucal. 2009;14(5):E222–8. PMID: 19218906
27. Cisternino A, Asaad F, Fusco N, Ferrero S, Rasperini G. Role of multidisciplinary approach in a case of Langerhans cell histiocytosis with initial periodontal manifestations. Int J Clin Exp Pathol. 2015;8(10):13539–45. PMID: 26722570; PMCID: PMC4680515
28. Wang YC, Li ZZ, Yin CY, et al. Langerhans cell histiocytosis involving the oral and maxillofacial region: an analysis of 12 cases. Zhongguo Dang Dai Er Ke Za Zhi. 2019;21(5):415–20. https://doi.org/10.7499/j.issn.1008-8830.2019.05.003. PMID: 31104654; PMCID: PMC7389420

Part VII

Other Lesions, Tumors and Cysts Affecting Periodontal Tissues

44 Reactive Lesions

Contents

Pyogenic Granuloma

Definition Pyogenic granuloma is a common reactive lesion of oral mucosa.

Etiology It is not a true neoplasm but a reactive overgrowth of vascular tissue (capillary neoangiogenesis) to topical irritation or mild trauma.

Gingival Involvement Common. Dental biofilm may be associated.

Other Sites of Involvement Tongue, lips, buccal mucosa, palate.

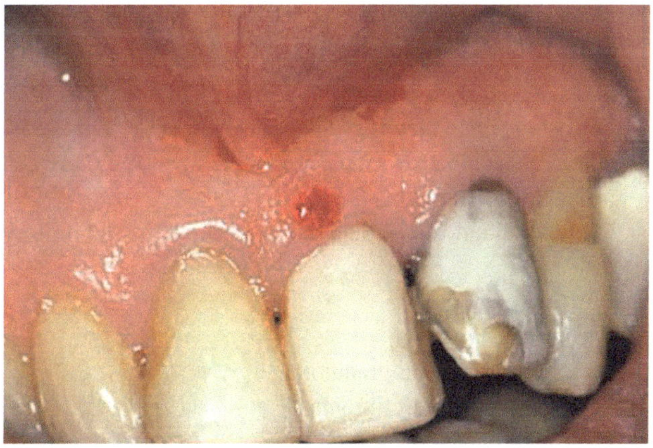

Fig. 44.1 Pyogenic granuloma, small lesion on the gingiva

Clinical Features

- It is more common in females (ratio 2:1) and can affect any age group. However, over 60% of patients are between 11 and 40 years of age. It shows a marked predilection for the gingiva (75% of all cases).
- Clinically, gingival pyogenic granuloma appears as a painless, sessile, or pedunculated exophytic nodule with smooth or slightly lobulated surface and deep red color (Figs. 44.1, 44.2 and 44.3) Often, the surface is ulcerated

G. Laskaris et al., *Periodontal Manifestations of Local and Systemic Diseases*, https://doi.org/10.1007/978-3-031-10828-0_44

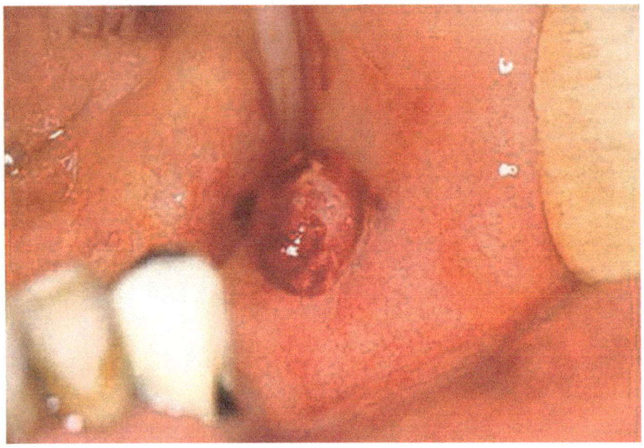

Fig. 44.2 Pyogenic granuloma on the alveolar mucosa of the mandible

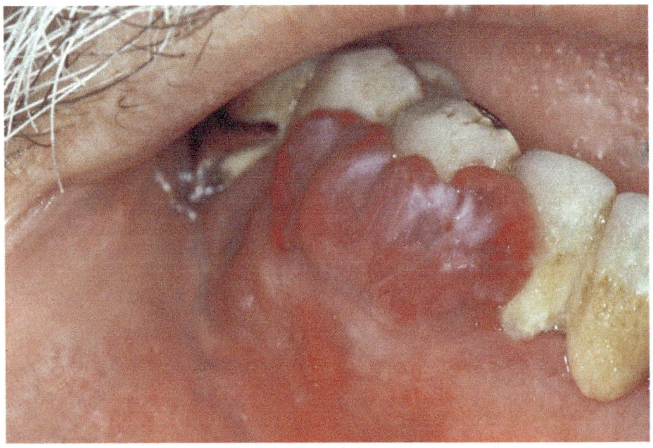

Fig. 44.3 Pyogenic granuloma, large exophytic multilobulated red nodule on the gingiva

and covered by a white-yellow membrane. It has elastic consistency and bleeds spontaneously or under light pressure. The lesion grows rapidly, and the size varies between a few millimeters to 1–2 cm.
- Clinical diagnosis should be confirmed by laboratory tests.

Differential Diagnosis
- Peripheral giant cell granuloma
- Peripheral ossifying fibroma
- Hemangioma
- Leiomyoma
- Kaposi sarcoma
- Hemangioendothelioma
- Hemangiopericytoma
- Angiosarcoma

Laboratory Tests Histopathologic examination.

Treatment The treatment of choice is conservative surgical excision.

Variations of Pyogenic Granuloma

Pregnancy Tumor Pregnancy granuloma or pregnancy tumor develops during pregnancy and has the same clinical and histological characteristics as pyogenic granuloma. It is believed to be caused by high estrogen levels in combination with local mechanical factors. It most commonly occurs during the second trimester of pregnancy, usually on the gingiva (Fig. 44.4).
- The recommended treatment is excision usually following childbirth. However, excision should be carried out during pregnancy in cases where the tumor causes irritation.

Postextraction Granuloma
- Postextraction granuloma is a variant of pyogenic granuloma that characteristically develops in the socket following recent dental extraction (Fig. 44.5).
- It is caused by dental, or osseous remnants or remnants of restoration materials left in the socket following the extraction of the tooth.
- Extraction socket debridement and curettage are the treatment of choice.

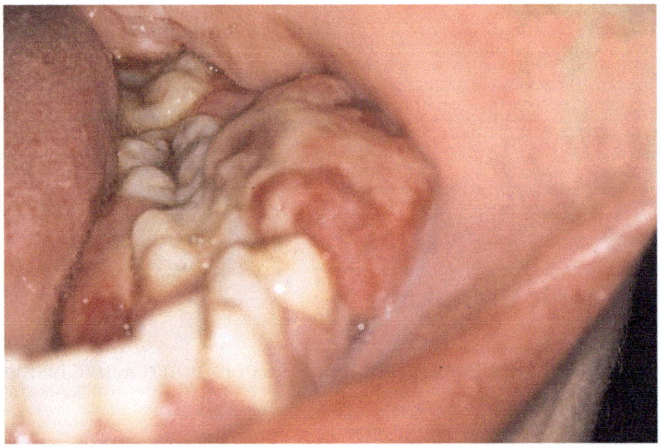

Fig. 44.4 Pregnancy granuloma on the gingiva

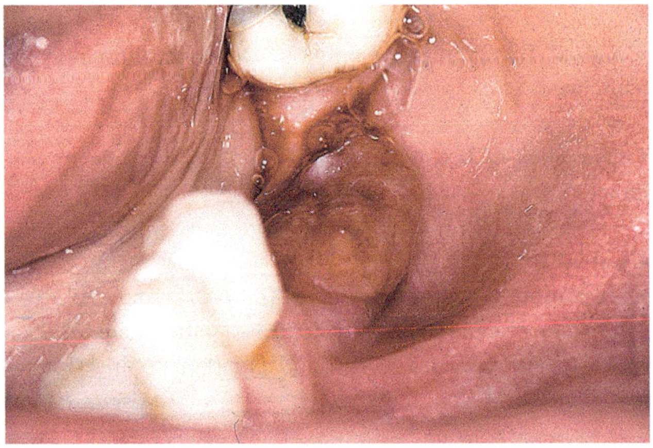

Fig. 44.5 Postextraction granuloma on the gingiva of the mandible

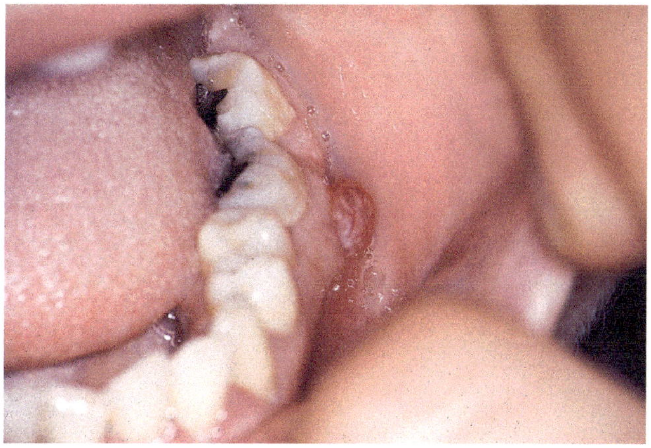

Fig. 44.6 Fistula granuloma on the gingiva of the mandible

Fistula Granuloma

- It characteristically develops at the opening of a dental or periodontal fistula (Fig. 44.6).
- Endodontic treatment of the responsible tooth or periodontal treatment/scaling is recommended.

Plasma Cell Granuloma

Definition Plasma cell granuloma is a rare reactive lesion composed of polyclonal plasma cells.

Etiology Unknown. It may be idiopathic or may represent an altered antigen-antibody reaction of the host or an alteration of blood flow imposing congestive vasodilation.

Gingival Involvement Rare. Possibly, a dental biofilm coinduced lesion.

Other Sites of Involvement In oral mucosa rare (tongue, lip, buccal mucosa). Primarily, lungs, brain, kidney, stomach, heart.

Clinical Features

- Clinically, plasma cell granuloma of the gingiva presents as a slowly growing tumor, usually asymptomatic, erythematous, well-circumscribed, and sessile covered by intact normal mucosa. Upon palpation, it is soft but not fluctuant (Fig. 44.7). The size varies from 0.5 to 2 cm. When it interferes with oral hygiene practice, it may become inflamed and hemorrhagic.
- The clinical characteristics are not pathognomonic since it resembles other lesions. Therefore, the final diagnosis will be placed after immunohistochemical testing that will reveal polyclonal plasma cells.
- Diagnosis should be confirmed by further laboratory investigation.

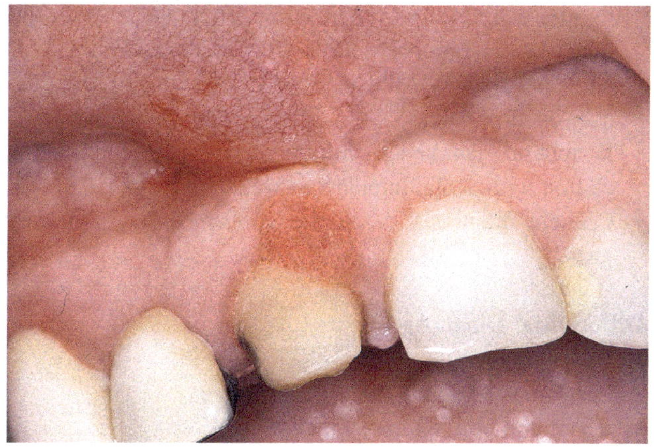

Fig. 44.7 Plasma cell granuloma, erythematous small nodule on the gingiva

Differential Diagnosis

- Localized juvenile spongiotic gingivitis
- Soft tissue plasmacytoma
- Pyogenic granuloma
- Peripheral giant cell granuloma
- Peripheral ossifying fibroma
- Fibroma

Laboratory Tests Histopathologic examination, immunohistochemical tests, in situ hybridization.

Treatment Conservative surgical excision.

Peripheral Giant Cell Granuloma

Definition Peripheral giant cell granuloma is a relatively common, reactive, tumor-like lesion with characteristic clinical and histologic features.

Etiology The lesion may represent a reactive process of the marginal gingiva to chronic mechanical irritation, dental biofilm, or mild trauma originating from mononuclear phagocytes or osteoclasts.

Gingival Involvement Exclusively. Usually dental biofilm-related lesions.

Other Sites of Involvement None.

Clinical Features

- It occurs exclusively on the gingiva and the alveolar mucosa of an edentulous ridge. It is the most prevalent of all reactive lesions.
- Clinically, peripheral giant cell granuloma appears as an asymptomatic, well-defined exophytic and circumscribed soft tumor of deep red to purple color with a relatively

rapid growth rate, an elastic consistency, and smooth surface that easily bleeds and is often ulcerated (Figs. 44.8, 44.9 and 44.10). Mild osseous destruction of the jaws may occur.
- Peripheral giant cell granuloma seems to develop in association with dental implants as well.
- Clinical diagnosis should be confirmed by laboratory tests.

Differential Diagnosis
- Pyogenic granuloma
- Peripheral ossifying fibroma
- Peripheral brown tumor
- Peripheral odontogenic neoplasms
- Kaposi sarcoma
- Hemangioendothelioma
- Hemangiopericytoma
- Malignant melanoma

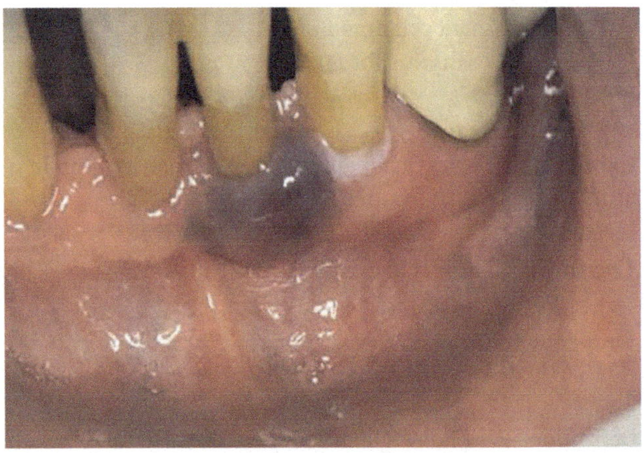

Fig. 44.8 Peripheral giant cell granuloma, bluish tumor on the mandibular gingiva

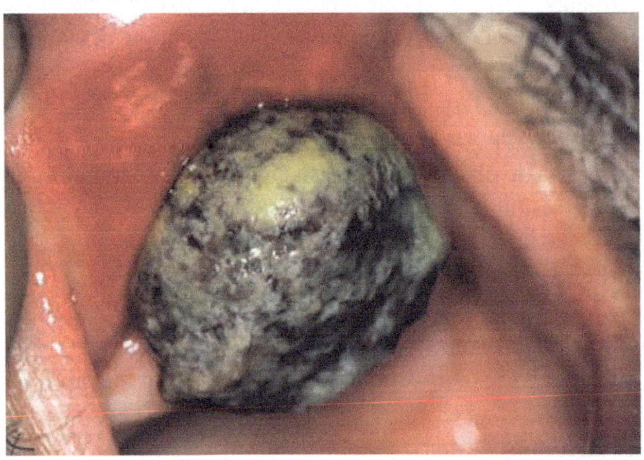

Fig. 44.9 Peripheral giant cell granuloma, large black tumor on the maxillary gingiva

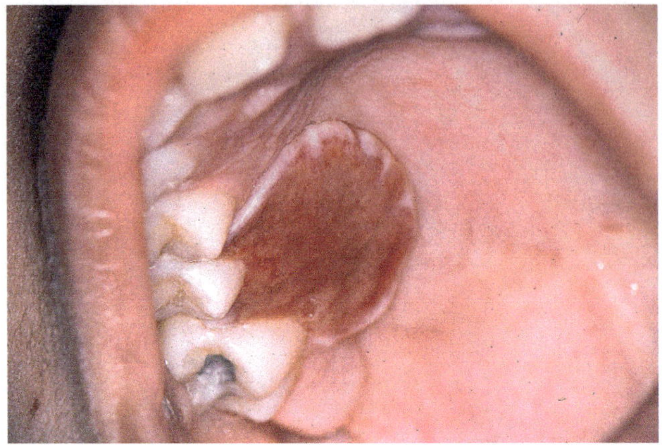

Fig. 44.10 Peripheral giant cell granuloma, large red exophytic tumor on the gingiva of the palate

Laboratory Tests Histopathologic examination and periapical radiographs.

Treatment The treatment of choice is conservative surgical excision.

"Brown" Giant Cell Tumor of Hyperparathyroidism

Definition "Brown" giant cell tumor is a rare non-neoplastic bone lesion associated with *primary* and, more commonly, *secondary* hyperparathyroidism.

Etiology The excessively secreted parathyroid hormone (PTH) which is caused by hyperfunction of parathyroid gland, causes bone resorption through overactive osteoclasts and "brown" giant cell tumor formation.

Gingival Involvement Rare.

Other Sites of Involvement Jaws usually mandible (rare), other bones.

Clinical Features
- The primary form of parathyroidism affects more often women over 60 years of age.
- Clinically, in the oral cavity, "brown" giant cell tumors may present in the jaws, sometimes being the early sign of the disease. Rarely the tumor may protrude as a soft painless, well-circumscribed mass on the gingiva due to bone destruction (Fig. 44.11). It can cause microfractures, hemorrhage, and calcification.
- In addition to tumors, hyperparathyroidism presents with polydipsia, polyuria hypertension, bone pain, fatigue,

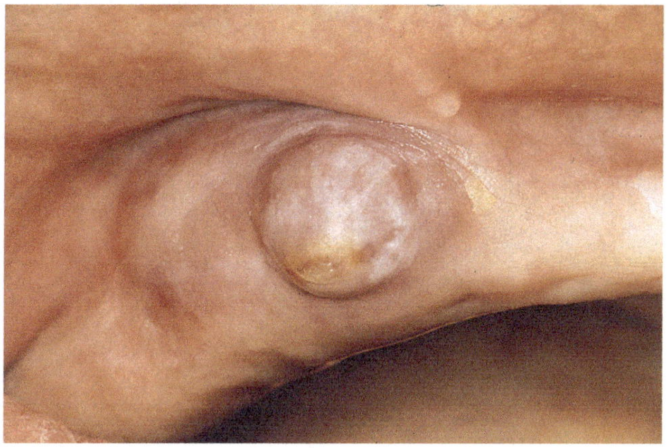

Fig. 44.11 "Brown" giant cell tumor of hyperparathyroidism, tumor on the alveolar mucosa of the maxilla

muscular weakness, osteoporosis, renal calculi, mental dysfunction.
- The clinical manifestations depend on the severity and the chronicity.
- The diagnosis of "brown" giant cell tumor is based on history, clinical and laboratory criteria.

Differential Diagnosis
- Central giant cell granuloma
- Peripheral giant cell granuloma
- Pyogenic granuloma
- Leiomyoma
- Kaposi sarcoma
- Hemangioendothelioma
- Hemangiopericytoma

Laboratory Tests Histopathologic examination, blood tests (serum calcium and phosphate, alkaline phosphatase, serum levels of intact PTH), skeletal and dental radiographs, CT scan, radioisotope scan.

Treatment Excision of the "brown" tumor is curative only if the underlying disease is treated simultaneously. With the PTH status corrected, "brown" tumors regress with normal ossification resumed.

Denture-Induced Fibrous Hyperplasia

Definition It is a denture-induced reactive lesion arising from excessive and continued mechanical pressure on the vestibular oral mucosa.

Etiology Pressure from denture flange areas causes chronic irritation and hyperplastic response.

Gingival Involvement Relatively rare. Non-dental biofilm-related lesion.

Other Sites of Involvement Vestibules and buccal sulcus.

Clinical Features
- Clinically, multiple (rarely solitary) and painless folds of tissue with a smooth, soft and pink surface, usually in the vestibule and the buccal sulcus (Figs. 44.12, 44.13 and 44.14).
- On the gingiva, exophytic and fibrous masses with a smooth, pink surface and firm in consistency are noticed.
- Lesion/s may be associated with discomfort and pain when inflammation and ulceration occur.
- Clinical diagnosis should be confirmed by laboratory tests.

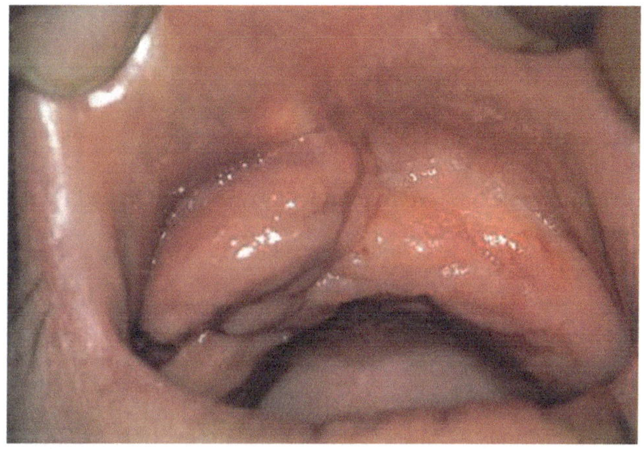

Fig. 44.12 Denture induced fibrous hyperplasia on the alveolar mucosa of the maxilla of an edentulous patient

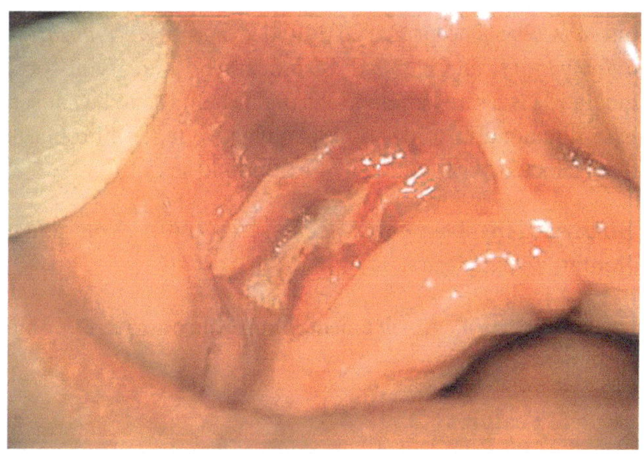

Fig. 44.13 Denture induced fibrous hyperplasia on the alveolar mucosa of the maxilla of an edentulous patient

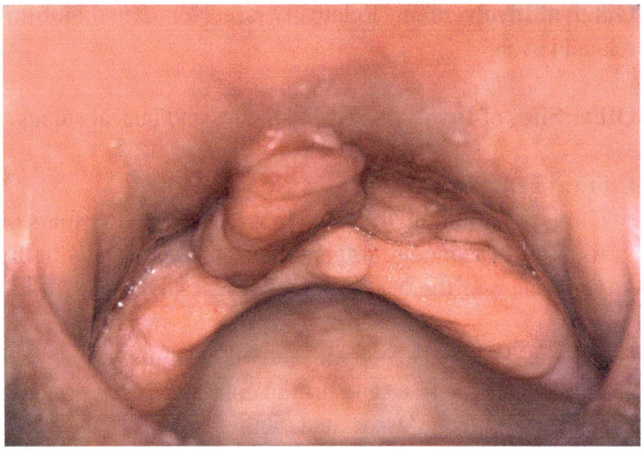

Fig. 44.14 Denture induced multifocal fibrous hyperplasia on the anterior alveolar mucosa of the maxilla

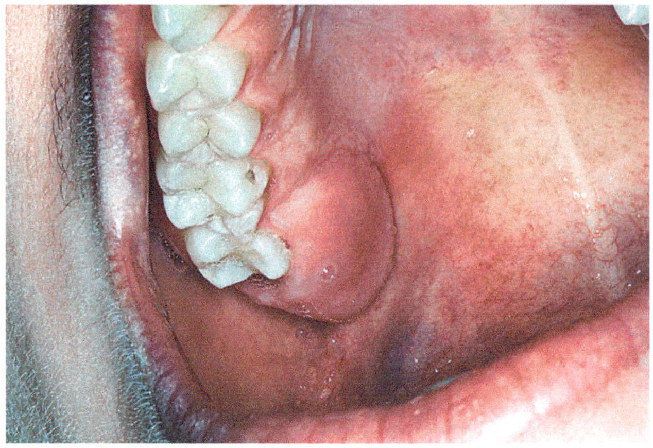

Fig. 44.15 Oral focal mucinosis, elevated mass of normal color on the palatal gingiva

Differential Diagnosis

- Multiple fibromas
- Neurofibromatosis
- Squamous cell carcinoma

Laboratory Tests Histopathologic examination.

Treatment Conservative surgical excision, followed by the construction of new dentures.

Oral Focal Mucinosis

Definition Mucinoses are a heterogenous group of disorders presenting with increased mucus production and deposition mainly on the skin.

Etiology The exact etiology is unknown.

Classification Mucinoses are classified into a. *primary;* and b. *secondary.* The primary is divided into a. *degenerative-inflammatory;* and b. *hamartomatous-neoplastic*. Oral focal mucinosis is a rare benign lesion and is believed to be caused by a functional disorder of the connective tissue fibroblasts that leads to overproduction of hyaluronic acid.

Gingival Involvement Common (>70%). Non-dental biofilm-induced lesion.

Other Sites of Involvement Oral mucosa (rare), skin (common).

Clinical Features

- Clinically, gingival or oral lesion presents as a well-circumscribed, painless tumor that might be sessile or pedunculated and is covered by smooth normal mucosa (Fig. 44.15). The size varies between 0.5 and 2.0 cm. It is more common in females between 30 and 50 years of age.
- Clinical diagnosis should be confirmed by laboratory tests.

Differential Diagnosis

- Fibroma
- Peripheral ossifying fibroma
- Lipoma
- Myxoma
- Cystadenoma

Laboratory Tests Histopathologic and histochemical examination.

Treatment Conservative surgical excision.

Angiolymphoid Hyperplasia with Eosinophilia

Definition Angiolymphoid hyperplasia with eosinophilia is a rare reactive and benign vascular disorder.

Etiology The exact etiology remains unknown, although mechanical trauma may be responsible.

Gingival Involvement Rare. Non-dental biofilm-induced lesions.

Other Sites of Involvement Skin (common), oral mucosa (rare), salivary glands, muscles.

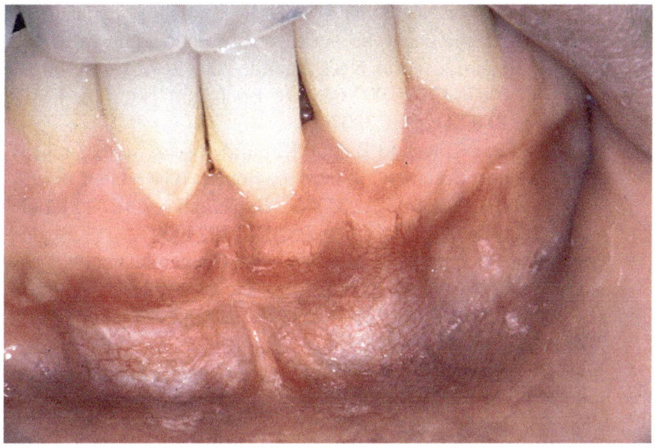

Fig. 44.16 Angiolymphoid hyperplasia with eosinophilia, flat lesion on the gingiva of the mandible

Clinical Features

- Clinically, the lesion appears as a red, painless nodule or papule with flat surface (Fig. 44.16). The gingiva, buccal mucosa, tongue, palate, and lips may be affected.
- It is more common in females between 30 and 50 years of age.
- Clinical diagnosis should be confirmed by laboratory tests.

Differential Diagnosis

- Pyogenic granuloma
- Hemangioma
- Benign lymphoid hyperplasia
- Angiosarcoma
- Kaposi sarcoma
- Kimuradisease

Laboratory Tests Histopathologic and histochemical examination.

Treatment Conservative surgical excision.

Granular Cell Tumor of the Newborn

Definition Granular cell tumor of the newborn, or congenital epulis of the newborn, is a reactive tumor exclusively seen in newborns.

Etiology Of unclear histogenesis. It may originate from primitive mesenchymal stem cells.

Gingival Involvement Rare. Non-dental biofilm-induced lesion.

Other Sites of Involvement None.

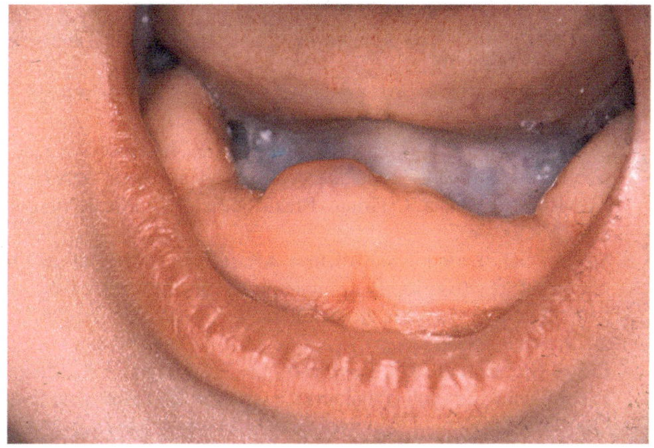

Fig. 44.17 Granular cell tumor of the newborn, multilobulated tumor on the alveolar mucosa

Clinical Features

- It occurs on the alveolar mucosa, most commonly seen in the maxilla than the mandible with a predilection for women (80–90%).
- Clinically, it usually appears as a solitary, asymptomatic, erythematous or normal in color, tumor with smooth or slightly papillomatous surface (Fig. 44.17). Its size varies between 0.5 and 2 cm.
- Clinical diagnosis should be confirmed by laboratory tests.

Differential Diagnosis

- Melanotic neuroectodermal tumor of infancy
- Hamartomas
- Gingival cyst of the newborn
- Hemangioma
- Pyogenic granuloma

Laboratory Tests Histopathologic examination, immunohistochemical analysis (cells positive for the S-100 protein).

Treatment Conservative surgical excision is recommended.

References

1. Naderi NJ, Eshghyar N, Esfehanian H. Reactive lesions of the oral cavity: a retrospective study on 2068 cases. Dent Res J (Isfahan). 2012;9(3):251–5. PMID: 23087727; PMCID: PMC3469888
2. Sharma S, Chandra S, Gupta S, Srivastava S. Heterogeneous conceptualization of etiopathogenesis: Oral pyogenic granuloma. Natl J Maxillofac Surg. 2019;10(1):3–7. https://doi.org/10.4103/njms.NJMS_55_18. PMID: 31205381; PMCID: PMC6563641
3. Kamal R, Dahiya P, Puri A. Oral pyogenic granuloma: various concepts of etiopathogenesis. J Oral Maxillofac Pathol. 2012;16:79–82.4.
4. Akdogan N, Yalçin B, Aksoy GG, et al. A case of plasma cell granuloma located on the gingiva. Am J Dermatopathol. 2017;39(5):393.

5. Kanteti AP, Kelsey WP, Duarte EM. Case report. A rare case of plasma cell granuloma. Case Reports in Dentistry. 2020;2020:8861918.
6. Pandav AB, Gosavi AV, Lanjewar DN, Jagadale RV. Gingival plasma cell granuloma. J Dent Res. 2012;9:816–20.
7. Dutra KL, Longo L, Grando LJ, Rivero ER. Incidence of reactive hyperplastic lesions in the oral cavity: a 10year retrospective study in Santa Catarina; Brazil. Braz J Otorhinolaryngol. 2019;85:399–407.
8. Soyele OO, Ladeji AM, Adebiyi KE, et al. Pattern of distribution of reactive localised hyperplasia of the oral cavity in patients at a tertiary health institution in Nigeria. Afr Health Sci. 2019;19(1):1687–94.
9. Lester SR, Cordell KG, Rosebush MS, Palaiologou AA, Maney P. Peripheral giant cell granulomas: a series of 279 cases. Oral Surg Oral Med Oral Pathol Oral Radiol. 2014;118(4):475–82.
10. Gual-Vaqués P, Jané-Salas E, Egido-Moreno S, et al. Inflammatory papillary hyperplasia: a systematic review. Med Oral Patol Oral Cir Bucal. 2017;22(1):e36–42.
11. Firoosmand LM, Almeide JD, Cabral LA. Study of denture-induced fibrous hyperplasia cases diagnosed from 1979-2001. Quintessence Int. 2005;36:825–9.
12. Silva Cunha JL, Leite AA, de Castro AT, et al. Oral focal mucinosis: a multi-institutional study and literature review. J Cutan Pathol. 2021;48(1):24–33. https://doi.org/10.1111/cup.13813. Epub 2020 Sep 8. PMID: 33410541
13. Tobouti PL, Horikawa FK, Matuck BF, et al. Oral focal mucinosis of the hard palate and gingiva. Autops Case Rep. 2018;8(4):e2018044. https://doi.org/10.4322/acr.2018.044. PMID: 30775321; PMCID: PMC6360821
14. Bartralot R, Garcia-Patos V, Hueto J, et al. Angiolymphoid hyperplasia with eosinophilia affecting the oral mucosa: report of a case and a review of the literature. Br J Dermatol. 1996;134(4):744–8. PMID: 8733384
15. Naqvi J, Ordonez NG, Luna MA, et al. Epithelioid hemangioendothelioma of the head and neck: role of podoplanin in the differential diagnosis. Head Neck Pathol. 2008;2(1):25–30. https://doi.org/10.1007/s12105-007-0035-0. Epub 2007 Oct 26. PMID: 20614338; PMCID: PMC2807604
16. Okubo A, Fujii K, Kondo T, et al. Kimura's disease in the oral cavity: a rare manifestation of immunoglobulin G4-related disease. J Dermatol. 2017;44(12):e357–8. https://doi.org/10.1111/1346-8138.14021. Epub 2017 Sep 19. PMID: 28925000
17. Kokubun K, Matsuzaka K, Akashi Y, et al. Congenital epulis. A case and review of the literature. Bull Tokyo Dent Coll. 2018;59(2):127–32. https://doi.org/10.2209/tdcpublication.2017-0028. PMID: 29962420
18. Silva GC, Vieira TC, Vieira JC, et al. Congenital granular cell tumour (congenital epulis): a lesion of multidisciplinary interest. Med Oral Patol Cir Bucal. 2007;12:E428–30.
19. Kumar R, Jaiswal S, Singhal A, Garg R. Congenital granular cell lesion: a rare tumor of new born. J Oral Maxillofac Pathol. 2013;17(3):440–2.
20. Lee JC, Huang HY. Soft tissue special issue: Giant cell-rich lesions of the head and neck region. Head Neck Pathol. 2020;14(1):97–108. https://doi.org/10.1007/s12105-019-01086-2. Epub 2020 Jan 16. PMID: 31950466; PMCID: PMC7021864
21. Gosavi S, Kaur H, Gandhi P. Multifocal osteolytic lesions of jaw as a road map to diagnosis of brown tumor of hyperparathyroidism: a rare case report with review of literature. J Oral Maxillofac Pathol. 2020;24(Suppl 1):S59–66. https://doi.org/10.4103/jomfp.JOMFP_319_19. Epub 2020 Feb 28. PMID: 32189907; PMCID: PMC7069142
22. Yigit B, Tanal M, Citgez B. Giant parathyroid adenoma diagnosed by brown tumour, a clinical manifestation of primary hyperparathyroidism: a case report. J Pak Med Assoc. 2021;71(4):1266–9. https://doi.org/10.47391/JPMA.393. PMID: 34125787

Fibro-Osseous Lesions

45

Contents

Fibrous Dysplasia

Definition Fibrous dysplasia is a benign, developmental disorder of bone, in which the normal architecture of bone is replaced by fibrous tissue containing varying amounts of mineralized foci.

Etiology The exact etiology remains unknown. Mutation in *GNAS 1* gene is common.

Classification Two forms of the disease are recognized: (a) the *monostotic*, which is limited to a single bone and accounts for 80–90% of cases; and (b) the *polyostotic* with involvement of two or more bones, where two types are described: (a) *Jaffe-Lichtenstein syndrome*; and (b) *McCune-Albright syndrome.*

Gingival Involvement Common. Dental biofilm-related lesion modified by the jaw bone lesions.

Other Sites of Involvement Long bones of extremity, ribs, femur, and shin are most often affected, bones of the skull, cranial and jaw bones.

Clinical Features

- It appears most commonly in the second or third decade of life.
- Clinically, in the *monostotic* form the jaw lesions present as painless and slow-growing bone swellings, usually unilateral and rarely bilateral. The swellings may be firm, elastic, or hard to palpation and may cause intraoral bone deformity and tooth displacement with resultant malocclusion (Fig. 45.1). In children, teeth in the affected area may fail to erupt. The maxilla is more often affected.
- Due to bone expansion decreased width of attached gingiva is observed as well as thin gingival tissue and occasionally frenum displacement. Severe malocclusion causes dental plaque accumulation that leads to caries and gingivitis (Fig. 45.2).
- The *polyostotic* form is characterized by the involvement of multiple bones, skin pigmentation or *café-au-lait macules*, endocrine dysfunction, and hormonal changes similar to those in pregnancy (Fig. 45.3).
- Clinical diagnosis should be confirmed by laboratory tests.

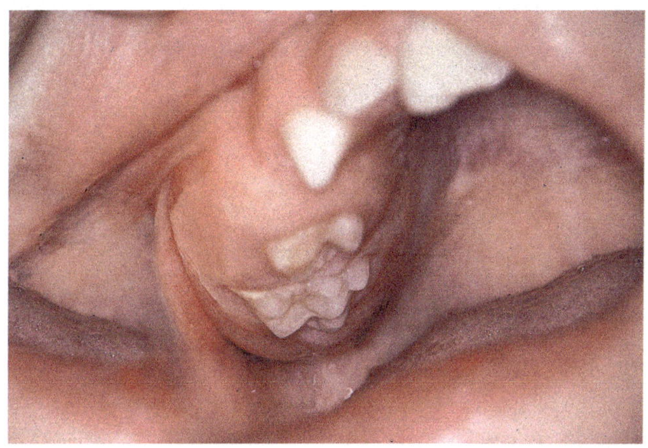

Fig. 45.1 Fibrous dysplasia, swelling of the bone and gingivar

G. Laskaris et al., *Periodontal Manifestations of Local and Systemic Diseases*, https://doi.org/10.1007/978-3-031-10828-0_45

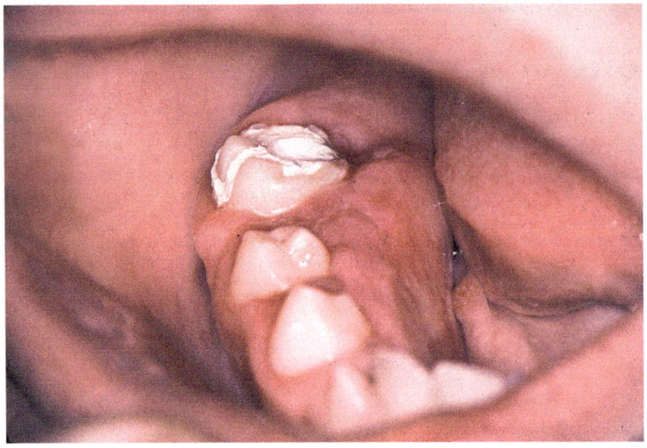

Fig. 45.2 Fibrous dysplasia, swelling of the bone and gingiva of the mandible

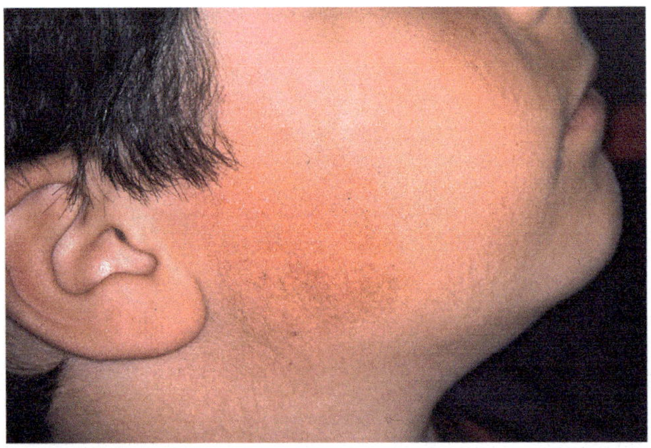

Fig. 45.3 Fibrous dysplasia, skin pigmentation

Differential Diagnosis

- Cherubism
- Odontogenic tumors
- Ossifying fibroma
- Paget disease
- Exostoses
- Osteosarcoma
- Chondrosarcoma
- Cemento osseous dysplasia
- Hyperparathyroidism
- Chronic sclerosing osteomyelitis

Laboratory Tests Histopathologic and radiographic examination. Computed tomography (CT) and magnetic resonance imaging (MRI). A slight elevation of serum alkaline phosphatase may be found.

Treatment Conservative surgical excision. Systemic bisphosphonates. Small and inactive jaw bone lesions do not require treatment.

Paget Disease

Definition Paget disease of bone or osteitis deformans is a progressive chronic metabolic disorder characterized by focal areas of accelerated bone remodeling activity.

Etiology The etiology is unknown. However, viral and hereditary (recurrent mutation of the gene encoding sequestosome 1-SQSTM1/p62) causes have been implicated.

Classification (a) *monostotic form*; and (b) *polyostotic* form.

Gingival Involvement Uncommon. Non-dental biofilm-induced lesion.

Other Sites of Involvement Long bones, pelvis, spine, and skull.

Clinical Features

- Aside from osteoporosis, Paget disease is the most common bone disorder with an increased incidence in persons 50 years or older.
- The jaws are affected in about 15–20% of cases with the maxilla being involved more often than the mandible. Progressive expansion of both the maxilla and mandible leads to symmetrical thickening of the alveolar ridges (Figs. 45.4 and 45.5). Complications include teeth mobility, difficult tooth extractions, delayed wound healing, postoperative bleeding, osteomyelitis after tooth extraction, postoperative infection, and ill-fitting denture. Due to bone expansion the gingiva may become thin and pale. Extensive contiguous erythematous and erosive gingivae may be observed in rare cases. Due to bite misalignment, gingivitis may develop.
- In the skull, bone enlargement can cause nerve compression leading to deafness, headaches, or vision loss.

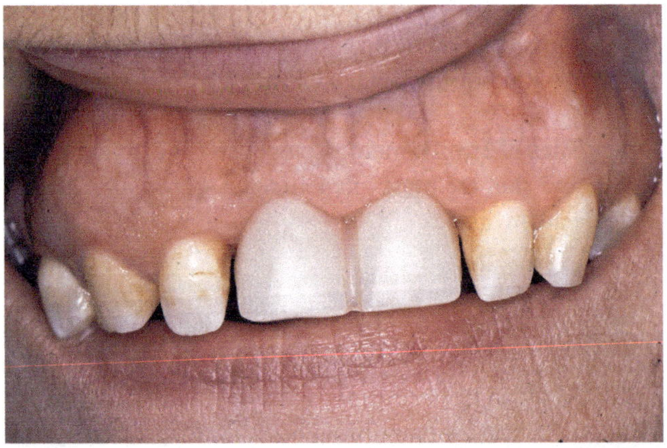

Fig. 45.4 Paget disease, expansion of the maxillary bone and thin pale gingiva

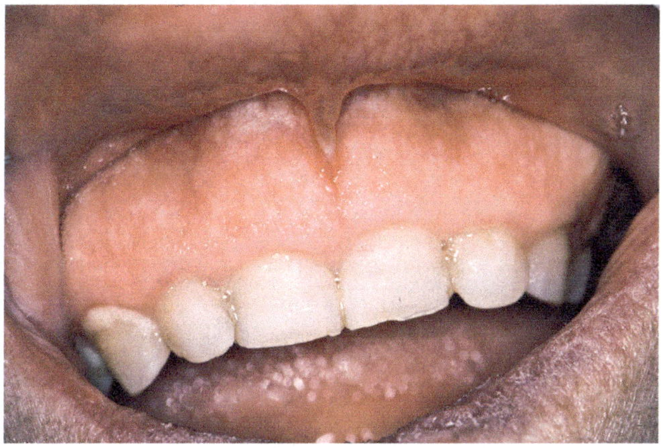

Fig. 45.5 Paget disease, expansion of the maxilla

Patients usually complain that their hats no longer fit. Other bone deformities are common.

- Symptoms of the disease are dull bone pain, joint pain, stiffness and swelling, numbness and tingling, and loss of movement affecting one part of the body.
- Complications include cranial neuropathies, malignant change (osteosarcoma), cardiac failure, increased skin temperature around the affected bones.
- Clinical diagnosis should be confirmed by laboratory tests.

Differential Diagnosis

- Fibrous dysplasia
- Other fibro-osseous lesions
- Multiple exostoses
- Multiple myeloma
- Osteosarcoma
- Hyperparathyroidism

Laboratory Tests Histopathologic examination. Radiographic imaging, computed tomography (CT) scan, MRI, scintigraphy, genetic testing, biochemical markers (serum alkaline phosphatase, N-telopeptide, C-telopeptide, urinary hydroxyproline).

Treatment Most cases require no treatment. Bisphosphonates, calcitonin or plicamycin may slow the pathological process. Analgesics and nonsteroidal anti-inflammatory drugs are also used. Surgical intervention is advised in cases with great osseous deformities.

References

1. Yang XD, Xu G, Song LH, et al. Comparison of radiological and clinicopathological features of craniofacial fibro-osseous lesions. Zhonghua Bing Li Xue Za Zhi. 2020;49(2):122–8. Chinese. https://doi.org/10.3760/cma.j.issn.0529-5807.2020.02.004.
2. Burke AB, Collins MT, Boyce AM. Fibrous dysplasia of bone: craniofacial and dental implications. Oral Dis. 2017;23(6):697–708. https://doi.org/10.1111/odi.12563. Epub 2016 Sep 1. PMID: 27493082; PMCID: PMC5292317
3. Hartley I, Zhadina M, Collins MT, Boyce AM. Fibrous dysplasia of bone and McCune-Albright syndrome: a bench to bedside review. Calcif Tissue Int. 2019;104(5):517–29. https://doi.org/10.1007/s00223-019-00550-z. Epub 2019 Apr 29. PMID: 31037426; PMCID: PMC6541017
4. Mac Donald DS. Maxillofacial fibro-osseous lesions. Clin Radiol. 2015;70(1):25–36.
5. Wang X, Wu L, Shi X, et al. Extramammary Paget's disease of the oral mucosa and perioral skin. Oral Surg Oral Med Oral Pathol Oral Radiol. 2017;124(2):e157–63. https://doi.org/10.1016/j.oooo.2017.05.473. Epub 2017 May 11
6. Galson DL, Roodman GD. Pathobiology of Paget's disease of bone. J Bone Metab. 2014;21:85–98.
7. Kang H, Park Y-C. Kyu Hyun Yang Paget's disease: skeletal manifestations and effect of bisphosphonates. J Bone Metab. 2017;24:97–103.
8. Al-Rashid M, Ramkumar DB, Raskin K, et al. Paget disease of the bone. Orthop Clin North Am. 2015;46(4):577–85.

Benign Peripheral Odontogenic Tumors

46

Contents

Ameloblastoma

Definition Ameloblastoma is the most common tumor of odontogenic epithelial origin.

Etiology The *extraosseous* or *peripheral* ameloblastoma may originate from dental lamina remnants or from basal cells of the surface epithelium. Recurrent activating mutations in FGFR2, BRAF, and RAS, leading to defective regulation of the MAPK pathway, may also be implicated.

Classification Ameloblastomas are classified into (a) *intraosseous* or *central*; and (b) *extraosseous* or *peripheral*.

Gingival Involvement Rare. Non-dental biofilm-related lesion.

Other Sites of Involvement Base of the tongue and floor of the mouth.

Clinical Features

- Ameloblastoma represents 1–2% of all cases and arises nearly always in the posterior tooth-bearing mucosa. It is more common between 30 and 60 years of age and affects males and females equally.
- Clinically, it develops in the gingiva and in the alveolar process of the jaws as a painless, slow growing, exophytic, solid, and erythematous mass with a smooth, granular, or papillary surface that rarely ulcerates (Fig. 46.1).
- It is a benign tumor, but occasionally can be locally aggressive, causing osseous destruction. Extremely rarely, it can undergo malignant transformation that gives metastases.
- Most commonly, there are no radiographic findings as the tumor may or may not cause mild osseous destruction.
- Clinical diagnosis should be confirmed by laboratory tests.

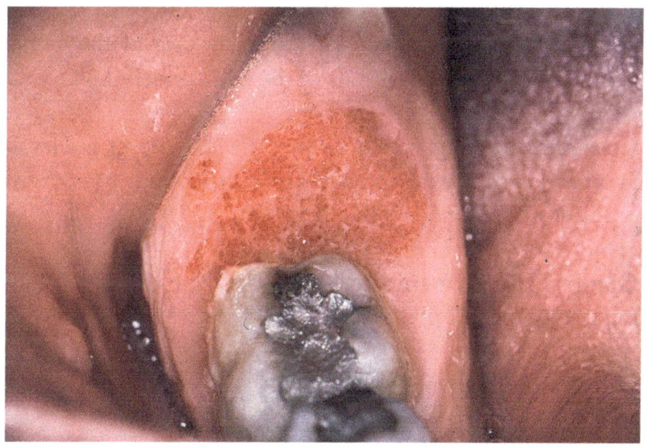

Fig. 46.1 Peripheral ameloblastoma, unusual red mass on the posterior alveolar mucosa

G. Laskaris et al., *Periodontal Manifestations of Local and Systemic Diseases*, https://doi.org/10.1007/978-3-031-10828-0_46

Differential Diagnosis

- Pyogenic granuloma
- Peripheral giant cell granuloma
- Fibroma
- Calcifying odontogenic tumor
- Non-Hodgkin lymphoma
- Squamous cell carcinoma

Laboratory Tests Histopathologic and radiographic examinations. Immunohistochemical examination (positive reactivity for cytokeratins AE1/AE3, KL1, 34beta E12, and MNF116).

Treatment A conservative supraperiosteal surgical excision. Continuous follow-up is necessary as late recurrence may occur.

Calcifying Epithelial Odontogenic Tumor

Definition The calcifying epithelial odontogenic tumor (CEOT), or Pindborg tumor, is a benign odontogenic tumor.

Etiology The tumor may arise from the rest of the dental lamina or from the basal cells of the oral epithelium.

Classification Depending on the affected site, it is classified into (a) *intraosseous* (94%) or *central*; and (b) *extraosseous* or *peripheral* (3–6%).

Gingival Involvement Relatively rare. Non-dental biofilm-related lesion.

Other Sites of Involvement None.

Clinical Features

- It is a slow growing, but locally invasive tumor that accounts for 0.4–3% of all odontogenic tumors and most commonly, occurs in the anterior part of the mouth of tooth-bearing and edentulous areas of the jaws. Mandible is affected twice as much as maxilla. The peripheral type demonstrates a less aggressive behavior and good prognosis.
- Clinically, gingival lesions present as single, painless, non-bleeding, and superficial soft tissue swellings that may be ulcerated or not (Fig. 46.2).
- Clinical diagnosis should be confirmed by laboratory tests.

Differential Diagnosis

- Other peripheral odontogenic tumors
- Peripheral ossifying fibroma

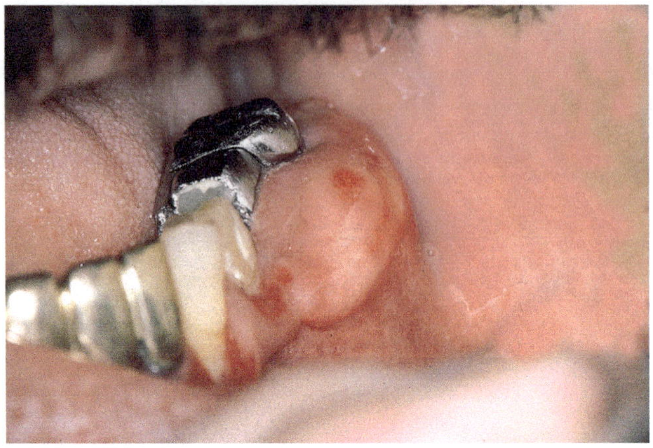

Fig. 46.2 Peripheral calcifying epithelial odontogenic tumor, soft gingival swelling

- Peripheral giant cell granuloma
- Chondrosarcoma
- Non-Hodgkin lymphoma
- Squamous cell carcinoma
- Metastatic neoplasms

Laboratory Tests Histopathologic and radiographic examination.

Treatment The treatment ranges from simple enucleation or curettage to radical and extensive resection.

Odontogenic Myxoma

Definition Odontogenic myxoma is a rare benign odontogenic tumor.

Etiology It is believed to be of mesenchymal, from the tooth germ or ectomesenchymal origin.

Gingival Involvement Rare. Non-dental biofilm-related lesion.

Other Sites of Involvement Jaws.

Clinical Features

- Odontogenic myxoma most commonly affects the molar region of the mandible of both sexes between the ages 20 and 30 years.
- Clinically, the gingival odontogenic myxoma appears, due to the bone destruction and expansion of the intraosseous lesion, as a painless, soft, exophytic, and elevated gingival mass with a pink/reddish color (Fig. 46.3). It lacks specific characteristics, mimicking a nonspecific gingival enlargement.
- Clinical diagnosis should be confirmed by laboratory tests.

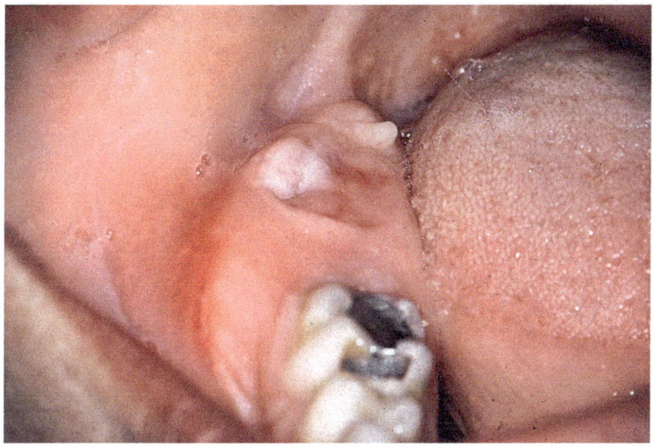

Fig. 46.3 Peripheral odontogenic myxoma, expanding bone mass, extending to the gingiva

Differential Diagnosis

- Peripheral giant cell granuloma
- Peripheral ossifying fibroma
- Calcifying epithelial odontogenic tumor
- Peripheral ameloblastoma
- Hemangioma

Laboratory Tests Radiographic, histopathologic, and immunohistochemical examination.

Treatment Surgical excision.

References

1. Beena VT, Choudhary K, Heera R, et al. Peripheral ameloblastoma: a case report and review of literature. Case Reports in Dentistry. 2012;2012:571509.
2. Vezhavendhan N, Vidyalakshmi S, Muthukumaran R, et al. Peripheral ameloblastoma of the gingiva. Autops Case Rep. 2020;10(1):e2019127.
3. Houston GD, Fowler CB. Extraosseous calcifying epithelial odontogenic tumor: report of two cases and review of the literature. Oral Surg Oral Med Oral Pathol Oral Radiol Endod. 1997;83:577e583.
4. Soares ECS, Costa FWG, Esses DFS, et al. Gingival calcifying epithelial odontogenic tumor: case report and review of the literature comprising a period of 44 years. J Clin Exp Dent. 2011;3(5):e491ee496.
5. Feitosa SG, et al. Peripheral calcifying epithelial odontogenic tumor: case report. Oral Surg Oral Med Oral Pathol Oral Radiol. 2020;129(1):e102.
6. Shenoy VS, et al. Soft tissue myxoma- a rare differential diagnosis of localized oral cavity lesions. J Clin Diagn Res. 2014;8(12):KD01–2. https://doi.org/10.7860/JCDR/2014/10189.5288. Epub 2014 Dec 5. PMID: 25653975; PMCID: PMC4316281
7. Chrcanovic BR, Gomez RS. Odontogenic myxoma: an updated analysis of 1,692 cases reported in the literature. Oral Dis. 2019;25(3):676–83. https://doi.org/10.1111/odi.12875. Epub 2018 Jun 8. PMID: 29683236
8. Kanitkar S, Kamat M, Tamagond S, Varekar A, Datar U. Peripheral odontogenic myxoma in a 12-year-old girl: a rare entity. J Korean Assoc Oral Maxillofac Surg. 2017;43(3):178–81. https://doi.org/10.5125/jkaoms.2017.43.3.178. Epub 2017 Jun 28. PMID: 28770159; PMCID: PMC5529192

Soft Tissue Cysts

47

Contents

Cysts are epithelium-lined, pathological cavities, usually filled with fluid, semi-solid material, or cellular debris. Cysts of the oral cavity are a histologically and genetically heterogenous group of disorders. They are mainly located in the soft tissues of the oral cavity. Clinically, they present as a soft or fluctuant swelling. The cysts that are included in this group may be developmental, odontogenic, and non-odontogenic, traumatic in origin, located on the gingival tissue.

Eruption Cyst

Definition Eruption cyst is a variant of dentigerous cyst arising from the follicle of an erupting deciduous or permanent tooth, located just above the tooth crown.

Etiology It is due to separation of the dental follicle from around the crown of the tooth.

Gingival Involvement Exclusively. Non-dental biofilm-induced lesion.

Other Sites of Involvement None.

Clinical Features

- It usually occurs at the site of eruption of the maxillary central incisors and first permanent molars in children younger than 10 years.
- Clinically, eruption cyst appears as well-demarcated, soft fluctuant swelling directly overlying the crown of an erupting deciduous or permanent tooth (Figs. 47.1, 47.2).
- They often burst spontaneously before eruption of the associated tooth. Usually, the color is blue or dark red, depending on the amount of blood in the cystic fluid.
- Clinical diagnosis should be confirmed by laboratory tests.

Differential Diagnosis

- Other odontogenic cysts
- Hematoma
- Hemangioma
- Oral pigmented nevi
- Malignant melanoma
- Amalgam tattoo
- Melanotic neuroectodermal tumor of infancy*

Laboratory Tests Histopathologic and radiographic examination.

G. Laskaris et al., *Periodontal Manifestations of Local and Systemic Diseases*, https://doi.org/10.1007/978-3-031-10828-0_47

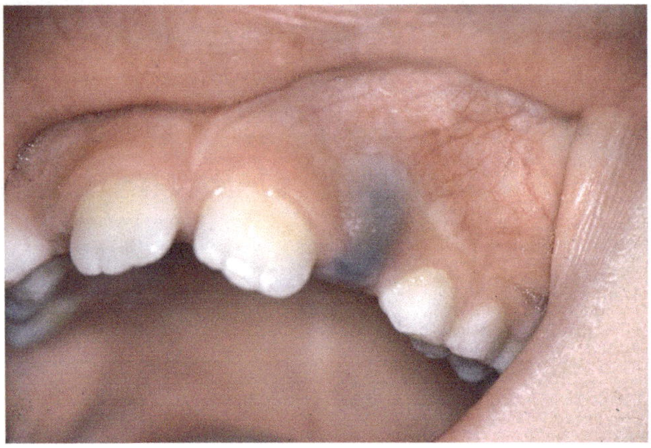

Fig. 47.1 Eruption cyst, blue swelling at the site of erupting tooth

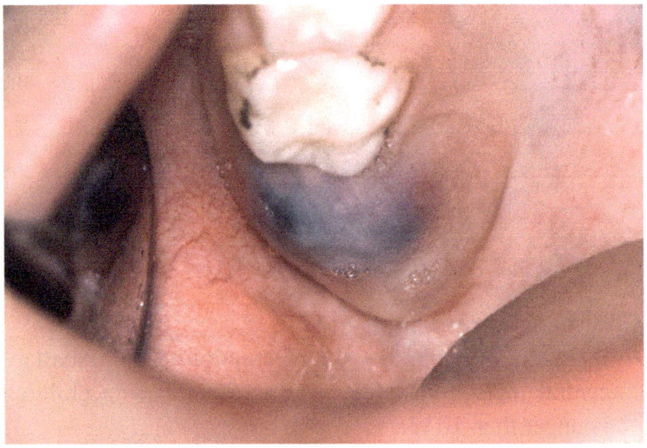

Fig. 47.2 Eruption cyst, blue swelling at the site of erupting tooth

Treatment Usually none. Rarely, they require excision if impeding normal eruption. In cases with symptoms or secondary infection, a simple excision of the roof of the cyst is recommended.

Gingival Cysts of the Newborn

Definition Gingival cysts of newborns are small and keratin-filled cysts on the alveolar mucosa of infants that appear at birth or soon thereafter.

Etiology They arise from remnants of the dental lamina.

Gingival Involvement Relatively common. Non-dental biofilm-related lesion. They appear on alveolar mucosa before tooth eruption and gingival formation.

Other Sites of Involvement Similar lesions may occur along the median palatal raphe (*Epstein's pearls*) or scattered in the hard palate (*Bohn's nodules*).

Clinical Features

- Clinically, they appear as multiple or solitary, asymptomatic, superficial, and raised whitish nodules with a diameter of 1–3 mm. They usually occur in the maxillary alveolar mucosa (Figs. 47.3, 47.4).
- The cysts contain keratin and regress spontaneously within a few weeks.
- Diagnosis is mainly based on clinical features.

Differential Diagnosis

- Lymphangioma
- Hamartomas
- Granular-cell tumor of the newborn
- Other odontogenic cysts

Laboratory Tests Histopathologic examination may be required for a definitive diagnosis.

Treatment No treatment is required as the lesions regress spontaneously.

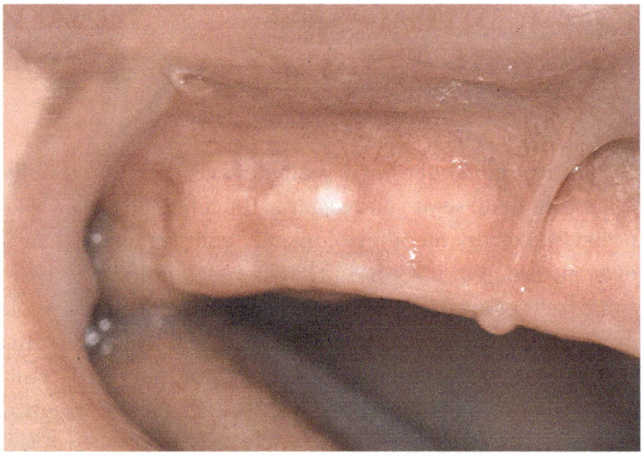

Fig. 47.3 Gingival cyst of the newborn, white nodule on the alveolar mucosa

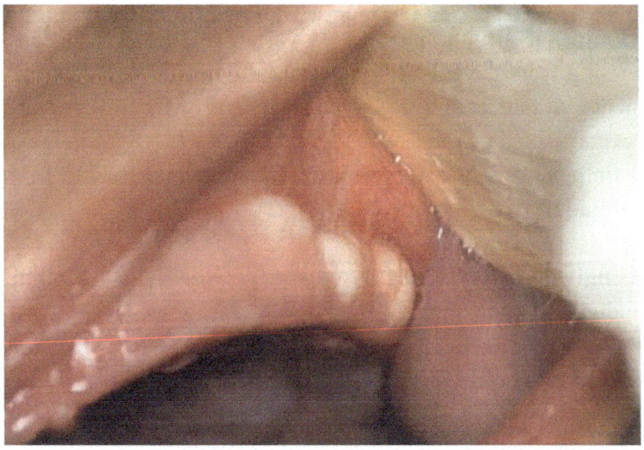

Fig. 47.4 Multiple gingival cysts of the newborn on the maxilla

Gingival Cyst of the Adult

Definition Gingival cyst of the adult is an uncommon lesion located on free or attached gingiva.

Etiology It originates from remnants of the dental lamina.

Gingival Involvement Exclusively, non-dental biofilm-induced lesion.

Other Sites of Involvement None.

Clinical Features

- The condition is more frequent in patients over 40 years of age.
- It is found on the free or attached gingiva, usually between the mandibular lateral incisor, canine, and premolar (70–80%).
- Clinically, it appears as a painless, spherical, and well-circumscribed swelling, 0.5–1 cm in diameter, and of normal color (Figs. 47.5, 47.6, 47.7). The adjacent teeth are vital.
- Clinical diagnosis should be confirmed by laboratory test.

Differential Diagnosis

- Other odontogenic cysts
- Lateral periodontal cyst
- Dental or periodontal abscess
- Fibroma
- Peripheral ossifying fibroma
- Neurofibroma

Laboratory Tests Histopathologic examination. There are no radiographic findings.

Treatment Conservative surgical removal.

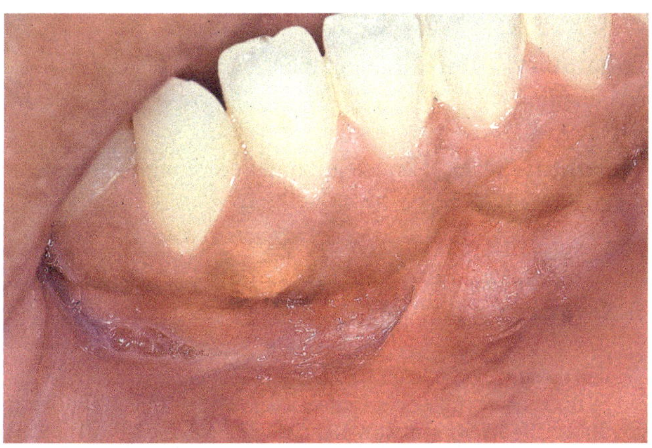

Fig. 47.5 Gingival cyst of the adult on the anterior gingiva of the mandible

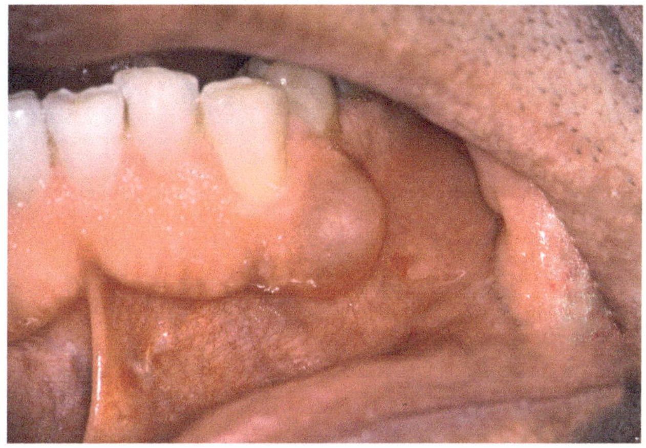

Fig. 47.6 Gingival cyst of the adult on the mandible

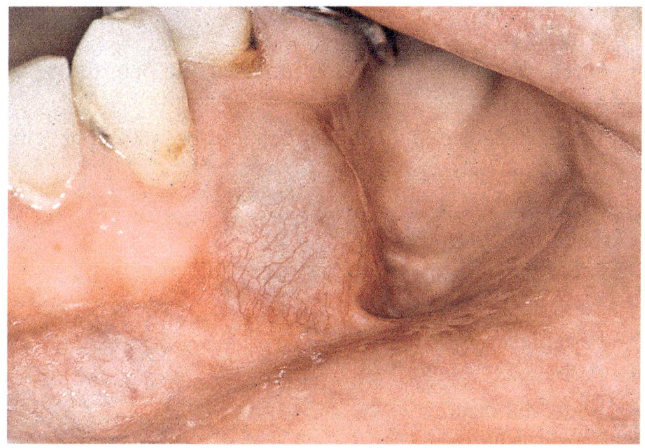

Fig. 47.7 Gingival cyst of the adult on the mandible

Incisive Papilla Cyst

Definition A relatively rare non-odontogenic cyst in the palatine papilla.

Etiology A developmental cyst that is believed to arise from epithelial remnants of the nasopalatine duct.

Gingival Involvement Rare. Non-dental biofilm-induced lesion.

Other Sites of Involvements None.

Clinical Features

- It may occur either within the nasopalatine canal or in the soft tissues of the palate, at the opening of the canal, usually after the age of 40.
- Clinically, it appears as a spherical and soft swelling of incisive papilla and surrounding gingiva, covered by normal mucosa (Fig. 47.8). It grows slowly and is usually

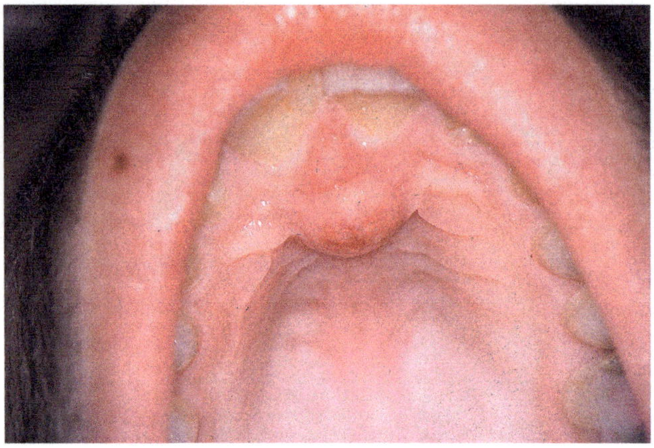

Fig. 47.8 Incisive papilla cyst

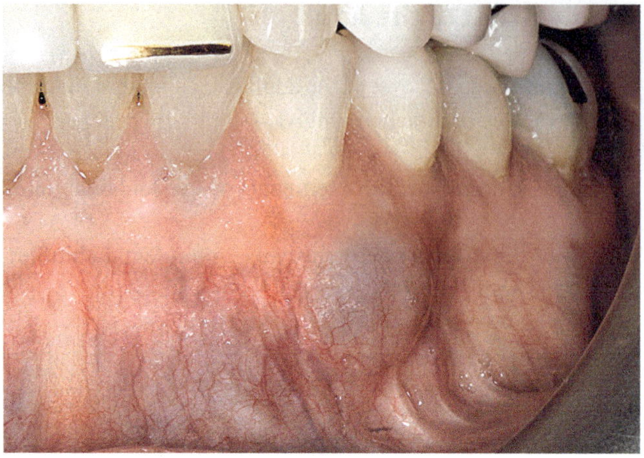

Fig. 47.9 Lateral periodontal cyst at the area of the canine protruding on the gingiva as the result of bone destruction

asymptomatic or it may discharge into the mouth giving a salty taste.
- Often, the cyst may become inflamed and painful due to infection.
- Diagnosis is based on clinical features but should be confirmed by laboratory tests.

Differential Diagnosis
- Other odontogenic cysts
- Periapical granuloma
- Periapical cyst
- Periodontal abscess
- Radicular cyst

Laboratory Tests Radiography, pulp vitality test of teeth adjacent to the lesion, histopathologic examination.

Treatment Conservative surgical excision.

Lateral Periodontal Cyst

Definition Lateral periodontal cyst is a non-keratinized and non-inflammatory developmental cyst located adjacent or lateral to the root of a vital tooth.

Etiology Developmental cyst that originates from either the remnants of dental lamina, reduced enamel epithelium, or rest of Malassez.

Gingival Involvement Rare. Non-dental biofilm-induced lesion.

Other Sites of Involvement Alveolar bone.

Clinical Features
- Lateral periodontal cyst is more prevalent in adults in the fifth to seventh decades of life—with mean age of 52 years—without preference for race or sex. The most frequently reported location is the mandibular premolar area, followed by the anterior region of maxilla.
- It is an intraosseous lesion that is usually asymptomatic. The cyst is often discovered during routine radiographic examination. The associated teeth are vital. Radiographs of the lateral periodontal cyst show a well-circumscribed, round or ovoid radiolucent area, usually with a sclerotic margin.
- Clinically, on the gingiva it presents as a small swelling due to cortical expansion or secondary inflammation, or as a swelling of the alveolar mucosa, followed by tenderness (Fig. 47.9).
- The final diagnosis should be based on clinical, radiologic, and histopatologic examination.

Differential Diagnosis
- Odontogenic cyst
- Lateral radicular cyst
- Lesions of endodontic and periodontal origin
- Gingival cyst of the adult
- Other cysts

Laboratory Tests Radiographic and histopathologic examination.

Treatment Surgical enucleation with thorough curettage is the treatment of choice.

References

1. de Oliveira AJ, Silveira ML, Duarte DA, Diniz MB. Eruption cyst in the neonate. Int J Clin Pediatr Dent. 2018;11(1):58–60. https://doi.org/10.5005/jp-journals-10005-1485. Epub 2017 Feb 1. PMID: 29805237; PMCID: PMC5968165
2. Dhawan P, Kochhar GK, Chachra S, et al. Eruption cysts: a series of two cases. Dent Res J (Isfahan). 2012;9(5):647–50.

3. Nagaveni NB, Umashankara KV, Radhika NB, Maj Satisha TS. Eruption cyst: a literature review and four case reports. Indian J Dent Res. 2011;22:148–51.
4. Diaz de Ortiz LE, Mendez MD. Epstein pearls. In: Stat Pearls [Internet]. Treasure Island (FL): Stat Pearls Publishing; 2021. PMID: 29630229.
5. Moda A. Gingival cyst of newborn. Inter J Clin Ped Dent. 2011;4(1):83–4.
6. Chrcanovic BR, Gomez RS. Gingival cyst of the adult, lateral periodontal cyst, and botryoid odontogenic cyst: an updated systematic review. Oral Dis. 2019;25(1):26–33. https://doi.org/10.1111/odi.12808. Epub 2018 Feb 8. PMID: 29156092
7. Viveiros SK, Pinho RFC, Custódio M, et al. A rare odontogenic cyst: gingival cyst of the adult. A series of 20 new cases from a single center. J Craniomaxillofac Surg. 2019;47(4):647–50. https://doi.org/10.1016/j.jcms.2019.01.048. Epub 2019 Feb 2. PMID: 30773330
8. Houston GD. Incisive canal cyst. J Okla Dent Assoc. 2011;102(8):47. PMID: 22216592
9. Barros CCDS, Santos HBP, Cavalcante IL, et al. Clinical and histopathological features of nasopalatine duct cyst: a 47-year retrospective study and review of current concepts. J Craniomaxillofac Surg. 2018;46(2):264–8. https://doi.org/10.1016/j.jcms.2017.11.014. Epub 2017 Dec 2. PMID: 29248496
10. Friedrich RE, Scheuer HA, Zustin J. Lateral periodontal cyst. In Vivo. 2014;28(4):595–8. PMID: 24982228
11. Kerezoudis NP, Donta-Bakoyianni C, Siskos G. The lateral periodontal cyst: aetiology, clinical significance and diagnosis. Endod Dent Traumatol. 2000;16(4):144–50. https://doi.org/10.1034/j.1600-9657.2000.016004144.x. PMID: 11202873
12. das Chagas LF, de Carvalho S, Lima CF, Cabral LAG, et al. Lateral periodontal cyst: a case report and literature review. J Oral Maxillofac Res. 2010;1(4):e5.
13. Ramesh R, Sadasivan A. Lateral periodontal cyst a diagnostic dilemma: report of a rare case with CBCT and histological findings. Int J Surg Case Rep. 2020;75:454–7.
14. Menditti D, Laino L, Di Domenico M, et al. Review cysts and pseudocysts of the oral cavity: revision of the literature and a new proposed classification. In Vivo. 2018;32:999–1007. https://doi.org/10.21873/invivo.11340.

Appendix: Classification of Gingival Lesions by Color and Morphology

Color (Tables A.1, A.2, and A.3)

Table A.1 White Lesions

Keratinizing, attached to the gingiva	Non-keratinizing, scraped off from the gingiva
Frictional keratosis	Materia alba
Smoker's keratosis	Chemical burns
Leukoplakia	Thermal burn
Leukoplakia due to sanguinaria	Necrotic epithelium after erosions or ulcerations
Hairy leukoplakia	Pseudomembranous candidiasis
Candidal leukoplakia	Syphilitic mucous patches
Chronic mucocutaneous candidiasis	Necrotizing gingivitis
White sponge nevus	Others
Focal palmoplantar and oral mucosa hyperkeratosis syndrome	
Darier's disease	
Lichen planus	
Lichenoid reaction	
Discoid lupus erythematosus	
Psoriasis	
Squamous cell carcinoma	
Verrucous carcinoma	
Cinnamon contact stomatitis	
Uremic stomatitis	
Others	

Table A.2 Red lesions

Dental biofilm-induced gingivitis	Erythroplakia
Spongiotic gingivitis	Squamous cell carcinoma
Periodontitis	Leukemia
Traumatic lesions	Cyclic neutropenia
Allergic reactions	Thrombocytopenic purpura
Drug-influenced gingivitis	Soft tissue plasmacytoma
Plasma cell gingivitis	Capillary hemangioma
Granulomatous gingivitis	Sturge-weber syndrome
Desquamative gingivitis	Klippel-Trénaunay-weber syndrome
Erythematous candidiasis	Cystic fibrosis
Linear gingival erythema	Hereditary hemorrhagic telangiectasia
Herpetic gingivitis	Sjögren syndrome
Melkersson-Rosenthal syndrome	Porphyria
Sarcoidosis	Reiter disease
Crohn disease	Peripheral ameloblastoma
Glycogen storage disease type I b	Aplastic anemia
Gonococcal infection	Plasminogen deficiency
Scurvy	Von-Willebrand disease
Gingivitis due to radiation	Others

Table A.3 Black and Brown lesions

Racial pigmentation	Lentigo simplex
Bismuth deposition	Freckles
Lead deposition	Nevi
Silver deposition	Melanoacanthoma
Amalgam tattoo	Nevus of Ota
Other tattoo	Kaposi sarcoma
Smoker's melanosis	Lentigo maligna
Pencil peel deposition	Malignant melanoma
Eruption cyst	Peutz-Jenger syndrome
Drug-induced pigmentation	Addison disease
	Others

G. Laskaris et al., *Periodontal Manifestations of Local and Systemic Diseases*, https://doi.org/10.1007/978-3-031-10828-0

Morphology (Elementary Lesions) (Tables A.4, A.5, A.6, and A.7)

Table A.4 Ulcers and erosions

Traumatic lesions	Familial neutropenia
Thermal burns	Cyclic neutropenia
Necrotizing gingivitis	Agranulocytosis
Necrotizing periodontitis	Aplastic anemia
Desquamative gingivitis	Leukemias
Drugs (gold and others)	Multiple myeloma
Streptococcal gingivitis	Non-Hodgkin lymphoma
Herpetic gingivitis	Erythema multiforme
Aphthous ulcer	Stevens-Johnson syndrome
Adamandiades-Behcet disease	Toxic epidermal necrolysis
Tuberculosis	Pemphigus vulgaris
Syphilis	Mucous membrane pemphigoid
Measles	Bullous pemphigoid
Chickenpox	Linear IgA disease
Herpes zoster	Pemphigoid gestations
Gonococcal infection	Epidermolysis bullosa acquisita
Cytomegalovirus infection	Hereditary epidermolysis bullosa
Histoplasmosis	Dermatitis herpetiformis
Mucormycosis	Chronic ulcerative stomatitis
Paracoccidioidomycosis	Lichen planus
Langerhans cell histiocytosis	Lupus erythematosus
Squamous cell carcinoma	Mixed connective tissue disease
Other neoplasms	Graft-versus-host disease
Pyostomatitis vegetans	Crohn disease
	Glycogen storage disease, type 1b

Table A.5 Vesiculobullous Lesions

Herpetic gingivitis	Hereditary epidermolysis bullosa
Desquamative gingivitis	Pemphigoid gestationis
Herpes zoster	Dermatitis herpetiformis
Chickenpox	Pemphigus vulgaris
Erythema multiforme	Paraneoplastic pemphigus
Stevens-Johnson syndrome	Lichen planus (bullous type)
Toxic epidermal necrolysis	Primary systemic amyloidosis
Mucous membrane pemphigoid	Pyostomatitis vegetans
Bullous pemphigoid	
Linear IgA disease	
Epidermolysis bullosa acquisita	

Table A.6 Lumps and Swellings-Localized

Gingival abscess	
Periodontal abscess	Bacillary angiomatosis
Pericoronal abscess	Kaposi sarcoma
Periodontal fistula	Non-Hodgkin lymphoma
Exostoses	Burkitt lymphoma
Eruption cyst	Cutaneous T cell lymphoma
Gingival cyst of newborn	Multiple myeloma
Gingival cyst of adult	Langerhans cell histiocytosis
Palatine papilla cyst	Other neoplasms
Odontogenic cysts	Granulomatous gingivitis
Condyloma acuminatum	Tuberous sclerosis
Verruca vulgaris	Cowden disease
Papilloma	Gardner syndrome
Focal epithelial hyperplasia	Focal dermal hypoplasia syndrome
Pyogenic granuloma	Actinomycosis
Pregnancy granuloma	Crohn disease
Peripheral giant cell granuloma	Others
Peripheral ossifying fibroma	
Traumatic fibroma	
Squamous cell carcinoma	
Verrucous carcinoma	
Granular cell tumor of the newborn	
Oral myiasis	

Table A.7 Lumps and Swellings-Generalized

Multiple exostoses	
Mouth breathing gingivitis	
Gingival enlargement during pregnancy	Sarcoidosis
Granulomatous gingivitis	Pyostomatis vegetans
Scurvy	Amyloidosis
Drug-induced gingival enlargement due to phenytoin, calcium channel blockers, ciclosporin	A-Mannosidosis
Monoclonal antibodies	Malignant acanthosis nigricans
Hereditary gingival fibromatosis	Familial acanthosis nigricans
Zimmermann–Laband syndrome	Leukemia
Hurler syndrome	Wegener granulomatosis
Sturge-Weber syndrome	Others
Klippel-Trénaunay-Weber syndrome	
Soft tissue plasmacytoma	
Melkersson-Rosenthal syndrome	
Crohn disease	
Plasminogen deficiency	
Von-Willebrand disease	

Index

G. Laskaris et al., *Periodontal Manifestations of Local and Systemic Diseases*, https://doi.org/10.1007/978-3-031-10828-0

GPSR Compliance

The European Union's (EU) General Product Safety Regulation (GPSR) is a set of rules that requires consumer products to be safe and our obligations to ensure this.

If you have any concerns about our products, you can contact us on ProductSafety@springernature.com

In case Publisher is established outside the EU, the EU authorized representative is:

Springer Nature Customer Service Center GmbH
Europaplatz 3
69115 Heidelberg, Germany

Batch number: 09255836

Printed by Printforce, the Netherlands